CT of Non-Traumatic Body Emergencies

Luigia Romano
Marco Di Serafino
Francesca Iacobellis
Gianluca Ponticiello
Editors

CT of Non-Traumatic Body Emergencies

Springer

Editors
Luigia Romano
Department of General and Emergency Radiology
"Antonio Cardarelli" Hospital
Naples, Italy

Marco Di Serafino
Department of General and Emergency Radiology
"Antonio Cardarelli" Hospital
Naples, Italy

Francesca Iacobellis
Department of General and Emergency Radiology
"Antonio Cardarelli" Hospital
Naples, Italy

Gianluca Ponticiello
Department of General and Emergency Radiology
"Antonio Cardarelli" Hospital
Naples, Italy

ISBN 978-3-031-84848-3 ISBN 978-3-031-84849-0 (eBook)
https://doi.org/10.1007/978-3-031-84849-0

This Springer imprint is published by the registered company Springer Nature Switzerland AG
The registered company address is: Gewerbestrasse 11, 6330 Cham, Switzerland

Preface

In recent decades, radiological imaging has utilized increasingly advanced diagnostic technologies, offering faster, higher spatial, temporal, and contrast resolution. Among these, Computed Tomography (CT) plays a pivotal role in emergency diagnostics due to its ability to perform high-precision scans in a matter of seconds. Its use enables radiologists to provide accurate, timely diagnoses, allowing clinicians to make targeted and critical therapeutic decisions, ultimately guiding the medical or surgical management of the patient. This significantly improves outcomes and reduces hospitalization times.

Non-traumatic emergency conditions affecting the body region can present with highly variable and complex clinical pictures, often characterized by subtle, misleading, or even mild symptoms, despite being potentially life-threatening. To support clinicians in navigating these challenging situations, we aimed to develop a comprehensive text on the use of CT in non-traumatic body emergencies. This text offers both theoretical foundations and practical advice derived from field experience, with the goal of assisting radiologists working in the Emergency Department.

This book was created to provide a complete and up-to-date guide on CT applications, utilizing optimal protocols, acquisition techniques, and software to ensure the highest diagnostic accuracy with minimal radiation exposure. It follows a structured and clinically oriented approach to diagnosing the major non-traumatic emergency conditions of the body.

Naples, Italy — Marco Di Serafino
Naples, Italy — Francesca Iacobellis
Naples, Italy — Gianluca Ponticiello
Naples, Italy — Luigia Romano

Contents

Part II Abdomen

Part III Bowel Inflammations and Infections

Patient Approach in Emergency Settings: Imaging Protocols

1

Luigia Romano, Sonia Fulciniti, Tiziana Capussela, Teresa Cinque, Stefania Daniele, and Massimo Silva

1.1 Introduction

The diagnosis of urgent non-traumatic thoraco-abdominal pathologies includes a wide spectrum of clinical entities ranging from non-deferrable alterations to deferrable alterations, with possible lethal evolution, for which a timely evaluation with an immediate therapeutic program is necessary. Currently, CT plays an important role in emergency patient evaluation [1–3]. The progressive improvement of the hardware and software of modern equipment has limited the acquisition time to a few minutes, expanding the study volumes, improving spatial and contrast resolution, and diagnostic accuracy, with a low exposure dose [4, 5]. The CT exam is useful for diagnosing the disease, demonstrating its complications, providing essential information to undertake the most appropriate treatment strategy, allowing to differentiate patients who need immediate or deferrable surgery, endovascular treatment, from those who can be treated conservatively, placing them in a short and intensive observation program. By promoting the appropriateness of therapeutic treatment and hospitalization in the most suitable Care Departments, it reduces short and long-term complications and hospitalization times, limiting the total cost of both hospital, and post-discharge care. The goal of any CT examination is to obtain high diagnostic accuracy in studies with limited quantities of contrast medium (CM). With current CT equipment, it is possible to obtain optimal image quality by reducing the CM volume and exposure to ionizing radiation, using iterative software.

1.2 Exposure Dose

To obtain high-quality CT studies it is necessary to refer to optimal scanning parameters (tube voltage of 80–120 kVp; reference mA with automatic current modulation; rotation time 0.5 s; slice thickness 1–2.5 mm; low noise index). It is important to balance the risk of radiation exposure with the benefit of making a clinically accurate diagnosis. An incomplete or suboptimal CT study can lead to repeat examinations or the need for study volumes additional to the initial one, which increases the total exposure dose for the patient. The greater exposure to the radiation dose, determined by a multiphasic and volumetrically complete CT

L. Romano (✉) · S. Fulciniti · T. Cinque
S. Daniele · M. Silva
Department of General and Emergency Radiology, "Antonio Cardarelli" Hospital, Naples, Italy
e-mail: sonia.fulciniti@aocardarelli.it; massimo.silva@aocardarelli.it

T. Capussela
Emergency and General Radiological Department, Cardarelli Hospital, Naples, Italy

Departmental Health Physics Unit, Cardarelli Hospital, Naples, Italy
e-mail: tiziana.capussela@aocardarelli.it

L. Romano et al. (eds.), *CT of Non-Traumatic Body Emergencies*,
https://doi.org/10.1007/978-3-031-84849-0_1

study, is counterbalanced by greater diagnostic accuracy with the consequent notable advantages in the clinical management of the patient [6]. Therefore, every effort should be made to reduce the exposure dose without compromising the diagnostic capacity of the CT study [7–9]. There are new strategies applied to current CT technologies, indicated by the various manufacturing companies, which include the use of iterative reconstruction algorithms such as "Admire", "Safire", "iDose", "Asir", "Iris", "Veo", etc. which significantly reduce the exposure dose by up to 80% [10] without compromising image quality. Technological advances in the field of CT equipment, have also led to the development of technologies based on the use of dual-energy (DE) which offers further advantages compared to traditional CT, scanning the same anatomical structures with two different kilovoltages (e.g. 80 kV and 120 kV) improving contrast resolution, with lower quantities of intravenous CM (about 50% less, compared to a conventional CT) [11, 12]. In addition to highlighting the density of iodine, with DE it is possible to detect minimal differences in density based on the different attenuation coefficients and it is possible to improve the visibility of lesions or anatomical components with intrinsic low contrast [13]. It is also possible to create images with iodine subtraction and skeletal structures [14]. The use of DE does not involve an increase in the exposure dose and allows the quantity of CM administered to be reduced [15, 16].

1.3 Contrast Material Injection

The identification and characterization of the different emergency pathologies is strictly dependent not only on the CT scan parameters but also on the injection of CM. To obtain optimal vascular and parenchymal enhancement, some parameters must be taken into consideration: patient-related factors (sex, age, body weight, and cardiac output) and CM injection protocols (iodine dose and CM administration rate). Post-contrast vascular and parenchymal enhancement, are influenced by different administration kinetics of the contrast agent. The vascular one is essentially determined by the dose of iodine delivered per unit of time, while the parenchymal one is determined by the total administered dose of iodine. However, both are dependent on patient-related factors such as body volume of distribution and cardiac output [17–19]. In particular, two parameters determine the temporal trend of vascular enhancement: the rate of iodine delivery (IDR: gI/sec.) which depends on the concentration of the CM and the injection flow rate (FR), and the injection duration (ID). Injection duration (ID) influences vascular enhancement in acquisitions of longer duration (>10 s) that are applied to larger study volumes: the higher the ID, the greater the arterial enhancement. This is due to the phenomenon of recirculation of the contrast bolus which contributes to an increase, quantified at around 10–20%, in the peak arterial enhancement [20]. The maximum peak intensity of the aorta increases in patients with reduced cardiac output. A 60% reduction in cardiac output increases the magnitude of aortic peak enhancement by approximately 30% [21]. To optimize the arterial phase and determine the start of the volumetric scan after the injection of the CM, the "bolus tracking" technique, based on the automatic calculation of the CT numbers in a selected region of the aorta lumen, must be systematically used, with the start of the acquisition when it has reached an increase in the threshold level of 100–120 HU. Parenchymal enhancement does not depend on cardiac output but is influenced by the relationship between the total dose of iodine administered (mg.I) and the total volume of distribution, corresponding to the intravascular and interstitial spaces of the organs and tissues of the anatomical district to be examined [21]. The IDR is then also calculated, based on the patient's body volume (TWB) [22]. It has been shown that it is necessary to administer a quantity of iodine equal to 500–600 mg. per kg of TBW, to obtain optimal parenchymal enhancement (approximately 50–60 HU) [23].

1.4 Study Protocol

Multiphasic acquisitions are used to obtain precise diagnostic information necessary to differentiate various emergency pathologies. The pre-contrastographic phase is used to identify the presence of stones or calcifications, to highlight hemorrhagic lesions (hemorrhagic cysts, hematomas, clots, free or sac collections with partial or total blood content), and to determine any difference in attenuation before and after the administration of the CM. It is also useful for detecting any high-density material pre-existing the administration of the contrast, which could lead to interpretation difficulties if evaluated only in the contrastographic phases. With an appropriate selection of scanning parameters, the precontrast CT phase can be obtained with a reduction in exposure dose of approximately 80% [24, 25]. In the contrastographic study, although the portal phase is the most used [26] for the diagnosis of various pathologies of the thorax and abdomen, there is however an improvement in diagnostic accuracy when using a multiphasic study [27, 28]. In this case, the arterial phase and the portal phase are obtained with the administration, with the automatic injector, of a single injection of CM (60–130 ml of CM depending on the study volume and the patient's weight), for high CM concentration (370–400 mg.I/ml), with a flow of 3.5–5 ml/s, followed by a bolus of 40 ml of physiological solution at the same flow, to obtain compactness of the contrast bolus. The two acquisitions are in sequence: the arterial phase is obtained with bolus tracking and the portal is programmed at 60–70 s. From the beginning of arterial acquisition (Fig. 1.1). In selected cases, may be an additional study phase (late phase) at around 120 s of delay from the start of the injection, to detect any pathologies of the caval venous system, bleeding at very low pressure, or to evaluate urinary extravasation, in patients with suspected lesions of the renal excretory tract (Fig. 1.2) [29]. The arterial phase is used to evaluate the anatomy, anatomical variants, and pathologies of both the main arteries and the afferents of the organs. It allows the identification of hypervascularized, inflammatory, typically hyperemic lesions in this study phase [30] and of any active bleeding [31]. Arterial lesions such as aneurysms, pseudoaneurysms, and arteriovenous fistulas are therefore clearly evident in the arterial phase. In the portal and late phases, it is possible

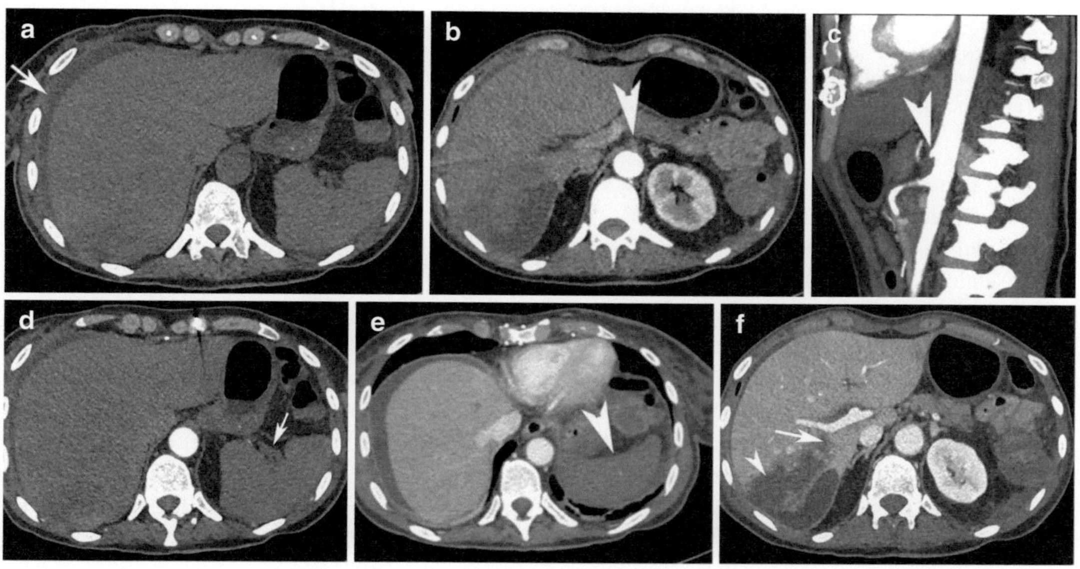

Fig. 1.1 Patient with systemic lupus erythematosus undergoes CT for sudden abdominal pain, fever, with increased liver enzymes and lactates. The baseline CT acquisition (**a**) shows the presence of a perihepatic ascitic layer (arrow). The contrast acquisition in the arterial phase shows the thrombotic occlusion of the celiac artery (arrowheads) (**b** and **c**) and of its hepatic and splenic branches (arrow) (**d**). The acquisition in the portal phase shows an extensive infarction of the spleen (arrowhead) (**e**), thrombosis of the portal branch for the VII hepatic segment (arrow) (**f**), and an extensive infarction of the corresponding hepatic parenchyma (arrowhead) (**f**)

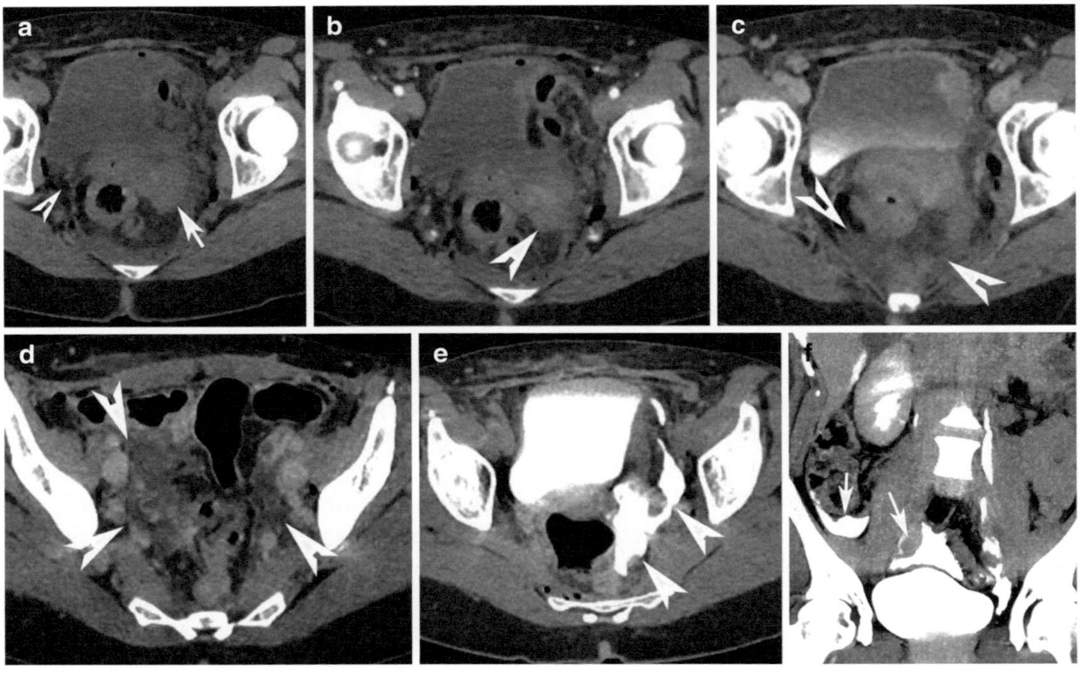

Fig. 1.2 Patient undergoing hysteroanexectomy. In the post-operative period, she presents a modest drop in hematocrit, abdominal pain, fever, and neutrophilic leukocytosis. The pre-contrast CT shows a dense blood collection (arrow) in the pelvis, to the left of the vaginal sac cul, and a non-bloody fluid layer (arrowhead) to the right (**a**). In the arterial post-contrast phase, no signs of active hemorrhage are seen in the blood collection (arrowhead) (**b**), a finding also confirmed in the portal phase (**c**) where a non-bloody fluid layer is seen also in the pre-sacral area (arrowheads) with extension into the extraperitoneal iliac recesses of the pelvis (arrowheads) (**d**). In the late phase, a leakage of iodized urine from iatrogenic laceration of the pre-vesical tract of the left ureter is seen (arrowheads) (**e**); in the coronal reconstruction, iodine-containing urine also expands in the supravesical area and in the right parieto-colic gutter (arrows) (**f**)

to differentiate stable, non-bleeding lesions from unstable, bleeding ones [32].

The diagnosis of vascular lesions, both stable (i.e., pseudoaneurysms or arteriovenous fistulas) (Fig. 1.3) and unstable (i.e., associated with active bleeding) (Fig. 1.4) is therefore dependent on the multiphase study [33].

On arterial phase CT images, active bleeding is typically identified as a focal area of high attenuation caused by a collection of extravasated CM mixed with blood. Active arterial extravasation can be differentiated from clotted blood by measuring the densitometric attenuation of the collection.

Willmann et al. [34] reported that the attenuation level of active arterial extravasation on varied CT has a mean attenuation level of 155 HU, whereas that of clotted blood has a mean attention level of 54 HU.

Furthermore, active bleeding appears on CT images as an area of CM extravasation that is typically larger and more irregular than contained vascular lesions. The volume of hemorrhagic extravasation typically increases in images from sequential acquisitions and does not show the wash-out, characteristic of a contained arterial lesion, although the apparent attenuation of extravasated blood may also decrease, due to dilution related to mixing with blood pre-existing in hematoma (Fig. 1.5) [35]. Therefore, multiphasic CT is useful, and in many cases necessary, for an accurate characterization of vascular pathology (Figs. 1.3 and 1.4) [36, 37].

For the detection of acute bleeding, CT has a sensitivity of 90.9% and a specificity of 99% [36, 37]. Detection of active bleeding and vascular lesions is crucial for planning an optimal thera-

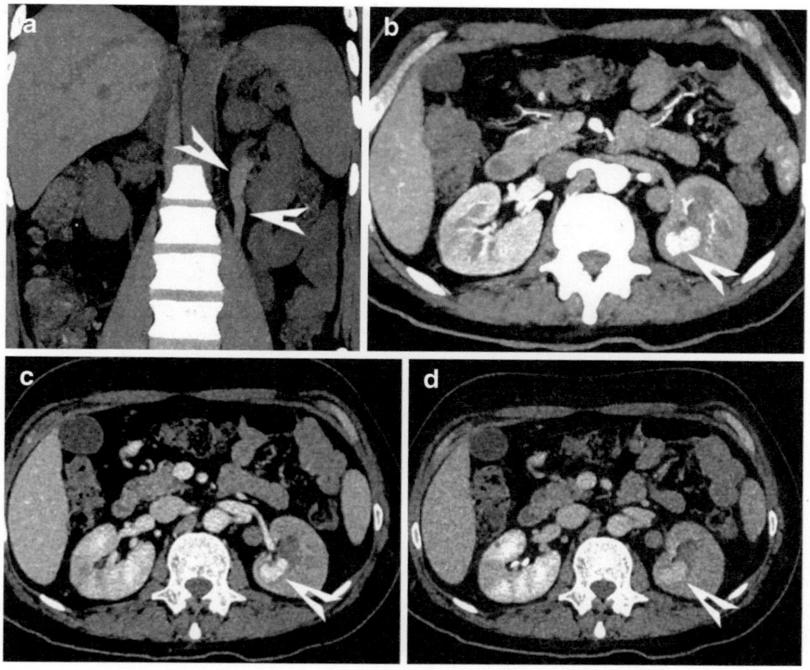

Fig. 1.3 Patient with intermittent post-lithotripsy hematuria and with pain in the left lumbar region. Precontrast CT shows the presence of blood in the lumen of the left ureter (arrowheads) (**a**). In the arterial contrast phase, a pseudoaneurysm is observed located in the medulla of the left kidney (arrowhead) (**b**); in the portal phase (**c**) and in the late phase (**d**), a progressive wash-out of the pseudoaneurysm is appreciated, stable, without signs of active hemorrhage (arrowheads)

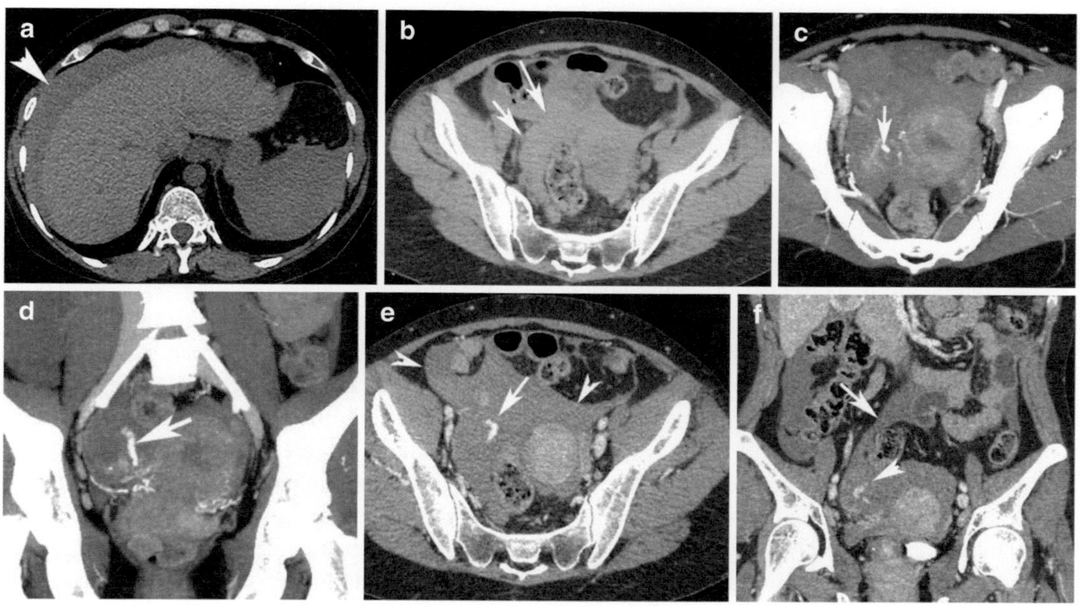

Fig. 1.4 Patient with abdominal pain and hypovolemic shock. The pre-contrast CT study documents the presence of hemoperitoneum in the perihepatic area (arrowhead) (**a**) and in the pelvis, especially in the right adnexal area (arrows) (**b**). The contrast study in the arterial phase shows a small right ovarian cyst with parietal rupture and active bleeding in the context (arrow) (**c**). The coronal reconstruction of the same study phase shows that the active bleeding comes from a branch of the right uterine artery (arrow) (**d**). In the portal phase, a spread of the active bleeding (arrow) is observed within the pelvic peritoneal blood collection (arrowheads) (**e**). The coronal reconstruction in the same study phase shows the extension of the blood collection in the root of the mesentery (arrow) (**f**)

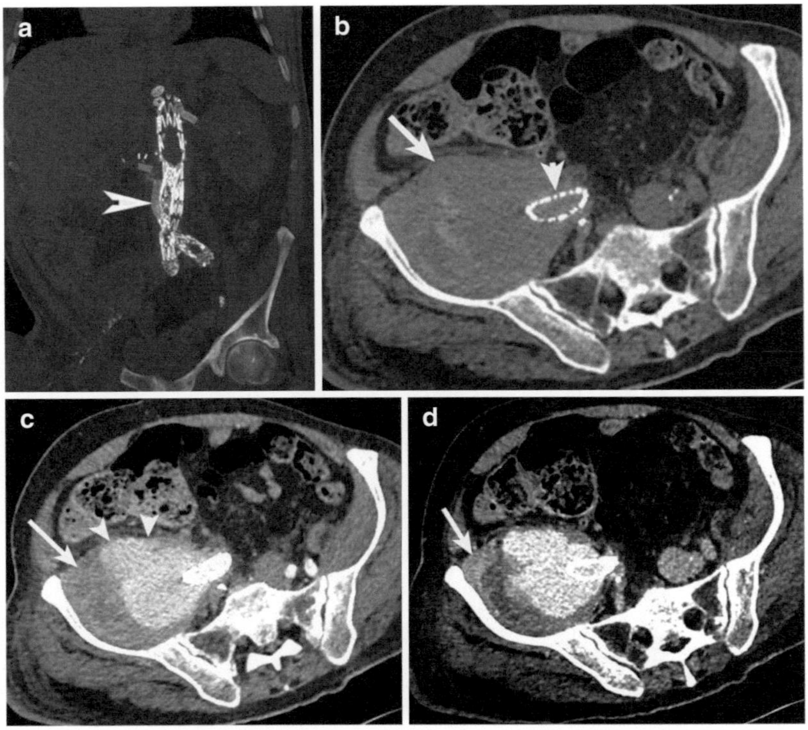

Fig. 1.5 Patient with aorto-bisiliac endoprosthesis, with abdominal pain extending to the right lumbar region and a sharp drop in hematocrit. Coronal reconstruction of the baseline CT shows the endoprosthesis (arrowhead) (**a**) and the axial scan in the pelvic region shows that the right iliac extension (arrowhead) is surrounded by a large hematoma (arrow) (**b**). Contrast study in the arterial phase shows a large periprosthetic pseudoaneurysm (arrowheads) surrounded by a portion of blood (arrow) (**c**). In the portal phase, within the blood portion, active low-flow bleeding (arrow) from the periprosthetic pseudoaneurysm is seen (**d**)

peutic intervention (surgery or transcatheter embolization) [38].

In fact, the pre-procedural detection of the site of contrast extravasation can lead to the execution of a targeted and superselective angiography with rapid occlusion of the hemorrhagic source.

Portal phase scans can be useful in determining the cause of non-arterial bleeding, especially due to hypervascularized lesions.

Identification of the origin of arterial or venous bleeding impacts patient management. When CT is limited to the portal phase, adequate differentiation between the two types of hemorrhage cannot be achieved [39, 40]. Arterial bleeding in most cases requires emergency treatment (embolization or surgery), while venous bleeding can be treated conservatively due to the low pressure which allows it to be self-limited.

In some cases, active bleeding may appear only on portal phase images, with a negative arterial phase (Fig. 1.5), due to intermittent hemorrhage, a venous source of bleeding, or as a reflection of decreased arterial perfusion related to failure. Cardiovascular disease, vasospasm, or hypotension [41]. The acquisition of images in the portal phase therefore provides additional information based on parenchymographic enhancement, that is necessary for the identification of pathologies of the organs and the hollow viscus.

1.5 Conclusions

An accurate diagnosis of emergency clinical conditions can be made on the basis of medical history, physical examination, and laboratory test results in only a small percentage of patients who access the Emergency Department. The clinical manifestations of the various causes of acute non-traumatic thoraco-abdominal pathologies are often subtle, but potentially fatal.

For adequate treatment, a diagnostic workup that allows for a precise diagnosis is important and emergency imaging plays a very important role in this process.

CT is an extremely rapid and effective method for evaluating patients with emergency-urgent thoraco-abdominal pathologies. Precision in the study techniques and the CM injection protocol, allows for optimization of the examination, reducing the exposure dose and maximizing diagnostic accuracy, allowing timely and accurate therapeutic procedures that impact significantly on the morbidity and mortality of patients.

References

1. Tsushima Y, Yamada S, Aoki J, et al. Effect of contrast-enhanced computed tomography on diagnosis and management of acute abdomen in adults. Clin Radiol. 2002;57:507–13. https://doi.org/10.1053/crad.2001.0925.
2. Novelline RA, Rhea JT, Rao PM, et al. Helical CT in emergency radiology. Radiology. 1999;213:321–39. https://doi.org/10.1148/radiology.213.2.r99nv01321.
3. Rosen MP, Sands DZ, Longmaid HE III, et al. Impact of abdominal CT on the management of patients presenting to the emergency department with acute abdominal pain. AJR. 2000;174:1391–6. https://doi.org/10.2214/ajr.174.5.1741391.
4. Howard SA, Rosenthal MH, Qin L, et al. Quantifying decreased radiation exposure from modern CT scan technology and surveillance programs of germ cell tumors. Am J Clin Oncol. 2018;41(10):949–52. https://doi.org/10.1097/COC.0000000000000399.
5. Gottumukkala RV, Kalra MK, Tabari A, et al. Advanced CT techniques for decreasing radiation dose reducing sedation requirements and optimizing image quality in children. Radiographics. 2019;39(3):709–26. https://doi.org/10.1148/rg.2019180082.
6. Griffey RT, Jeffe DB, Bailey T. Emergency physicians' attitudes and preferences regarding computed tomography radiation exposure and imaging decision support. Acad Emerg Med. 2014;21:768–77. https://doi.org/10.1111/acem.12410.
7. Booij R, Dijkshoorn ML, van Straten M. Efficacy of adynamic collimator for overranging dose reduction in a second and third generation dual source CT scanner. Eur Radiol. 2017;27(9):3618–24. https://doi.org/10.1007/s00330-017-4745-8.
8. Alagic Z, Eriksson A, Drageryd E, et al. A new low-dose multiphase trauma CT protocol and its impact on diagnostic assessment and radiation dose in multitrauma patients. Emerg Radiol. 2017;24:509–18. https://doi.org/10.1007/s10140-017-1496-4.
9. Yaniv G, Portnoy O, Simon D, et al. Revised protocol for whole-body CT for multitrauma patients applying triphasic injection followed by a single-pass scan on a 64-MDCT. Clin Radiol. 2013;68:668–75. https://doi.org/10.1016/j.crad.2012.12.011.
10. Gangadhar K, Kielar A, Dighe MK, et al. Multimodality approach for imaging of non-traumatic acute abdominal emergencies. Abdom Radiol. 2016;41(1):136–48. https://doi.org/10.1007/s00261-015-0586-6.
11. Meier A, Wurnig M, Desbiolles L, et al. Advanced virtual monoenergetic images: improving the contrast of dual-energy CT pulmonary angiography. Clin Radiol. 2015;70(11):1244–51. https://doi.org/10.1016/j.crad.2015.06.094.
12. Lira D, Padole A, Kalra MK, et al. Tube potential and CT radiation dose optimization. AJR. 2015;204(1):W4–W10. https://doi.org/10.2214/AJR.14.13281.
13. Vlahos I, Chung R, Nair A, et al. Dual-energy CT: vascular applications. AJR. 2012;199:S87–97. https://doi.org/10.2214/AJR.12.9114.
14. Heye T, Nelson RC, Ho LM, et al. Dual-energy CT applications in the abdomen. AJR. 2012;199:S64–70. https://doi.org/10.2214/AJR.12.9196.
15. Sun EX, Wortman JR, Uyeda JW, et al. Virtual monoenergetic dual-energy CT for evaluation of hepatic and splenic lacerations. Emerg Radiol. 2019;26(4):419–25. https://doi.org/10.1007/s10140-019-01687-y.
16. Di Serafino M, Iacobellis F, Schillirò ML, et al. The role of CT-angiography in the acute gastrointestinal bleeding: a pictorial essay of active and obscure findings. Tomography. 2022;8(5):2369–402. https://doi.org/10.3390/tomography8050198.
17. Caruso D, Rosati E, Panvini N, et al. Optimization of contrast medium volume for abdominal CT in oncologic patients: prospective comparison between fixed and lean body weight-adapted dosing protocols. Insights Imaging. 2021;12(1):40. https://doi.org/10.1186/s13244-021-00980-0.
18. Yap LPP, Wong JHD, Muhammad Gowdh NF, et al. Customised weight-based volume contrast media protocol in CT of chest abdomen and pelvis examination. J Med Imaging Radiat Sci. 2021;52(2):257–64. https://doi.org/10.1016/j.jmir.2021.01.003.
19. Kitadate M, Kondou T, Yokota H, et al. Depiction of hypervascular hepatocellular carcinoma with 64-MDCT: comparison of moderate and high concentration contrast material with and without saline flush. AJR. 2009;193:738–44. https://doi.org/10.2214/AJR.08.2028.

20. Fleischmann D. How to design injection protocols for multiple detector-row CT angiography (MDCTA). Eur Radiol. 2005;15:60–5. https://doi.org/10.1007/s10406-005-0166-x.
21. Bae KT, Heiken JP, Brink JA. Aortic and hepatic contrast medium enhancement at CT. Part II. Effect of reduced cardiac output in a porcine model. Radiology. 1998;207:657–62. https://doi.org/10.1148/radiology.207.3.9609887.
22. Lell MM, Fleischmann U, Pietsch H, et al. Relationship between low tube voltage (70 kV) and the iodine delivery rate (IDR) in CT angiography: an experimental in-vivo study. Eur Radiol. 2017;27(3):e0173592. https://doi.org/10.1371/journal.pone.0173592.
23. Kondo H, Kanematsu M, Goshima S, et al. Body size indexes for optimizing iodine dose for aortic and hepatic enhancement at multidetector CT: comparison of total body weight lean body weight and blood volume. Radiology. 2010;254:163–9. https://doi.org/10.1148/radiol.09090369.
24. Rampado O, Depaoli A, Marchisio F, et al. Effects of different levels of CT iterative reconstruction on low-contrast detectability and radiation dose in patients of different sizes: an anthropomorphic phantom study. Radiol Med. 2021;126(1):55–62. https://doi.org/10.1007/s11547-020-01228-5.
25. Pooler BD, Lubner MG, Kim DH, et al. Prospective trial for the detection of urolithiasis at ultra-low-dose (sub-mSv) non-contrast CT: direct comparison against routine low-dose reference standard. J Urol. 2014;192(5):1433–9. https://doi.org/10.1016/j.juro.2014.05.089.
26. Johnson PT, Fishman EK. Routine use of precontrast and delayed acquisitions in abdominal CT: time for change. Abdom Imaging. 2013;38:215–23. https://doi.org/10.1007/s00261-012-9964-5.
27. Konno Y, Hiraka T, Kanoto M, et al. Pancreatic perfusion imaging method that reduces radiation dose and maintains image quality by combining volumetric perfusion CT with multiphasic contrast enhanced-CT. Pancreatology. 2020;20(7):1406–12. https://doi.org/10.1016/j.pan.2020.08.010.
28. Wang J, Zhong L, Zhou X, et al. Value of multiphase contrast-enhanced CT with three-dimensional reconstruction in detecting depth of infiltration lymph node metastasis and extramural vascular invasion of gastric cancer. J Gastrointest Oncol. 2021;12(4):1351–62. https://doi.org/10.21037/jgo-21-276.
29. Yoon W, Jeong YY, Shin SS, et al. Acute massive gastrointestinal bleeding: detection and localization with arterial phase multidetector row helical CT. Radiology. 2006;239:160–7. https://doi.org/10.1148/radiol.2383050175.
30. Arai K, Kawai K, Kohda W, et al. Dynamic CT of acute cholangitis: early inhomogeneous enhancement of the liver. AJR. 2003;181:115–8. https://doi.org/10.2214/ajr.181.1.1810115.
31. Dobritz M, Engels HP, Schneider A, et al. Detection of intestinal bleeding with multi-detector row CT in an experimental setup. How many acquisitions are necessary? Eur Radiol. 2009;19:2862–9. https://doi.org/10.1007/s00330-009-1510-7.
32. Tew K, Davies RP, Jadun CK, et al. MDCT of acute lower gastrointestinal bleeding. AJR. 2004;182:427–30. https://doi.org/10.2214/ajr.182.2.1820427.
33. Al Qahtani AR, Satin R, Stern J, et al. Investigative modalities for massive lower gastrointestinal bleeding. World J Surg. 2002;26:620–5. https://doi.org/10.1007/s00268-001-0279-x.
34. Willmann JK, Roos JE, Platz A, et al. Multidetector CT: detection of active hemorrhage in patients with blunt abdominal trauma. AJR. 2002;179:437–44. https://doi.org/10.2214/ajr.179.2.1790437.
35. Kuhle WG, Sheiman RG. Detection of active colonic hemorrhage with use of helical CT: findings in a swine model. Radiology. 2003;228:743–52. https://doi.org/10.1148/radiol.2283020756.
36. Dreizin D, Liang Y, Dent J, et al. Diagnostic value of CT contrast extravasation for major arterial injury after pelvic fracture: a meta-analysis. Am J Emerg Med. 2020;38(11):2335–42. https://doi.org/10.1016/j.ajem.2019.11.038.
37. Wells ML, Hansel SL, Bruining DH, et al. CT for evaluation of acute gastrointestinal bleeding. Radiographics. 2018;38(4):1089–107. https://doi.org/10.1148/rg.2018170138.
38. Sommer CM, Stampfl U, Bellemann N, et al. Patients with life-threatening arterial renal hemorrhage: CT angiography and catheter angiography with subsequent superselective embolization. Cardiovasc Intervent Radiol. 2010;33:498–508. https://doi.org/10.1007/s00270-009-9787-0.
39. Jaeckle T, Stuber G, Hoffmann M, et al. Detection and localization of acute upper and lower gastrointestinal (GI) bleeding with arterial phase multidetector row helical CT. Eur Radiol. 2008;18(7):1406–13. https://doi.org/10.1007/s00330-008-0907-z.
40. Gaiani F, De'Angelis N, Kayali S, et al. Clinical approach to the patient with acute gastrointestinal bleeding. Acta Biomed. 2018;89(8-S):12–9. https://doi.org/10.23750/abm.v89i8-S.7861.
41. Jaeckle T, Stuber G, Hoffmann MH, et al. Acute gastrointestinal bleeding: value of multidetector CT. Abdom Imaging. 2008;33(3):285–93. https://doi.org/10.1007/s00261-007-9263-8.

Part I

Neck and Chest

Inflammatory and Infectious Process of the Neck and Mediastinum

2

Vittorio Sabatino, Gianluca Ponticiello, Luigi Barbuto, Gaspare Oliva, Elena Nappa, and Marco Di Serafino

2.1 Introduction

Mediastinal syndromes encompass a set of signs and symptoms caused by the compression or infiltration of mediastinal structures, such as edema, dyspnea, and dysphagia. These syndromes have an acute cause in approximately 20% of cases and represent clinical conditions characterized by the impairment of mediastinal structures, which, while not common, have a mortality rate of up to 40% if not promptly treated [1]. Infectious and inflammatory processes involving the neck and mediastinum often present as chest pain, which is the most common cause of emergency room visits (5–9%) and is associated with a high mortality rate (2–4%). The underlying cause is often initially unrecognized, leading to a significant rate of diagnostic errors (25–50%) [2]. Chest pain has many possible causes and imaging plays a critical role in correctly identifying its source. Radiologists must be familiar with all potential differential diagnoses, including rare ones, and the best techniques for their identification. Acute mediastinitis has various etiologies, with the most common being esophageal lacerations, which may be iatrogenic, traumatic, caustic, or spontaneous. Other causes include post-surgical complications related to procedures in the mediastinal area, mainly cardiac surgeries or post-thymectomy. Less frequent but equally concerning are descending necrotizing mediastinitis types, which arise from infections in the neck that spread downward into the mediastinum due to the continuity of fascial spaces. This type of mediastinitis is typically associated with cervical infections, such as abscesses, and may also result from conditions like septic arthritis involving nearby structures [3–5].

Descending necrotizing mediastinitis (DNM) is primarily caused by odontogenic abscesses (40–60% of cases), retropharyngeal abscesses (14%), peritonsillar abscesses (11%). Less common are sternocleidomastoid muscle abscesses, foreign body-induced mediastinitis, sternoclavicular septic arthritis, and other causes (cervical lymphadenitis, clavicular osteomyelitis, intravenous drug injection, parotid or thyroid infections) (Table 2.1) [6]. DNM is classified into two types according to Endo Classification: type 1 (focal) and type 2 (diffuse). Type 2 can be further divided into type 2a if the infection remains supracarinal or type 2b if it extends into the subcarinal compartments. The treatment strategy depends on this classification (Table 2.2) [7].

V. Sabatino (✉) · G. Ponticiello · L. Barbuto
G. Oliva · E. Nappa · M. Di Serafino
Department of General and Emergency Radiology, "Antonio Cardarelli" Hospital, Naples, Italy
e-mail: vittorio.sabatino@aocardarelli.it; gianluca.ponticiello@aocardarelli.it; luigi.barbuto@aocardarelli.it; gaspare.oliva@aocardarelli.it; elena.nappa@aocardarelli.it; marco.diserafino@aocardarelli.it

L. Romano et al. (eds.), *CT of Non-Traumatic Body Emergencies*,
https://doi.org/10.1007/978-3-031-84849-0_2

Table 2.1 Causes and incidence of descending necrotizing mediastinitis

Causes	Incidence
Odontogenic abscesses	40–60%
Retropharyngeal abscesses	14%
Peritonsillar abscesses	11%
Sternocleidomastoid muscle abscesses	Less common, significant in immunocompromised patients
Foreign body-induced mediastinitis	Rare, but significant in undiagnosed cases
Sternoclavicular septic arthritis	<1% of all septic arthritis cases
Other causes (cervical lymphadenitis, clavicular osteomyelitis, intravenous drug injection, parotid or thyroid infections)	Rare

Table 2.2 Types of descending necrotizing mediastinitis (according to Endo et al. 1999)

Types	Mediastinal extension
Type 1 (focal)	Located in the pre-carinal upper mediastinum
Type 2a (diffuse)	Extended to the anterior sub-carinal mediastinum
Type 2b (diffuse)	Extended to the anterior mediastinum and the posterior inferior mediastinum

2.2 Anatomy and Pathways of Spread

2.2.1 Anatomy

Understanding the anatomy of the mediastinum is crucial to identifying the pathways through which infections spread from the neck to the mediastinum. The mediastinum has traditionally been divided into various compartments: superior, anterior, middle, and posterior, according to schemes by Fraser et al. (1977) (Fig. 2.1a) [8]. These divisions were primarily based on lateral chest X-ray images rather than actual anatomical boundaries. However, due to the lack of true anatomical limits between these compartments, a more modern classification, the ITMIG 2017 (International Thymic Malignancy Interest Group), has been proposed [9]. This classification is based on modern cross-sectional imaging modalities such as CT and MRI, allowing for better localization of both neoplastic and inflammatory diseases by considering the displacement of fascial planes, adipose tissue, and adjacent organs. To enhance the understanding of mediastinal anatomy and improve diagnostic accuracy, the ITMIG 2017 classification divides the mediastinum into three main compartments: prevascular, visceral, and paravertebral compartments. Each compartment is defined by specific anatomical landmarks and contains distinct structures, which are crucial for identifying the pathways of infection spread and for localizing both neoplastic and inflammatory processes (Fig. 2.1b). Prevascular compartment: corresponds to the superior and anterior mediastinum in the traditional classification. It is bounded superiorly by the thoracic inlet, inferiorly by the diaphragm, anteriorly by the sternum, laterally by the parietal mediastinal pleura, and posteriorly by the anterior surface of the pericardium and the great vessels (aorta, aortic arch, and its branches, superior vena cava). It contains structures such as the thymus, adipose tissue, lymph nodes, and the left brachiocephalic vein. Visceral compartment: substantially corresponds to the middle mediastinum and includes a portion of the posterior mediastinum, specifically the esophagus. It extends from the thoracic inlet to the diaphragm, is anteriorly bordered by the posterior surface of the pericardium and great vessels, and posteriorly by a plane passing 1 cm behind the anterior margin of the thoracic spine. This compartment contains both non-vascular structures (e.g., trachea, carina, esophagus, lymph nodes) and vascular structures (e.g., heart, ascending thoracic aorta, aortic arch, descending thoracic aorta, superior vena cava, and intrapericardial

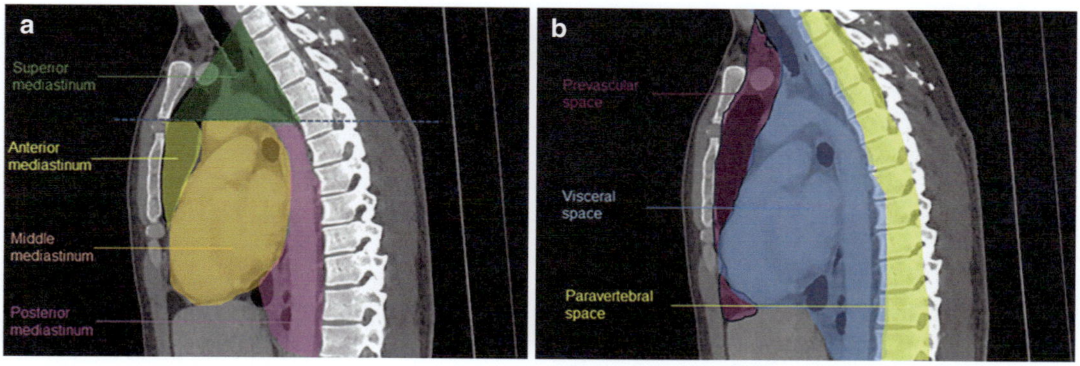

Fig. 2.1 Mediastinal spaces. (**a**) Traditional classification of mediastinal spaces, delineating the superior mediastinum (green), anterior mediastinum (yellow), middle mediastinum (orange), and posterior mediastinum (purple). (**b**) ITMIG 2017 classification of mediastinal compartments, featuring the prevascular space (purple), visceral space (blue), and paravertebral space (yellow)

pulmonary arteries, thoracic duct). Paravertebral compartment: corresponds to the remaining part of the posterior mediastinum. It is bounded superiorly by the thoracic inlet, inferiorly by the diaphragm, anteriorly by a plane passing 1 cm behind the anterior margin of the thoracic spine, and posteriorly by a plane passing through the lateral margins of the transverse processes of the thoracic vertebrae. It contains structures such as the posterior ribs, transverse processes, thoracic vertebrae, and paravertebral soft tissues. By understanding these compartments and their interconnections, radiologists can better assess the spread of infectious processes from the neck to the mediastinum (Fig. 2.1).

The neck spaces are diverse and interconnected, including the parapharyngeal space, masticatory space, carotid space, parotid space, mucosal pharyngeal space, visceral space, retropharyngeal space, and paravertebral space [10]. Some of these spaces have direct communication with the mediastinum and are referred to as vertically oriented spaces, which have a higher risk of complications. These vertically oriented spaces include the pretracheal space, parapharyngeal space, retropharyngeal space, paravertebral space, and carotid space. The deep cervical fascia is crucial in understanding the spread of infections from the neck to the mediastinum [11]. The superficial layer extends from the base of the skull to the lower cervical vertebrae, while the deep layer is further divided into the prevertebral and alar fasciae. The prevertebral fascia extends from the skull base to the coccyx, compartmentalizing the spine and paraspinal muscles and forming the anterior boundary of the prevertebral space. The alar fascia, located between the prevertebral fascia and the middle layer of the deep cervical fascia, extends from the skull base to the mediastinum. The retropharyngeal space, located anterior to the alar fascia, forms the "danger space," which provides a direct route from the skull base to the mediastinum. This space is typically a potential or virtual space without an actual cavity but can open up during inflammatory or infectious processes, creating a direct pathway for infections to spread from the neck to the posterior mediastinum. Due to the absence of anatomical barriers, the danger space allows for the rapid and unimpeded extension of infections and is the most common route for the spread of odontogenic infections to the posterior mediastinum and pleural space (Fig. 2.2) [12].

2.2.2 Pathways of Infection Spread

An infectious process affecting the pretracheal space typically extends into the prevascular mediastinal compartment, reaching the superior mediastinum above the trachea. This configuration characterizes a type I descending necrotizing mediastinitis, which may be managed with conservative pharmacological treatment or transcervical drainage. Conversely, an infectious process involving the parapharyngeal space may spread to the subcarinal prevascular compartment and the visceral compartment within the anterior and middle mediastinum, resulting in a type IIa diffuse infection that necessitates transcervical drainage. Finally, an infection impacting the retropharyngeal space, commonly referred to as the "danger space", can involve both the visceral and paravertebral compartments, potentially extending to the lower portion of the posterior mediastinum, thus representing a type IIb diffuse infection with a worse prognosis, which requires mediastinal drainage [13]. Additionally, the parapharyngeal space serves as a central conduit for infections because it has direct communication with the submandibular space, the retropharyngeal space, and the carotid space. This underscores the critical importance of recognizing inflammatory processes of the neck as potentially dangerous due to their complex anatomical interconnections, which can facilitate the rapid spread of infection into the mediastinum and other thoracic structures (Fig. 2.3) [14].

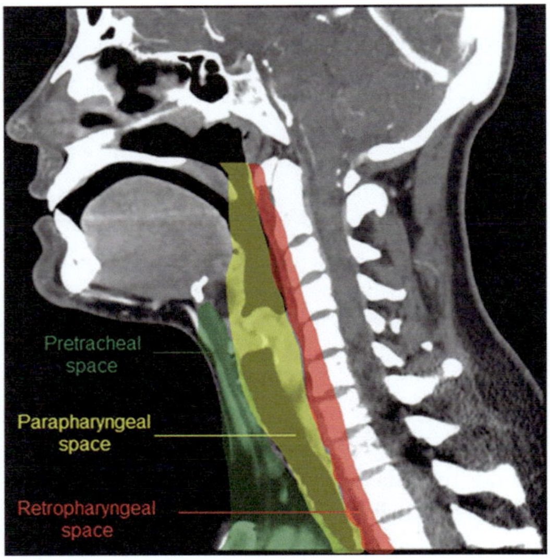

Fig. 2.2 Main neck spaces connected to mediastinal spaces. The pretracheal space (green), parapharyngeal space (yellow), and retropharyngeal space (red) are depicted

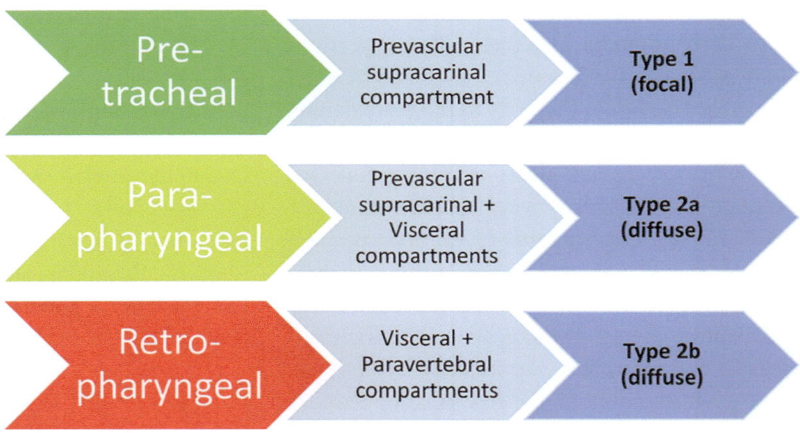

Fig. 2.3 Main pathways of infection spread from neck spaces to mediastinal compartments, according to ITMIG, and correlated with the classification of descending necrotizing mediastinitis

2.3 Odontogenic and Retropharyngeal Abscesses

Odontogenic abscesses arise from infections in the oral cavity, typically originating from a dental element. These infections are often self-limiting, but their spread to interconnected neck spaces poses a risk for severe complications. Approximately 40–60% of descending necrotizing mediastinitis cases originate from odontogenic abscesses [6]. In some instances, these abscesses can extend into the retropharyngeal space, forming a retropharyngeal abscess, which occurs in about 14% of such cases and carries a high risk of descending into the mediastinum [15]. Clinically, odontogenic abscesses present with swelling in the oral cavity, and advanced cases may show external manifestations in the angular-mandibular region. Non-contrast CT of the maxillofacial region can detect dental erosions, but contrast-enhanced CT of the neck is essential for identifying fluid collections, hyperemia, and the involvement of neck spaces. Retropharyngeal abscesses require thorough CT imaging due to their potential to progress to mediastinitis. A comprehensive evaluation should include chest CT to identify signs of mediastinitis, as this can significantly influence treatment strategy and prognosis. Careful assessment for fluid collections and air pockets between the neck and mediastinal spaces is crucial (Fig. 2.4).

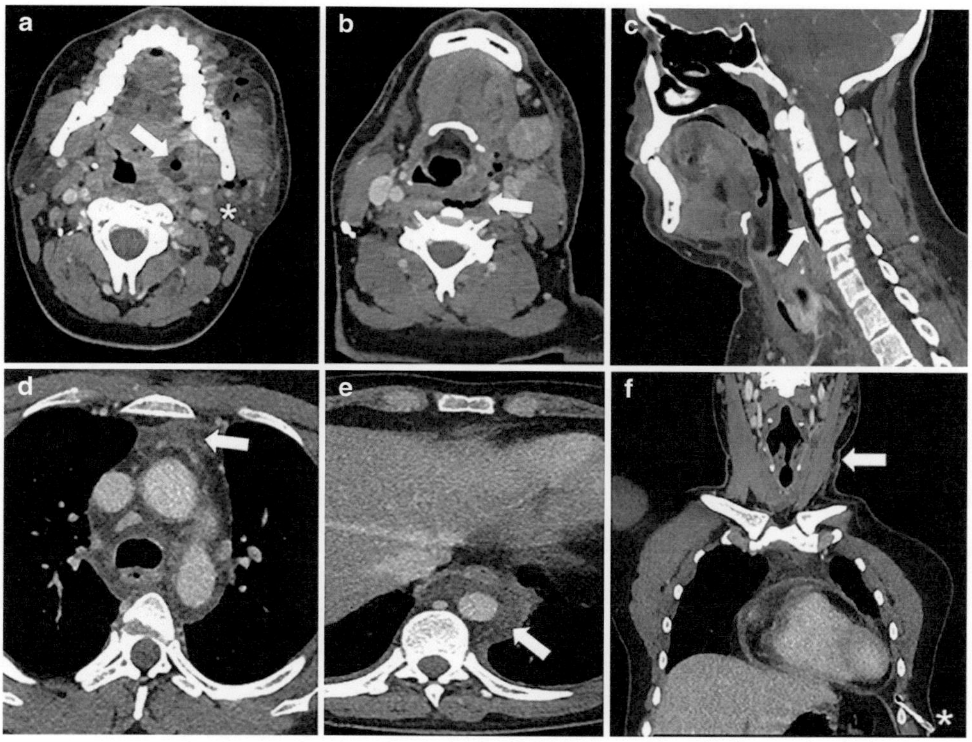

Fig. 2.4 Odontogenic abscess in an 18-year-old male patient presenting with left submandibular swelling, pain, and fever. (**a**) Fluid collection with hyperaemic walls (asterisk) and air bubbles (arrow) involving the left submandibular space, extending externally to the parotid space and medially to the parapharyngeal space. (**b**) Axial and (**c**) coronal reconstructions showing air bubbles (arrow) in the retropharyngeal space, extending caudally. (**d**) The collection involves the prevascular compartment, the superior mediastinum (arrow). (**e**) The collection also extends to the visceral and paravertebral mediastinal spaces, reaching the inferior portion of the posterior mediastinum (arrow), classified as type 2b. (**f**) Coronal reconstruction at 2-week follow-up, after medical therapy and mediastinal drainage, shows resolution of cervical abscesses (arrow), with persistent mediastinal involvement necessitating continued placement of the mediastinal drainage tube (asterisk)

2.4 Peritonsillar Abscess

Peritonsillar abscesses are infectious complications of acute tonsillitis, characterized by the accumulation of pus in the peritonsillar space, located between the palatine tonsil capsule and the pharyngeal constrictor muscles. These abscesses are common in adolescents and young adults and account for approximately 11% of cases of descending necrotizing mediastinitis [6]. Clinically, they often present as an initial enlargement of one of the palatine tonsils. Contrast-enhanced imaging can reveal a fluid collection with parietal hyperemia indicative of abscess formation. While peritonsillar abscesses are generally self-limiting, more severe cases can extend horizontally into the submandibular space or, more critically, spread vertically through the retropharyngeal space toward the mediastinum. The parapharyngeal space serves as a central conduit for the spread of these infections, underscoring the importance of extending imaging studies to include the chest to detect any signs of mediastinitis. Special attention should be given to evaluating the retropharyngeal space, the main route for potentially life-threatening mediastinitis [16]. It is important to note that peritonsillar abscesses are typically found in adolescents and young adults. In these patients, the thymic lodge in the superior mediastinum may also contain residual thymic tissue, characterized by solid Hounsfield unit (HU) values on imaging. This finding should not be mistaken for mediastinal involvement, which would instead present as edematous infiltration with fluid HU values or evidence of fluid collections (Fig. 2.5).

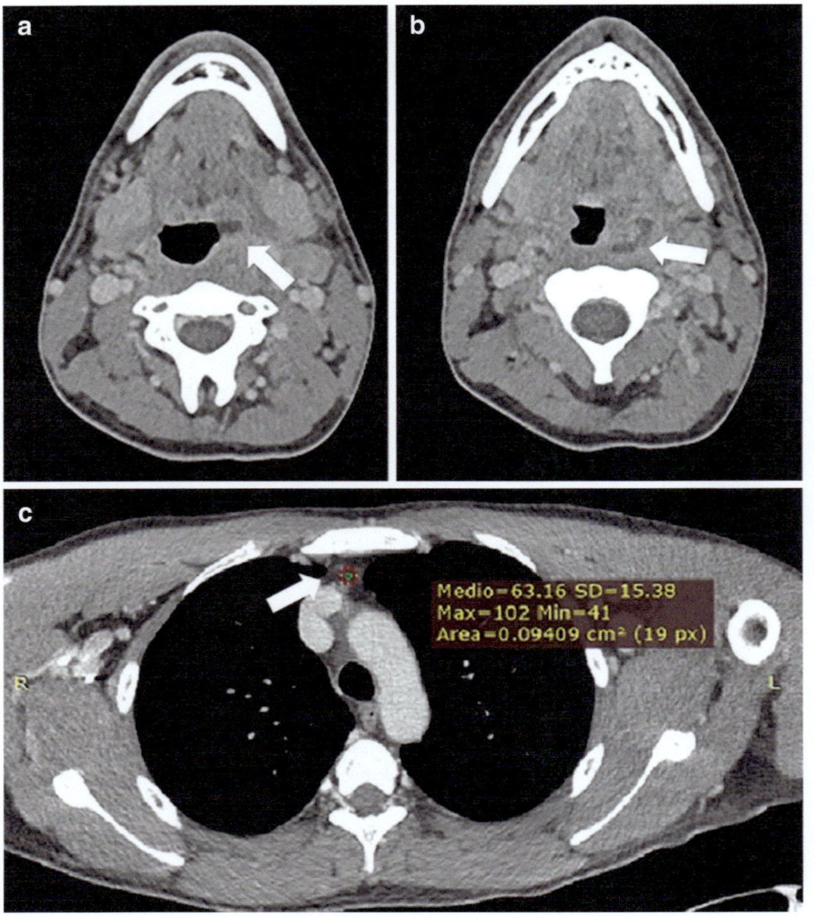

Fig. 2.5 Peritonsillar abscess in a 16-year-old boy presenting with throat pain. (**a**) Enlargement of the left palatine tonsil with asymmetry compared to the contralateral side, showing a fluid collection in the left palatine region (arrow). (**b**) Further caudally, there is a collection developing in the parapharyngeal space, closely approaching the retropharyngeal space without affecting it (arrow). (**c**) Mediastinal imaging reveals the prevascular compartment, the superior mediastinum occupied by tissue with a density of 63 HU, consistent with a thymic remnant rather than a mediastinal collection (arrow)

2.5 Sternocleidomastoid Muscle Abscesses

Infections originating from the neck's muscular structures, especially the sternocleidomastoid muscle, can lead to extensive abscess formation with mediastinal involvement. These abscesses are relatively uncommon but are more frequently observed in immunocompromised patients. The sternocleidomastoid muscle extends from the upper part of the sternum's manubrium and the middle third of the clavicle to the mastoid process of the temporal bone and the superior nuchal line of the occipital bone. Although it does not directly extend into the mediastinum, it has indirect anatomical relationships through the continuity of the superficial (pretracheal) and deep (prevertebral) cervical fascia. Indicators of a muscle abscess include fluid collections with hyperemic walls, air pockets, involvement of cervical fascia, and potential associated venous thrombosis. These abscesses account for a small percentage of descending necrotizing mediastinitis cases, often arising due to skin infections, infections of other neck structures, or hematogenous spread, particularly in patients with compromised immune systems (Fig. 2.6) [17].

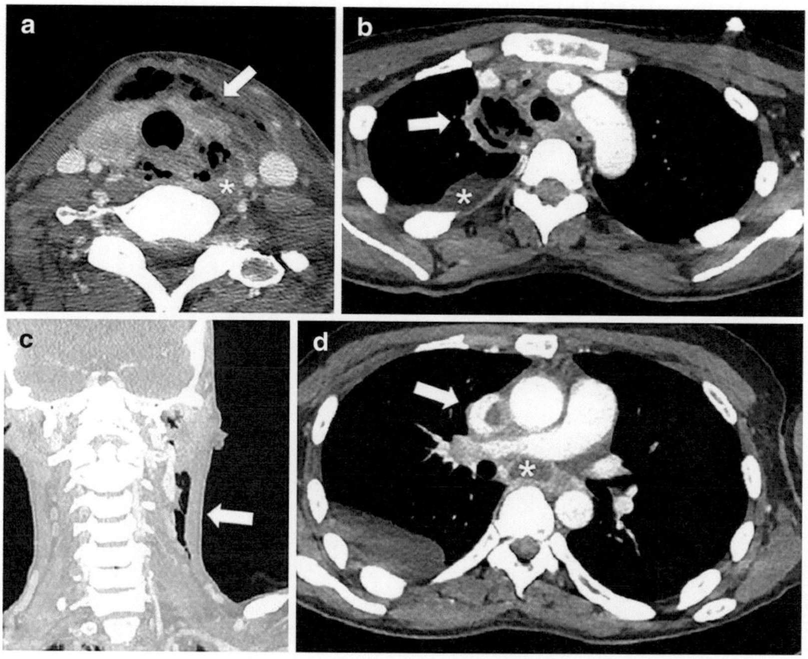

Fig. 2.6 Sternocleidomastoid abscess in an immunocompromised 53-year-old patient presenting with neck swelling, dysphonia, and dysphagia. (**a**) Fluid collection with air bubbles involving the belly of the sternocleidomastoid muscle, extending to the sternohyoid muscle (arrow). The infection reaches the parapharyngeal space, with initial involvement of the retropharyngeal space (asterisk). (**b**) The infection extends into the supracarinal prevascular space of the mediastinum (arrow), with associated right pleural effusion (asterisk). (**c**) Coronal reconstruction with lung window shows widespread involvement of the sternocleidomastoid muscle with visible air bubbles (arrow). (**d**) Thrombosis of the superior vena cava (arrow) and fluid distension of the esophageal lumen (asterisk) are also evident. The collection remains confined to the superior mediastinum, within the prevascular space, and is classified as type 1

2.6 Foreign Body-Induced Mediastinitis

A foreign body lodged in the airways or digestive tract can trigger a significant inflammatory response, which may spread both horizontally across the neck spaces and vertically, depending on the location of the obstruction. The incidence of foreign body-induced mediastinitis is relatively low, but it is more common in older adults and children. Chicken or fish bones are the most frequently implicated, often becoming lodged in the hypopharynx, esophagus, or bronchi. These objects can occasionally migrate deeper into the bronchi or even into the mediastinum, leading to severe complications. It is essential to thoroughly evaluate all potential sites where a foreign body may be retained, starting from the shared passageway between the respiratory and digestive tracts, the pharyngeal space, and extending to both contiguous and less common adjacent sites. Non-contrast CT imaging is mandatory to accurately identify small fragments and distinguish them from areas of contrast-induced enhancement. Multiplanar reconstruction (MPR) on several planes can provide more precise localization of the foreign body. Particular attention should be given to reviewing imaging if an endoscopic examination is negative but symptoms persist, as foreign bodies may lodge in less common adjacent sites that are easily missed. It is important to note that foreign bodies often cause only initial discomfort, depending on their location. However, if not promptly removed, they can lead to extensive abscess formation and suppuration, potentially extending into the deepest regions of the mediastinum and posing a significant life-threatening risk (Fig. 2.7) [18].

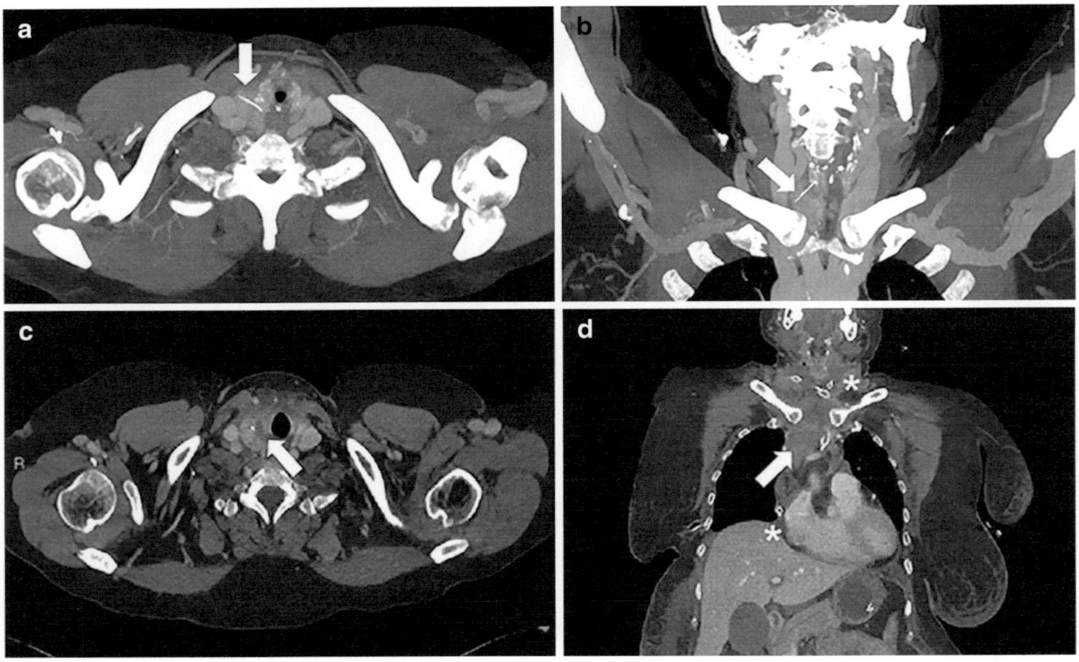

Fig. 2.7 A 60-year-old woman presenting with a persistent sensation of a foreign body in the throat, 3 days after a large meal. (**a**) MIP axial and (**b**) coronal reconstructions reveal a fishbone embedded in the right thyroid lobe (arrow). (**c**) There is evident fluid infiltration of the thyroid gland near the bone, with a perithyroidal fluid collection confined to the parathyroid space (arrow). (**d**) Unfortunately, the inflammatory and infectious process progresses despite thyroidectomy surgery, with a mediastinal abscess visible in the superior mediastinum extending from the prevascular compartment to the visceral compartment (arrow); multiple mediastinal drainage tubes are evident, and necessary for treatment (asterisks)

2.7 Sternoclavicular Septic Arthritis

Joint infections are rare, typically occurring in immunocompromised patients or following intravenous injections of substances or drugs, although they can also arise spontaneously. The most concerning location for mediastinal involvement is septic arthritis of the sternoclavicular joint due to its anatomical proximity to the mediastinum. When the left sternoclavicular joint is affected, it can cause angina-like chest pain, which should be considered in the differential diagnosis of chest pain [2]. This is particularly important because imaging studies optimized exclusively for pulmonary embolism, such as those involving contrast injection from the left arm, may fail to identify sternoclavicular septic arthritis and its associated mediastinal involvement. Sternoclavicular septic arthritis is very rare, accounting for only 1% of all septic arthritis cases. It can be caused by several factors, including intravenous drug use, distant infections, diabetes mellitus, trauma, or infected central venous catheters (CVCs). The infection may spread from a distant source (hematogenous spread) or from nearby infected tissues (contiguous spread). It presents insidiously and can be easily overlooked, especially in healthy adults. It may also occur spontaneously, particularly in young athletes, due to repetitive microtraumas. Management generally includes a prolonged course of intravenous antibiotics, and in some cases, surgical intervention, particularly when extensive osteomyelitis or mediastinal involvement is present. Initial empirical therapy should begin with antistaphylococcal antibiotics, which can be adjusted based on culture results [19]. Due to the proximity of the sternoclavicular joint to vital structures, early diagnosis, and appropriate management are essential to minimize morbidity and prevent complications like descending necrotizing mediastinitis, which can spread to the mediastinum. Complications of sternoclavicular septic arthritis can include osteomyelitis, muscle abscesses, and, in severe cases, descending necrotizing mediastinitis, predominantly affecting the prevascular space (Fig. 2.8).

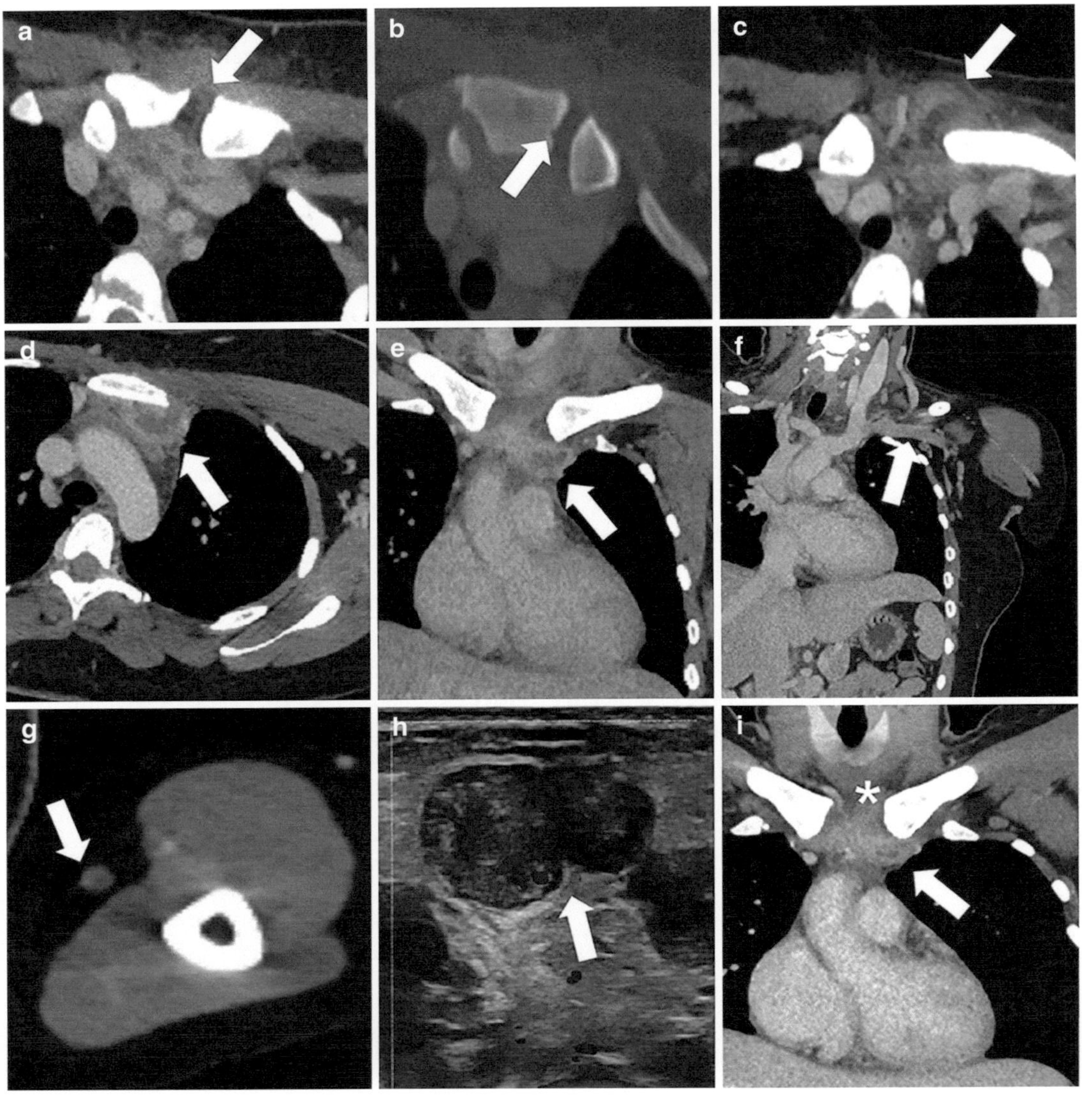

Fig. 2.8 Sternoclavicular septic arthritis in a 22-year-old woman presenting with left arm and neck pain, angina-like symptoms, following recent intravenous administration of the COVID-19 vaccine. (**a**) Fluid distension of the left sternoclavicular joint (arrow). (**b**) Cortical erosion of the clavicular profile (arrow), suggestive of osteomyelitis foci. (**c**) Myositis with abscess formation at the caudal insertion of the sternocleidomastoid muscle (arrow). (**d**) Axial and (**e**) coronal reconstructions showing a superior mediastinal abscess (arrow). (**f**) Coronal and (**g**) axial reconstructions showing compressive venous thrombosis in the venous axis of the left arm, (**h**) confirmed by ultrasound with color-Doppler imaging (arrow). (**i**) One-week follow-up after conservative pharmacological therapy, following isolation of methicillin-sensitive Staphylococcus (MSSA) in blood culture: resolution of myositis and arthritis (asterisk), with a significant reduction of the mediastinal abscess affecting the prevascular compartment (arrow)

Bibliography

1. Carter BW, Muse VV, Mansouri M. Imaging of non-traumatic mediastinal and pulmonary processes. In: Emergency radiology. Springer; 2017. p. 387–402.
2. Gulati M, Levy PD, Mukherjee D, Amsterdam E, Bhatt DL, Birtcher KK, Blankstein R, Boyd J, Bullock-Palmer RP, Conejo T, Diercks DB, Gentile F, Greenwood JP, Hess EP, Hollenberg SM, Jaber WA, Jneid H, Joglar JA, Morrow DA, Shaw LJ. 2021 AHA/ACC/ASE/CHEST/SAEM/SCCT/SCMR guideline for the evaluation and diagnosis of CHEST pain: a report of the American College of Cardiology/American Heart Association Joint Committee on Clinical Practice Guidelines. Circulation. 2021;144(22) Ovid Technologies (Wolters Kluwer Health) https://doi.org/10.1161/cir.0000000000001029.
3. Carter BW, Muse VV, Mansouri M. Imaging of non-traumatic mediastinal and pulmonary processes. In: Emergency radiology. Springer; 2017. p. 387–402. https://doi.org/10.1007/978-3-319-65397-6_23.
4. Giannitto C, Esposito AA, Casiraghi E, Biondetti PR. Epidemiological profile of non-traumatic emergencies of the neck in CT imaging: our experience. Med Radiol. 2014;119(10):784–9). Springer. https://doi.org/10.1007/s11547-014-0389-9.
5. Katabathina VS, Restrepo CS, Martinez-Jimenez S, Riascos RF. Nonvascular, nontraumatic mediastinal emergencies in adults: a comprehensive review of imaging findings. Radiographics. 2011;31(4):1141–60). Radiological Society of North America (RSNA). https://doi.org/10.1148/rg.314105177.
6. Sumi Y. Descending necrotizing mediastinitis: 5 years of published data in Japan. Acute Med Surg. 2014;2(1):1–12). Wiley. https://doi.org/10.1002/ams2.56.
7. Endo S, Murayama F, Hasegawa T, Yamamoto S, Yamaguchi T, Sohara Y, Fuse K, Miyata M, Nishino H. Guideline of surgical management based on diffusion of descending necrotizing mediastinitis. Jpn J Thorac Cardiovasc Surg. 1999;47(1):14–9). Springer. https://doi.org/10.1007/bf03217934.
8. Fraser RG, Paré JA. Diagnosis of diseases of the chest. W.B. Saunders Co; 1977.
9. Carter BW, Benveniste MF, Madan R, Godoy MC, de Groot PM, Truong MT, Rosado-de-Christenson ML, Marom EM. ITMIG classification of mediastinal compartments and multidisciplinary approach to mediastinal masses. Radiographics. 2017;37(2):413–36. Radiological Society of North America (RSNA). https://doi.org/10.1148/rg.2017160095.
10. Mansouri M, Singh A. Imaging of neck emergencies. In: Singh A, editor. Emergency radiology. Cham: Springer; 2018. https://doi.org/10.1007/978-3-319-65397-6_15.
11. Raghavan P, Mukherjee S, Jameson MJ, Wintermark M. Manual of head and neck imaging. Springer; 2014. https://doi.org/10.1007/978-3-642-40377-4.
12. Kamalian S, Avery L, Lev MH, Schaefer PW, Curtin HD, Kamalian S. Nontraumatic head and neck emergencies. Radiographics. 2019;39(6):1808–23). Radiological Society of North America (RSNA). https://doi.org/10.1148/rg.2019190159.
13. Yano M, Numanami H, Akiyama T, Taguchi R, Furuta C, Ogawa T, Kishimoto M, Okamoto H, Inukai D, Haniuda M. Distribution of descending necrotizing mediastinitis and efficacy of distribution-specific drainage. Journal of Thoracic Disease. 2020;12(5):2380–7). AME Publishing Company. https://doi.org/10.21037/jtd.2020.03.82.
14. Scaglione M, Pinto A, Giovine S, Di Nuzzo L, Giuliano V, Romano L. CT features of descending necrotizing mediastinitis—a pictorial essay. Emerg Radiol. 2007;14(2):77–81). Springer. https://doi.org/10.1007/s10140-007-0606-0.
15. Neal TW, Schlieve T. Complications of severe odontogenic infections: a review. Biology. 2022;11(12):1784. https://doi.org/10.3390/biology11121784.
16. Ullah A, Ambreen A, Gul Z. Complications of Peritonsillar abscess. Ann Clin Microbiol Antimicrob. 2022;21(1):84. https://doi.org/10.1186/s12941-022-00484-6.
17. Gosnell EJ, Anwar B, Varadarajan V, Freeman S. Sternocleidomastoid pyomyositis. Eur Ann Otorhinolaryngol Head Neck Dis. 2016;133(4):273–5. https://doi.org/10.1016/j.anorl.2015.02.003.
18. Athanassiadi K, Gerazounis M, Metaxas E, Kalantzi N. Management of esophageal foreign bodies: a retrospective review of 400 cases. Eur J Cardiothorac Surg. 2002;21(4):653–6. https://doi.org/10.1016/S1010-7940(02)00047-0.
19. Ross JJ, Shamsuddin H. Sternoclavicular septic arthritis: review of 180 cases. Medicine (Baltimore). 2004;83(3):139–48. https://doi.org/10.1097/01.md.0000126761.83417.29.

Dysphagia

3

Maria Febi, Salvatore Claudio Fanni,
Claudio Giardina, Stefania Tamburrini,
and Michele Tonerini

3.1 Introduction

Dysphagia, derived from the Greek roots "dys" (difficulty) and "phagein" (to eat), is a symptom characterized by the sensation of experiencing difficulty in swallowing [1]. Dysphagia is a common condition, about one in six adults experience dysphagia in their lifetime, which, however, often remains untreated [2]. Any disorder disrupting the passage of food from the mouth, through swallowing, down the esophagus into the stomach can cause dysphagia [3]. Dysphagia can be classified according to the location of the symptoms (oropharyngeal or esophageal), the types of food or liquids that are involved, and the duration of symptoms (acute, chronic, intermittent, or persistent) [4].

Oropharyngeal Dysphagia refers to pathologies of the first digestive tract including the mouth, the pharynx, and the swallowing process. Causes of oropharyngeal dysphagia can be structural, due to anatomical, mechanical or obstructive causes [4]. Some examples are Zenker diverticulum, esophageal webs, lymphadenopathy, abscess, neoplasms, and post-treatment alterations [4]. In the elderly, it is commonly related to chronic neurologic conditions, such as Parkinson's disease, stroke, and dementia [3]. The prevalence of dysphagia after a stroke is 42–67% and half of the patients suffering from Parkinsonism have dysphagia [4]. Dysphagia can also occur due to multiple sclerosis, contractile disturbances such as myasthenia gravis, and after radiation therapy for head and neck cancer [4].

Esophageal Dysphagia is the term for swallowing difficulty referred to conditions involving the esophagus. The most common condition associated with esophageal dysphagia is gastroesophageal reflux disease (GERD) [3]. The main differential diagnosis is neoplasia, with esophageal cancer ranks seventh in global cancer incidence [5]. Dysphagia is the predominant initial manifestation observed in patients affected and it is attributable to the tumor-induced obstruction of the esophageal passage [5]. Other causes of esophageal dysphagia are esophageal webs and rings, eosinophilic esophagitis, infectious esophagitis, achalasia, spasm, hypercontractile motility disorders, rheumatologic diseases (scleroderma), extrinsic compression, radiation, and postsurgical injuries [3, 4].

Caustic ingestion is a less common cause of esophageal dysphagia, but it remains a life-

M. Febi · S. C. Fanni
Department of Translational Research, Academic Radiology, University of Pisa, Pisa, Italy

C. Giardina
Service Department, A.O. Papardo, Messina, Italy

S. Tamburrini
Department of Radiology, Ospedale del Mare-ASL NA1 Centro, Naples, Italy

M. Tonerini (✉)
Department of Emergency Radiology, University Hospital of Pisa, Pisa, Italy

L. Romano et al. (eds.), *CT of Non-Traumatic Body Emergencies*,
https://doi.org/10.1007/978-3-031-84849-0_3

threatening condition for patients admitted to the emergency room. Caustic exposure can be accidental, especially in young children, or intentional, often seen as self-harm attempts [4, 6]. Food impaction or the ingestion of foreign bodies can also determine acute-onset dysphagia and it is commonly seen in children from 6 months to 6 years old; in adults, instead they are usually ingested accidentally together with food [3, 7].

Dysphagia may also pose a critical concern, potentially indicating severe underlying conditions such as stroke, neurological disorders, or obstructive lesions in the upper gastrointestinal tract.

This chapter will address dysphagia from the emergency radiologist's perspective, focusing on the predominant diagnoses identified through computed tomography (CT).

3.2 Diagnostic Imaging Techniques

Several diagnostic techniques can be used to assess the patient suffering from dysphagia. These techniques may assist in identifying structural abnormalities, functional impairments, and underlying causes contributing to swallowing difficulties.

The *modified barium swallow study (MBSS)* is the gold standard for evaluating oropharyngeal dysphagia [4]. Video-fluoroscopy allows the swallowing process to be visualized in real-time, detecting potential impairment to the swallowing mechanism. The evaluation is made while the patient is swallowing a bolus of contrast agent made of a barium sulfate suspension, available in liquid, solid, and semisolid form to simulate different real meal consistencies [8]. The MBSS has been demonstrated to be useful in evaluating oral and pharyngeal swallowing function and airway protection, allowing the diagnosis of neurological disorders in the elderly, tumors or masses in the tongue, pharynx, larynx, or in the retropharyngeal region, and suspected aspiration [9].

The American College of Radiology (ACR) guidelines differentiate the MBSS from the so-called *esophagram*. Esophagram is used to evaluate esophageal motility and morphology, but also to assess the GE junction. Two techniques should be distinguished: single-contrast or double-contrast. The single-contrast is similar to the MBSS with a video-fluoroscopic observation of the esophagus after a bolus of barium. The double-contrast uses an effervescent agent releasing carbon dioxide into the lumen of the stomach. The exam must be tailored to the patient's disease, and it is indicated in all the causes of esophageal dysphagia such as GERD or motility disorders [10]. An exception should be made in cases where, according to patient history and symptomatology, esophageal perforation is suspected. Guidelines for investigating nontraumatic esophageal perforations typically recommend initiating the examination with a water-soluble contrast agent (Gastrografin/diatrizoate) due to the potential risks associated with barium extravasation into the mediastinum leading to the risk of inflammation. Conversely, if there is any sign of a concomitant tracheal injury, it must be noted that Gastrografin/diatrizoate is known to cause more severe pneumonitis than Barium sulfate [11].

Computed tomography (CT) is not the initial imaging technique suggested in oropharyngeal and esophageal dysphagia considering the high dose of radiation and the poor evaluation of the motility in real time [12]. However, due to its spatial resolution, speed, ease of acquisition, and availability worldwide, CT is an important imaging modality for the evaluation, diagnosis, and staging of multiple oropharyngeal and esophageal pathologies that can present with the main symptom of dysphagia [13]. In particular, CT is fundamental in the emergency setting. The administration of an intravenous contrast agent is recommended during the CT scan to better define all the anatomical structures of the neck and chest. To ensure the integrity of the esophagus an oral contrast administration immediately before the examination may be helpful [12].

3.3 Pathologies

The subsequent sections will address the predominant and significant pathologies associated with oropharyngeal and esophageal dysphagia in emergency and urgent care settings, with a particular focus on CT imaging.

3.3.1 Foreign Bodies

Ingestion of objects that get stuck in the esophagus creating obstruction can lead to a range of symptoms including dysphagia, odynophagia, chest pain, and vomiting [14]. Usually, the patient is stable and has no further symptoms [15]. The swallowing of objects can be involuntary, which is more common in children, or voluntary such as in psychiatric patients or prisoners [14]. Sometimes patients who have esophageal foreign body obstruction have underlying predisposing pathology, such as eosinophilic esophagitis, previous esophageal surgery, or motility disorders [14]. Obstruction can occur with different types of ingested objects, the most common include: food boluses, chicken bones, fish bones, and coins (Fig. 3.1) [15].

However, some objects such as batteries, multiple magnets, and sharp or pointed objects may create greater risk, such as mucosal damage, esophageal perforation, and damage to surrounding structures [15]. It is critical to understand and localize the problem, also by asking adults and older children to verbally explain the type of object [14]. Imaging helps for anatomical identification, as radiopaque objects are identifiable by chest X-ray in the two projections. However, for radiolucent objects, the X-ray may help in detecting possible complications such as aspiration of material or perforation [16]. European Society of Gastrointestinal Endoscopy (ESGE) does not advise radiological assessment if there is a non-bony food bolus impaction without complications, however, an X-ray is needed if a radiopaque object is suspected or the type of object is unknown [16]. CT can be of great help as it has

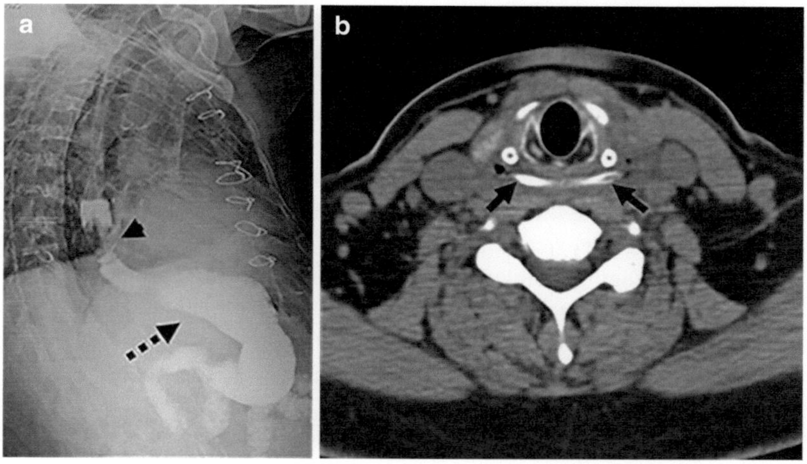

Fig. 3.1 (**a**) A 74-years-old man was admitted to the emergency room due to the rapid onset of dysphagia after the ingestion of a meat bolus that remained stuck in the lower third of the thoracic esophagus; the fluoroscopic examination (anterior left oblique view), performed in the emergency setting, after the assumption of an oral water-soluble contrast, showed a filling defect in the esophageal lumen, determined by the meat bolus (arrowhead); the luminal obstruction however was not complete and oral contrast could flow downstream (dashed arrow). The bolus was removed during the emergency endoscopic examination. (**b**) A 45-year-old old woman with pain and difficulty swallowing after an accidental chicken bone ingestion; the plain axial neck CT image shows a little chicken bone, looking like a drumstick, that remained crossed in the hypopharynx (straight arrows). There was no sign of pharyngeal perforation and of subcutaneous emphysema. The bone was promptly removed by the otolaryngology physician

greater accuracy and sensitivity ensuring three-dimensional reconstructions [16]. CT generally is recommended in all patients with suspected perforation and in all cases when surgery can be required [16]. Oral contrast should not be administered because it can compromise endoscopy and the risk of contrast aspiration [16].

3.3.2 Chemical Injury

Chemical injury of the esophagus is caused by the ingestion of dangerous substances, in particular by caustic ingestion. This pathology is uncommon and the majority are due to unintentional ingestion of this type of substance by children, or intentional ingestion by adults who suffer from psychiatric diseases or who are attempting suicide [17]. The substances can be alkaline, producing colliquative necrosis with immediate and severe damage to the entire gastrointestinal tract, or acidic, producing instead coagulative necrosis with less tissue penetration and damage [18]. Alkaline materials, such as bleach, are usually thicker, viscose substances that remain in contact with the esophagus longer, leading to progressive thinning of the esophageal lining and consequent damage from colliquative necrosis that can take several days to manifest [17, 19]. The substance then is neutralized by the acidity of the stomach [19]. Acid materials instead, for the unpleasant odor and taste are quickly ingested in a smaller dose, and being more fluid they pass rapidly through the esophagus damaging primarily the stomach [17, 19]. The patient usually presents with dysphagia, odynophagia, and hematemesis. There is the risk of perforation and death that varies depending on the type of substance and amount of substance ingested [19]. Chronically, there is an increased risk of the formation of strictures and obstructions, but also a higher risk of malignant transformation [19]. X-ray can be used to exclude perforation [19]. Esophagogastroduodenoscopy, instead, is capable of measuring the luminal extension and severity. However, the primary risk of endoscopy is perforation, particularly within 5–15 days post-procedure when the tissue begins to heal. In addition, endoscopy is not capable of seeing the depth of necrosis [17, 19].

CT allows for evaluation of the severity of the disease, and then categorizes patients between emergency, surgery, and nonoperative management, helping to improve patient survival [17]. The CT protocol includes a baseline acquisition of the neck, thorax, and abdomen, the administration of an intravenous contrast agent, and the acquisition of an arterial and a venous phase (Fig. 3.2).

If a perforation is suspected, after the baseline and before intravenous administration, 100–150 ml of water-soluble iodine-based oral contrast agent can be given. Bruzzi et al. [20] suggested a classification of esophageal wall injury to predict the risk of stricture formation: grade I is normal appearing organs; in grade II there is wall edema, surrounding soft tissue inflammation with increased postcontrast wall enhancement; the transmural necrosis corresponds to grade III, it is shown by the absence of postcontrast wall enhancement, and requires esophagectomy. Edema results in the thickening of the esophageal wall, it can be focal (more common distally) or diffuse [21]. Esophageal perforation is the first and most frequent acute complication to look for in CT. In this case, the administration of an oral contrast agent can identify the perforation site. Pneumomediastinum is another sign of esophageal perforation that must be searched for [21]. Communication with the airway in an esophago-respiratory fistula is another rather rare complication that can lead to aspiration or infectious pneumonia. It is pathognomonic if the contrast agent reaches the airway. Similarly, if the oral contrast agent reaches the pleura space an esophago-pleura fistula can be diagnosed [21].

3.3.3 Oncologic and Iatrogenic Diseases

Oncologic emergencies are an extensive range of conditions including any acute up to life-threatening events in oncologic patients, either caused by the malignancy itself or its treatment

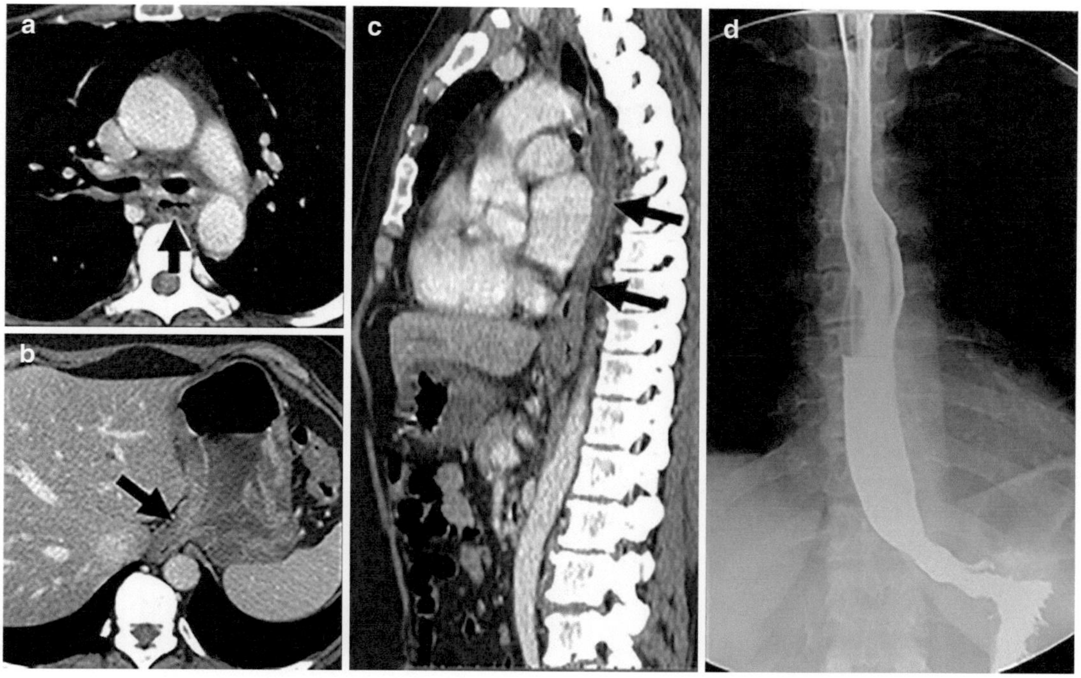

Fig. 3.2 (**a–d**) A 51-year-old woman after the intentional ingestion of a small amount of bleach in a self-harm attempt. (**a** and **b**) The contrast-enhanced CT shows an internal esophageal mucosal thickening and enhancement below the tracheal carina (arrow) and at the esophago-gastric junction (arrow). In this case, a "target" aspect may appear. Mediastinal fat stranding is however absent. In the coronal MPR reconstruction (arrows in **c**) the esophageal wall edema appears hypodense. (**d**) A month later, an esophago-gastric fluoroscopic examination, after the assumption of oral water-soluble contrast, displayed a regular passage of contrast in the esophageal lumen without residual mucosal damage and fibrotic strictures

[22]. All tumors and lymphadenopathy in the head-neck and thoracic region may create a mass effect in various tracts of the mouth, pharynx, or esophagus leading to dysphagia (Fig. 3.3) [23].

Pre-treatment dysphagia was observed in 28.2% of patients with stage T2 oral cancer, 50.9% with pharyngeal cancer, and 28.6% with laryngeal cancer [24]. In these patients, dysphagia may result also from the consequence of radiotherapy, chemotherapy, or surgery [1]. Tumors involving the mouth may require demolition surgery, for example of the tongue or of the bone structures resulting in swallowing deficits. It has been reported that patients undergoing total laryngectomy had a risk of developing dysphagia ranging from 10% to 80% [1]. Radiation therapy, likewise, irradiates and damages not only the tumor but also all the structures deputed to swallowing. Dysphagia, xerostomia, and swallowing impairment are the more common side effects, and their severity depends on the dose, duration of treatment, and irradiated area. These side effects can appear also years after treatment due to collagen transformation (Fig. 3.4) [1].

Considering esophageal cancer, dysphagia can be a consequence of tumor growth obstructing the esophageal lumen. It may be a symptom at onset or a symptom in inoperable patients to be treated in palliative care [25, 26]. Lung cancer causes dysphagia in 1–2% of patients [27] due to mediastinal or cervical lymphadenopathy, brainstem lesions, gastrointestinal tract metastasis, or esophageal stenosis from radiation therapy (Fig. 3.4) [28].

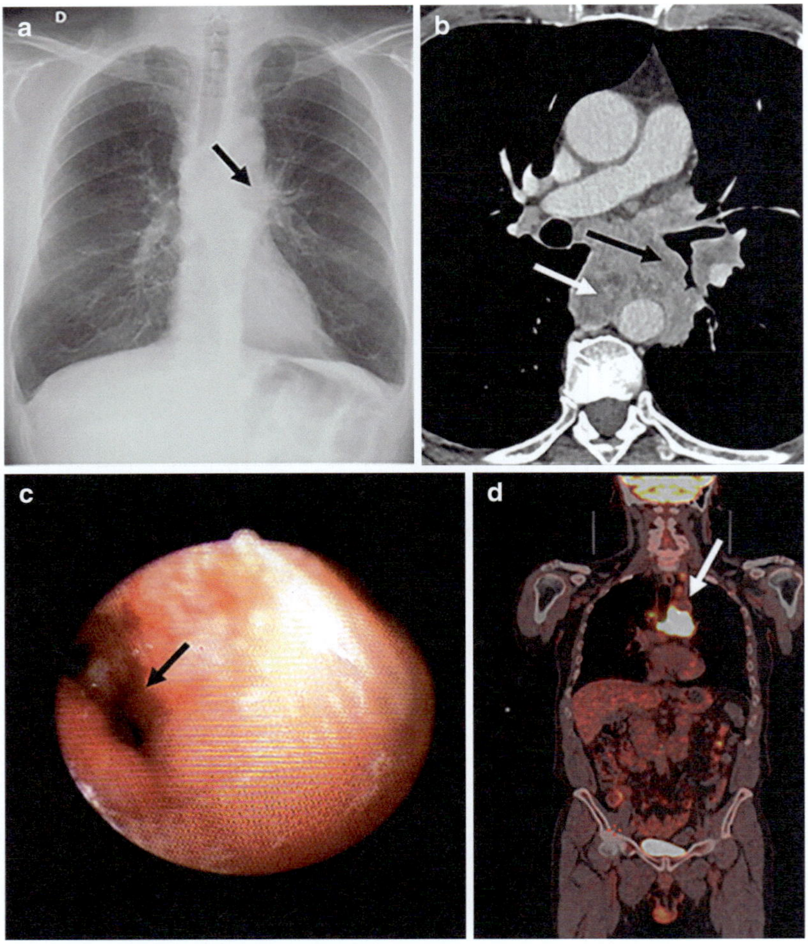

Fig. 3.3 (**a**–**d**) A 57-year-old man was admitted to the emergency room for chest pain and difficulty in swallowing both solids and liquids. The chest plain film showed a middle mediastinal enlargement, especially in the left hilar region (arrow in **a**). A chest contrast-enhanced CT (**b**) was immediately performed and it revealed a middle mediastinal neoplastic mass, caused by a primary lung carcinoma, that narrows left main bronchus (black arrow), completely infiltrates the esophageal lumen and surrounds descending aorta (white arrow). A bronchoscopy examination (**c**), performed after 2 days, confirmed the neoplastic lesion narrowing the left main bronchus (black arrow in **c**). The FDG PET-CT (**d**) displayed a high uptake (22 SUV Max) in the middle mediastinum and the left hilum (white arrow)

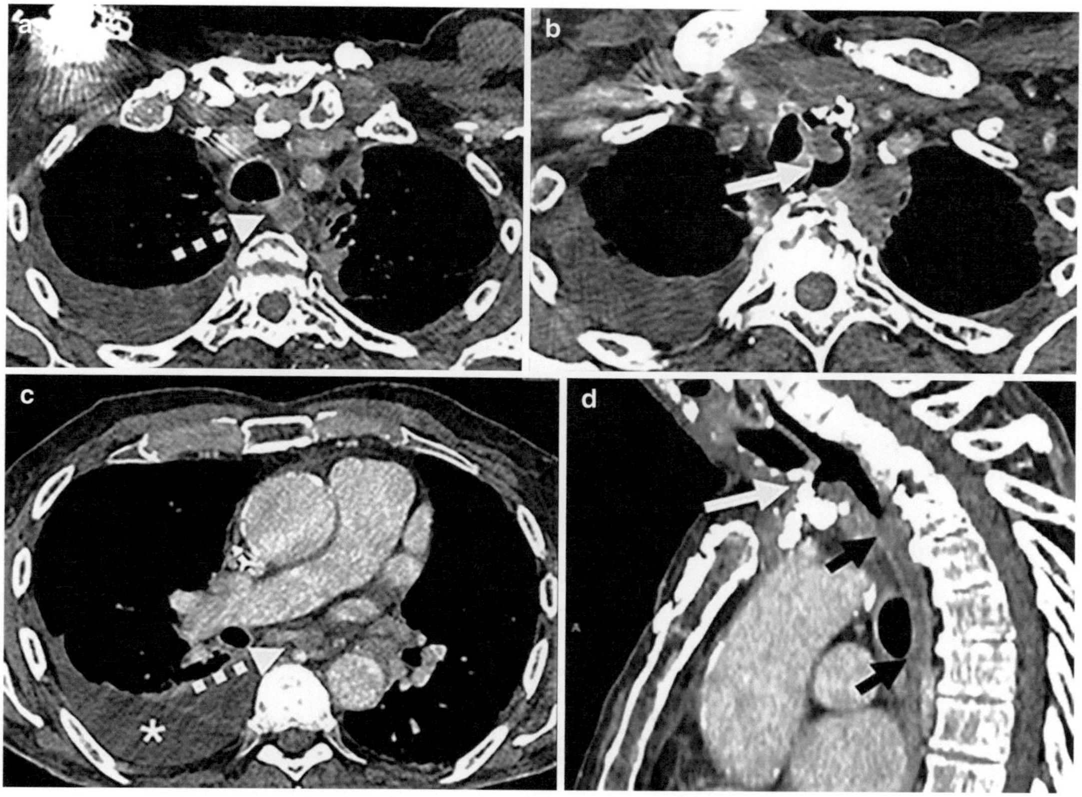

Fig. 3.4 (**a–d**) A 76-year-old man developed dysphagia 12 months after the end of the radiation therapy for left upper lobe lung cancer. There were signs of esophagitis, characterized by mild thickening and contrast enhancement of the esophageal wall (dashed arrows in **a** and **c**). The longitudinal extension of the esophageal inflammatory reaction was better displayed in the sagittal MPR CT reconstruction (black arrows in **d**). The chronic esophagitis was complicated by a fistulous tract originating from the anterior wall of the third superior of the thoracic esophagus, from the left of the tracheal wall to a group of mediastinal calcifications (white arrows in **b** and **d**). The patient was also dyspnoeic due to a right pleural effusion (asterisk in **c**)

3.3.4 Inflammatory, Infectious, and Motility Diseases

Inflammation of the wall of the esophagus, i.e., esophagitis, is most commonly caused by GERD. Frequent exposure to acid results in chronic mucosal damage, but also impaired motility and strictures [3]. Other causes of esophagitis are eosinophilic esophagitis and infectious esophagitis. Eosinophilic esophagitis, caused by food allergens, is increasingly prevalent among young people, particularly in the United States [4]. The most common form of infectious esophagitis in immunocompromised patients is candida esophagitis. CT findings of esophagitis usually include a circumferential wall thickening of at least 5 mm. with the so-called "target sign." The "target sign" is composed of esophageal mucosal enhancement internally and submucosal hypodensity externally [13]. However, CT alone is not enough in the diagnosis of these diseases, and clinical integration and other diagnostic techniques such as endoscopy or esophagram are required. CT can also evaluate complications such as strictures, fistulas, dilatations, bleeding, and perforations (Fig. 3.5) [13].

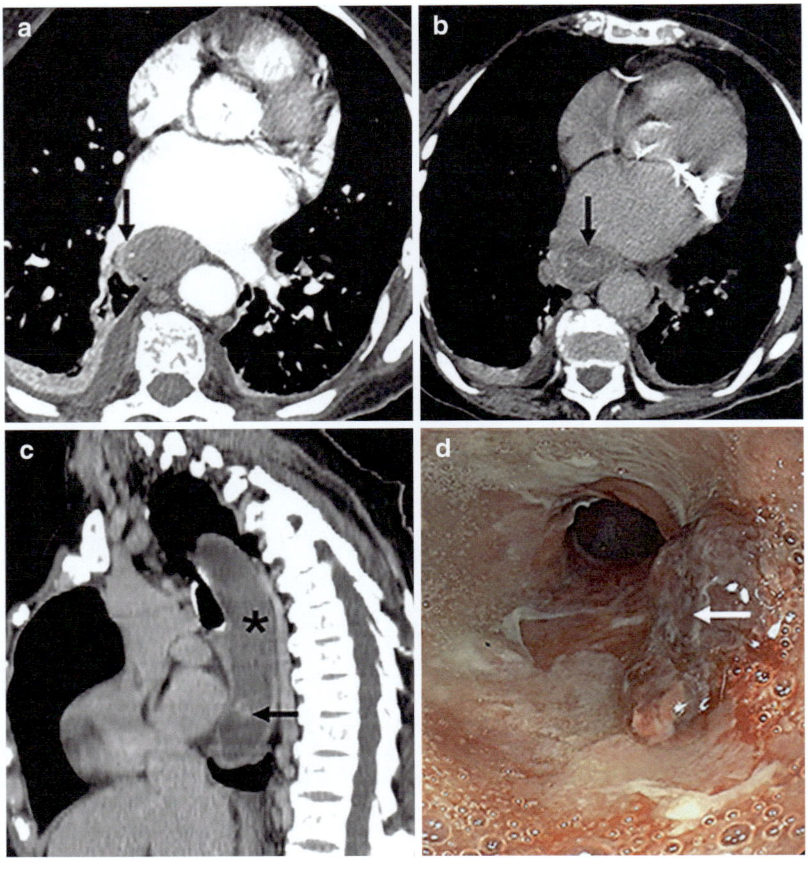

Fig. 3.5 (**a**–**d**) A 74-year-old woman, the suffering of GERD, was admitted to the emergency department owing to the sudden onset of dysphagia and hematemesis. The contrast-enhanced CT scan revealed signs of ongoing bleeding from the thoracic esophageal wall (arrows) both in the arterial phase (**a**) and in the venous one (**b**), characterized by contrast blushes in the visceral lumen, which was distended by refluxed gastric content (asterisk **c**). The sagittal MPR CT reconstruction clearly displayed the extravasation of intravenously administered contrast in the enlarged esophageal lumen (arrow in **c**). An urgent endoscopic examination was performed and confirmed the signs of esophagitis and the mucosal acute bleeding (arrow in **d**)

Rare causes of dysphagia, and even more infrequently observed on CT in an urgent setting, are esophageal motility disorders. These are for example achalasia, systemic sclerosis (scleroderma), and distal esophageal spasm [3]. On CT the typical findings in these diseases are the enlarged transverse diameter (over 10 mm) and the presence of air-fluid levels [13].

3.4 Conclusions

Dysphagia can occur alone or alongside other symptoms. In emergency settings, it is not uncommon and must be promptly recognized and investigated due to the wide range of underlying conditions, varying in severity, that can cause it. CT imaging can aid in diagnosis and patient management. Identifying severe complications, such as perforation or bleeding, is crucial for guiding patient care.

References

1. Manikantan K, Khode S, Sayed SI, Roe J, Nutting CM, Rhys-Evans P, Harrington KJ, Kazi R. Dysphagia in head and neck cancer. Cancer Treat Rev. 2009;35:724–32. https://doi.org/10.1016/j.ctrv.2009.08.008.
2. Adkins C, Takakura W, Spiegel BMR, Lu M, Vera-Llonch M, Williams J, Almario CV. Prevalence and characteristics of dysphagia based on a population-based survey. Clin Gastroenterol Hepatol. 2020;18:1970–1979.e2. https://doi.org/10.1016/j.cgh.2019.10.029.
3. Wilkinson JM, Codipilly DC, Wilfahrt RP. Dysphagia: evaluation and collaborative management. Am Fam Physician. 2021;103:97–106.
4. Malagelada J-R, Bazzoli F, Boeckxstaens G, et al. World gastroenterology organisation global guidelines: dysphagia–global guidelines and cascades update September 2014. J Clin Gastroenterol. 2015;49:370–8. https://doi.org/10.1097/MCG.0000000000000307.
5. Mohapatra S, Santharaman A, Gomez K, Pannala R, Kachaamy T. Optimal management of dysphagia in patients with inoperable esophageal cancer: current perspectives. Cancer Manag Res. 2022;14:3281–91. https://doi.org/10.2147/CMAR.S362666.
6. Bielecki JE, Recio-Boiles A, Chen RJ, Gupta V. Caustic Ingestions. In: StatPearls [Internet]. Treasure Island (FL): StatPearls Publishing; 2024.
7. Ambe P, Weber SA, Schauer M, Knoefel WT. Swallowed foreign bodies in adults. Dtsch Arztebl Int. 2012;109:869–75. https://doi.org/10.3238/arztebl.2012.0869.
8. Martin-Harris B, Canon CL, Bonilha HS, Murray J, Davidson K, Lefton-Greif MA. Best practices in modified barium swallow studies. Am J Speech-Language Pathol. 2020;29:1078–93. https://doi.org/10.1044/2020_AJSLP-19-00189.
9. American College of Radiology (ACR), the Society for Pediatric Radiology (SPR). ACR—SPR practice parameter for the performance of the modified barium; 2023, pp. 0–12.
10. American College of Radiology (ACR). ACR practice parameter for the performance of esophagrams and upper gastrointestinal examinations in adults; 2019. 1076, pp. 1–11.
11. Chen A, Tafti D, Tuma F. Barium Swallow. [Updated 2023 Jul 24]. In: StatPearls [Internet]. Treasure Island (FL): StatPearls Publishing; 2024. Available from: https://www.ncbi.nlm.nih.gov/books/NBK493176/.
12. Levy AD, Carucci LR, Bartel TB, et al. ACR appropriateness criteria(®) dysphagia. J Am Coll Radiol. 2019;16:S104–15. https://doi.org/10.1016/j.jacr.2019.02.007.
13. Buchanan ME, Fishman EK, Azadi JR. CT evaluation of the esophagus: the role of CT imaging and CT imaging findings in diagnosing esophageal abnormalities. Curr Probl Diagn Radiol. 2023;52:289–99. https://doi.org/10.1067/j.cpradiol.2023.03.002.
14. Pfau PR. Removal and management of esophageal foreign bodies. Tech Gastrointest Endosc. 2014;16:32–9. https://doi.org/10.1016/j.tgie.2013.10.004.
15. Schaefer TJ, Trocinski D. Esophageal Foreign Body. [Updated 2023 Jan 30]. In: StatPearls [Internet]. Treasure Island (FL): StatPearls Publishing; 2024. Available from: https://www.ncbi.nlm.nih.gov/books/NBK482131/16. Fung BM, Sweetser S, Wong Kee Song LM, Tabibian JH. Foreign object ingestion and esophageal food impaction: an update and review on endoscopic management. World J Gastrointest Endosc 2019;11:174–92.
16. Birk M, Bauerfeind P, Deprez PH, Häfner M, Hartmann D, Hassan C, Hucl T, Lesur G, Aabakken L, Meining A. Removal of foreign bodies in the upper gastrointestinal tract in adults: European Society of Gastrointestinal Endoscopy (ESGE) Clinical Guideline. Endoscopy. 2016;48:489–96. https://doi.org/10.1055/s-0042-100456.
17. Kluger Y, Ben IO, Sartelli M, et al. Caustic ingestion management: world society of emergency surgery preliminary survey of expert opinion. World J Emerg Surg. 2015;10:48. https://doi.org/10.1186/s13017-015-0050-5.
18. Chirica M, Bonavina L, Kelly MD, Sarfati E, Cattan P. Caustic ingestion. Lancet. 2017;389:2041–52. https://doi.org/10.1016/S0140-6736(16)30313-0.
19. De Lusong MAA, Timbol ABG, Tuazon DJS. Management of esophageal caustic injury. World J Gastrointest Pharmacol Ther. 2017;8:90–8. https://doi.org/10.4292/wjgpt.v8.i2.90.
20. Bruzzi M, Chirica M, Resche-Rigon M, Corte H, Voron T, Sarfati E, Zagdanski AM, Cattan P. Emergency computed tomography predicts caustic esophageal stricture formation. Ann Surg. 2019;270(1):109–14. https://doi.org/10.1097/SLA.0000000000002732.
21. Cutaia G, Messina M, Rubino S, et al. Caustic ingestion: CT findings of esophageal injuries and thoracic complications. Emerg Radiol. 2021;28:845–56. https://doi.org/10.1007/s10140-021-01918-1.
22. Fanni SC, Greco G, Rossi S, Aghakhanyan G, Masala S, Scaglione M, Tonerini M, Neri E. Role of artificial intelligence in oncologic emergen-

cies: a narrative review. Explor Target Anti-Tumor Ther. 2023;4:344–54. https://doi.org/10.37349/etat.2023.00138.
23. Raber-Durlacher JE, Brennan MT, Verdonck-de Leeuw IM, et al. Swallowing dysfunction in cancer patients. Support Care Cancer. 2012;20:433–43. https://doi.org/10.1007/s00520-011-1342-2.
24. Logemann JA, Rademaker AW, Pauloski BR, et al. Site of disease and treatment protocol as correlates of swallowing function in patients with head and neck cancer treated with chemoradiation. Head Neck. 2006;28:64–73. https://doi.org/10.1002/hed.20299.
25. Sadaps M, Bhatt A, Chevalier C, Sohal D, Videtic G, McNamara MJ. A practical guide to the management of dysphagia in patients with metastatic esophageal cancer. Ann Esophagus. 2018;1 https://doi.org/10.21037/aoe.2018.03.01.
26. Hanna WC, Sudarshan M, Roberge D, David M, Waschke KA, Mayrand S, Alcindor T, Ferri LE. What is the optimal management of dysphagia in metastatic esophageal cancer? Curr Oncol. 2012;19:e60–6. https://doi.org/10.3747/co.19.892.
27. Le Roux BT. The presentation of bronchial carcinoma. Scott Med J. 1968;13:31–7. https://doi.org/10.1177/003693306801300201.
28. Camidge DR. The causes of dysphagia in carcinoma of the lung. J R Soc Med. 2001;94:567–72. https://doi.org/10.1177/014107680109401104.

4 Dyspnea

Giacomo Bonito, Silvia Gigli, Laura Corso, Lucia Malzone, Monica Mattone, and Paolo Ricci

4.1 Introduction

According to a consensus statement of the American Thoracic Society (ATS), dyspnea is defined as "a subjective experience of breathing discomfort that consists of qualitatively distinct sensations that vary in intensity" [1]. The term dyspnea, encompasses, therefore, a range of breath-related sensations, such as the sensation of air hunger, chest oppression, and exertion/work, which occur at rest or at lower-than-expected levels of exertion [2]. The intensity, duration, and severity of dyspnea depend on the underlying pathophysiologic mechanism but the resulting perception is influenced by the social, cultural, and psychological characteristics of the patient. Therefore, self-report is critical in the assessment of dyspnea [1].

Dyspnea is a major reason for admission to the emergency department (ED) [3].

The differential diagnosis includes a variety of disorders, classified into obstructive, parenchymal, cardiac, neuromuscular, psychogenic, systemic illness, or a combination of these.

Several blood biomarkers are helpful in diagnostic evaluation, such as arterial blood gas analysis, B-type natriuretic peptide, troponins, creatine kinase, and D-dimer [3].

According to the American College of Radiology (ACR) appropriateness criteria, chest X-ray (CXR) represents the first-level examination in a diagnostic flowchart [4, 5]. Computed Tomography (CT) is considered the gold standard, both for its high specificity and sensitivity; however, it is not appropriate in the first assessment of dyspnoic patients, except in the suspicion of pulmonary embolism. Therefore CT should be preferred when clinical, X-ray, and laboratory study results are inconclusive [6]. Unlike cardiac ultrasound, the use of which is validated by many studies and guidelines [7], the employ of lung ultrasound (LUS) in dyspnoic patients, is relatively recent [8].

G. Bonito
Emergency Radiology Unit, Policlinico Umberto I Hospital, Rome, Italy

Department of Radiology, Oncology and Pathology, Sapienza University of Rome, Rome, Italy
e-mail: giacomo.bonito@alice.it

S. Gigli
Department of Diagnostic Imaging, Sandro Pertini Hospital, Rome, Italy
e-mail: silvia.gigli@aslroma2.it

L. Corso · L. Malzone · M. Mattone
Department of Radiology, Oncology and Pathology, Sapienza University of Rome, Rome, Italy
e-mail: laura.corso@uniroma1.it; lucia.malzone@uniroma1.it; monica.mattone@uniroma1.it

P. Ricci (✉)
Emergency Radiology Unit, Policlinico Umberto I Hospital, Rome, Italy

Department of Radiology, Oncology and Pathology, Sapienza University of Rome, Rome, Italy
e-mail: paolo.ricci@uniroma1.it

L. Romano et al. (eds.), *CT of Non-Traumatic Body Emergencies*,
https://doi.org/10.1007/978-3-031-84849-0_4

4.2 Imaging Methods

Due to its widespread availability, low cost, and feasibility CXR represents the first-line imaging exam in a patient presenting to the ED complaining of acute dyspnea. In suspicion of cardiac origin dyspnea, CXR is recommended as a first-line method, followed by transthoracic echocardiography (TTE) and ECG, to exclude, congestive heart failure [9]. In evaluating patients with suspected pulmonary origin of dyspnea, CXR allows to exclude pneumonia and to detect other pulmonary diseases [10].

Although not recommended for the first assessment of dyspnoic patients, CT represents the gold standard in assessing lung disorders with a sensitivity and specificity ranging from 90% to 100%. However, CT employ is limited in critically ill patients, whose transport is not always feasible. Therefore CT plays a significant role as a second second-level modality, in patients who have already had a normal or equivocal chest X-ray, with positive physical examination, abnormal vital signs, or risk factors as elderly [4]. Another drawback of this method is represented by radiation exposure: thus, several low-dose and ultra-low-dose protocols are proposed to optimize the radiation exposure, without compromising the diagnostic quality of the image [11, 12].

In case of suspected pulmonary embolism with a positive D-dimer, even with a low or intermediate pre-test probability, CT pulmonary angiography with intravenous contrast medium is the first-line imaging method, considering its high sensitivity and specificity [13]. A diagnostic CTPA should result in adequate opacification of the pulmonary arteries, such that a thrombus can be readily distinguished from intraluminal contrast material [14].

If the presence of pulmonary embolism is highlighted, the study can be extended to the venous phase of the lower limbs to search for deep vein thrombosis (DVT). In this case, a further scan positioned on the pelvis up to the popliteal fossa should be acquired [13].

In the past, the role of lung ultrasound (LUS) was mainly employed for detecting of pleural effusion and guiding thoracentesis. However, in the last decade, LUS in critically ill patients has emerged as a practical diagnostic tool for several lung diseases such as pneumonia, pleural and pericardial effusion, pneumothorax, and heart failure. LUS arouses particular interest due to its many inherent advantages such as the lack of ionizing radiation, the wide availability, and the relatively low cost. The major drawback of this method is the poor penetration of the US beam due to the overlying thoracic cage and air content within the lung, leading to artifacts. Lichtenstein utilized these artifacts to propose the BLUE–protocol (bedside LUS examination), which provides a standardized technique for performing and interpreting LUS in critically ill patients [15].

4.3 Airways Diseases

4.3.1 Bronchiolitis

Bronchiolitis is a disease of the small airways caused by inflammation of the membranous and respiratory bronchioles, associated with progressive airflow obstruction. Bronchiolitis recognizes several causes such as infection, toxic exposure, collagen vascular disease, post-lung and stem cell transplant, and idiopathic etiology. Clinical manifestations include dyspnea, productive cough, and wheezing [16]. Chest radiographic findings can be normal or show non-specific findings, such as hyperinflation. Bronchioles are distal airways within secondary pulmonary lobules that are only recognizable on CT when abnormal. Direct signs of acute bronchiolitis include centrilobular nodules and linear opacities (tree-in-bud), sometimes associated with alveolar-interstitial opacities (Fig. 4.1) [17]. Centrilobular nodules should spare the pleural and fissural surfaces, thus differentiating them from random and perilymphatic nodules. Moreover, the obstruction of the small airways causes reflex vasoconstriction with redistribution of blood flow: these changes result in a combination of air trapping and oligoemia (mosaic attenuation pattern). Other findings include bronchial wall thickening and bronchiectasis [18].

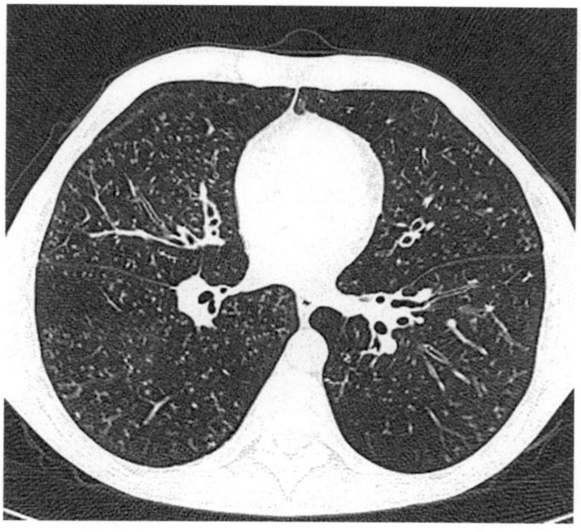

Fig. 4.1 CT image of an immunocompromised 37-year-old man affected with infectious bronchiolitis from adenovirus. Extensive branching, soft tissue attenuation opacities, so-called tree-in-bud nodules, are present throughout both lungs. Note how these parenchymal changes spare the subpleural regions and fissures, as expected from a disease arising from secondary pulmonary lobules

4.3.2 Asthma

Asthma is a common disease due to chronic inflammation of the lower respiratory tract and is characterized by recurrent episodes of airway obstruction and reversible airflow limitation [19]. Imaging plays a minor role in diagnosing acute asthma. Radiographic features associated with asthma are non-specific, including increased lung volume, pulmonary hyperlucency, slight thickening of the bronchial walls, and mild prominence of the hilar vessels due to transient pulmonary hypertension [20]. There is usually poor correlation between the severity of radiographic findings and the intensity or reversibility of an asthma attack [21].

In patients with uncomplicated asthma, CT may reveal mild parietal thickening or dilation of the small bronchi in about half of the cases [22]. Approximately 20% of cases show mucus plugs and a tree-in-bud pattern, which generally resolve with treatment. Mosaic perfusion is seen in 20–30% of cases on inhalation scans. Expiratory CT may demonstrate airway trapping in up to 50% of asthmatic patients [22]. Bronchiectasis and bronchial wall thickening have been associated with worse lung function and longer disease duration [23]. CT is especially helpful in severe asthmatics with acute decompensation, in diagnosing diseases associated with asthma (allergic bronchopulmonary aspergillosis, eosinophilic pneumonia), and in assessing complications (pneumothorax, pneumomediastinum) [20].

Pneumomediastinum can complicate asthma alone or in combination with pneumothorax due to intense coughing and forceful inhalation/exhalation. Radiographically, the air in the mediastinum appears as a thin linear or curvilinear lucency in areas usually occupied by the confluence of the heart, great vessels, bronchial walls, and esophagus shadows. This is often most noticeable along the left heart border. CT assesses the extent of the pneumomediastinum (ie., mild, moderate, or severe), confirming the diagnosis in suspicious cases with an indeterminate plain chest X-ray (Fig. 4.2) [21].

4.3.3 Foreign Body Ingestion or Aspiration

Foreign body ingestion or aspiration is one of the most common emergencies in pediatric patients younger than 3 years while is an uncommon clinical entity in adults (often observed in psychiatric patients or after iatrogenic procedures) [24]. Foreign bodies can either be organic (eg, peanuts, peas) or inorganic (coins, teeth). The clinical presentation varies depending on the location of FB in the airway and can range from an asymptomatic presentation to a life-threatening emergency. Patients may present with acute onset cough, chest pain, breathlessness or dyspnea, hemoptysis, and recurrent post-obstructive pneumonia [25].

Guidelines recommend performing bronchoscopy on any suspected or confirmed foreign body aspiration [26]. However, when the patient is stable, other diagnostic tests may be performed during pre-procedural planning to reduce the complications and enhance the outcomes. As bronchoscopy often requires general anesthesia

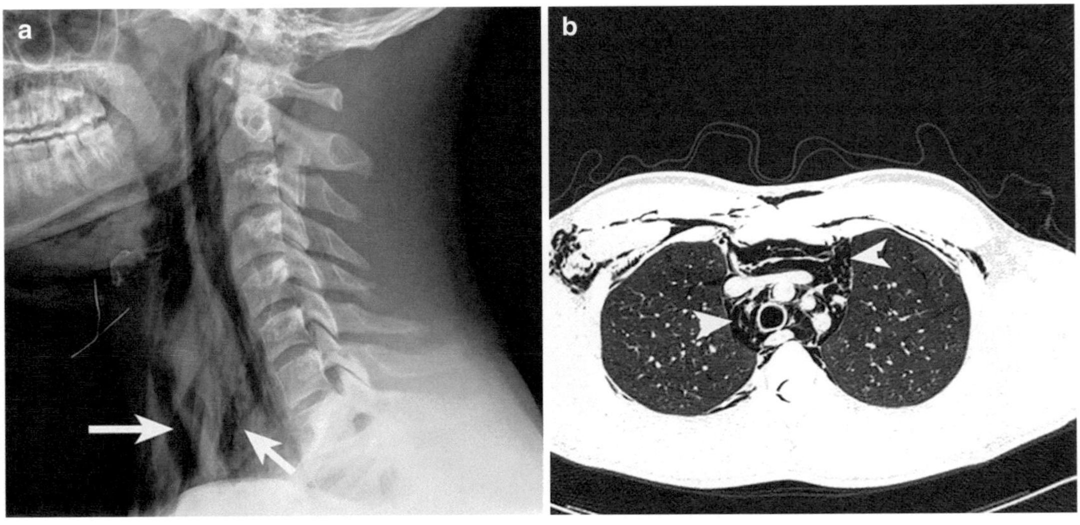

Fig. 4.2 (**a–b**) A 27-year-old man with a history of asthma, was admitted to the Emergency Department with sudden-onset dyspnea associated with neck welling and chest pain. (**a**) Plain radiographs revealed striated lucencies within the soft tissue of the supraclavicular area and the laterocervical regions; findings consistent with subcutaneous emphysema (arrows). (**b**) CT scan showed extensive pneumomediastinum (arrowheads) and soft tissue enphisema extending from the chest wall to the soft tissue of the neck

for children, it is important to avoid this procedure if it is not needed [27].

The initial diagnostic evaluation of patients with suspected FB aspiration includes obtaining a postero-anterior and lateral chest radiograph. It is estimated that only around 26% of the aspirated FBs are radio-opaque and visible on chest radiographs [28]. Inspiratory and expiratory phase films may show hyperinflation of air-trapping, which suggests an aspirated foreign body [24].

Imaging findings include visualization of the foreign body in the case of radiopaque foreign bodies or indirect signs (representing airway obstruction) such as hyper-lucency suggesting air trapping, atelectasis, non-resolving pneumonia, or localized bronchiectasis, especially in those with organic foreign bodies [29].

Computed tomography (CT) of the chest helps in detecting the FB and provides more information compared to a plain chest radiograph. CT identifies consolidation, atelectasis, pleural effusion, and bronchial wall abnormalities [30].

CT can also be useful in the assessment of a missed or retained foreign body after initial bronchoscopy [31].

4.4 Pulmonary Embolism

Pulmonary embolism (PE) is a frequent and life-threatening condition representing the third most common cause of cardiovascular death worldwide after stroke and heart attack with a reported incidence of 50–200 per 100,000 and an overall mortality of 10–30% [32, 33].

PE refers to the migration of solid, liquid, or gas emboli into a vessel of the pulmonary arterial circulation causing a total or partial deficit in blood flow with secondary respiratory and circulatory alterations [34]. In 95% of cases, PE is caused by detached thrombus material from deep vein thrombosis (DVT) of the lower extremity [35]. Risk factors include immobilization for prolonged periods, recent orthopedic surgery, malignancy, indwelling venous catheter, obesity, pregnancy, smoking, and oral contraceptive use [35, 36].

Clinical symptoms of PE are often nonspecific, so establishing a prompt diagnosis can be challenging. Common presentations include acute onset of dyspnea (80%), chest pain (60%) tachycardia (40%), and hemoptysis (9%). In a minority of cases arrhythmias, syncope, and hemodynamic collapse are reported.

Hemodynamic instability is rare, indicating central or extensive PE with severely reduced hemodynamic reserve [33].

Risk stratification is one of the cornerstones of the management of acute pulmonary embolism, determining the choice of both diagnostic and therapeutic strategies.

Diagnosis of PE often requires a sequential strategy combining a pre-test probability assessment, D-dimers levels measurement, and thoracic imaging [36].

Wells criteria are the most used scoring system to estimate the pretest probability of PE. This allows to classification of patients with suspected PE into pretest probability categories to rule out PE-avoiding imaging [37].

Once the diagnosis of acute PE has been established, further classifications are used to establish the severity of PE to optimize management [38].

The most widely used systems to stratify the severity of PE are those of the American Heart Association (AHA) and the European Society of Cardiology (ESC) [39, 40].

4.5 Imaging Features

4.5.1 Chest Radiography

Chest radiography is the first imaging method of choice in an emergency setting. Chest radiography has relatively low specificity and sensitivity in the diagnosis of PE and it is aimed to exclude other diseases such as pneumonia and pneumothorax that may mimic clinically PE [34].

Imaging findings of PE include [41]:

Fleischner Sign: enlarged pulmonary artery.

Hampton Hump: a peripheral wedge of airspace opacity and implies lung infarction (sensitivity 22%, specificity 82%, PPV 28%, NPV 76%).

Westermark Sign: regional oligemia has 14% sensitivity, 92% specificity, 38% positive predictive value (PPV), and 76% negative predictive value (NPV) in the diagnosis of PE.

Knuckle Sign: abrupt tapering or cutoff of a pulmonary artery secondary to a pulmonary embolus (PE).

Palla Sign: enlarged right descending pulmonary artery.

Chang Sign: dilated right descending pulmonary artery with sudden cut-off.

Elevated Diaphragm: (sensitivity 22%, specificity 82%, PPV 28%, NPV 76%).

Pleural Effusions: described in 35% of cases.

4.5.2 CT Pulmonary Angiography

Multidetector CT pulmonary angiography (CTPA) represents the cornerstone of PE diagnosis, due to its wide availability, relatively low cost, and very short scan time [42].

CTPA allows the analysis both of the pulmonary arteries and the pulmonary parenchyma and other chest structures allowing a prompt early identification of PE and excluding alternative diagnoses [43].

CTPA shows high sensitivity (83%) and specificity (96%), as demonstrated in PIOPED II trial. PIOPED II also highlighted the pretest clinical probability influence on the predictive value of CTPA. A normal CTPA had a high negative predictive value for PE at 96% and 89% in patients with a low or intermediate clinical probability, respectively [44].

Acute pulmonary thromboemboli can rarely be detected on non-contrast CT as intraluminal hyperdensities [45].

CTPA directly shows filling defects within the pulmonary arterial tree. Diagnostic criteria for acute pulmonary embolism include:

- Complete arterial occlusion with failure to enhance the entire lumen due to a large filling defect; the artery may be enlarged compared with adjacent patent vessels (Fig. 4.3).
- When the artery is viewed in its axial plane the central filling defect is surrounded by a thin rim of contrast, producing the "polo mint" sign.

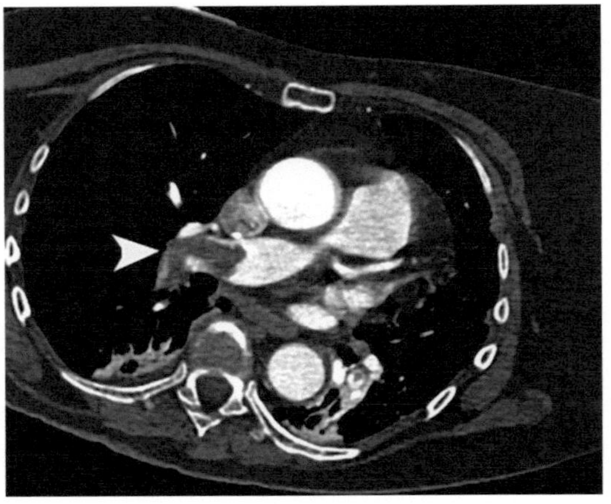

Fig. 4.3 A 74-year-old woman presented to the emergency department with a hypertensive crisis, acute shortness of breath, and desaturation. CT scan revealed an extensive filling defect in the right pulmonary artery (arrowhead), which appears enlarged; findings consistent with pulmonary embolism. Further filling defect is detectable in the lumen of the lower left lobar artery

- A peripheral intraluminal filling defect that forms acute angles with the arterial wall [46, 47].

In submassive or massive PE, the clot may have a saddle component (so-called "saddle embolus") that lodges at the bifurcation of the pulmonary artery obstructing blood flow to both lungs [48].

A possible consequence of acute PE is a pulmonary infarct, presenting as wedge-shaped, peripheral opacity commonly with a "reverse-halo" or "atoll" appearance. Pleural effusions can also be associated with acute PE [49].

These findings are different from chronic PE, which manifests as intraluminal webs, calcification, thrombus recanalization, and filling defects adherent to the wall that form obtuse angles and concave surfaces. In chronic PE, the vessels are typically smaller than normal, exhibit abnormal tapering, and may show complete cut-off of the segmental vessel. Parenchymal changes of chronic PE include mosaic perfusion, band-like opacities, and bronchial dilation in abnormal areas [50].

CT provides also several parameters for estimating the severity of PE and risk-stratification, such as right heart strain, clot burden and lung perfusion.

Right ventricular strain or failure is optimally monitored on echocardiography. However, some morphologic abnormalities that suggest right ventricular failure can be quantified on CT pulmonary angiography.

Imaging findings in right heart strain include [51]:

- Increased right ventricle (RV)/left ventricular (LV) ratio (>1 in axial plane associated with increased risk of death within 30 days, >0.9 in 4-chamber reconstruction combined with high-sensitivity-cardiac-troponin-I is associated with poor clinical outcome);
- Flattening of the interventricular septum and reflux of contrast medium into the IVC and hepatic veins.

In recent years, European and other international societies have proposed various algorithms for the assessment of suspected PE in pregnancy [40]. Compression ultrasound is the first step and is incorporated into the pregnancy-adapted algorithms of the YEARS algorithm (ARTEMIS study) [52]. The use of the pregnancy-adapted YEARS algorithm excludes PE in 80% of pregnant women without the need for radiation exposure. Chest X-ray is often recommended in the guidelines but appears not to be the imaging modality of choice for the diagnosis of PE in pregnant women. It should be noted that the radiation dose from chest radiography to the fetus is <0.1 mGy, well below the threshold dose for fetal malformations, and should not be withheld for this reason [40].

If the chest X-ray is abnormal or non-diagnostic, CTPA should be performed and preferred to ventilation-perfusion lung scanning in an emergency setting, being aware of some methodological limitations, such as poor pulmonary arterial opacification and artifacts due to respiratory motion, which is more common in pregnants [53].

Different technical approaches have been developed to increase image quality, gain additional functional information, and, ideally, simultaneously reduce the radiation dose. In this setting with the implementation of multidetector

CT scanners with two X-ray tubes (dual-source CT) and a single tube with two focal spots (dual-energy), additional functional information compared with single-energy CT for evaluations of PE should be obtained [54, 55]. DECT enables the characterization and quantification of iodine within tissues via imaging at different X-ray energies and analysis of attenuation differences and is more sensitive for subsegmental emboli compared with conventional CTA (96% vs. 24%) albeit at the cost of specificity (76% vs. 96%) [56].

Particularly the area of perfused lung can be directly assessed and quantified in addition to the standard documentation of clot burden and presence of right heart strain.

The distribution of iodine represents the distribution of pulmonary blood perfusion. Regarding acute PE, the relative volume of perfusion defects is associated with an increased risk of death from any cause within 30 days (HR: 1.04) and pulmonary embolism-related death (HR: 1.05) [57].

4.5.3 Lower Extremity Ultrasound

Thanks to its availability, lack of ionizing radiation, and low-cost, lower extremity ultrasound (US) represent the first step imaging method for suspected VTE. However diagnostic accuracy of US is highly dependent on technique and operators.

Imaging US findings include the presence of the clot manifesting as fully occlusive or non-occlusive hypoechoic material into the venous lumen, non-compressible venous segment, loss of phasic flow on Valsalva maneuver, absent color flow on Color Doppler and increased flow in superficial veins [58].

4.5.4 Diffuse Parencymal Diseases

Patients with acute respiratory symptoms often exhibit similar parenchymal changes. When radiography is interdeterminate, CT may be crucial to provide information, particularly if there is a mismatch between radiographic features, the patient's clinical history, and symptoms. While edema in patients with heart failure or pneumonia in patients with fever and consolidations may be straightforward clinical cases, there are other scenarios that present greater challenges for clinicians.

In this case, imaging plays a pivotal role in narrowing the differential diagnosis. Conversely, imaging features are rarely pathognomonic for a particular diagnosis, making the clinical history, symptoms, and laboratory findings essential for a correct interpretation.

4.5.5 Pulmonary Edema

Pulmonary edema is a common clinical entity caused by the abnormal fluid build-up into the pulmonary interstitium and alveoli, leading to dyspnea. The clinical scenario of pulmonary edema includes acute breathlessness, orthopnea, paroxysmal nocturnal dyspnea (PND), and foaming at the mouth [59]. Pulmonary edema is classified as hydrostatic (cardiogenic) or due to increased capillary permeability (non-cardiogenic) [59, 60]. However, it must be considered that it is not always possible or appropriate to make a differential diagnosis between these two entities. A classification that better adapts to pathology and physiology, provides the following types:

(a) Hydrostatic edema (cardiogenic);
(b) Edema due to increased permeability associated with diffuse alveolar damage;
(c) Edema of increased permeability without associated damage;
(d) Mixed-type edema.

Although these types of edema cannot always be distinguished based on an X-ray or CT scan alone, imaging findings usually tend to differ in the various types. Accurate radiographic diagnosis is crucial for proper management of this common condition. Although a CT scan represents the gold standard for radiological assessment of pulmonary edema, it requires to transport of a critically ill patient to the radiology department:

therefore it is performed in a minority of cases [61]. Consequently, chest X-ray remains essential as a first-line method for detecting, quantifying, and following pulmonary edema [62, 63]. Lung US is an accessible technique and represents a promising tool for diagnosis and monitoring pulmonary edema in ICU patients [64]; it could serve also as the main diagnostic method in low-resource settings where access to CT scanners is limited. CT is a key tool to detect complications, that may occur during pulmonary edema management, and that may not be easily recognizable on chest X-ray.

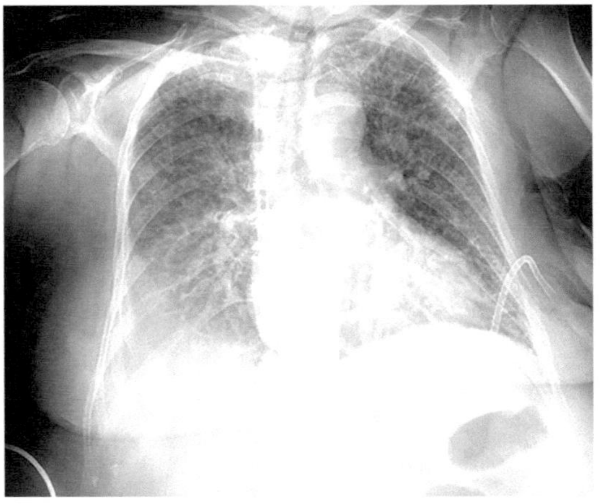

Fig. 4.4 An 83-year-old woman with a new diagnosis of acute renal failure developed dyspnea. CXR demonstrated an increased cardiothoracic ratio, diffuse perihilar airspace and septal lines (Kerley lines)

4.6 Cardiogenic Edema

In most cases, the main cause is the increase in intravascular pressure due to pulmonary venous hypertension. This condition can occur in cases of left hearth failure, obstruction of the left atrium or pulmonary veins, volume overload to renal failure, or hyperhydration [3]. Even low intravascular oncotic pressure, as in cases of hypoalbuminemia or hepatorenal failure, can cause an abnormal accumulation of fluid into the interstitium [59, 65]. Findings useful for broadly assessing cardiogenic pulmonary edema on a plain chest radiograph include:

- Features of pulmonary interstitial edema (Fig. 4.4):
  - Increased vascular diameter;
  - Enlargement of the vascular pedicle;
  - Cephalization of pulmonary vessels;
  - Septal Kerley lines;
  - Peribronchial cuffing;
  - Thickening of interlobar fissures.
- Increased cardiothoracic ratio/cardiac silhouette size.
- Pleural effusion in interlobar fissures.
- Features of pulmonary alveolar edema: air space opacification classically in a batwing distribution.

The earliest findings of cardiogenic pulmonary edema (hearth failure) on CXR include the enlargement and blurred appearance of the pulmonary hila, the widening of the vascular pedicle, defined as the superior mediastinum just above the aortic arch, and the cephalization of pulmonary vessels. Cephalization is defined as the redistribution of blood into the upper lobe vessels and can be identified when the upper lobe veins are the same or larger in diameter relative to the lower lobe veins: on CT this sign may be better depicted in coronal reconstructed images [63, 66, 67].

Kerley B lines visible on radiographs represent engorgement of the subpleural interlobular septa. These are horizontal thin lines (1–2 cm in length), identified peripherally and oriented perpendicular to the pleural surface, usually seen at lung bases [68].

Kerley A lines are found less frequently on CXR. These are 2–6 cm long oblique lines and less than 1 mm thick, that have a different appearance than the B lines, extending radially from the hilum to the upper lobes. They represent the thickening of the interlobular septa containing lymphatic connections between the perivenous and broncho-arterial lymphatics deep within the lung parenchyma. On CT, Kerley lines appear as a smooth reticular thickening of the interlobular septa (Fig. 4.5).

The subpleural interstitial space is continuous with the peripheral interlobular septa. When a

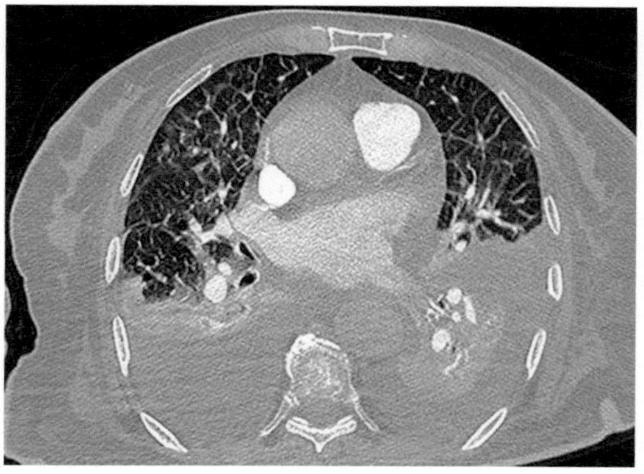

Fig. 4.5 Axial CT scan of a 78-year-old man with cardiogenic pulmonary edema. Smooth interlobular septal thickening and bilateral pleural effusions with underlying segmental basal consolidations are depicted

thickening of the interlobular septa and Kerley lines are present, a thickening of the subpleural interstitium can often also be demonstrated on X-ray or CT. This finding may also be related to pleural effusion within the fissure [67].

The so-called "peribronchial cuffing" describes haziness or increased density around the bronchial walls in the hilar region, due to the accumulation of fluid in the connective tissue surrounding the bronchi. When viewed tangentially, it can give the appearance of tram tracks [66, 67].

While the aforementioned imaging features are commonly detected in cardiogenic pulmonary edema they are rarely seen in permeability edema.

Moreover in cardiogenic edema, cardiomegaly is found with a prevalence of left sections, whereas in permeability edema there are no volumetric changes in the heart or the right ventricle may be enlarged due to an increase in pulmonary vascular resistance [69].

If interstitial pressure increases and the edema worsens, the fluid overloads the interstitial space and oozes in the alveoli: bilateral and symmetric ground-glass opacities (GGOs) and consolidations with central or gravity-dependent distribution appear. In 10% of cases, these parenchymal changes show a pattern of bilateral perihilar lung shadowing sparing the subpleural region, also known as "bat wing appearance", due to a rapid increase in fluid as seen in sever cardiac failure or in mitral insufficiency [62]. It must be considered that the patient's positioning significantly affects the distribution of pulmonary edema.

Both interstitial and alveolar pulmonary edema regress rapidly in response to therapy. Typically complete radiographic resolution occurs in less than 3 days and is late compared to the normalization of blood pressure values [59].

Lung US can play a key role in the diagnosis and assessment of pulmonary edema, avoiding exposure to ionizing radiation. The thickening of interalveolar septa and alveolar flooding result in a short path reverberation artefact, defined as B lines [70]. The finding of three or more B lines in anterior or lateral regions is always pathological. When spaced 7 mm apart they are caused by thickened interlobular septa characterizing interstitial edema (correlating with radiographic Kerley B lines). Conversely, when spaced 3 mm apart they are caused by GGO areas, characterizing alveolar edema. In the most severe conditions, a white lung is demonstrated [70, 71].

Pulmonary edema is mostly symmetric, but asymmetry can be found in approximately 2%, with predilection for the right upper lobe; it can be due to patient position, mitral regurgitation, or congenital heart disease. Patients with reduced unilateral blood flow may develop edema in the contrateral lung. This condition may occur in cases of pulmonary embolism or Swyer-James syndrome [72].

4.7 Permeability Edema/ARDS

Acute respiratory distress syndrome (ARDS) is an important cause of respiratory failure, with a mortality rate of around 40% [73]: ARDS is characterized by increased permeability edema and rapid onset of dyspnea and hypoxemia, triggered by direct or indirect lung injury [74]. It is not a primary pathology but rather a complication that occurs when several clinical disorders (including pneumonia, sepsis, aspiration of gastric contents, major trauma and metabolic/neurologic disorders) precipitate in a severe systemic inflammatory response [73]. Despite the different pathological triggers, similar histopathologic changes consistent with diffuse alveolar damage (DAD) are recognized. Radiographic features are often normal, within 12–24 h after the injury, even in the presence of dyspnea [67]. This latency period is suggestive of ARDS. Bilateral patchy consolidation areas appear beyond the 24-h time-point, often with a peripheral distribution (unlike cardiogenic edema). These consolidations areas increase becoming confluent. The air bronchogram is found more frequently than in hydrostatic edema. Interstitial changes may be found, but Kerley lines are unusual. Pleural effusion is much less frequent than in hydrostatic edema [75].

CT features correlate with the disease phase (Fig. 4.6). In the acute setting, scattered or diffuse areas of GGO and/or dependent consolidations are depicted, reflecting interstitial and alveolar edema and haemorrhage [76]. A longitudinal gradient with increasing parenchymal density from the apices to the lung bases is recognizable. Different CT patterns may correlate with the different etiology of ARDS: in cases of pulmonary etiology (primary lung injuries), consolidations and GGO are both depicted with asymmetric distribution, while in cases of extrapulmonary etiology, bilateral and symmetrical GGO are the main finding [75, 76]. In fat embolism syndrome, a possible cause of ARDS, nodular opacities are typically associated with GGO with geographic distribution and consolidations [77].

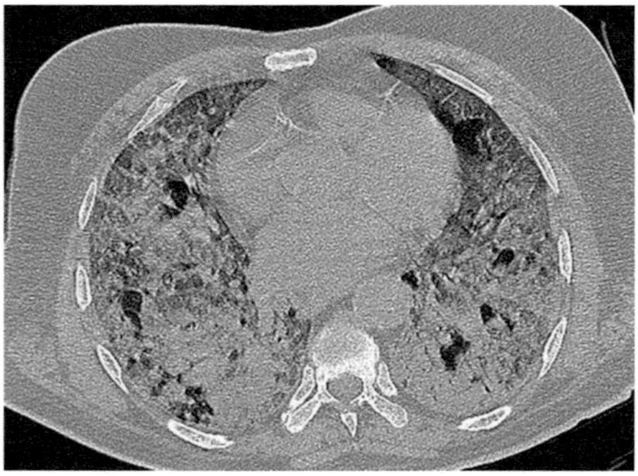

Fig. 4.6 A 79-year-old man affected with H1N1 pneumonia presenting at the Emergency Department with dyspnea, hemoptysis and fever. CT scan demonstrated bilateral and confluent ground-glass opacity (GGO) associated with more focal consolidation and air bronchograms dependently

Parenchymal changes regress more slowly than in hydrostatic edema. After a week, consolidations should start to resolve, taking on a patchy appearance or being replaced by reticular opacities. Conversely, the progression of consolidation after a week may be indicative of overlapping pneumonia. GGO may persist after resolution of consolidations [74].

A subset of ARDS survivors develops pulmonary fibrosis, showing reticular opacities, septal and interlobar thickening, architectural distortion and traction bronchiectasis; findings more clearly depicted on CT [78]. Fibrotic changes may be related to mechanical ventilation, especially if prolonged with a high concentration of oxygen. These findings show a predominantly anterior distribution, as in the posterior regions atelectasis and consolidations protect the lung parenchyma from the side effects of mechanic ventilation [73].

The application of CT in critically ill patients may be limited. Lung US is a bedside, safe and radiation-free method that as been extensively employed in ARDS assessment [79].

Sonographic features suggestive of ARDS include:

- Three or more B-lines per intercostal sonographic field, adjacent to the surface of the visceral pleura, heterogeneously distributed on both sides. Specifically "spared areas" of normal sonographic lung are interposed with lung fields in which the B-lines are present;
- Pleural interface abnormalities (thickening and/or irregularity; reduction or disappearance of "lung sliding", in regions with B-lines merged) [80];
- Absence of significant pleural effusion.

The main imaging features of cardiogenic and permeability edema, are summarized in Table 4.1.

Permeability edema can develop event without associated DAD. This condition occurs in cases of drug reactions, transfusion reactions, air embolism and toxic shock syndrome. The

Table 4.1 Key imaging features of cardiogenic edema vs permeability edema

Findings	Cardiogenic edema	Permeability edema
Cardiothoracic ratio/cardiac silhouette size	Increased	Normal
Vascular pedicle width	Increased	Normal
Cephalization of pulmonary vessels.	Common	Absent
Kerley lines	Common	Unusual
Peribronchial cuffing	Common	Absent
Air bronchogram	Unusual	Common
Distribution	Predominantly central	Patchy/Periferal
Pleural effusion	Common	Rare

absence of pulmonary epithelial damage, in these patients, reduces the extent of alveolar edema. In these cases, imaging findings are typically similar to hydrostatic edema, with thickening of interlobular septa as the main feature. The edema resolves rapidly due to the absence of epithelial damage [67, 81].

4.8 Mixed Type Edema

Mixed type, hydrostatic and permeability, occur in diseases that cause both an increase in intravascular pressure and damage to the capillary endothelium. These conditions occur in neurogenic pulmonary edema, expansion edema, high-altitude illness, reperfusion edema, post-partum and post-transplant edema, in some drug reactions, and in patients with ARDS, which are hyperhydrated. The imaging features of these different types of edema are variable [60].

4.8.1 Pneumonia

Lower respiratory tract infections are a major cause of mortality worldwide, especially among children and the elderly; infectious organisms can colonize the airways (tracheitis, bronchitis, and bronchiolitis) or spread to the lung parenchyma (pneumonia) [82]. Usually, chest X-ray is adequate to detect pneumonia, but in many cases, such as atypical infections or bronchiolar involvement, further investigation with CT scan and bronchiolo-alveolar lavage (BAL) are required. Early recognition and treatment are essential to reduce morbidity and mortality [83].

Pneumonia can be broadly classified on the basis of the radiographic appearance into lobar pneumonia, bronchopneumonia and interstitial pneumonia.

Lobar Pneumonia: Lobar pneumonia represents the most common radiographic pattern of community-acquired pneumonia. Usually due to *S.Pneumoniae*, lobar pneumonia has its pathogenetic background in a rapid production of edema with a modest cellular reaction [83].

Imaging shows a non-segmental homogenous consolidation. The opacification can be sharply defined at the fissures, although more commonly there is segmental consolidation. Consolidation initially affects the subpleural region, with later spread of edema from one acinus to the other through Kohn's pores. The larger bronchi remain pervious (air bronchogram) and there is no loss of volume (unlike in atelectasis), indeed sometimes there may be an increase in volume due to oedema (scissure displacement) (Fig. 4.7) [84].

Bronchopneumonia: It is distinguished from lobar pneumonia by the rapid production and spread of exudate that collects in the small respiratory and membranous bronchi (peribronchiolar distribution): consequently the inflammatory reaction extends from the airways to the adjacent pulmonary lobules (lobular pneumonia). Bronchopneumonia is most commonly caused by *S.Aureus* (mostly nosocomial pneumonias), *H.Iinfluentae* and fungi. The main imaging features include multiple small areas of patchy coalescent opacification, associated with peribronchial cuffing and ill-defined nodules. As it affects the airways, it may be associated with atelectasis and lung volume loss. Other findings may include cavitation and pneumatoceles (Fig. 4.8) [83].

Interstitial pneumonia: It is characterized by edema and inflammatory infiltrate in the lung interstitium. Chest X-ray shows extensive peribronchial thickening and ill-defined reticulonodular opacities. Diffuse bilateral interstitial and/or interstitial-alveolar opacities are commonly associated with viruses and *M.Pneumoniae* [83]. CT can show bilateral GGO interspersed by normal lung parenchyma (Figs. 4.9 and 4.10) [85].

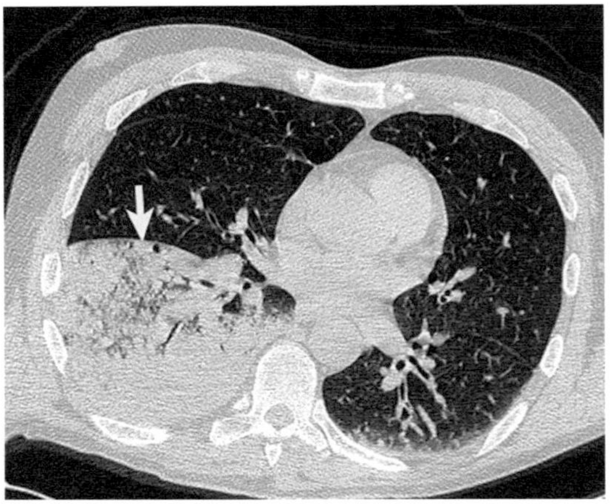

Fig. 4.7 A 57-year-old man presented to the emergency department with severe fatigue associated with dyspnea, tachypnea, and fever (39 °C). Unenhanced chest CT scan in the axial plane showed consolidation involving most of the right lower lobe (arrow), associated with an air bronchogram. The urinary antigen test was positive for *Legionella Pneumophila*

4.8.2 Acute Interstitial Pneumonia

Acute interstitial pneumonia (AIP), also known as Hamman-Rich syndrome, is a rapidly advancing non-infectious interstitial lung disease with unknown etiology. AIP includes three phases: first an acute exudative phase, then a subsequent organizing phase and a final fibrotic phase. It presents clinically and histologically similarly to acute respiratory distress syndrome (ARDS), exhibiting extensive diffuse alveolar damage (DAD). The disease generally advances to respiratory failure necessitating mechanical ventilation and corticosteroid therapy. Despite these interventions, the prognosis is poor [86].

Conventional radiography shows nonspecific findings with bilateral patchy or diffuse opacities in the airspace [87]. HRCT is valuable in distinguishing between infectious and noninfectious acute parenchymal lung diseases [88], but CT characteristics of AIP closely resemble those of adult respiratory distress syndrome, reflecting DAD [87]. The exudative (early) phase is marked by diffuse asymmetrical ground-glass opacities

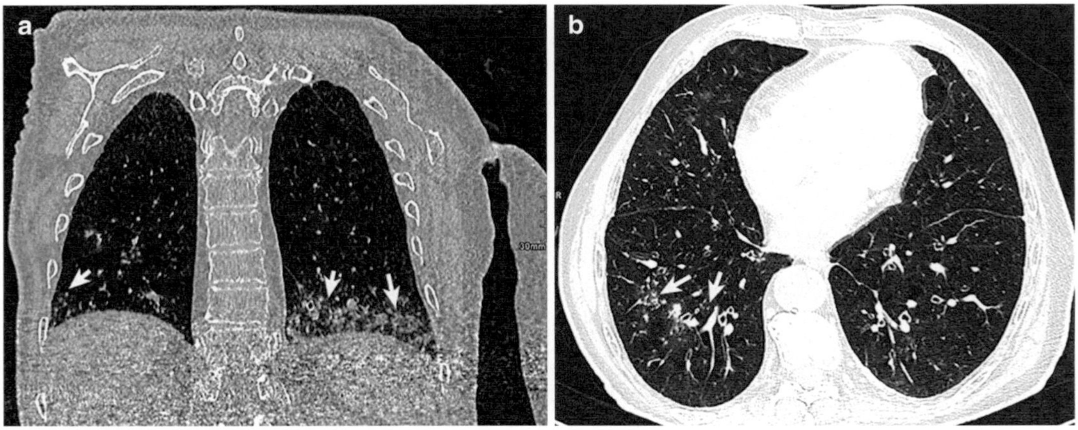

Fig. 4.8 (**a** and **b**) Coronal (**a**) and axial (**b**) CT scan of a 75-year-old man complaining of dyspnea, cough and fever (38 °C). Multiple, bilateral and patchy confluent nodular opacities are depicted (arrows). Findings are consistent with bronchopneumonia

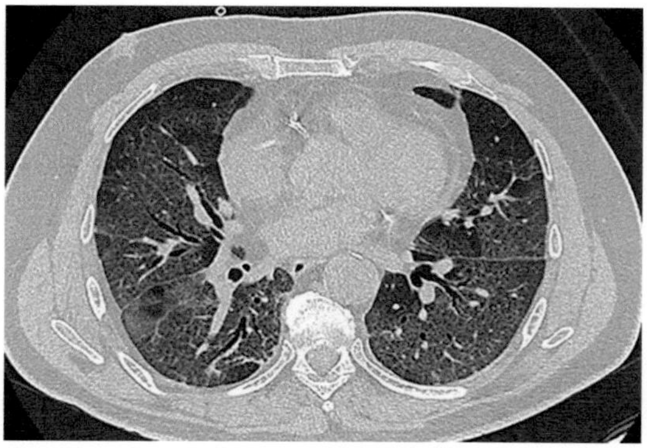

Fig. 4.9 A 63-year-old was admitted to the Emergency Department, with severe dyspnea, desaturation, myalgia, general malaise and fever (40 °C). CT showed widespread, bilateral, and symmetrical areas of ground-glass opacity (GGO) with overlying interlobular septal thickening, consistent with a crazy paving pattern. No pericardial or pleural effusion was detected. The nasopharyngeal swab confirmed the diagnosis of COVID-19 pneumonia

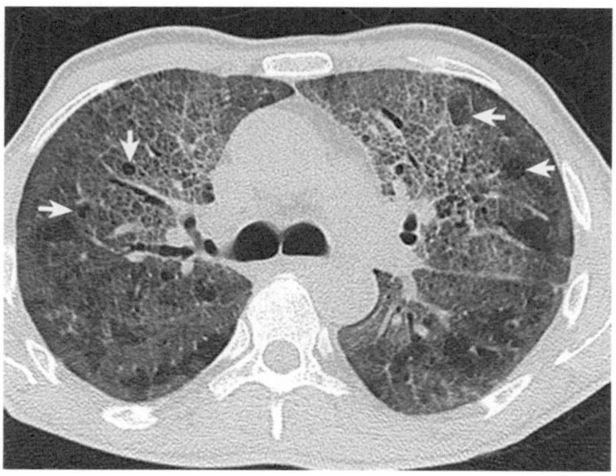

Fig. 4.10 A 57-year-old HIV positive patient, presented to the Emergency department with dyspnea and a dry cough. CT scan revealed patchy ground-glass opacities in the upper lobes, associated with septal thickening (crazy paving), and small pneumatoceles (arrows)

(GGO) and dependent consolidation. In the organizing (chronic) phase, which usually begins about 1 week after the initial injury, lung architectural distortion and traction bronchiectasis may appear [89]. The extent of GGO, consolidation and bronchiectasis correlate with disease duration [90]. Usually, these changes resolve over time, but in some cases, they can result in persistent lung fibrosis.

4.8.3 Acute Exacerbation of Chronic Diseases

Even though quantitative CT studies demonstrated the severity of emphysema and airway wall thickness with the frequency of chronic obstructive pulmonary disease (COPD) exacerbations [91], diagnosis and treatment of these conditions do not heavily rely on imaging. Acute exacerbations of COPD symptoms can be caused by pneumonia, bulla infection, or pneumothorax, which can be diagnosed through imaging. However, exacerbations often reflect changes that are not associated with distinct imaging features (ie. increased pathogen burden in respiratory tract infections).

A life-threatening complication in patients with idiopathic pulmonary fibrosis (IPF) is its acute exacerbation (AE-IPF), often described as diffuse alveolar damage (DAD) of unknown etiology; this condition is associated with a drastic decrease in respiratory function and a mortality rate of up to 85% [92]. In these patients CT demonstrates a rapid increase in ground-glass opacities and/or airspace consolidation, overlaying a background of the usual interstitial pneumonia (UIP) pattern. CT has been shown to be predictive of mortality, in these cases [93, 94].

Acute exacerbations are being increasingly reported in non-idiopathic interstitial pneumonia (NSIP), associated with connective tissue disorders (i.e. Scleroderma, Systemic Lupus Erythematosus) [95]. In these patients, a sudden worsening of the respiratory parameters, with characteristics imaging features (background of bilateral and peripheral GGO, reticular opacities, traction bronchiectasis), points towards this diagnosis. Before beginning treatment, it is crucial to rule out infections (ie. *Pneumocystis jirovecii*), or drug-related lung damage (i.e. Methotrexate-induced pneumonitis), by bronchoalveolar lavage (BAL) and laboratory tests [96].

4.8.4 Diffuse Alveolar Haemorrage

Diffuse alveolar hemorrhage (DAH) is a life-threatening emergency caused by widespread damage of the alveolar-capillary basement membrane, that results in intralveolar hemorrhage [97]. Diagnosis of DAH often requires endoscopic evaluation and BAL, as clinical features are non-specific including dyspnea, cough, anemia, hemoptysis (absent in up to 33% of patients), and acute respiratory failure, which can be severe leading to death. Therefore prompt diagnosis and treatment are crucial for survival [98]. BAL can detect DAH and rule-out infection, but its usefulness in determining the cause is limited. A lung biopsy is not commonly recommended but can be performed if the etiology remains uncertain [97].

DAH is associated with several clinical entities: the most common causes are autoimmune diseases, including Goodpasture Syndrome, antineutrophil cytoplasmatic autoantibodies (ANCA)-associated vasculitides, connective tissue disorders (systemic lupus erythematosus or mixed connective tissue disease) antiphospholipid syndrome [99]. Diseases causing nonimmunologic injury are less common including coagulation disorders, antiplatelet therapy inhaled toxins (trimellitic anhydride, isocyanates, cocaine, pesticides, vaping), pulmonary veno-occlusive disease, hematopoietic stem cell transplant and idiopathic pulmonary hemosiderosis [100, 101]. Radiological assessment with chest X-ray and CT is useful in the evaluation of DAH: however, imaging features are non-specific and similar to other acute alveolar filling processes: therefore adjudicating a cause based primarily on imaging usually is not possible. In about 80% of patients at onset, plain radiograph show diffuse bilateral opacifications predominantly in central and lower lung fields (with peripheral and apical sparing), evolving to a more reticular pattern over several days [102].

Focal or unilateral distribution does not exclude DAH. CT confirms radiographic features and more accurately assesses the extent of pulmonary involvement (Fig. 4.11). In the acute phase, CT reveals diffuse non-specific GGOs and consolidations with air bronchograms, commonly 1 cm. and less from the pleural surface. In the subacute phase, the smooth thickening of the interlobular septa may overlap with areas of ground-glass opacity, giving rise to "crazy-paving" pattern [102, 103].

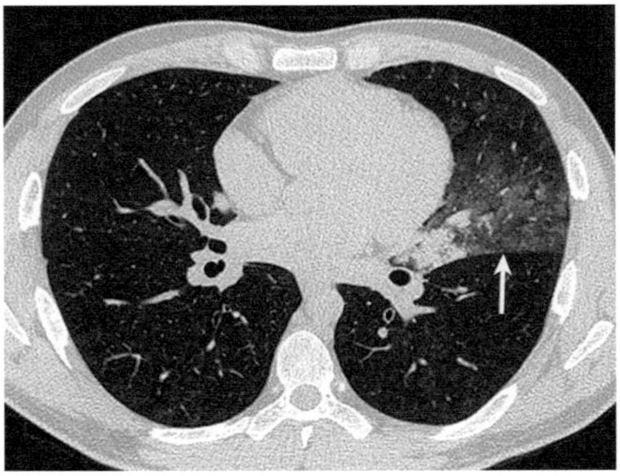

Fig. 4.11 A 24-year-old student with a history of cocaine abuse, presented to the emergency room, complaining of streaky hemoptysis and dyspnea. He had tachycardia (heart rate 138/min), and tachypnea (respiratory rate 39/min) with blood pressure of 160/90 mmHg and room air oxygen saturation of 58%. CXR was indeterminate (not showed), therefore CT scan was performed, showing diffuse GGO and scattered consolidations in the lingular segment (arrow)

Multiple bilateral centrilobular nodules or irregular cavitary masses with no zonal predominance are typically observed in ANCA-associated vasculitides. Within 3 days consolidations start to resolve, remaining irregular opacification or septal thickening. Complete radiographic resolution is usually observed in 2–3 weeks. Severe repeated hemorrhagic events can lead to organizing pneumonia and interstitial fibrosis, easily depicted on CT [102, 103]. Pleural effusion is uncommon and in most cases DPH is associated with SLE [104].

4.9 Pleural Effusion

Pleural effusion refers to the abnormal accumulation of fluid within the pleural cavity, due to many different underlying pulmonary, pleural or extrapulmonary diseases [105]. The most common causes of pleural effusion in the Intensive Care Unit (ICU), include volume overload, congestive heart failure and pleuropulmonary infection. The etiological diagnosis depends on a combination of clinical history, physical examination, imaging methods and pertinent pleural fluid analyses. If pleural effusion remains undiagnosed even after the analysis of one or more pleural fluid samples, invasive procedures (thoracentesis) may be required. Pleural effusions are broadly split into transudate, exudate and chylothorax [106].

Small amounts of pleural fluid may be asymptomatic. Even significant fluid accumulations can remain unnoticed depending on the patient's respiratory reserve.

Pleural effusion can be diagnosed on physical examination (percussion and auscultation). Chest X-ray (CXR) is the first imaging test to detect pleural effusion. The sensitivity of CXR depends on the patient's position. In ICU the assessment of pleural effusion relies mostly on the antero-posterior CXR acquired at the bedside, in the supine position [107]: technical limitations and coexisting parenchymal diseases could result in poor quality plain radiograph, underdiagnosing pleural effusion.

On a routine erect CXR about 250 mL of fluid, is required before it becomes detectable [108]. Effusion accumulates in the most dependent areas of the pleural cavity. The appearance varies with the patient's position.

- Lateral Decubitus (with the affected side down): to depict small fluid amounts layering against the dependent parietal pleura and differentiate between free-flowing and loculated effusions.
- Erect Position: effusion gathers in the postero-basal regions, showing as a meniscus-shaped opacity in the costophrenic angle and fluid within fissures. A postero-anterior (PA) view may show indirect signs, such as elevation and lateralization of the hemidiaphragm dome (pseudo-diaphragm sign).
- Supine Position: large amounts of fluid can be masked as the fluid collects posteriorly, making only subtle signs, such as the loss of the hemidiaphragm silhouette or blunting of the lateral costophrenic angle. Large effusion may push structures in the chest away from it, causing a mediastinal shift.

Both US and CT are more sensitive in detecting only few ml of pleural effusions and characterizing fluid composition, in comparison to CXR [109]. CT represents the gold standard but is not always feasible to perform on ICU patients [110]. CT can recognize underlying pulmonary causes, such as primary lung neoplasm, showing nodular or enhancing pleural thickening. Moreover CT differentiates between pleural effusion and pleural empyema [111].

Empyema appears as a fluid density collection, with a lenticular shape, forming an obtuse angle with the pleural surface [112]. The so-called "pleural split sign" consists of both thickened, contrast-enhancing pleural layers, separated by fluid collection: this finding allows confident distinction of loculated empyema from a peripheral lung abscess [113]. However other diseases associated with pleuritic, such as hemothorax and malignant pleural effusion, can also result in this appearance on CT [114]. The employ of lung US is increasing in ICU because of its high accuracy, its suitability for bedside application, and its role in aiding treatment (thoracentesis, insertion chest drain). Several studies demonstrated that US was able to detect pleural effusions smaller than 15 mm [115]: therefore the employ of US in ICU has been implemented, decreasing X-ray examinations, not only to reduce exposure to ionizing radiations but also to provide more diagnostic information.

A prospective study by Lichtenstein et al., including 32 patients, compared the accuracy of physical examination, lung US and chest X-ray with that of chest CT. Lung US showed a sensitivity of 92%, a specificity of 93% and a diagnostic accuracy of 93% for pleural effusion. Bedside chest X-ray and physical examination had poor percentages of sensitivity, specificity and diagnostic accuracy for pleural effusion [116]. A prospective study by Xirouchaki et al. compared the diagnostic performance of lung US and bedside chest X-ray, for different pathologic entities. The sensitivity, specificity and diagnostic accuracy of bedside CXR were 65,81,69% for pleural effusion respectively; the corresponding values for lung US were 100,100,100% for pleural effusion respectively [117]. Therefore, the International Consensus Conference of LUS stated: "for the detection of pleural effusion lung US is more accurate than supine radiography and is accurate as CT" [118].

4.10 Pneumothorax

Pneumothorax is defined as the abnormal presence of air within the pleural cavity.

Although it is most frequently caused by traumatic injuries, pneumothorax can occur and is often associated with various underlying conditions [119]. Patients with pneumothorax may exhibit a broad spectrum of clinical manifestations ranging from no symptoms to cardiovascular collapse. The most common symptoms are pleuritic chest pain and acute onset of dyspnea. The severity of symptoms of pneumothorax may not be related to its size and are usually more evident in patients with decreased pulmonary reserve [120].

When pneumothorax is suspected, CXR represents the first-line imaging test [121]. In a standing CXR, the diagnosis is confirmed by identifying the outer visceral pleural border, which appears as a thin, sharp white line. This pleural line is bordered by gas in the pleural space, seen as a crescent-shaped area of radiolucency devoid of lung markings [122]. In severe cases, the lung may be completely collapsed. Small pneumothoraces can be challenging to detect, as soft tissue folds and scapular borders can mimic pleural lines [121, 122]. In supine patients, bedside antero-posterior (AP) CXR is performed: pneumothorax might present as an air collection in the costo-phrenic angles, which appear deepened and more lucent (deep sulcus sign). However, the sensitivity of bedside CXR for pneumothorax is poor (20%), whereas upright PA radiographs show a sensitivity of 90% [109, 122]. There is no need to acquire expiratory radiographs, as they do not show higher sensitivity in the detection of pneumothorax [123]. The presence of a mediastinal shift or compression of thoracic structures suggests tension pneumothorax, although this diagnosis is primarily clinical [124].

CT represents the gold standard for the diagnosis of pneumothorax (Fig. 4.12), and is recommended when CXR results are inconclusive or in cases of recurrent pneumothorax with unknown causes: however, CT is not always feasible in critically ill patients [121]. One important, well-established application of US is the detection of pneumothorax. In a prospective study, US showed a sensitivity of 95.3% and a specificity of 91.1% for identifying pneumothorax in ICU [125, 126]. The most important sonographic features include:

- The absence of lung sliding: the typical to-and-fro movement or shimmering of the pleural line is not recognizable. The same technique using M-mode can confirm a lack of sliding, showing the "stratosphere sign": parallel horizontal lines above and below the pleural line, resembling a barcode. The negative predictive value (NPV) of this sign is reported as 99.2–100% [121, 127]. The absence of lung sliding is not specific to pneu-

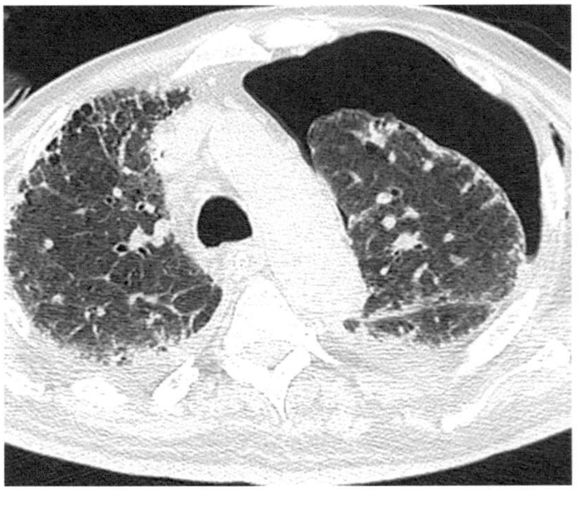

Fig. 4.12 A 71-year-old man with known usual interstitial pneumonia (UIP) was admitted to the emergency room with acute respiratory failure and dyspnea. CT scan showed a large pneumothorax on the left side, extending from the base to the apex of the lung, predominantly located in the anterior dependent position, leading to a reduction in lung volume on that side. On the right lung, fibrotic changes are detectable

mothorax, and being associated with several diseases, including ARDS, pulmonary fibrosis, consolidations and atelectasis [127];

- Loss of "comet tail artifacts" or "B-lines": these reverberation artifacts, generated by the visceral pleura, are lost due to air accumulating within the pleural space. Detection of even one comet-tail sign rules out a pneumothorax (NPV 98–100%) [121, 128];
- A-lines: horizontal reverberation artifacts, appearing as equally spaced hyperchoic lines, originating from the pleural line. In the normal patients, A-lines are erased by the B-lines [127].
- Lung point sign is the most specific sign of pneumothorax (specificity 100%), occurring at its border. It is due to sliding lungs intermittently touching the chest wall during inspiration and is useful in assessing the size of the pneumothorax. This sign can be further demonstrated by employing M-mode: the "seashore" and "stratosphere sign" are depicted over time [129].

References

1. Parshall MB, Schwartzstein RM, Adams L, et al. An official American thoracic society statement: update on the mechanisms, assessment, and management of dyspnea. Am J Respir Crit Care Med. 2012;185:435–52.
2. Elliott MW, Adams L, Cockcroft A, Macrae KD, Murphy K, Guz A. The language of breathlessness: use of verbal descriptors by patients with cardiopulmonary disease. Am Rev Respir Dis. 1991;144:826–32.
3. Santus P, Radovanovic D, Saad M, Zilianti C, Coppola S, Chiumello DA, Pecchiari M. Acute dyspnea in the emergency department: a clinical review. Intern Emerg Med. 2023;18:1491–507.
4. McComb BL, Ravenel JG, Steiner RM, et al. ACR appropriateness criteria® chronic dyspnea-noncardiovascular origin. J Am Coll Radiol. 2018;15:S291–301.
5. Vogel-Claussen J, Elshafee ASM, Kirsch J, et al. ACR appropriateness criteria ® dyspnea—suspected cardiac origin. J Am Coll Radiol. 2017;14:S127–37.
6. DeVos E, Jacobson L. Approach to adult patients with acute dyspnea. Emerg Med Clin North Am. 2016;34:129–49.
7. Lancellotti P, Price S, Edvardsen T, et al. The use of echocardiography in acute cardiovascular care: recommendations of the European Association of Cardiovascular Imaging and the Acute Cardiovascular Care Association. Eur Heart J Acute Cardiovasc Care. 2015;4:100–32.
8. Bicci E, Grazzini G, Cozzi D, et al. Non-traumatic non-cardiovascular thoracic emergencies: role of imaging. Eur Rev Med Pharmacol Sci. 2022;26:3249–60.
9. Milos R-I, Bartha C, Röhrich S, et al. Imaging in patients with acute dyspnea when cardiac or pulmonary origin is suspected. BJR|Open. 2023;5:20220026.
10. Self WH, Courtney DM, McNaughton CD, Wunderink RG, Kline JA. High discordance of chest x-ray and computed tomography for detection of pulmonary opacities in ED patients: implications for diagnosing pneumonia. Am J Emerg Med. 2013;31:401–5.
11. Kim Y, Kim YK, Lee BE, Lee SJ, Ryu YJ, Lee JH, Chang JH. Ultra-low-dose CT of the thorax using iterative reconstruction: evaluation of image quality and radiation dose reduction. Am J Roentgenol. 2015;204:1197–202.
12. Park JE, Kim Y, Lee SW, Shim SS, Lee JK, Lee JH. The usefulness of low-dose CT scan in elderly patients with suspected acute lower respiratory infection in the emergency room. BJR. 2016;89:20150654.
13. Kirsch J, Wu CC, Bolen MA, et al. ACR appropriateness criteria® suspected pulmonary embolism: 2022 update. J Am Coll Radiol. 2022;19:S488–501.
14. Palacio D, Benveniste MF, Betancourt-Cuellar SL, Gladish GW. Multidetector computed tomography pulmonary angiography pitfalls in the evaluation of pulmonary embolism with emphasis in technique. Semin Roentgenol. 2015;50:217–25.
15. Lichtenstein DA, Mezière GA. Relevance of lung ultrasound in the diagnosis of acute respiratory failure*: the BLUE protocol. Chest. 2008;134:117–25.
16. Dalziel SR, Haskell L, O'Brien S, Borland ML, Plint AC, Babl FE, Oakley E. Bronchiolitis. Lancet. 2022;400:392–406.
17. Rodriguez K, Hariri LP, VanderLaan P, Abbott GF. Imaging of small airways disease. Clin Chest Med. 2024;45:475–88.
18. Lee GM, Carroll MB, Galvin JR, Walker CM. Mosaic attenuation pattern. Radiol Clin North Am. 2022;60:963–78.
19. Mims JW. Asthma: definitions and pathophysiology. Int Forum Allergy Rhinol. 2015;5 https://doi.org/10.1002/alr.21609.
20. Niedbalski PJ, Choi J, Hall CS, Castro M. Imaging in asthma management. Semin Respir Crit Care Med. 2022;43:613–26.
21. Trivedi A, Hall C, Hoffman EA, Woods JC, Gierada DS, Castro M. Using imaging as a biomarker for asthma. J Allergy Clin Immunol. 2017;139:1–10.

22. Ash SY, Diaz AA. The role of imaging in the assessment of severe asthma. Curr Opin Pulm Med. 2017;23:97–102.
23. Gupta S, Siddiqui S, Haldar P, Raj JV, Entwisle JJ, Wardlaw AJ, Bradding P, Pavord ID, Green RH, Brightling CE. Qualitative analysis of high-resolution CT scans in severe asthma. Chest. 2009;136:1521–8.
24. Karišik M. Foreign body aspiration and ingestion in children. ACC. 2023;62:105. https://doi.org/10.20471/acc.2023.62.s1.13.
25. Sutherland J, Bowen L. Ingestion of foreign bodies and caustic substances in children. BJA Educ. 2023;23:2–7.
26. Oliva S, Romano C, De Angelis P, et al. Foreign body and caustic ingestions in children: a clinical practice guideline. Dig Liver Dis. 2020;52:1266–81.
27. Kendigelen P. The anaesthetic consideration of tracheobronchial foreign body aspiration in children. J Thorac Dis. 2016;8:3803–7.
28. Bajaj D, Sachdeva A, Deepak D. Foreign body aspiration. J Thorac Dis. 2021;13:5159–75.
29. Won HS, Cha YK, Kim JS, Jang SJ, Bak SH, Yoon HJ. A pictorial review of radiologic findings of foreign bodies in the thorax. J Korean Soc Radiol. 2022;83:293.
30. Yang X-J, Xing G-F, Shi C-W, Li W. Value of 3-dimensional CT virtual anatomy imaging in complex foreign body retrieval from soft tissues. Korean J Radiol. 2013;14:269.
31. Guelfguat M, Kaplinskiy V, Reddy SH, DiPoce J. Clinical guidelines for imaging and reporting ingested foreign bodies. Am J Roentgenol. 2014;203:37–53.
32. Essien E-O, Rali P, Mathai SC. Pulmonary embolism. Med Clin North Am. 2019;103:549–64.
33. Kulka HC, Zeller A, Fornaro J, Wuillemin WA, Konstantinides S, Christ M. Acute pulmonary embolism: its diagnosis and treatment from a multidisciplinary viewpoint. Dtsch Arztebl Int. 2021;118:618. https://doi.org/10.3238/arztebl.m2021.0226.
34. Moore AJE, Wachsmann J, Chamarthy MR, Panjikaran L, Tanabe Y, Rajiah P. Imaging of acute pulmonary embolism: an update. Cardiovasc Diagn Ther. 2018;8:225–43.
35. Di Nisio M, Van Es N, Büller HR. Deep vein thrombosis and pulmonary embolism. Lancet. 2016;388:3060–73.
36. Becattini C, Agnelli G. Risk stratification and management of acute pulmonary embolism. Hematology. 2016;2016:404–12.
37. Wells PS, Anderson DR, Rodger M, Stiell I, Dreyer JF, Barnes D, Forgie M, Kovacs G, Ward J, Kovacs MJ. Excluding pulmonary embolism at the bedside without diagnostic imaging: management of patients with suspected pulmonary embolism presenting to the emergency department by using a simple clinical model and D -dimer. Ann Intern Med. 2001;135:98.
38. Carlon TA, Goldman DT, Marinelli BS, Korff RA, Watchmaker JM, Patel RS, Lipson SD, Bishay VL, Lookstein RA. Contemporary management of acute pulmonary embolism: evolution of catheter-based therapy. Radiographics. 2022;42:1861–80.
39. Giri J, Sista AK, Weinberg I, et al. Interventional therapies for acute pulmonary embolism: current status and principles for the development of novel evidence: a scientific statement from the American Heart Association. Circulation. 2019;140:e774. https://doi.org/10.1161/CIR.0000000000000707.
40. Konstantinides SV, Meyer G, Becattini C, et al. 2019 ESC Guidelines for the diagnosis and management of acute pulmonary embolism developed in collaboration with the European Respiratory Society (ERS). Eur Heart J. 2020;41:543–603.
41. Worsley DF, Alavi A, Aronchick JM, Chen JT, Greenspan RH, Ravin CE. Chest radiographic findings in patients with acute pulmonary embolism: observations from the PIOPED Study. Radiology. 1993;189:133–6.
42. Han D, Lee KS, Franquet T, Müller NL, Kim TS, Kim H, Kwon OJ, Byun HS. Thrombotic and nonthrombotic pulmonary arterial embolism: spectrum of imaging findings. Radiographics. 2003;23:1521–39.
43. Ghaye B, Ghuysen A, Bruyere P-J, D'Orio V, Dondelinger RF. Can CT pulmonary angiography allow assessment of severity and prognosis in patients presenting with pulmonary embolism? What the radiologist needs to know. Radiographics. 2006;26:23–39.
44. Stein PD, Woodard PK, Weg JG, et al. Diagnostic pathways in acute pulmonary embolism: recommendations of the PIOPED II investigators. Radiology. 2007;242:15–21.
45. Kaykisiz EK, Unluer EE, Eser U. The diagnosis of pulmonary embolism without contrastis not always challenging: be aware of hyperdense lumen sign. Pan Afr Med J. 2018;30:279. https://doi.org/10.11604/pamj.2018.30.279.16283.
46. Wittram C, Maher MM, Yoo AJ, Kalra MK, Shepard J-AO, McLoud TC. CT angiography of pulmonary embolism: diagnostic criteria and causes of misdiagnosis. Radiographics. 2004;24:1219–38.
47. Leitman EM, McDermott S. Pulmonary arteries: imaging of pulmonary embolism and beyond. Cardiovasc Diagn Ther. 2019;9:S37–58.
48. Rali PM, Criner GJ. Submassive pulmonary embolism. Am J Respir Crit Care Med. 2018;198:588–98.
49. Revel M-P, Triki R, Chatellier G, Couchon S, Haddad N, Hernigou A, Danel C, Frija G. Is it possible to recognize pulmonary infarction on multisection CT images? Radiology. 2007;244:875–82.
50. Haramati A, Haramati LB. Imaging of chronic thromboembolic disease. Lung. 2020;198:245–55.
51. Mohebali D, Heidinger BH, Feldman SA, Matos JD, Dabreo D, McCormick I, Litmanovich D, Manning WJ, Carroll BJ. Right ventricular strain in patients with pulmonary embolism and syncope. J Thromb Thrombolysis. 2020;50:157–64.
52. Van Der Pol LM, Tromeur C, Bistervels IM, et al. Pregnancy-adapted YEARS algorithm for diagnosis

of suspected pulmonary embolism. N Engl J Med. 2019;380:1139–49.
53. Tromeur C, Van Der Pol LM, Le Roux P-Y, Ende-Verhaar Y, Salaun P-Y, Leroyer C, Couturaud F, Kroft LJM, Huisman MV, Klok FA. Computed tomography pulmonary angiography *versus* ventilation-perfusion lung scanning for diagnosing pulmonary embolism during pregnancy: a systematic review and meta-analysis. Haematologica. 2019;104:176–88.
54. Petritsch B, Kosmala A, Gassenmaier T, Weng A, Veldhoen S, Kunz A, Bley T. Diagnosis of pulmonary artery embolism: comparison of single-source CT and 3rd generation dual-source CT using a dual-energy protocol regarding image quality and radiation dose. Fortschr Röntgenstr. 2017;189:527–36.
55. Tao SM, Li X, Schoepf UJ, Nance JW, Jacobs BE, Zhou CS, Gu HF, Lu MJ, Lu GM, Zhang LJ. Comparison of the effect of radiation exposure from dual-energy CT versus single-energy CT on double-strand breaks at CT pulmonary angiography. Eur J Radiol. 2018;101:92–6.
56. Jawad S, Ulriksen PS, Kalhauge A, Hansen KL. Acute pulmonary embolism severity assessment evaluated with dual energy CT perfusion compared to conventional CT angiographic measurements. Diagnostics. 2021;11:495.
57. Im DJ, Hur J, Han KH, Lee H-J, Kim YJ, Kwon W, Choi BW. Acute pulmonary embolism: retrospective cohort study of the predictive value of perfusion defect volume measured with dual-energy CT. Am J Roentgenol. 2017;209:1015–22.
58. Gianesini S, Obi A, Onida S, et al. Global guidelines trends and controversies in lower limb venous and lymphatic disease: narrative literature revision and experts' opinions following the winter international meeting in Phlebology, Lymphology & Aesthetics, 23–25 January 2019. Phlebology. 2019;34:4–66.
59. Assaad S, Kratzert WB, Shelley B, Friedman MB, Perrino A. Assessment of pulmonary edema: principles and practice. J Cardiothorac Vasc Anesth. 2018;32:901–14.
60. Glaus MT, Schellenberg S, Lang J. Kardiales und nicht kardiales Lungenödem: Pathomechanismen und Ursachen. Schweiz Arch Tierheilkd. 2010;152:311–7.
61. Maw AM, Hassanin A, Ho PM, et al. Diagnostic accuracy of point-of-care lung ultrasonography and chest radiography in adults with symptoms suggestive of acute decompensated heart failure: a systematic review and meta-analysis. JAMA Netw Open. 2019;2:e190703.
62. Tsuchiya N, Griffin L, Yabuuchi H, Kawanami S, Shinzato J, Murayama S. Imaging findings of pulmonary edema: part 1. Cardiogenic pulmonary edema and acute respiratory distress syndrome. Acta Radiol. 2020;61:184–94.
63. Lindow T, Quadrelli S, Ugander M. Noninvasive imaging methods for quantification of pulmonary edema and congestion. JACC Cardiovasc Imaging. 2023;16:1469–84.
64. Wooten WM, Shaffer LET, Hamilton LA. Bedside ultrasound versus chest radiography for detection of pulmonary edema: a prospective cohort study. J Ultrasound Med. 2019;38:967–73.
65. Dobbe L, Rahman R, Elmassry M, Paz P, Nugent K. Cardiogenic pulmonary edema. Am J Med Sci. 2019;358:389–97.
66. Kobayashi M, Bercker M, Huttin O, et al. Chest X-ray quantification of admission lung congestion as a prognostic factor in patients admitted for worsening heart failure from the ICALOR cohort study. Int J Cardiol. 2020;299:192–8.
67. Gluecker T, Capasso P, Schnyder P, Gudinchet F, Schaller M-D, Revelly J-P, Chiolero R, Vock P, Wicky S. Clinical and radiologic features of pulmonary edema. Radiographics. 1999;19:1507–31.
68. Loebelenz LI, Ebner L, Obmann VC, Huber AT, Christe A. Kerley B lines in the lung apex—a distinct CT sign for pulmonary congestion. Swiss Med Wkly. 2019;149:w20119. https://doi.org/10.4414/smw.2019.20119.
69. Siwik D, Apanasiewicz W, Żukowska M, Jaczewski G, Dąbrowska M. Diagnosing lung abnormalities related to heart failure in chest radiogram, lung ultrasound and thoracic computed tomography. Adv Respir Med. 2023;91:103–22.
70. Lichtenstein DA. Lung ultrasound in the critically ill. Ann Intensive Care. 2014;4(1):1.
71. Dong L-J, Li J, Liu W, Ankaerjiang A-W, Li B, Chen Y-T, Yu Z-X. Diagnostic efficacy of lung ultrasound in cardiogenic pulmonary edema: a systematic review and meta-analysis. Eur Rev Med Pharmacol Sci. 2023;27:6947–55.
72. Nishimura Y, Komatsu J, Sugane H, et al. Unilateral pulmonary edema in patients with acute mitral regurgitation caused by chordal rupture. Circ Rep. 2022;4:571–8.
73. Bellani G, Laffey JG, Pham T, et al. Epidemiology, patterns of care, and mortality for patients with acute respiratory distress syndrome in intensive care units in 50 countries. JAMA. 2016;315:788.
74. Huang X, Zhang R, Fan G, et al. Incidence and outcomes of acute respiratory distress syndrome in intensive care units of mainland China: a multicentre prospective longitudinal study. Crit Care. 2020;24:515.
75. Bitker L, Talmor D, Richard J-C. Imaging the acute respiratory distress syndrome: past, present and future. Intensive Care Med. 2022;48:995–1008.
76. Chung JH, Kradin RL, Greene RE, Shepard J-AO, Digumarthy SR. CT predictors of mortality in pathology confirmed ARDS. Eur Radiol. 2011;21:730–7.
77. Qi M, Zhou H, Yi Q, Wang M, Tang Y. Pulmonary CT imaging findings in fat embolism syndrome: case series and literature review. Clin Med. 2023;23:88–93.

78. Sturgill JL, Mayer KP, Kalema AG, Dave K, Mora S, Kalantar A, Carter DJ, Montgomery-Yates AA, Morris PE. Post-intensive care syndrome and pulmonary fibrosis in patients surviving ARDS-pneumonia of COVID-19 and non-COVID-19 etiologies. Sci Rep. 2023;13:6554.
79. Chen W-T, Wang H-Y, Ye Q-H, Tang M, Wang Y-W. The diagnostic values of lung ultrasound for ARDS. Eur Rev Med Pharmacol Sci. 2022;26:6642–6.
80. Chiumello D, Mongodi S, Algieri I, Vergani GL, Orlando A, Via G, Crimella F, Cressoni M, Mojoli F. Assessment of lung aeration and recruitment by CT scan and ultrasound in acute respiratory distress syndrome patients*. Crit Care Med. 2018;46:1761–8.
81. Barile M. Pulmonary edema: a pictorial review of imaging manifestations and current understanding of mechanisms of disease. Eur J Radiol Open. 2020;7:100274.
82. Reynolds JH, Mcdonald G, Alton H, Gordon SB. Pneumonia in the immunocompetent patient. BJR. 2010;83:998–1009.
83. Franquet T. Imaging of community-acquired pneumonia. J Thorac Imaging. 2018;33:282–94.
84. Reynolds JH, Banerjee AK. Imaging pneumonia in immunocompetent and immunocompromised individuals. Curr Opin Pulm Med. 2012;18:194–201.
85. Koo HJ, Lim S, Choe J, Choi S-H, Sung H, Do K-H. Radiographic and CT features of viral pneumonia. Radiographics. 2018;38:719–39.
86. Bouros D, Nicholson AC, Polychronopoulos V, du Bois RM. Acute interstitial pneumonia. Eur Respir J. 2000;15:412–8.
87. Primack SL, Hartman TE, Ikezoe J, Akira M, Sakatani M, Müller NL. Acute interstitial pneumonia: radiographic and CT findings in nine patients. Radiology. 1993;188:817–20.
88. Tomiyama N, Müller NL, Johkoh T, Honda O, Mihara N, Kozuka T, Hamada S, Nakamura H, Akira M, Ichikado K. Acute parenchymal lung disease in immunocompetent patients: diagnostic accuracy of high-resolution CT. AJR Am J Roentgenol. 2000;174:1745–50.
89. Wittram C, Mark EJ, McLoud TC. CT-histologic correlation of the ATS/ERS 2002 classification of idiopathic interstitial pneumonias. Radiographics. 2003;23:1057–71.
90. Johkoh T, Müller NL, Taniguchi H, Kondoh Y, Akira M, Ichikado K, Ando M, Honda O, Tomiyama N, Nakamura H. Acute interstitial pneumonia: thin-section CT findings in 36 patients. Radiology. 1999;211:859–63.
91. Han MK, Kazerooni EA, Lynch DA, et al. Chronic obstructive pulmonary disease exacerbations in the COPDGene study: associated radiologic phenotypes. Radiology. 2011;261:274–82.
92. Biondini D, Balestro E, Sverzellati N, Cocconcelli E, Bernardinello N, Ryerson CJ, Spagnolo P. Acute exacerbations of idiopathic pulmonary fibrosis (AE-IPF): an overview of current and future therapeutic strategies. Expert Rev Respir Med. 2020;14:405–14.
93. Luppi F, Cerri S, Taddei S, Ferrara G, Cottin V. Acute exacerbation of idiopathic pulmonary fibrosis: a clinical review. Intern Emerg Med. 2015;10:401–11.
94. Song JW, Hong S-B, Lim C-M, Koh Y, Kim DS. Acute exacerbation of idiopathic pulmonary fibrosis: incidence, risk factors and outcome. Eur Respir J. 2011;37:356–63.
95. Palmucci S, Galioto F, Fazio G, et al. Clinical and radiological features of lung disorders related to connective-tissue diseases: a pictorial essay. Insights Imaging. 2022;13:108.
96. Yoo H, Hino T, Hwang J, Franks TJ, Han J, Im Y, Lee HY, Chung MP, Hatabu H, Lee KS. Connective tissue disease-related interstitial lung disease (CTD-ILD) and interstitial lung abnormality (ILA): evolving concept of CT findings, pathology and management. Eur J Radiol Open. 2022;9:100419.
97. Lara AR, Schwarz MI. Diffuse alveolar hemorrhage. Chest. 2010;137:1164–71.
98. Park JA. Treatment of diffuse alveolar hemorrhage: controlling inflammation and obtaining rapid and effective hemostasis. IJMS. 2021;22:793.
99. Martínez-Martínez MU, Oostdam DAH, Abud-Mendoza C. Diffuse alveolar hemorrhage in autoimmune diseases. Curr Rheumatol Rep. 2017;19:27.
100. Alexandre AT, Vale A, Gomes T. Diffuse alveolar hemorrhage: how relevant is etiology? Sarcoidosis Vasc Diffuse Lung Dis. 2019;36:47–52.
101. Thakrar PD, Boyd KP, Swanson CP, Wideburg E, Kumbhar SS. E-cigarette, or vaping, product use-associated lung injury in adolescents: a review of imaging features. Pediatr Radiol. 2020;50:338–44.
102. Reisman S, Chung M, Bernheim A. A review of clinical and imaging features of diffuse pulmonary hemorrhage. Am J Roentgenol. 2021;216:1500–9.
103. Cortese G, Nicali R, Placido R, Gariazzo G, Anrò P. Radiological aspects of diffuse alveolar haemorrhage. Radiol Med. 2008;113:16–28.
104. Capobianco J, Grimberg A, Thompson BM, Antunes VB, Jasinowodolinski D, Meirelles GSP. Thoracic manifestations of collagen vascular diseases. Radiographics. 2012;32:33–50.
105. Beaudoin S, Gonzalez AV. Evaluation of the patient with pleural effusion. CMAJ. 2018;190:E291–5.
106. Light RW. Pleural effusions. Med Clin North Am. 2011;95:1055–70.
107. Brogi E, Gargani L, Bignami E, Barbariol F, Marra A, Forfori F, Vetrugno L. Thoracic ultrasound for pleural effusion in the intensive care unit: a narrative review from diagnosis to treatment. Crit Care. 2017;21:325.
108. Craig Blackmore C, Black WC, Dallas RV, Crow HC. Pleural fluid volume estimation: a chest radiograph prediction rule. Acad Radiol. 1996;3:103–9.
109. Hassan M, Mercer RM, Rahman NM. Thoracic ultrasound in the modern management of pleural disease. Eur Respir Rev. 2020;29:190136.

110. Baldi G, Gargani L, Abramo A, D'Errico L, Caramella D, Picano E, Giunta F, Forfori F. Lung water assessment by lung ultrasonography in intensive care: a pilot study. Intensive Care Med. 2013;39:74–84.
111. Satoto B, Budi WS, Khumaeni A, Yueniwati Y, Noorhamdani N. Comparative estimation of pleural effusion volume based on lateral decubitus position of chest x-ray and CT scan imaging. Biomed Phys Eng Express. 2022;8:055028.
112. Raju S, Ghosh S, Mehta AC. Chest CT signs in pulmonary disease. Chest. 2017;151:1356–74.
113. Tsujimoto N, Saraya T, Light RW, Tsukahara Y, Koide T, Kurai D, Ishii H, Kimura H, Goto H, Takizawa H. A simple method for differentiating complicated parapneumonic effusion/empyema from parapneumonic effusion using the split pleura sign and the amount of pleural effusion on thoracic CT. PLoS One. 2015;10:e0130141.
114. Algin O, Gokalp G, Topal U. Signs in chest imaging: a pictorial review. Diagn Interv Radiol. 2009; https://doi.org/10.4261/1305-3825.DIR.2901-09.1.
115. Kocijančič I, Vidmar K, Ivanovi-Herceg Z. Chest sonography versus lateral decubitus radiography in the diagnosis of small pleural effusions. J Clin Ultrasound. 2003;31:69–74.
116. Lichtenstein D, Goldstein I, Mourgeon E, Cluzel P, Grenier P, Rouby J-J. Comparative diagnostic performances of auscultation, chest radiography, and lung ultrasonography in acute respiratory distress syndrome. Anesthesiology. 2004;100:9–15.
117. Xirouchaki N, Magkanas E, Vaporidi K, Kondili E, Plataki M, Patrianakos A, Akoumianaki E, Georgopoulos D. Lung ultrasound in critically ill patients: comparison with bedside chest radiography. Intensive Care Med. 2011;37:1488.
118. International Liaison Committee on Lung Ultrasound (ILC-LUS) for the International Consensus Conference on Lung Ultrasound (ICC-LUS), Volpicelli G, Elbarbary M, et al. International evidence-based recommendations for point-of-care lung ultrasound. Intensive Care Med. 2012;38:577–91.
119. Dahmarde H, Parooie F, Salarzaei M. Accuracy of ultrasound in diagnosis of pneumothorax: a comparison between neonates and adults—a systematic review and meta-analysis. Can Respir J. 2019;2019:1–16.
120. Huan N-C, Sidhu C, Thomas R. Pneumothorax. Clin Chest Med. 2021;42:711–27.
121. Kanne JP, Rother MDM. Pneumothorax: imaging diagnosis and etiology. Semin Roentgenol. 2023;58:440–53.
122. Omar HR, Abdelmalak H, Mangar D, Rashad R, Helal E, Camporesi EM. Occult pneumothorax, revisited. J Trauma Manage Outcomes. 2010;4:12.
123. Butler H, Chrisanthopoulos V, Harous A, Eattimoottil SS, Senthilkumaran D, Tanious P, Wang B, Arruzza E. A scoping review of clinical practice guidelines for the diagnosis of primary spontaneous pneumothorax. J Med Imaging Radiat Sci. 2022;53:728–36.
124. Roberts DJ, Leigh-Smith S, Faris PD, et al. Clinical presentation of patients with tension pneumothorax: a systematic review. Ann Surg. 2015;261:1068–78.
125. Husain L, Hagopian L, Wayman D, Baker W, Carmody K. Sonographic diagnosis of pneumothorax. J Emerg Trauma Shock. 2012;5:76.
126. Turner JP, Dankoff J. Thoracic ultrasound. Emerg Med Clin North Am. 2012;30:451–73.
127. Volpicelli G. Sonographic diagnosis of pneumothorax. Intensive Care Med. 2011;37:224–32.
128. Hassan M, Touman AA, Grabczak EM, Skaarup SH, Faber K, Blyth KG, Pochepnia S. Imaging of pleural disease. Breathe. 2024;20:230172.
129. Skulec R, Parizek T, David M, Matousek V, Cerny V. Lung point sign in ultrasound diagnostics of pneumothorax: imitations and variants. Emerg Med Int. 2021;2021:1–7.

5 Hemoptysis

Antonio Raucci, Vittorio Sabatino, Giovanna Russo, Francesco Muto, Angelo Masella, and Francesca Iacobellis

5.1 Introduction

Hemoptysis is a pathologic sign commonly referred to as the "coughing up of blood," but better defined as the expectoration of blood from the lungs or lower respiratory tract. Hemoptysis must be differentiated from pseudo-hemoptysis, which is blood that originates from nasopharyngeal or gastrointestinal sources. Hemoptysis is a concerning symptom that can range from blood-streaked sputum (non-massive or hemoptoe) to a large volume of blood expectoration (massive). However, as the severity of hemoptysis cannot be accurately defined by blood volume alone because a significant amount can be retained, the definition of "massive" has now shifted to "a condition that places the patient at high risk of asphyxiation or exsanguination." The initial assessment of hemoptysis focuses on the severity of bleeding and the patient cardiovascular stability. Most cases are classified as mild hemoptysis and have a good prognosis, while massive hemoptysis is more rare but associated with high mortality. Hemoptysis can occur in a multitude of diseases. Medical history and physical examination can often guide the diagnosis, but diagnostic testing is usually required. Chest radiography is a good initial test, but it has limited sensitivity for the site and etiology of the bleeding. Computed tomography (CT) and CT-Angiography of the chest with intravenous contrast are the preferred modalities to determine the etiology of bleeding. Bronchoscopy may also be needed for diagnostic or airway protection purposes. Bronchial arterial embolization is used in cases of massive hemoptysis, especially when a bleeding artery is visible on CTA. Surgery is reserved for those who do not respond to medical management and embolization [1–3].

5.2 Etiology

Hemoptysis is a manifestation that can be associated with a wide range of diseases.

The differential diagnosis is broad and some causes are summarized in Table 5.1.

The etiology of hemoptysis varies depending on geographic location and healthcare setting. In developed countries, common causes of hemoptysis in outpatient settings include acute respiratory infections, chronic obstructive pulmonary disease (COPD), malignancies and bronchiectasis. Specialized centers report bronchiectasis, respiratory infections and lung cancers as the primary causes. In developing countries, tuberculosis and

A. Raucci (✉) · V. Sabatino · G. Russo · F. Muto
A. Masella · F. Iacobellis
Department of General and Emergency Radiology, "Antonio Cardarelli" Hospital, Napoli, Italy
e-mail: antonio.raucci2@aocardarelli.it; vittorio.sabatino@aocardarelli.it; giovanna.russo@aocardarelli.it; francesco.muto@aocardarelli.it; angelo.masella@aocardarelli.it; francesca.iacobellis@aocardarelli.it

L. Romano et al. (eds.), *CT of Non-Traumatic Body Emergencies*,
https://doi.org/10.1007/978-3-031-84849-0_5

Table 5.1 Most common differential diagnosis of hemoptysis

Category	Causes
Infectious	Acute respiratory infections Tuberculosis (common in developing countries)
Chronic lung diseases	Chronic obstructive pulmonary disease (COPD) Bronchiectasis
Malignancies	Lung cancer Metastatic cancers
Vascular disorders	Pulmonary arteriovenous malformations Pseudoaneurysms Artery aneurysms
Autoimmune/Inflammatory	Sarcoidosis Autoimmune diseases (e.g., causing capillaritis or cavitation)
Coagulation disorders	Coagulation abnormalities (e.g., due to anticoagulant therapy, hemophilia)
Pulmonary embolism	Rare cause of hemoptysis
Sequelae of respiratory infections	Scarring or damage post-infection, including abscesses
Cryptogenic (idiopathic)	No identifiable cause in approximately 20% of cases

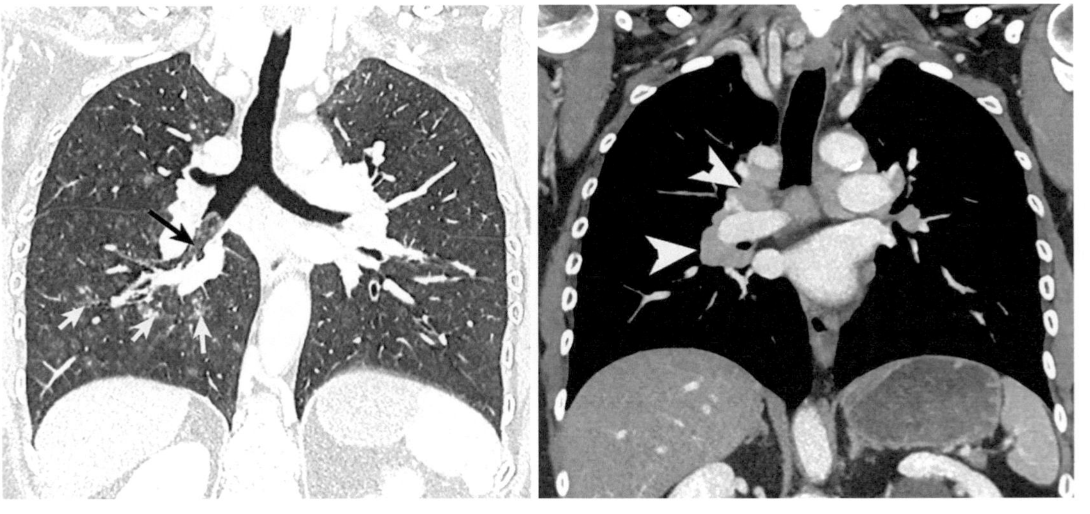

Fig. 5.1 Blood clot in right main lower bronchus (black arrow) associates with diffuse ground glass opacities (white arrows); mediastinal lymph node enlargement is also noted (white arrowheads). The alteration was later diagnosed as sarcoidosis

its sequelae remain the leading cause of hemoptysis. Other potential causes of hemoptysis encompass sarcoidosis (Fig. 5.1), autoimmune disorders leading to capillaritis or cavitation (Figs. 5.2 and 5.3), coagulation abnormalities, sequelae from pulmonary biopsy (Figs. 5.4 and 5.5) respiratory infections and vascular disorders such as pulmonary arteriovenous malformations (Figs. 5.6 and 5.7), pseudoaneurysms or rupture of an intramediastinal aortic segment (Fig. 5.8). Pulmonary embolism rarely results in hemoptysis. Despite extensive investigations, approximately 20% of hemoptysis cases remain "cryptogenic" meaning that the cause cannot be identified even with advanced imaging and procedures like CT scans and bronchoscopies [1–3].

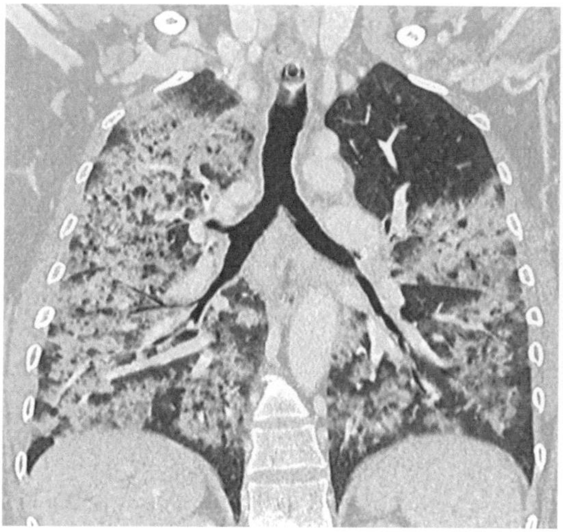

Fig. 5.2 Diffuse bilateral ground glass opacities in a patient with severe hemoptysis. The radiological picture is compatible with diffuse alveolar hemorrhage

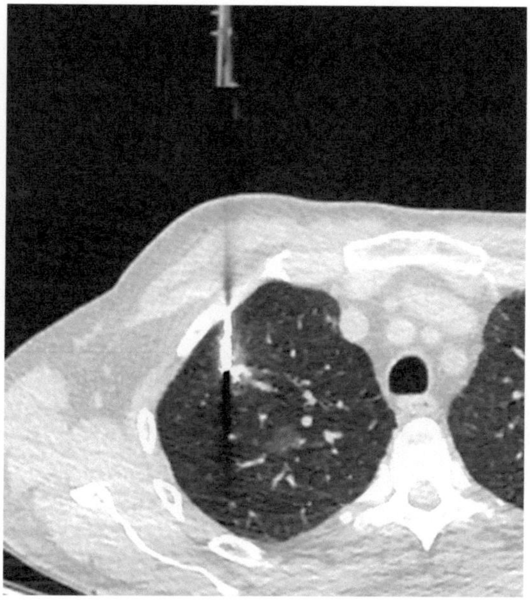

Fig. 5.4 CT-guided biopsy of a little pulmonary nodule

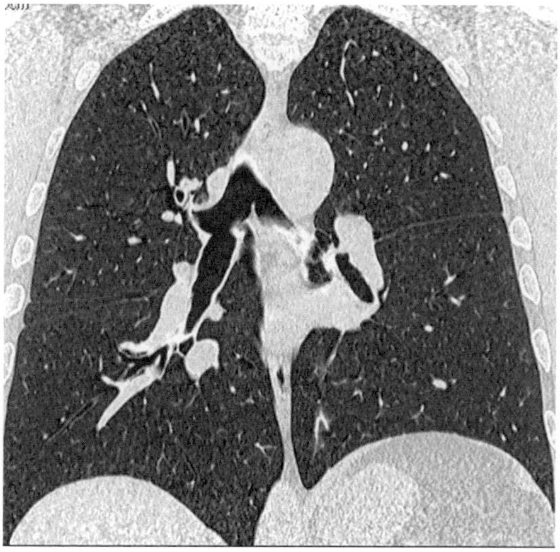

Fig. 5.3 In the same case (Fig. 5.2), a CT scan obtained 40 days later shows a complete resolution of alveolar hemorrhage

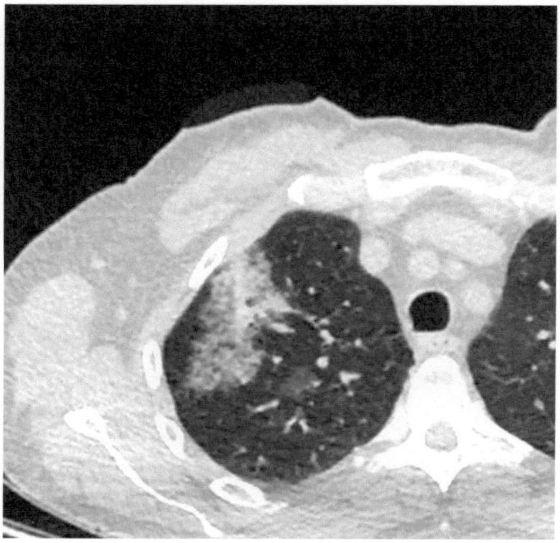

Fig. 5.5 In the same case there is a post-biopsy alveolar hemorrhage manifesting with hemoptysis, usually self-limited

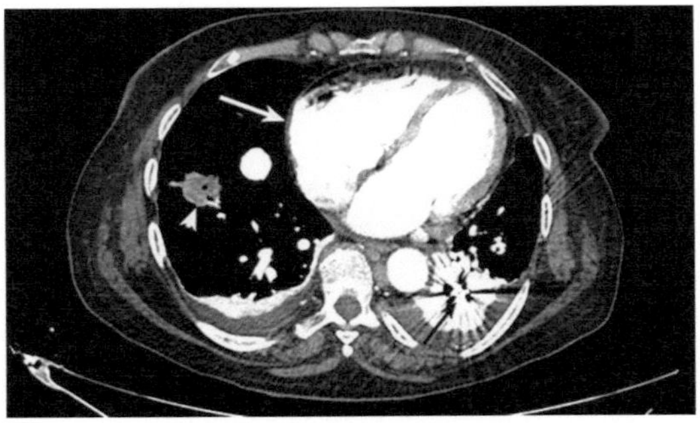

Fig. 5.6 Hereditary hemorrhagic telangiectasia (HTT or Rendu-Osler disease), which is a rare genetic disorder: there is a coil from previous embolization in the left lower lobe (black arrow) and an incidental nodule in keeping with lung cancer (white arrowhead). Right ventricular enlargement (white arrow) due to volume overload from pulmonary artero-venous shunting, is also present

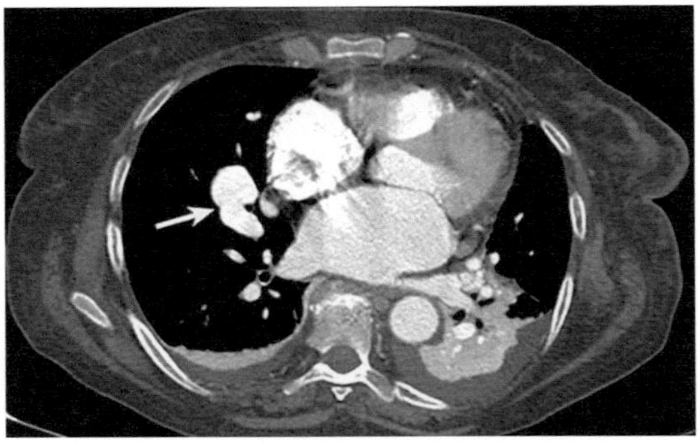

Fig. 5.7 In the same case (Fig. 5.6), a large artero-venous fistula is shown in the right lower lobe (arrow)

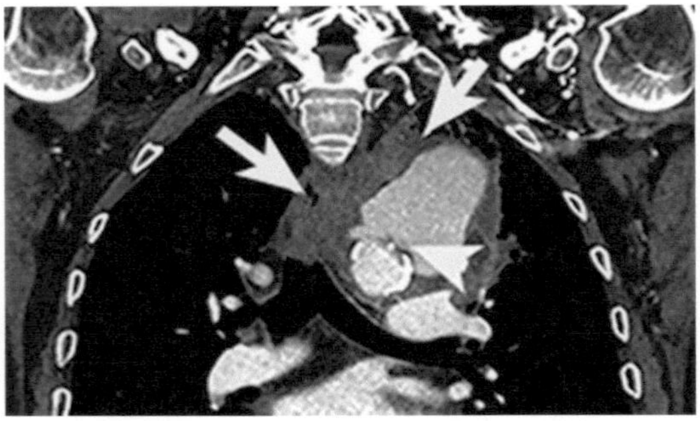

Fig. 5.8 Rupture of the anterior wall of the ascending aorta (arrowhead) with large contrast leak and presence of a mediastinal hematoma (arrows)

5.3 Pathophysiology

The mechanisms leading to hemoptysis can be categorized according to the vascular involvement in primary or secondary. However, hemoptysis may even result from more than a single pathophysiological mechanism. Mechanisms of primary vascular involvement are chronic hypertrophy of systemic vascular supply, vascular damage, pseudoaneurysms, dysplastic lung parenchyma with systemic supply, arteriovenous malformations, fistulas and capillary-level bleeding. Mechanisms of secondary vascular involvement are conditions that directly affect lung tissue such as infections, infarcts or tumors or benign processes invading the airways. Treatment strategies vary according to the pathophysiology: for instance, chronic systemic vascular hypertrophy might be managed with regional endovascular therapy, typically bronchial artery embolization. Damaged vessels developing pseudo-aneurysms may require local endovascular therapy or surgical intervention. Airway erosion typically necessitates bronchoscopic or surgical intervention [1, 2].

5.4 Diagnostic Work-Up

The initial management of hemoptysis necessitates a rapid assessment of the patient's hemodynamic and respiratory stability to identify a life-threatening hemorrhage. Signs of airway compromise, respiratory failure or hemodynamic instability may need an appropriate critical care setting for stabilization and further evaluation.

In hemodynamically stable patients, a comprehensive history and physical examination are imperative. The primary objectives of this initial assessment are to confirm the presence of hemoptysis, localize the site of bleeding and determine the underlying etiology. Physical findings may aid in establishing the diagnosis and reveal concomitant systemic pathologies. It is crucial to identify the etiology of bleeding even in cases of cessation. Laboratory assessment should include evaluation for underlying coagulopathy with additional testing guided by clinical suspicion.

For non-massive hemoptysis, the American College of Radiology (ACR) Appropriateness Criteria suggests initial imaging with chest X-Ray, Computed Tomography (CT) of the chest with intravenous (IV) contrast or CT Angiography of the chest (CTA with IV contrast) [4].

Chest X-Ray is wide accessible and cost-effective, even though may not detect malignancy and demonstrates a lower sensitivity compared to CT in identifying the bleeding source and etiology. Portable AP (antero-posterior) radiography, frequently employed in unstable patients, has demonstrated clinical utility in localizing the side of bleeding. In the absence of definitive findings on chest radiography, further investigation with CT or bronchoscopy is indicated [5].

CT and bronchoscopy has comparable efficacy in localizing bleeding, however CT surpasses bronchoscopy in determining etiology. CT with IV contrast demonstrates superior sensitivity to radiography in identifying the site and cause of hemorrhage. CT Angiography accurately delineates potential bleeding arteries and aids in the diagnosis of pulmonary embolism; moreover, CTA proves invaluable for pre-procedural planning in cases where embolization is anticipated.

Bronchoscopy offers both diagnostic and therapeutic purposes, proving particularly advantageous in detecting endobronchial lesions which are prevalent in patients presenting with hemoptysis and normal chest radiography. Bronchoscopy facilitates tissue and microbial sampling. In massive hemoptysis, rigid bronchoscopy can secure the airway and ventilation. Additionally, it permits the removal of blood or foreign bodies and tumor debulking. The combined use of bronchoscopy and CT may enhance the sensitivity for localizing the bleeding site and determining the etiology in cases where CT alone is inconclusive [3, 6, 7].

5.5 Imaging

Computed tomography (CT) has emerged as a relevant non-invasive modality in the evaluation of hemoptysis, receiving a "usually appropriate" grade from the American College of Radiology (ACR) Appropriateness Criteria for both life-threatening and non-life-threatening cases [4].

In patients with established diagnoses known to precipitate hemoptysis, such as cystic fibrosis or neoplasms, CT serves to identify localized or treatable sources of hemorrhage, thereby optimizing therapeutic strategies. In patients presenting with hemoptysis as the initial manifestation of an underlying disease, CT also demonstrates significant utility as facilitates the localization of hemorrhage and contributes to determining the etiology. Overall, CT has proven to be an indispensable and versatile tool in the diagnostic workup and clinical management of hemoptysis across a broad spectrum of clinical presentations.

5.6 CT Scanning Technique

As CT imaging plays a crucial role in the assessment of hemoptysis, adherence to a standardized protocol is strongly recommended. The optimal acquisition phase in the systemic arterial phase is the contrast injection flow should be high (4–5 mL/s) with bolus tracking initiated at the descending thoracic aorta. The protocol is aimed to ensure an adequate opacification of the bronchial arteries, which are the predominant source of bleeding in hemoptysis necessitating intervention. A saline chaser should be omitted to prevent dilution of contrast within the pulmonary arterial tree. Additionally, a higher volume of iodinated contrast (100–120 mL) is recommended to maintain pulmonary artery opacification. The scan range should encompass the lower neck through the celiac axis as some bleeding sources may originate from upper abdominal vasculature. Image reconstruction with a 1 mm section thickness utilizing a standard kernel is recommended for the evaluation of vascular and soft-tissue structures. Dedicated lung windows with a proper kernel should be employed for the assessment of lung parenchyma. A single systemic arterial phase scan often suffices for most patients, however, a pre-contrast scan may be added in post-surgical or post-traumatic cases to differentiate dense materials from enhancing vessels or extravasated contrast. A venous phase acquisition could be beneficial in patients with known tumors or infections, while a prolonged bolus may be considered in those with pulmonary arterial anomalies [1, 2].

5.6.1 CT Findings of Hemorrhage

5.6.1.1 Assessment of Lung Parenchima

In CT evaluation of hemoptysis, the identification of findings indicative of intra-alveolar or intra-airway hemorrhage is paramount. Hemorrhage within the alveoli typically manifests as ground-glass opacity or consolidation, potentially accompanied by septal thickening in subacute cases due to macrophage infiltration (Figs. 5.2 and 5.5). Blood products within the bronchial tree may appear as filling defects on CT with higher attenuation observed in larger airways (Fig. 5.1), aiding in differentiation from mucus plugs. Obstruction of larger airways by blood products can lead to atelectasis.

Conversely, blood in the distal airways manifests as centrilobular nodules, often exhibiting a "tree-in-bud" configuration. The distribution of these findings can assist in localizing the source of hemorrhage, necessitating careful scrutiny for associated lesions or vascular abnormalities within the proximal bronchial tree. The distribution of hemorrhage is critical for therapeutic decision-making. A diffuse pattern of pulmonary parenchymal hemorrhage suggests a systemic etiology, rendering targeted interventions less viable. In contrast, focal parenchymal hemorrhage can guide localized interventions aimed at specific lesions or vascular territories. Differentiating parenchymal hemorrhage from aspirated blood, although challenging, can be valuable. Aspirated blood implies a more proximal or localized source, often characterized by clustered tree-in-bud nodules, while regional or diffuse ground-glass opacities favor parenchymal bleeding [1, 2].

The hemorrhage can obscure subtle underlying pathologies: blood filling the airway may mask small endobronchial tumors and blood clots can mimic nodules or masses. Therefore, a follow-up CT scan weeks after the hemoptysis episode is recommended for a comprehensive assessment.

Table 5.2 summarizes the CT findings of parenchymal alteration related to hemoptysis.

5.6.1.2 Assessment of Pulmonary Vasculature

The assessment of thoracic vasculature needs a comprehensive approach to evaluating pulmonary arteries as well as bronchial and non-bronchial systemic arteries.

Pulmonary Arteries

The pulmonary arteries should be carefully examined to rule out emboli, especially with subpleural enhancement indicating lung infarction, a common cause of non-massive hemoptysis that requires anticoagulation. In some cases, pulmonary arteries can be the source of bleeding due to direct invasion by cancer or necrotizing infections (like tuberculosis). Less frequently, life-threatening hemoptysis can result from ruptured pulmonary arteriovenous malformations (AVMs), which are abnormal connections between arteries and veins in the lungs.

Bronchial Arteries

In the vast majority of hemoptysis cases, the bleeding source lies within the systemic arterial circulation, most commonly the bronchial arteries. A direct correlation between bronchial artery dilatation and hemorrhage risk is not consistently observed, however, a diameter exceeding 2 mm is considered abnormal (Figs. 5.9 and 5.10). The bronchial arteries follow a predictable yet tortuous pathway. Bleeding often originates from these arteries, however the actual site of

Table 5.2 CT findings of parenchymal alterations associated with hemoptysis

Finding	Description	Clinical significance
Ground-glass opacity (GGO)	Hazy opacities without obscuration of bronchial structures	Indicative of intra-alveolar hemorrhage; may represent parenchymal bleeding
Consolidation	Dense opacification with obscured bronchial structures	Suggests blood filling the alveoli; associated with parenchymal hemorrhage
Septal thickening	Thickening of interlobular septa, often subacute	Can result from macrophage infiltration post-hemorrhage
Filling defects in airways	Low-density material in the bronchial tree with high attenuation	Represents blood within airways; differentiation from mucus plugs
Atelectasis	Collapse or volume loss of lung tissue	Caused by airway obstruction from blood clots in larger airways
Centrilobular nodules	Small nodules in a peribronchovascular distribution	Indicates blood in the distal airways; often seen in a "tree-in-bud" pattern
"Tree-in-bud" pattern	Small centrilobular opacities with branching linear structures	Suggests distal airway involvement; helps localize the source of bleeding
Diffuse ground-glass opacities	Widespread hazy opacities	Implies systemic or diffuse parenchymal hemorrhage
Clustered tree-in-bud nodules	Grouped centrilobular opacities	Suggests aspirated blood, usually from a more proximal or localized source
Obscuration of underlying pathology	Hemorrhage masking subtle lesions (e.g., nodules, masses)	Follow-up CT recommended to detect underlying conditions like tumors
Blood clots mimicking nodules/masses	Dense filling material mimicking solid lesions	May complicate diagnosis; follow-up imaging needed to reassess

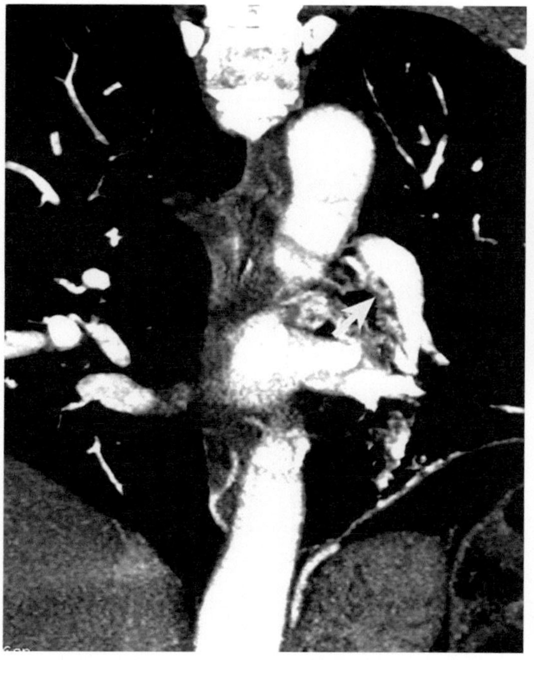

Fig. 5.9 Bronchial left artery (arrow) in a usual tortuous pathway, but abnormally dilatated

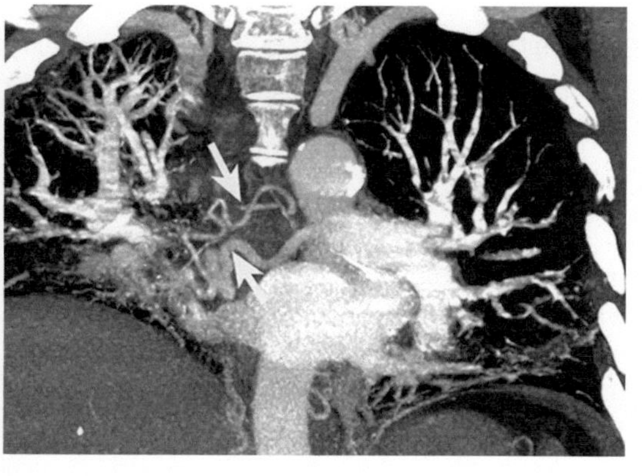

Fig. 5.10 Bronchial right arteries (arrows) in a usual tortuous pathway, but abnormally dilatated

hemorrhage usually occurs at fragile anastomoses between distal bronchial and pulmonary arterial branches, located in the airway submucosa. These anastomoses are too small for a direct visualization on CT and active bleeding is rarely visualized as the presence of contrast material in the airway lumen [1, 2, 8].

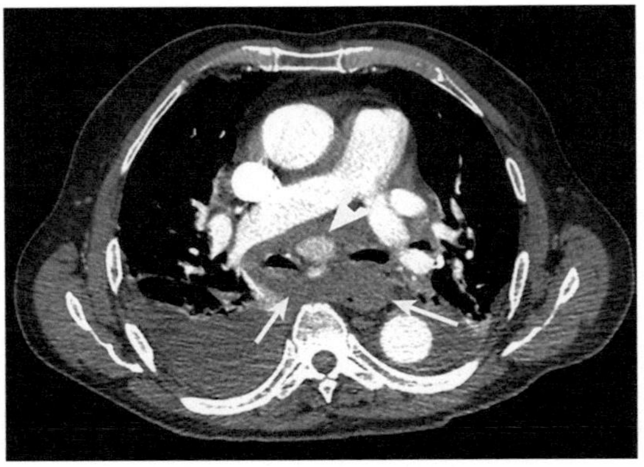

Fig. 5.11 Bronchial artery pseudoaneurysm (arrowhead) associated with mediastinal hematoma (arrows) and bilateral hemothoracs

Although uncommon, bronchial artery aneurysms can arise within the mediastinum (Fig. 5.11) or intrapulmonary regions.

Non-bronchial Arteries

Non-bronchial systemic arteries may represent a source of hemoptysis. Small arteries originating from anatomical locations such as the supra-aortic great vessels, axillary, internal mammary and infra-diaphragmatic branches may manifest as abnormally dilated and tortuous, frequently associated with pleural thickening exceeding 3 mm and enhancement within extrapleural fat; often -coexist-with radiologic signs of chronic pulmonary inflammatory disease and pleural adhesions. Failure to recognize these systemic arteries can result in recurrent hemoptysis after a bronchial artery embolization. Pseudo-sequestration, a rare vascular anomaly characterized by systemic arterial supply to normal lung parenchyma without bronchial involvement, can also manifest as hemoptysis.

Bronchial to Systemic Artery Communications and Embolization Risks

Bronchial and non-bronchial systemic artery embolization therapy for hemoptysis carries a risk of inadvertent spinal cord ischemia due to potential communication between the bronchial and spinal arterial systems: thus, the importance of careful identification of the anterior spinal artery and arteria radicularis magna (artery of Adamkiewicz) during bronchial angiography. Furthermore, communications between bronchial and coronary arteries can occur, particularly in conditions with reduced pulmonary blood flow: this can lead to coronary-to-bronchial arterial shunting and potentially contribute to the "pulmonary steal" syndrome, presenting as angina-like symptoms in patients with angiographically normal coronary arteries. Thoracic CT angiography is essential for identifying these anastomoses prior to bronchial artery embolization (Figs. 5.10 and 5.11). Cryptogenic hemoptysis, a diagnosis of exclusion with a higher prevalence in smokers, is associated with an increased risk of lung cancer: in patients with hemoptysis and no identifiable cause, it is strongly suggested to repeat CT exam several months later to monitor for potential occult tumor progression [9].

In conclusion, CT is invaluable for hemoptysis diagnosis and management. However, understanding relevant vascular anatomy and potential complications, such as spinal artery embolization or coronary-to-bronchial anastomoses, is essential for safe and effective treatment.

References

1. Marquis KM, Raptis CA, Rajput MZ, et al. CT for evaluation of hemoptysis. Radiographics. 2021;41(3):742–61. https://doi.org/10.1148/rg.2021200150.
2. Bruzzi JF, Rémy-Jardin M, Delhaye D, Teisseire A, Khalil C, Rémy J. Multi-detector row CT of hemoptysis. Radiographics. 2006;26(1):3–22. https://doi.org/10.1148/rg.261045726.
3. O'Gurek D, Choi HYJ. Hemoptysis: evaluation and management. Am Fam Physician. 2022;105(2):144–51.
4. Expert Panel on Thoracic Imaging, Olsen KM, Manouchehr-Pour S, et al. ACR appropriateness criteria® hemoptysis. J Am Coll Radiol. 2020;17(5S):S148–59. https://doi.org/10.1016/j.jacr.2020.01.043.
5. Colice GL. Haemoptysis with a normal chest radiograph: how concerned should we be? Thorax. 2009;64(10):829–30. https://doi.org/10.1136/thx.2009.113191.
6. Radchenko C, Alraiyes AH, Shojaee S. A systematic approach to the management of massive hemoptysis. J Thorac Dis. 2017;9(Suppl 10):S1069–86. https://doi.org/10.21037/jtd.2017.06.41.

7. Davidson K, Shojaee S. Managing massive hemoptysis. Chest. 2020;157(1):77–88. https://doi.org/10.1016/j.chest.2019.07.012.
8. Almeida J, Leal C, Figueiredo L. Evaluation of the bronchial arteries: normal findings, hypertrophy and embolization in patients with hemoptysis. Insights Imaging. 2020;11:70. https://doi.org/10.1186/s13244-020-00877-4.
9. Valentin LI, Walker TG. Bronchial artery embolization. In: Keefe N, Haskal Z, Park A, Angle J, editors. IR playbook. Cham: Springer; 2018. https://doi.org/10.1007/978-3-319-71300-7_21.

Chest Pain

6

Luca Gozzi, Diletta Cozzi, Giulia Grazzini,
Silvia Pradella, and Vittorio Miele

Acronyms

ACS	Acute coronary syndrome
AHA/ACC	American Heart Association/ American college of cardiology
AMI	Acute myocardial infarction
APE	Acute pulmonary embolism
CAC	Coronary artery calcification
CAD	Coronary artery disease
CAD-RADS	CAD-reporting and data system
CO	Cardiac output
CT	Computed tomography
CCTA	Coronary CT angiography
CTA	CT angiography
CTP	CT perfusion
CTPA	CT pulmonary angiography
CMRI	Cardiac magnetic resonance imaging
CNR	Contrast-to-noise ratio
CXR	Chest x-ray
DECT	Dual-energy computed tomography
DVT	Deep vein thrombosis
ED	Emergency department
ERS	European Respiratory Society
ESC	European society of cardiology
FFR_{CT}	CT fractional-flow-reserve
Hs-cTn	High-sensitivity cardiac troponin
ICA	Invasive coronary angiography
IDR	Iodine delivery ratio
IPD	Iodine perfusion defect
IVC	Inferior vena cava
LMWH	Low-molecular-weight heparin
LV	Left ventricle
MINOCA	Myocardial infarction with non-obstructive coronary arteries
MRI	Magnetic resonance imaging
NECT	Non-contrast enhanced computed tomography
NPV	Negative predictive value
NSTE	Non-ST elevation
PAD	Pulmonary artery diameter
PE	Pulmonary embolism
ROI	Region of interest
RV	Right ventricle
RVD	Right ventricular dysfunction
SIS	Segment involvement score
SVC	Superior vena cava
TRO	Triple-rule-out protocol
TTE	Transthoracic echocardiography
VTE	Venous thromboembolism

L. Gozzi · D. Cozzi · G. Grazzini · S. Pradella
V. Miele (✉)
Department of Emergency Radiology, Careggi University Hospital, Florence, Italy
e-mail: luca.gozzi@unifi.it; cozzid@aou-careggi.toscana.it; grazzinigi@aou-careggi.toscana.it; pradellas@aou-careggi.toscana.it; vmiele@sirm.org

L. Romano et al. (eds.), *CT of Non-Traumatic Body Emergencies*,
https://doi.org/10.1007/978-3-031-84849-0_6

6.1 Introduction

Chest pain is one of the major reasons for adults to seek medical advice, and after injuries, is one of the main causes for adults to reach Emergency Department (ED). Even after all these years, chest pain remains a diagnostic challenge. In fact, although the term "chest pain" is now commonplace in clinical practice, patients usually refer to it as a whole spectrum of symptoms or unpleasant sensations that may be experienced and better described as "chest discomfort," localized mainly in the anterior chest, that may arouse apprehension for something cardiac. For this reason, an accurate and comprehensive history of the patients, featuring all the characteristics of the unpleasant sensation (nature, onset, duration, location, radiations, precipitating and relieving factors, associated symptoms) is mandatory in order to better identify potential emergencies and cardiac causes.

Even though most of the times the cause of chest pain is non-cardiac, acute coronary syndrome (ACS) and pulmonary embolism (PE) are considered the two main cardiovascular emergencies (along with stroke) that must be recognized correctly and treated promptly. Failing to successfully diagnose these conditions may have major consequences, since ACS remains the leading cause of death accounting for >365.000 deaths annually and PE causes ≤300.000 deaths per year in the US [1].

6.2 Guidelines

6.2.1 ACS Guidelines

In the latest revised 2023 European guidelines of the European Society of Cardiology (ESC), major changes have occurred in interesting coronary computed tomography angiography (CCTA) in patients with suspected Non-ST elevation (NSTE) ACS. In fact, in comparison to the 2017–2020 versions (in which the Class of recommendation was I), in the 2023 version CCTA has been downgraded to a Class of recommendation IIa in patients with suspected ACS, non-elevated (or uncertain) hs-cTn (*high-sensitivity cardiac troponin*), no ECG changes and no recurrence of pain. This downgrading is mainly due to the introduction of hs-cTn. In this context, CCTA has a complementary role as demonstrated in many trials (BEACON, ROMICAT II and RAPID-CCTA) as a method capable of analyzing coronary plaques optimizing the patient's therapeutic path. CCTA does not play a role in patients with high suspect of an ongoing ACS, where invasive coronary angiography (ICA) remains the gold standard. Additionally, emergency transthoracic echocardiography (TTE) is indicated in those patients in which ACS is suspected presenting with cardiogenic shock or a mechanical complication (Class I) [2, 3].

However, CCTA has a high negative predictive value (NPV) to exclude ACS in patients in the observed zone in whom cTn and ECG results remain inconclusive or where a false positivity is suspected. Moreover, the use of CCTA in rule-out patients after hospital discharge may guide preventative medical therapies in identifying the presence of obstructive or non-obstructive plaque.

Regarding the most recent guidelines of the American Heart Association/American College of Cardiology (AHA/ACC) of 2021, the use of CCTA in acute chest pain is indicated as Class of Recommendation I for intermediate-risk patients with no known coronary artery disease (CAD) after a negative or inconclusive evaluation of ACS, to assess the presence of plaques or obstructive CAD. Otherwise, in intermediate-risk patients with acute chest pain, with no known CAD and evidence of mildly abnormal stress test within 1 year, CCTA may be useful (Class IIa). Moreover, for high and intermediate-risk patients with acute chest pain either with no known CAD or known CAD and inconclusive CCTA, stress tests (MRI, PET/SPECT, echocardiography) are indicated (Class Ia). In addition, stress tests are reasonable in intermediate-high-risk patients with known CAD with worsening symptoms or in patients in which CAD has been excluded by ICA or CCTA (Class IIa). If ACS is suspected in high-intermediate risk patients with known CAD, then ICA is preferred (Class I) [1, 4].

6.2.2 PE Guidelines

Regarding PE, the proposed diagnostic algorithm in the 2019 ESC/ERS (European Respiratory Society) guidelines requires a distinction between patients with or without hemodynamic instability. In patients with hemodynamic instability, bedside TTE should be carried out and when right ventricle dysfunction is encountered, CT pulmonary angiography (CTPA) must be performed (Class I). In patients without hemodynamic instability if PE probability is high in pre-tests (Geneva tests, Wells score) CTPA is recommended (Class I). On the other hand, if in hemodynamic stable patients' pre-clinical probability is low/intermediate, a D-dimer test must be performed. If D-dimer is positive, then CTPA is required, otherwise, if D-dimer is negative, due to its high negative predictive value, diagnosis of PE is excluded (Class I) [5]. Therefore, is recommended to reject the diagnosis of PE if CTPA is normal in low/intermediate/high clinical probability and to accept the diagnosis of PE if CTPA shows filling defects in patients with intermediate/high clinical probability (Class I). In pregnancy, ACS diagnostic criteria are the same as non-pregnant women while for suspected PE, if pre-test probability is high/intermediate/low with positive D-dimer, anticoagulation with LMWH has to be started, followed by chest x-ray and compression ultrasound to exclude DVT (distal vein thrombosis). If DVT is positive CTPA can be avoided, whereas if DVT is negative, with a high risk and positive D-dimer test, CTPA should be performed: in these cases, a multidisciplinary discussion is recommended.

6.3 Imaging and Protocols

When a patient with acute chest pain arrives in the ER, besides laboratory findings and a clinical evaluation of signs and symptoms, it is necessary to conduct an initial investigation through imaging. Chest x-ray (CXR) stands as the first imaging examination, often conducted in the emergency room whether the patient is unconscious or hemodynamic unstable to exclude major causes of chest pain such as pneumothorax, fractures, pneumonia, pleural effusion or heart failure. However, in the emergency context, CXR is usually performed in an anteroposterior projection (AP), in relation to the supine position of the patient. Moreover, poor inspiration, multiple devices in the radiogram, skin folds and scapulae covering some portions of the lungs might be further limitations to a correct interpretation of the radiogram. For all these reasons, Computed Tomography (CT) stands as the diagnostic examination of choice in emergency to evaluate patients. In particular, CCTA and CTPA, as seen above in the international guidelines, are the exams of choice to study in emergency patients with suspicion of ACS and PE.

Although protocols are different in some specifics, the ultimate purpose remains the same: to achieve maximum opacification after injection of iodinated contrast medium of coronary and pulmonary arteries to assess, respectively, the presence of stenosis and atheromatous plaques or filling defects compatible with embolism. The major parameters of an injection protocol affect intravascular contrast enhancement including contrast medium volume, contrast medium flow rate, contrast medium concentration and saline chaser bolus. High-concentration iodinated contrast medium, at least 370–400 mg/mL, is required to magnify the brightness of iodium in the vessels and has to be injected from a peripheral venous access (right antecubital vein is preferred) through an 18–20 G cannula at a flow rate of 4–5 mL/s, followed by the saline solution to push the bolus (40–50 mL). Contrast pressure must be maintained high throughout the acquisition so that contrast wash-out and flow artifacts can be avoided. The right venous access is favored to avoid beam-hardening artifacts from contrast medium flowing through the left brachiocephalic vein and superior vena cava (SVC) and in doing so making it difficult to visualize the mediastinum. Therefore, high iodine concentration and high flow rate are essential to obtain an optimal level of vascular contrast enhancement. The iodine delivery rate, IDR (i.e., the amount of iodine delivered per second) is an important factor in setting the optimal iodine concentration and flow rate for vascular enhancement in computed tomographic angiography. The IDR value in CTA must be 1.8–2 g/s. The obtain the same IDR must be used with higher contrast medium concentration and lower flow or higher flow and lower contrast medium concentration. Another important factor affecting the magnitude of vascular contrast enhancement is body weight. To maintain a consistent level of contrast enhancement in larger patients, one should consider increasing the overall iodine dose delivery by increasing contrast medium volume and/or concentration. In patients with BMI > 30, a higher IDR should be used (≥2.0 g iodine /s).

According to the latest guidelines, a 64-slices CT minimum is required to perform a diagnostic exam and the choice of kV should be tailored depending on the patient, where an optimal kV range is 80–100 kV, since the effective energy at this kV is really close to iodium k-edge (33 keV) so that the contrast-to-noise ratio (CNR) will be high. Another important technical parameter that must be considered when studying vascular structures is pitch, defined as the table distance traveled in a 360° gantry rotation divided by beam collimation. This ratio, especially in CCTA, is important to reduce both motion artifacts and patient dose so that the pitch should be >1.2. Slice thickness, for both CCTA and CTPA, must be reduced <1 mm with a reduction of CNR but with better visualization of coronary vessels and filling defects (Table 6.1) [1, 6].

To synchronize the start of the scan with contrast administration three techniques are used: *bolus tracking*, *care bolus* (smart prep) and *bolus test*. Scanning with a *bolus tracking* protocol consists of positioning an ROI (Region of Interest) in the lumen of a vessel with repeated scans at this level until the intraluminal contrast reaches a default threshold (usually set at 100 HU), at this point the scan starts automatically. *Care bolus* (smart prep) scanning refers to a protocol in which an ROI is positioned in a vessel and manually the operator decides when to start the scan by the time adequate opacification of the vessel is obtained. In *bolus test* protocol, a preliminary administration of a small amount of contrast medium is injected and a time-to-peak graph is calculated in order to determine the optimal scan delay.

6.3.1 How to Perform CCTA?

In order to reduce cardiac pulsation artifacts, CCTA protocols are ECG-gated so that the scan is triggered by heartbeat. In CCTA is essential a carefully preparation of patients to achieve high diagnostic accuracy with the lowest possible radiation dose. During the scan the heart rate must be possibly lower than 70 bpm, regular and the patient must cooperate with breathing. The essential steps in preparing patients for coronary CTA include: evaluation, education and medication. During the evaluation step, the staff should assess that no contraindications exist to the CT examination and assess heart rate variability and blood pressure. Patient education is breath-hold training because it is essential to minimize respiratory motion during image acquisition. Coronary CTA should be acquired during an inspiratory breath hold. CCTA should not be performed if a patient cannot adhere to breath-hold commands.

Table 6.1 Technical parameters to optimize CTA exams

High concentration contrast medium	400 mg/mL
Mdc ev.	70–100 mL
Saline	40–50 mL
Injection	Bolus tracking/Test bolus
Injection rate	4.5–5 mL/s through 18 G (cannula from right arm)
Slice thickness	0.6 mm (arterial phase)
Voltage	80–100 kV
Current (mA)	Optimized relative to body attenuation
IDR	1.8–2.0 g/s
Pitch	>1.2

Finally, patient medication aims to achieve heart-rate control because a low heart rate and a regular cardiac rhythm during the scan are essential in CCTA. The precise target heart rate depends on the scanner's temporal resolution, the method of image acquisition and the indication for imaging. Some studies demonstrated that the image quality of third-generation dual-source scanners is the same at a heart rate of up to 80/min compared to a heart rate ≤ 60/min. Beta-blockers or Ivabradine are generally recommended to achieve heart- rate control. Beta-blockers may be given orally one hour prior to the examination or intravenously directly before CCTA or in combination. The typical beta blocker dose in CCTA is 50–100 mg orally or 5–30 mg intravenously. Moreover, Nitrate is routinely administered 3–5 minutes before examination to obtain the maximum coronary artery dilatation. The typical dose of sublingual nitroglycerin in CCTA is 0.4–0.8 mg (1–2 sprays). The use of nitroglycerin should be the default protocol but should be avoided in the presence of contraindications such as patients with hypotension sever aortic stenosis or PDE-5 inhibitors usage in the previous 24–48 h.

CCTA protocols should provide the highest diagnostic quality with the lowest radiation dose. The CCTA ECG-gated protocols are tailored to the patient according to his heart rate and clinical suspicion and can be divided into two groups: prospective ECG triggering techniques or retrospective ECG gating acquisitions. Prospectively ECG-triggered axial acquisition (named step-and-shoot mode) is indicated in patients with good heart rate control, including patients with regular rhythms and heart rates less than 65 beats per minute. In prospective gating, the X-ray beam is turned only at a predefined time of the cardiac cycle, usually at 75% of the R-R interval (diastolic phase). Since the scan is stopped at the rest of the cardiac cycle, the savings in radiation exposure compared to retrospective ECG-gating can be substantial (up to 90%) but this scan mode is more susceptible to heart rate variability. At higher heart rates (i.e. 66–72 beats per minute), the acquisition window can be widened ("padding") to reduce the risk of a non-diagnostic exam at the expense of greater radiation exposure.

Retrospective ECG-gating in coronary CTA should be considered in patients with higher heart rates (> 70 beats/min) or significant heart rate variability. In addition, retrospective ECG-gating should be considered for the evaluation of ventricular or valvular function. In retrospectively ECG-gated coronary CTA, X-ray beam is turned on throughout the entire cardiac cycle while the patient table is subjected to constant, slow motion. This generates an x-ray data set which allows reconstruction of all phases of the cardiac cycle thus resulting in a higher delivered dose. If retrospectively-gated scans are necessary, ECG-gated tube current modulation should generally be used unless specific clinical situations exist. The prospective ECG-gated high-pitch CCTA is a high-pitch helical acquisition of the heart developed specifically for low-dose imaging and is currently available on dual-source CT scanner. Scan acquisition is usually triggered during early diastole (60% of the R-R interval) and the entire heart is scanned within a single beat. High-pitch spiral coronary CTA may be considered for cooperative patients with stable sinus rhythm, heart frequency lower than 60 bpm and BMI <30 kg/m^2. The great advantage of high-pitch spiral coronary CTA is the generation of images with a radiation dose often less than 2 mSv. The disadvantage of this protocol is that only one phase of the cardiac cycle is available for image reconstruction [6–8].

With the latest generation scanners, it is also possible to add a delayed enhancement cardiac CT phase to the standard protocol "Myocardial Delayed Enhancement CT." This is an advanced imaging technique used to evaluate myocardial tissue for the presence of scar tissue, fibrosis or areas of infarction. This method is similar in purpose to delayed enhancement magnetic resonance imaging (MRI), but it uses CT technology.

After the contrast injection, there is a waiting period (typically around 5–10 minutes) to allow the contrast to wash out of the normal myocardium but remain in the areas of scar or fibrosis.

Modern CT scanners with dual-energy or multi-detector capabilities can provide high-quality images with reduced radiation exposure.

Delayed enhancement cardiac CT can identify areas of myocardial ischemia. The damaged tissue retains the contrast longer than normal tissue, appearing as hyper enhanced (bright) areas in the images. Also, conditions such as myocarditis or cardiomyopathies can be assessed using delayed enhancement cardiac CT, helping to distinguish between active inflammation and chronic fibrosis. CT scanners are more widely available and faster than MRI scanners, making cardiac CT a more accessible option in many settings. Some patients who cannot undergo MRI due to contraindications (e.g., pacemakers, claustrophobia) may be suitable candidates for CT [9, 10].

6.3.2 How to Perform CTPA?

Performing CTPA is technically less complicated compared to CCTA, although some precautions need to be considered to obtain a diagnostic exam. The CT scan should be obtained in a supine position, from the apex to the lung bases, in caudo-cranial directions (to reduce the motion artefacts) and with arms up. The study protocol should consist of a baseline acquisition (without contrast media, in a correct inspiration, to study lung parenchyma and investigate potential differential diagnosis that can cause chest pain and dyspnea), followed by the arterial phase. After a scout image of the whole chest is obtained, an unenhanced cranio-caudal scan in deep-inspiration breath-hold is performed. The unenhanced scan is mandatory to discriminate hyper-attenuating images in the post-contrast scans and potentially identify fresh blood clots in pulmonary arteries (whiter image inside the grey vessel). Depending on the performance capabilities of the CT scan, ROI can be positioned either in the common pulmonary artery or in the right ventricle: if scanning speed is fast enough, ROI can be placed in the common pulmonary artery with a threshold of 100 HU, otherwise, if CT scan is not particularly performing, ROI is placed in the right ventricle. After that, with the injection of contrast bolus, the scan direction has to be changed into caudo-cranial in order to grant a better visualization of lower lobes whilst reducing beam-hardening artefacts from the contrast bolus injected in SVC. At the start of the scan, the patient needs to be advised to hold his breath, rather than making a deep inspiration. In fact, it has been proved that obtaining a breath-hold CTPA without deep inspirations helps in reducing artefact from venous return and transient interruption of contrast. If necessary, in skinny patients kV can be lower to 60-70 kV, this lead to a reduction of SNR however CNR will be high and iodine opacification is magnified [11].

6.3.3 Triple Rule Out Protocol (TRO)

TRO is an ECG-gated cardiac CT in which the aorta, coronary arteries and pulmonary arteries are evaluated with a single scan. TRO is stated to preclude further diagnostic testing in up to 75% of patients with low-intermediate risk of ACS and removes the necessity to separate single studies, reducing time for patient triage and more importantly, reducing the total radiation exposure to the patient.

For whom it may concern technical parameters, as kV, pitch, type of acquisition (retrospective/prospective), flow rate, type of contrast medium and premedication, reference is made to what was said for CCTA. ROI is usually placed in left atrium and the starting of the scan is set with a threshold of 100 HU synchronized with *bolus tracking* protocol. The main difference between TRO and CT angiogram is how contrast medium is injected. In fact, as demonstrated in several studies, a properly timed biphasic injection of contrast medium is necessary to obtain an opacification of coronary arteries and aorta with the first injection, while with the second injection enhancement of pulmonary arteries is obtained. This last point in particular is critical since the entire success of the exam depends on how scan and contrast medium injection are synchronized with each other. To summarize, TRO requires more individualized attention, careful selection of patients and correct timing injection of contrast medium than a standard CT angiogram, for these reasons many radiologists consider it too technically challenging to be performed in ED. Moreover, Burris et al. in their study on more than 12,000 patients with acute chest pain, compared the diagnostic yield of CTA and TRO protocols demonstrating that non-diagnostic or uninterpretable image quality was more frequent in TRO [12].

6.3.4 Cardiac Magnetic Resonance Imaging (CMRI)

CMRI has the great ability to characterize the myocardial tissue and has the advantage of not using ionizing radiation. Cine sequences in cardiac planes allow the evaluation of ventricular function and volumes. Sequences for the evaluation of edema, late gadolinium enhancement and mapping permit the highlighting of ischemic and non-ischemic alterations. CMR allows direct visualization of infarcted regions, providing information on scarring and viability. CMRI may help to understand the underlying cause of chest pain, permitting precise risk stratification and identifying different conditions such as myocarditis, MINOCA (myocardial infarction with non-obstructive coronary arteries), Takotsubo cardiomyopathy, which have different therapeutic approach and better prognosis than ACS [13].

In addition, rest and stress CMR perfusion, in recent years, has shown an accurate assessment of various aspects of CAD both in diagnosis and in therapy. Stress CMR perfusion can be used as an alternative to CCTA in the assessment of patients in the observed zone. However, CMRI in emergency still plays a marginal role in the assessment of ACS, mainly due to the long acquisition times and the lower availability of scanners compared to those for CT [14].

6.4 Pulmonary Embolism

Pulmonary embolism and venous deep thrombosis are two different clinical presentations of the same disease, known as venous thromboembolism (VTE). VTE is the third most frequent acute cardiovascular syndrome worldwide after myocardial infarction and stroke and typically affects people >80 years. Recent time trend analysis shows a rising tendency of VTE incidence rate, mainly due to an increased number of predisposing conditions (such as smoking, trauma, surgery, lower-limb fractures, spinal cord injury, cancer, oral contraceptive therapy) in addition to overdiagnosis, in particular subsegmental or even non-existent PE. On the other hand, recent studies showed that despite an increased number of PE/VTE diagnosed, the absolute number of fatalities related to acute PE is decreasing and this can be related to better adherence to guidelines and increased use of effective therapies. PE is defined as an occlusion of one or more pulmonary arteries by emboli originating primarily from the distal venous district or less frequently from right heart chambers in conditions such as atrial fibrillation, infarction or endocarditis. Alternatively, emboli may originate as a consequence of bone fracture (fat embolism), penetrating trauma, surgery or diving (air embolism).

In an acute setting, PE interferes with both circulation and gas exchange. The abrupt surge in pressure within the pulmonary artery leads to right ventricular (RV) failure, considered to be the primary cause of death related to acute PE. The RV pressure overload in fact causes an increased strain of the right heart, with a progressive RV dilatation and disfunction, leftward bowing of interventricular septum and reduction of left ventricular (LV) preload yielding to a decline of cardiac output (CO). This causes systemic hypotension, reduction of coronary blood supply and hypoxemia of an already suffering RV, which ultimately results in obstructive shock and death.

The diagnosis of PE is indeed essential, even though it can be challenging due to the lack of specific signs and symptoms, particularly in elderly individuals with comorbidities. The presentation of PE can vary widely, where the most common signs of acute PE are tachycardia and tachypnea, along with chest pain, dyspnea and in the worst cases syncope, shock and sudden death. For all these reasons, as already seen in the International Guidelines, an accurate clinical evaluation with pre-test probability (Wells score or Geneva score; Table 6.2) is mandatory in suspect of PE: clinical signs of DVT, tachycardia, history of PE/DVT, recent surgery or immobilization, hemoptysis, malignancy or less likely diagnosis than PE have to be questioned, as well as try to identify signs of RV disfunction (hypotension, distended neck veins, tricuspid regurgitation or a T-wave inversion on ECG in the anterior leads). Moreover, specific markers have to be studied to further stratify the prognosis: D-dimer, as already

Table 6.2 Preclinical scores to assess the likelihood of PE

Geneva score		Revised Geneva score		Wells score	
Items	Score	Items	Score	Items	Score
Heart	1	History of PE or DVT	3	Clinical signs of DVT	3
frequency > 100 bpm	2	Lower limb pain (unilateral)	3	Alternative diagnosis less	3
History of PE or DVT	3	Concurrent malignancy	2	likely than PE	1.5
Previous recent surgery	1	Fracture/surgery within 1 month	2	Heart frequency > 100 bpm	1.5
Age	2	Hemoptyisis	2	History of PE or DVT	1.5
60–79	2	Age > 65y	1	Immobilization or surgery	1
≥80	1	Heart frequency	3	Cancer	1
Arterial gases	4	75-94 bpm	5	Hemoptysis	
CO_2 (kPa)	3	≥95 bpm	4		
< 4.8	2	Unilateral lower limb edema			
4.8–5.19	1	with pain on deep vein			
O_2 (kPa)	1	palpation			
<6.5	1				
6.5–7.99					
8–9.49					
9.5–10.99					
CXR					
Atelectasis					
Elevated diaphragm					
Clinical probability		Clinical probability		Clinical probability	
Low	0–4	Low	0–3	Low	<2
Intermediate	2–6	Intermediate	4–10	Intermediate	2–6
High	≥9	High	≥11	High	>6
				PE unlikely	≤4
				PE likely	>4

seen, is the most useful one in relation to its high predictive negative value but other laboratory tests such as Troponin I (index of myocardial ischemia) and BNP (a peptide produced by cardiomyocytes under straining) may be valuable since if increased correlate with a worst prognosis. Clinicians have to rely on a combination of what emerges on both clinical examination and laboratory tests to stratify the risk and therefore guide the following studies to reach the correct diagnosis. As already seen, except for hemodynamically unstable patients, CTPA stands as the gold standard in diagnosis PE [5].

6.4.1 Imaging Findings

Acute pulmonary embolism (APE) in CTPA appears as an endoluminal filling defect within an opacified pulmonary artery. As already seen, a non-contrast-enhanced CT scan (NECT) is mandatory since sometimes APE is seen as an endoluminal hyperdensity due to fresh blood within the thrombus. After iodinated contrast medium is injected, the filling defect may be complete or incomplete. When complete, the iodinated contrast medium ends abruptly within a dilated vessel, whereas when incomplete on the axial plane the filling defect may be seen as a central ipodensity surrounded by a rim of contrast, the so-called *"Polo Mint sign"* (*"railway sign"* when observed parallel to the vessel long axis) or as an eccentric ipodensity that makes an acute angle with the wall of the vessel. In 20–35% of patients a round or wedge-shaped opacity (± ground glass) with a *"reverse-halo sign"* appearance is the most frequent parenchymal finding in APE, suggestive of the pulmonary infarct. Moreover, current literature shows that in pulmonary infarcts pleural effusion is quite a common finding, present in up to 60% of patients (Fig. 6.1).

In addition to direct signs of PE, CTPA plays a fundamental role in assessing the hemodynamic effects of APE at the cardiac level, in particular regarding the evaluation of afterload, the evaluation of preload and cardiac morphological changes.

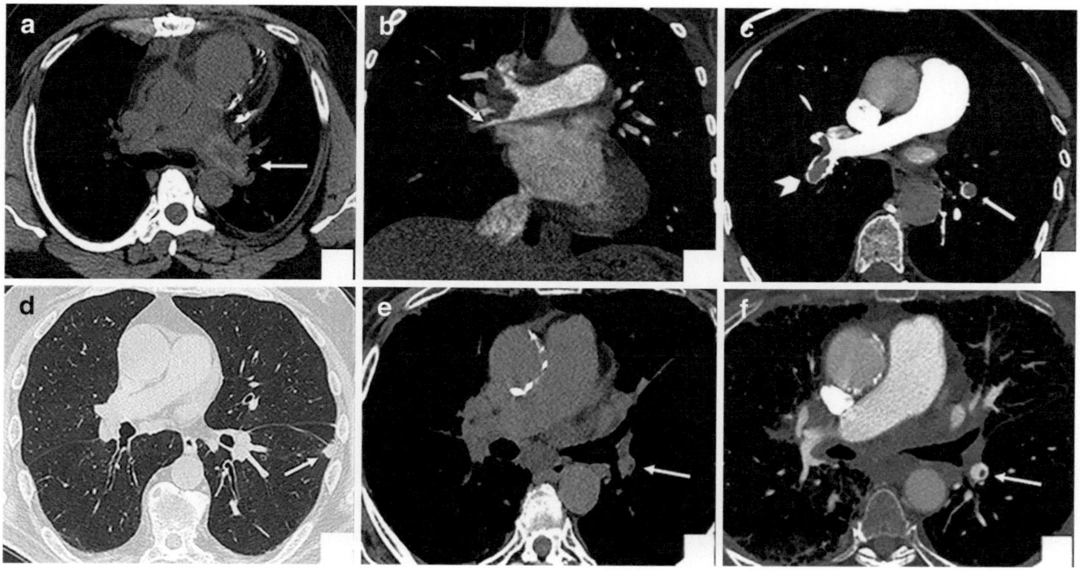

Fig. 6.1 Signs of pulmonary embolism. Axial NECT (**a**) showing spontaneous endoluminal hyperdensity representing a fresh blood clot. CTPA in coronal (**b**) and axial plane (**c**) showing endoluminal filling defects. Note in **c**, the "polo mint sign" (*arrow*) and "railway sign" (*arrowhead*). Lung window (**d**) showing a left triangular-shaped subpleural consolidation, sign of pulmonary infarct (*arrow*). In (**e**) and (**f**), NECT and CTPA of the same patient showing endoluminal filling defect with HU compatible with fat embolism (*arrow*)

To quantify the extension and degree of obstruction of pulmonary arteries, four scores can be used: Miller, Wals, Mastora and Qanadli. The Qanadli score, in particular, is the most used and considers how many arterial pulmonary segments are affected (up to 10 points per side) and whether the obstruction is partial or complete (respectively 1 or 2 points) for a total of 40 points. Moreover, as reported by several studies, such as the one by Kumar et al., the Qanadli score positively correlates with pulmonary hypertension and RV dysfunction with great sensitivity and specificity. Regardless of the scoring point method, all four present a very good correlation with each other and show that a central PE, interesting lobar or segmental arterial branches and thus with a greater score, correlate negatively with prognosis, with a higher percentage of 30-day mortality rather than distal subsegmental emboli [15, 16]. Moreover, CTPA is a reliable technique to measure pulmonary artery diameter (PAD), in particular, a PAD greater than 30 mm is associated with a higher pulmonary artery pressure; in addition, an increased pulmonary pressure shows a positive correlation with RV dilatation, septal bowing and RV remodeling, all parameters that contribute to RV dysfunction.

CTPA may be useful to assess preload dysfunction by evaluating vein size and retrograde reflux of contrast medium into inferior vena cava (IVC). Regarding the first one, CTPA is helpful in describing dilatation of systemic venous structure (azygos—jugulars veins, superior and inferior vena cava, coronary sinus) as a consequence of higher pressure in right heart chambers. None of these parameters is useful yet in CTPA to predict 30-days mortality, even though recently it has been described that a coronary sinus greater than 9 mm may have a prognostic value since correlates positively with short-term death, shows good interindividual reproducibility since it barely affected by cardiac motion. Regarding retrograde reflux of contrast in IVC, this sign can be found in ≈ 20% of patients with APE and has to be considered as a consequence of RV disfunction and tricuspid valve insufficiency [11].

About 45% of patients with acute PE will develop right ventricular dysfunction (RVD), mainly as a consequence of the increased pressure in pulmonary arteries. In fact, RV can compensate for this increased resistance due to embolic material by pumping against it, thus maintaining cardiac output. This compensatory mechanism is effective until approximately 50–70% of pulmonary arteries are obstructed or when pulmonary artery pressure rises above 40 mmHg. Moreover, hypoxia induced by emboli, in addition to increased arterial pressure, further worsens RV afterload until a critical level. Beyond that point, RV cannot compensate anymore and it dilates, with underfilling of LV and a decreased blood supply to the coronary arteries. This leads to myocardial hypoperfusion and thus to right ventricle ischemia. In that, CTPA plays a central role since it allows to measurement RV/LV diameter ratio, considered to be one of the major prognostic factors and predictor of short-term mortality when >0.9–1, with a mortality risk doubled in the first 30 days after diagnosis. Furthermore, quantification of RV/LV diameter, made on the axial plane, is considered a very reproducible parameter between radiologists to identify RVD. Along with the increased rising pressure in RV and thus its progressive exhaustion, septal bowing might be encountered. This sign is very specific (100%) but with poor sensitivity (26%) for RVD and is usually found in 1/5 of patients. Inter-observer reproducibility is worse than RV/LV ratio however, when positive, is a reliable indicator of severe APE and short-term death (Fig. 6.2) [17, 18].

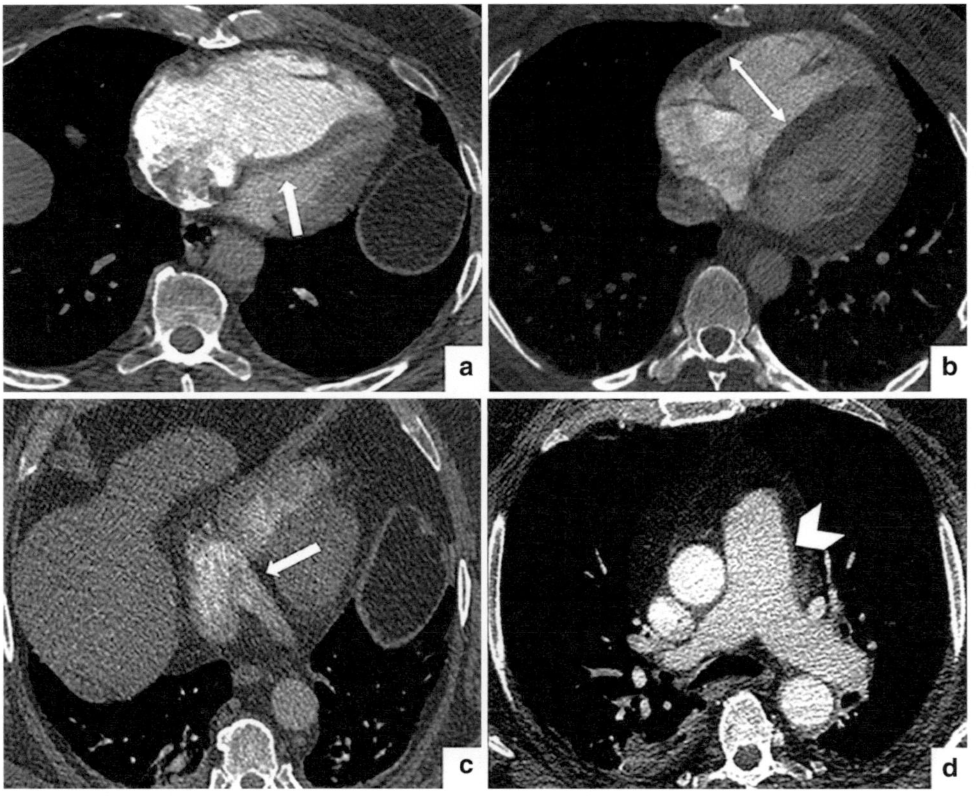

Fig. 6.2 Signs of RV dysfunction. In (**a**) left septal bowing (*arrow*); in (**b**) right ventricular enlargement with RV/LV ratio > 1 (*arrow*); in (**c**) dilatation of coronary sinus (*arrow*) and in (**d**) dilatation of common pulmonary artery (*arrowhead*)

6.4.2 Assessment of Pulmonary Perfusion on Dual Energy CTPA

Dual-energy computed tomography (DECT) is useful in providing both morphological and functional pulmonary information, particularly having the advantage of using two different X-rays energies through different commercial configurations (dual-source, rapid-switching, dual-layer detector, split-filter or sequential scanning) in particular to detect perfusion defects in lung parenchyma. This may bring additional information about the burden of PE without adding a significant dose compared to a normal CTPA. In fact, the reported sensitivity and specificity of DECT range respectively from 60–90% to 88–99%, with the major benefit of detecting subsegmental emboli in the form of regional iodine perfusion defect (IPD). However, the presence of IPD is not ubiquitous, in fact, occlusive PE presents IPD in 82–95% of cases compared to 6–9% in non-occlusive PE, leading to the consideration that IPD may be an indicator of more severe PE. This is consistent with several recent studies in which IPD correlates positively with RV/LV ratio, RVD, D-dimer and troponin level [19, 20] . Lastly, it is important to remember that not every defect in the perfusion map reflects a real IPD; in upper lobes in particular artifacts are common, mainly due to beam-hardening artifacts, that may cause a wrong interpretation of the image (Fig. 6.3). This can be resolved using a smaller quantitative of iodinated contrast media from right peripherical access with a caudo-cranial scan direction.

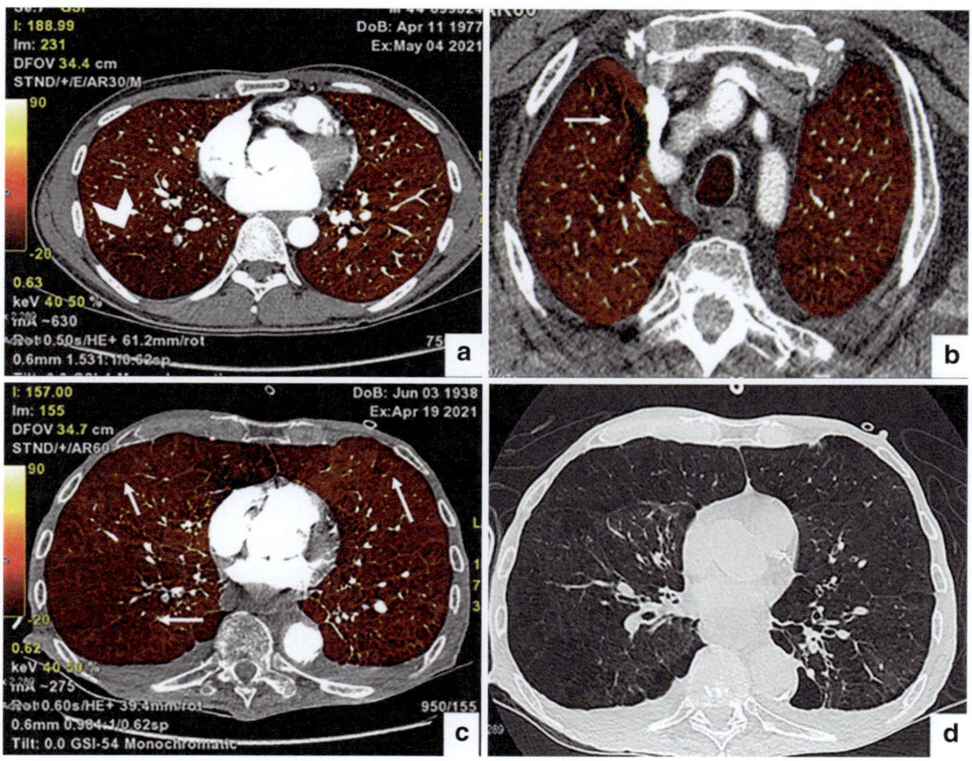

Fig. 6.3 Dual-Energy CT (DECT) showing a "*fan-shaped*" apical right lower lobe perfusion defect due to thromboembolic material (*arrowhead* in **a**) and beam-hardening artifacts in right upper lobe (*arrows in* **b**). In (**c**) e (**d**), comparison between DECT and HRCT of the same patient, showing multiple perfusion defects (*arrows* in **c**) caused by emphysematous changes, therefore not due to thromboembolic material

Pulmonary embolism: What to report then?
Pulmonary arteries filling defects
RV/LV ratio > 0.9/1
Coronary sinus >9 mm
Pulmonary artery diameter (PAD) > 30 mm
Vein dilatation and contrast medium retrograde reflux
Septal bowing
Parenchymal opacities
Iodine perfusion defects (IPD) in DECT

6.5 Acute Coronary Syndrome

Only 10–20% of patients with chest pain accessing the ED are diagnosed with ACS, and only in one-third of cases, the patient has an acute myocardial infarction (AMI). Patients with ACS may present a variety of symptoms as chest discomfort spread to mandibula, upper extremity or epigastrium either at rest or during exertion, dyspnea, fatigue and other non-specific signs such as excessive and algid sweating or anxiety. Therefore, the diagnosis can be difficult making it necessary to initiate diagnostic investigations based on a careful evaluation of the symptoms, the electrocardiographic trace, the increase of high-sensitivity troponin and the echocardiographic evaluation [21]. In this setting, CCTA plays a fundamental role in providing information about coronary atherosclerosis burden, plaque morphology and stenosis severity and assessing coronary anatomy. Despite not being the first-line examination in many clinical settings (as seen above in Guidelines) due to its temporal and spatial resolution, CCTA has become a alternative to invasive procedures (e.g. ICA) to evaluate coronary arteries. Additionally, a great strength of CCTA is its high sensitivity (≅ 95–100%) and high negative predictive value (NPV), close to 100%. In particular, according to the 2022 Society of Cardiovascular Computed Tomography Expert Consensus Document on Coronary Computed Tomographic Angiography, CCTA is usually appropriate to rule-out ACS in patients with no known CAD and low-to-intermediate risk for ACS in native vessels appropriate in stable coronary artery disease in patients with known/no known CAD with typical stable, atypical, or angina equivalent symptoms and may be appropriate for the evaluation of CAD after inconclusive functional testing in patients with no known CAD. Moreover, according to the Society of Cardiovascular Computed Tomography, CCTA is appropriate in symptomatic patients with known CAD and prior PCI with coronary stent >3-mm in diameter if the ECG is normal or nonischemic and if the baseline cTn or hs-cTn is normal or equivocal [4].

6.5.1 CAD-RADS

In order to standardize at best CCTA interpretation and to facilitate communication between Specialists, along with suggestions for following patient management, CAD-Reporting and Data System (CAD-RADS) has been introduced. In the latest 2022 CAD-RADS version, alongside with new methods to further categorize and describe overall coronary plaque burden and stenosis, a new option with modifiers to include ischemia evaluation by CT fractional-flow-reserve (FFR_{CT}) or myocardial CT perfusion (CTP) is introduced.

Since its first advent in 2016, CAD-RADS has been proven to be more accurate than traditional risk factors or other risk stratification systems in predicting ACS in patients presenting with chest pain and confirmed a good correlation with the degree of stenosis measured by ICA.

The CAD-RADS scoring system can be applied to two categories of patients: those with acute chest pain or those with stable chest pain. In this context, we will focus on patients coming to ED with acute chest pain. CAD-RADS categories are based on stenosis severity and plaque burden. The grading of degree luminal stenosis ranges from 0 to 5, where 0 means no plaques or stenosis and 5 means complete occlusion (100%). In patients assessed with CAD-RADS 1 (degree of stenosis 1–24%) and CAD-RADS 2 (degree 25–49%) the probability of ACS is respectively unlikely and less likely and no further action in evaluating ACS are generally required. In CAD-RADS from 3 to 5, the probability of ACS increases proportionally to coronary stenosis, ranging from 50–69% in CAD-RADS 3 (ACS possible), 70–99% degree in CAD-RADS 4 (ACS likely) or total occlusion (100% – ACS very likely) in CAD-RADS 5. Moreover, CAD-RADS 4 can be further divided into 4A, whether a single vessel presents severe stenosis, or 4B whether the presence of a left main stenosis ≥50% or three-vessel obstruction >70% is encountered (Figs. 6.4 and 6.5). Furthermore, in addition to an assessment of the degree of stenosis, the updated 2022 CAD-RADS version introduces the "P" parameter, indicating the overall amount of coronary plaque. In fact, it has been widely demonstrated that the overall amount of coronary plaque seen in CCTA, has a strong positive correlation with CAD and may significantly influence prognosis. Therefore, "P" categories range from P1 to P4, so that the overall amount of plaques may be categorized as mild (P1), moderate (P2), severe (P3) and extensive (P4). By now, there is not a universal method to quantify the amount of coronary plaques, thus in the Expert Consensus Document is suggested to use the technique considered most appropriate for the patient in according to local practice norms, considering that plaque evaluation based on CAC (Coronary Artery Calcification) testing or SIS (Segment Involvement Score) are the most used, the more reproducible and the ones supported by scientific evidence. Briefly, P1 refers to CAC 1–100 or SIS ≤2, P2 refers to CAC 101–300 or SIS 3–4, P3 refers to CAC 301–999 or SIS 5–7 and P4 refers to CAC >1000 or SIS ≥8. Further modifiers provided in CAD-RADS 2022 version, some of them recently introduced and other ones only revised, are: "N" for nondiagnostic study, "HRP" for high-risk plaque, "I" for ischemia, "S" for stent, "G" for graft and "E" for exceptions (non-atherosclerotic coronary abnormalities potentially causing coronary narrowing or stenosis as dissection or congenital malformations) [22].

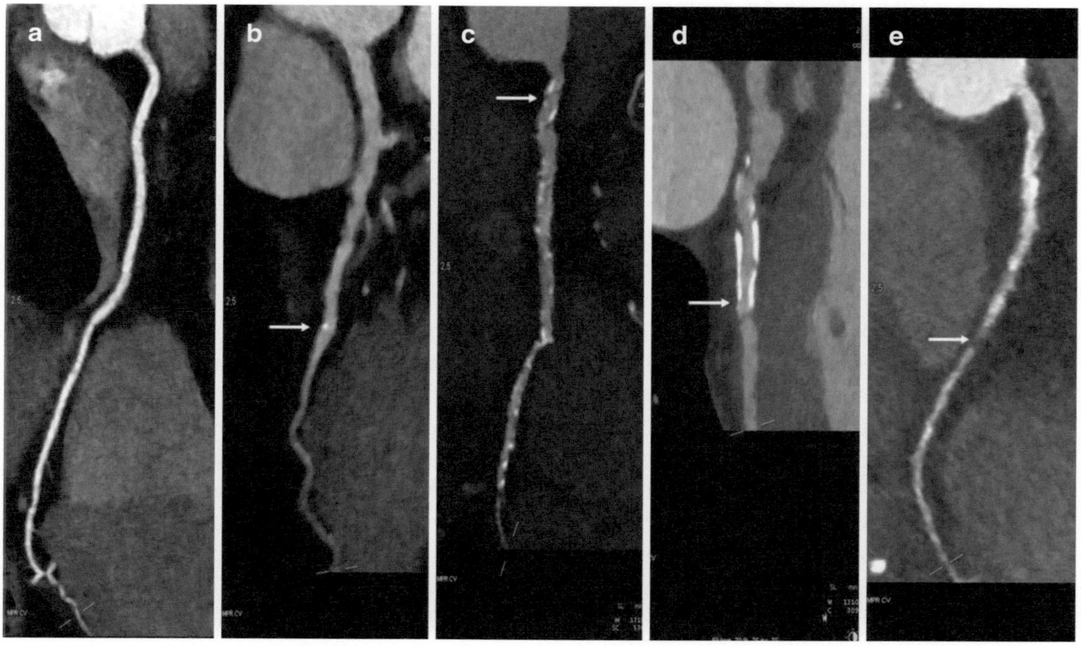

Fig. 6.4 CAD-RADS. In (**a**) no stenosis is reported: *CAD-RADS 0*. In (**b**) minimal stenosis, *CAD-RADS: 1 (1–24%)*. In (**c**) mild stenosis, *CAD-RADS: 2 (25–49%)*. In (**d**) moderate stenosis, *CAD-RADS: 3 (50–70%)*. In (**e**) severe stenosis, *CAD-RADS: 4A (in this case A because stenosis 70–99% in 1 vessel)*

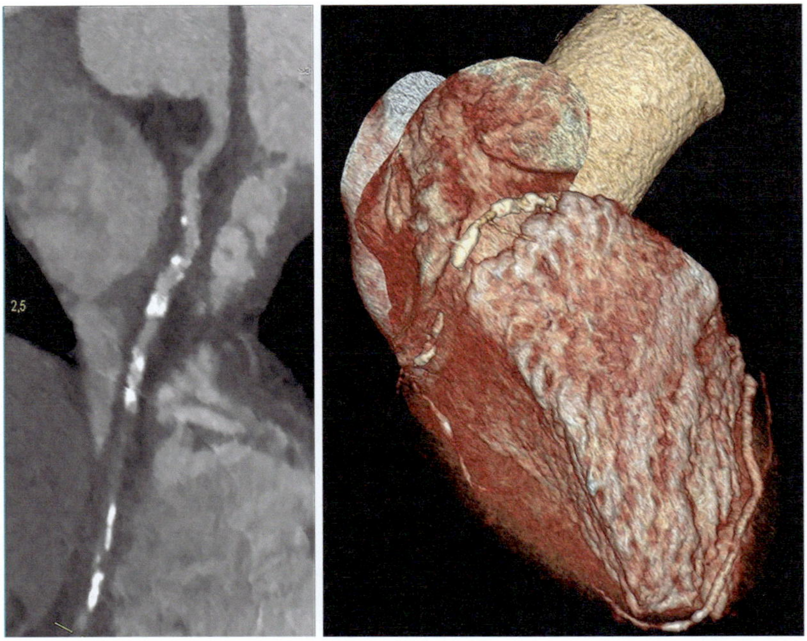

Fig. 6.5 CAD-RADS 5. On the *left*, total occlusion of RCA (*arrow*). VRT of the same patient on the *right*, showing interruption of RCA (*arrow*)

6.5.2 Functional Examinations in Intermediate-to-Severe Coronary Stenosis: CTP and FFR_{CT}

As said before, in the 2022 CAD-RADS version, the possibility of proceeding with cardiac investigation with further functional examination is introduced. This possibility must be considered in those patients with CAD-RADS categories 3 and 4 (A in particular), where using stress testing, CTP (CT Perfusion) or CT-FFR/FFR_{CT} (Fractional Flow Reserve) might be an option.

Although FFR_{CT} technology is a recent development, three multicenter trials (DISCOVER-FLOW, DEFACTO and NXT) have demonstrated promising results; in addition, according to the most recent cardiology guidelines, FFR is considered as the gold standard for functional assessment of CAD. Briefly, FFR_{CT} applies a computational fluid dynamic method allowing the creation of patient-specific anatomy, calculating fluid pressure and flow in coronary arteries from CCTA images, without further radiation exposure. This new technology has proven to be an effective diagnostic support in CAD-RADS 3 (50–69% stenosis) and CAD-RADS 4A (70–99% stenosis); in particular, FFR_{CT} values >0.80 are considered normal, indicating that the myocardium supplied by those vessels is unlikely to be ischemic, whereas values ≤0.75, are considered specific for ischemia. In those cases, in which FFR_{CT} values are between 0.76 and 0.80, further risk stratification is recommended [10].

The main limitation of this procedure is post-processing timing; in fact, despite not requiring additional scans, FFR_{CT} does require sophisticated computer hardware to run the software that effectively post-processes CCTA images. The entire post-processing procedure typically takes between 10 and 30 minutes.

CT perfusion may improve the overall diagnostic accuracy of cardiac CT, in particular in CAD-RADS 3–4, in-stent patency and in diffuse coronary atherosclerosis. CTP has proven to be a promising technique thanks to good sensitivity and specificity (compared to standards angiography, SPECT and MRI), respectively ranging from 75–89% to 78–95%, ensuring that this technique can play a significant role in an emergency context. Moreover, perfusion imaging can be acquired in static or dynamic; static CTP allows the evaluation of myocardial perfusion with a single stationary phase during the arterial first pass of iodinated contrast medium, permitting the assessment of coronary morphology and myocardial flow distribution based on differences in attenuation. Differently, dynamic CTP requires more advanced technology and post-processing software, with the major benefit of allowing the calculation of quantitative hemodynamic parameters, thus creating colored volumetric maps according to myocardial perfusion and permitting the detection of balanced ischemia in patients with multivessel disease or diabetic patients with microvascular disease. However, the major limit of CTP is radiation exposure, as it must be acquired as an additional scan to CCTA, with a minimum delay of 10 minutes between scans to ensure contrast medium and nitrate washout prior to CTP scan [23].

To summarize, through the continuous development of technologies, both CTP and FFR_{CT} could be valid techniques that in the next future should be routinely used to expand the diagnostic utility of CCTA.

Acute Coronary Syndrome: What to report then?
Coronary anatomy, with dominance and anatomical variants
Coronary arteries filling defects
CAD-RADS category
CAD-RADS modifiers, if present
If possible, CTP or FFR_{CT}

References

1. Gulati M, Levy PD, Mukherjee D, et al. AHA/ACC/ASE/ CHEST/SAEM/SCCT/SCMR guideline for the evaluation and diagnosis of CHEST pain: executive summary: a report of the American College of Cardiology/American Heart Association Joint Committee on Clinical Practice Guidelines. Circulation. 2021;144(22):e368–454. https://doi.org/10.1161/CIR.0000000000001030.
2. Byrne RA, Rossello X, Coughlan JJ, et al. ESC Scientific Document Group. 2023 ESC Guidelines for the management of acute coronary syndromes. Eur Heart J. 2023;44(38):3720–826. https://doi.org/10.1093/eurheartj/ehad191.
3. Patel MR, Calhoon JH, Dehmer GJ, et al. ACC/AATS/AHA/ASE/ ASNC/SCAI/SCCT/STS 2016 Appropriate Use Criteria for Coronary Revascularization in Patients With Acute Coronary Syndromes: A Report of the American College of Cardiology Appropriate Use Criteria Task Force, American Association for Thoracic Surgery, American Heart Association, American Society of Echocardiography, American Society of Nuclear Cardiology, Society for Cardiovascular Angiography and Interventions, Society of Cardiovascular Computed Tomography, and the Society of Thoracic Surgeons. J Am Coll Cardiol. 2017;69(5):570–91. https://doi.org/10.1016/j.jacc.2016.10.034.
4. Narula J, Chandrashekhar Y, Ahmadi A, et al. SCCT 2021 expert consensus document on coronary computed tomographic angiography: a report of the Society of Cardiovascular Computed Tomography. J Cardiovasc Comput Tomogr. 2021;15(3):192–217. https://doi.org/10.1016/j.jcct.2020.11.001.
5. Konstantinides SV, Meyer G, Becattini C, et al. ESC Scientific Document Group. 2019 ESC guidelines for the diagnosis and management of acute pulmonary embolism developed in collaboration with the European Respiratory Society (ERS). Eur Heart J. 2020;41(4):543–603. https://doi.org/10.1093/eurheartj/ehz405.
6. Ramjattan NA, Lala V, Kousa O, Shams P, Makaryus AN. Coronary CT Angiography. 2024 Jan 19. In: StatPearls [Internet]. Treasure Island: StatPearls Publishing; 2024. PMID: 29262000
7. Smettei OA, Sayed S, M Al Habib A, Alharbi F, Abazid RM. Ultra-fast, low dose high-pitch (FLASH) versus prospectively-gated coronary computed tomography angiography: comparison of image quality and patient radiation exposure. J Saudi Heart Assoc. 2018;30(3):165–71. https://doi.org/10.1016/j.jsha.2017.11.001.
8. Kapoor A, Mahajan G, Kapoor A. Evaluation of low-kVp low-volume iodinated contrast protocol for coronary CT angiography using retrospective ECG gating. Indian J Radiol Imaging. 2022;31(4):910–6. https://doi.org/10.1055/s-0041-1741102.
9. Tore D, Faletti R, Palmisano A, Salto S, et al. Cardiac computed tomography with late contrast enhancement: a review. Heliyon. 2024;10(11):e32436. https://doi.org/10.1016/j.heliyon.2024.e32436.
10. Yun CH, Hung CL, Wen MS, Wan YL, So A. CT assessment of myocardial perfusion and fractional flow reserve in coronary artery disease: a review of current clinical evidence and recent developments. Korean J Radiol. 2021;22(11):1749–63. https://doi.org/10.3348/kjr.2020.1277.
11. Cozzi D, Moroni C, Cavigli E, et al. Prognostic value of CT pulmonary angiography parameters in acute pulmonary embolism. Radiol Med. 2021;126(8):1030–6. https://doi.org/10.1007/s11547-021-01364-6.
12. Burris AC, Boura JA, Raff GL, Chinnaiyan KM. Triple rule out versus coronary CT angiography in patients with acute chest pain: results from the ACIC consortium. JACC Cardiovasc Imaging. 2015;8(7):817–25. https://doi.org/10.1016/j.jcmg.2015.02.023.
13. Pradella S, Zantonelli G, Grazzini G, et al. The radiologist as a gatekeeper in chest pain. Int J Environ Res Public Health. 2021;18(12):6677. https://doi.org/10.3390/ijerph18126677.

14. De Filippo M, Capasso R. Coronary computed tomography angiography (CCTA) and cardiac magnetic resonance (CMR) imaging in the assessment of patients presenting with chest pain suspected for acute coronary syndrome. Ann Transl Med. 2016;4(13):255. https://doi.org/10.21037/atm.2016.06.30. PMID: 27500156; PMCID: PMC4958724.
15. Kumar BS, Rajasekhar D, Vanajakshamma V. Study of clinical, radiological and echocardiographic features and correlation of Qanadli CT index with RV dysfunction and outcomes in pulmonary embolism. Indian Heart J. 2014;66(6):629–34. https://doi.org/10.1016/j.ihj.2014.10.405.
16. Qanadli SD, El Hajjam M, Vieillard-Baron A, et al. New CT index to quantify arterial obstruction in pulmonary embolism: comparison with angiographic index and echocardiography. AJR Am J Roentgenol. 2001;176:1415–20.
17. Bryce YC, Perez-Johnston R, Bryce EB, et al. Pathophysiology of right ventricular failure in acute pulmonary embolism and chronic thromboembolic pulmonary hypertension: a pictorial essay for the interventional radiologist. Insights Imaging. 2019;10(1):18. https://doi.org/10.1186/s13244-019-0695-9.
18. Zantonelli G, Cozzi D, Bindi A, et al. Acute pulmonary embolism: prognostic role of computed tomography pulmonary angiography (CTPA). Tomography. 2022;8(1):529–39. https://doi.org/10.3390/tomography8010042.
19. Hong YJ, Shim J, Lee SM, et al. Dual-energy CT for pulmonary embolism: current and evolving clinical applications. Korean J Radiol. 2021;22(9):1555–68. https://doi.org/10.3348/kjr.2020.1512.
20. Vlahos I, Jacobsen MC, Godoy MC, et al. Dual-energy CT in pulmonary vascular disease. Br J Radiol. 2022;95(1129):20210699. https://doi.org/10.1259/bjr.20210699.
21. Thygesen K, Alpert JS, Jaffe AS, et al. ESC Scientific Document Group, Fourth universal definition of myocardial infarction. Eur Heart J. 2018;40(3):237–69.
22. Cury RC, Leipsic J, Abbara S, et al. CAD-RADS™ 2.0–2022 Coronary artery disease-reporting and data system: an expert consensus document of the Society of Cardiovascular Computed Tomography (SCCT), the American College of Cardiology (ACC), the American College of Radiology (ACR), and the North America Society of Cardiovascular Imaging (NASCI). J Cardiovasc Comput Tomogr. 2022;16(6):536–57. https://doi.org/10.1016/j.jcct.2022.07.002.
23. Lee JH, Hartaigh BÓ, Han D, Rizvi A, Lin FY, Min JK. Fractional flow reserve measurement by computed tomography: an alternative to the stress test. Interv Cardiol. 2016;11(2):105–9. https://doi.org/10.15420/icr.2016:1:2.

7 Extrapulmonary Air

Luigi Barbuto, Antonio Raucci, Francesco Verde, Ornella Picascia, Maurizio Notorio, and Gianluca Ponticiello

7.1 Introduction

Extrapulmonary air can occur in various clinical conditions including both thoracic and non-thoracic pathologies. Thoracic pathologies certainly represent the vast majority, but extrapulmonary air can also derive from affections of the neck or abdomen. Anatomically, there are no barriers in the subcutaneous tissue or in the perivertebral space, allowing air to move freely. The visceral and retropharyngeal cervical spaces indeed connect with the mediastinum, and the thoracic cavity links to the abdomen through the diaphragmatic hiatus. Abnormal air in the thoracic cavity can collect in multiple spaces, including the pleural cavity, chest wall, mediastinum, and pericardium. Thus one of the most recognized classifications of extrapulmonary air is based on the localization: mediastinal, pericardial, pleural, or chest wall [1]. In Table 7.1, these conditions are reported, as well as the related CT findings that need to be described in the report, in addition to those of the determining conditions.

Table 7.1 Extrapulmonary air location & CT sign

Location	CT sign	What to report
Mediastinum	Pneumomediastinum	Extension
		Entity of cardio-vascular compression (if any)
		Entity of airway compression (if any)
Pericardium	Pneumopericardium	Entity of cardio-vascular compression (if any)
Pleural cavity	Pneumothorax	Extension
		Entity of pulmonary collapse
		Entity of mediastinal deviation (if any)
Chest wall	Subcutaneus emphysema	Extension

L. Barbuto (✉) · A. Raucci · F. Verde · O. Picascia
M. Notorio · G. Ponticiello
Department of General and Emergency Radiology, "Antonio Cardarelli" Hospital, Naples, Italy
e-mail: luigi.barbuto@aocardarelli.it; antonio.raucci@aocardarelli.it; francesco.verde@aocardarelli.it; ornella.picascia@aocardarelli.it; Maurizio.notorio@aocardarelli.it; gianluca.ponticiello@aocardarelli.it

L. Romano et al. (eds.), *CT of Non-Traumatic Body Emergencies*,
https://doi.org/10.1007/978-3-031-84849-0_7

7.2 Mediastinum Location

Pneumomediastinum refers to the presence of air outside the normal luminal spaces within the mediastinum. Excluding traumatic causes, which will not be covered here, gas can originate from the lungs, trachea, central bronchi, esophagus, or peritoneal cavity and may travel from the mediastinum to the neck or abdomen. The primary non-traumatic causes of pneumomediastinum include neck, thoracic, or retroperitoneal surgeries, esophageal perforation (such as from Boerhaave syndrome, endoscopic procedures, or esophageal cancer), tracheobronchial perforation, infections, pulmonary interstitial emphysema, asthma, barotrauma (from diving or mechanical ventilation), interstitial lung disease, and alveolar rupture. Pneumomediastinum can also occur spontaneously in a condition known as spontaneous pneumomediastinum. Pneumomediastinum is commonly seen after *laparoscopic esophageal surgeries* (Fig. 7.1) and often continues for more than 24 h. Following these procedures, the presence of pneumomediastinum does not necessarily signal esophageal perforation and generally does not lead to any clinically significant issues that would impact the patient's recovery [2].

Iatrogenic esophageal perforation is the most frequent cause of esophageal perforation and is associated with a high mortality rate of 19%. The most common symptom is an acute, sudden onset of pain following endoscopic procedures. Both CT scans and endoscopy are highly sensitive methods for diagnosing iatrogenic perforation (Fig. 7.2) [3].

Another potential cause of pneumomediastinum originating from the esophagus is *Boerhaave syndrome*. This condition involves an esophageal rupture caused by severe vomiting and retching. Although rare, it is a life-threatening emergency that necessitates prompt diagnosis and treatment.

If treatment is delayed, it can lead to severe and potentially fatal complications, such as mediastinitis, pleural empyema, septic shock, and multiple organ failure. Boerhaave syndrome is more common in males, with alcoholism being a notable risk factor. It is frequently associated with the clinical triad known as Mackler's triad, which includes vomiting, chest pain, and subcutaneous emphysem [4]. On unenhanced CT scans, signs of esophageal perforation typically include the presence of intramural hematoma with characteristic localization and peri-esophageal air collections. These features are indicative of an esophageal rupture [5]. Post-contrast CT imaging can reveal direct leakage of

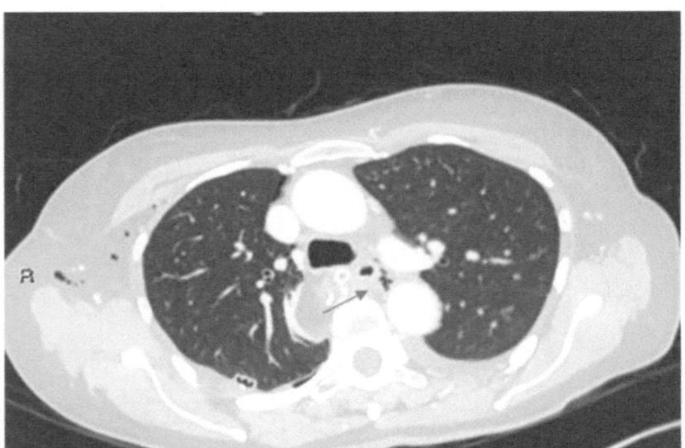

Fig. 7.1 Pneumomedastinum (blue arrow) following gastric esophagus resection surgery for adenocarcinoma of the cardias

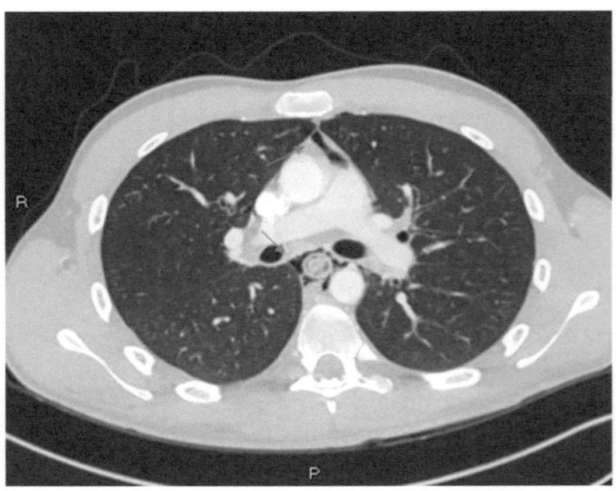

Fig. 7.2 Iatrogenic esophageal perforation and pneumomediastinum (blue arrows) after an endoscopic procedure due to ingestion of a foreign body

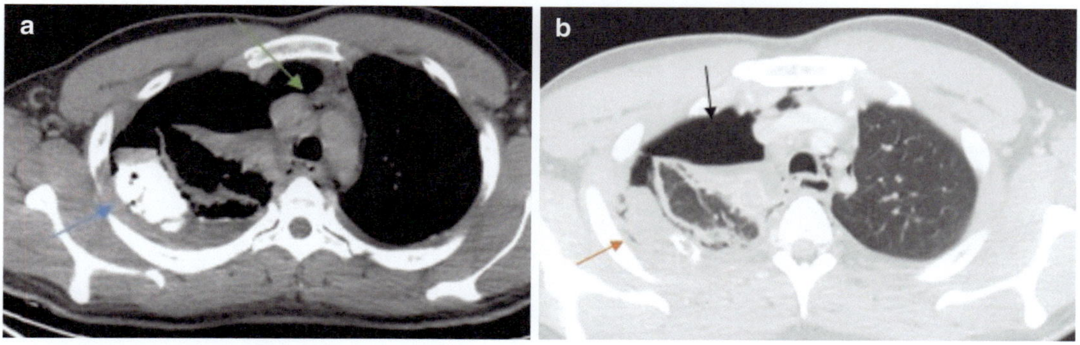

Fig. 7.3 (**a** and **b**) Twenty-two-year-old male with Boheerave syndrome in which esophageal perforation with pneumomediastinum (**a**, green arrow), idropneumotorax (**b**, orange and black arrow) and extravasation of oral contrast medium is documented (**a**, blue arrow)

contrast material or contrast tracks, as well as thickening of the esophageal wall (Fig. 7.3). Other findings that may be observed include periaortic air tracks, pneumothorax, pneumomediastinum, pleural effusion, mediastinal fluid collections, and extravasation of oral contrast from the esophagus [5].

Tracheobronchial tears are rare injuries involving lacerations or punctures anywhere in the tracheobronchial tree, usually resulting from penetrating or blunt trauma to the neck or chest, or due to iatrogenic procedures. These injuries are associated with significant morbidity and mortality. Increasingly, tracheobronchial injuries are being reported as complications of various medical interventions, including [6, 7]

- Airway instrumentation: Such as endotracheal intubation and rigid bronchoscopy.
- Diagnostic procedures: Including transbronchial needle aspiration (TBNA) using endobronchial ultrasound (EBUS).
- Therapeutic airway interventions: Such as tracheostomy (both open and percutaneous dilatational) and balloon bronchoplasty.
- Surgical procedures: Involving the head and neck, thyroid, and esophagus.

Most iatrogenic tracheobronchial injuries occur in the posterior membranous portion of the trachea. Injuries related to the endotracheal tube typically result in longitudinal tears in the membranous sections of both the cervical and thoracic trachea (Fig. 7.4a and b). In contrast, injuries from cuff inflation generally affect the proximal trachea (Fig. 7.4c). CT scans are both sensitive and specific for identifying tracheobronchial injuries and are the preferred non-invasive diagnostic method. They can reveal subtle pneumothoraces, mediastinal emphysema, and active bleeding in the injured airway. The presence of air within the wall of the trachea or bronchus, interrupting the wall profile, is a key diagnostic feature for tracheobronchial tears (Fig. 7.4). Additionally, CT scans are valuable for detecting associated severe injuries to the heart and major vessels.

Tracheoesophageal fistula (TOF) is another condition that can lead to pneumomediastinum. TOF involves an abnormal connection between the trachea and the esophagus and can arise from various underlying issues, including malignancies, infections, inhalation injuries, radiotherapy, and traumatic damage. TOF is classified into two main types: congenital and acquired. Congenital TOF is primarily associated with esophageal atresia. Acquired TOF is further divided into malignant and benign categories, with each type representing about half of the acquired cases. The most common malignancy linked to malignant TOF is esophageal cancer, affecting over 10% of patients during the course of the disease. For TOFs related to esophageal or tracheal malignancies, a thorough understanding of airway and digestive tract anatomy, the dimensions of the fistula, stent character-

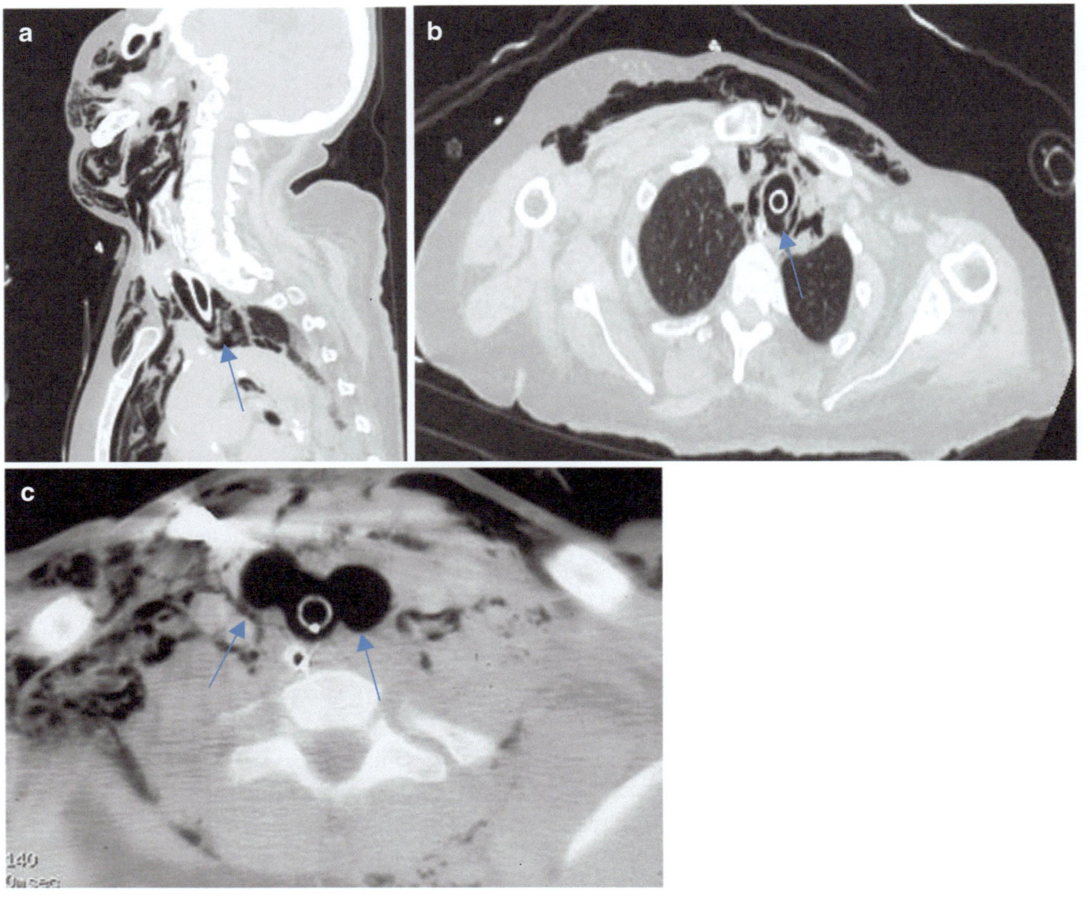

Fig. 7.4 (**a**–**c**) Tracheobronchial injury due to endotracheal intubation with laceration of the posterior membranous portion of the trachea (**a** and **b**, blue arrows) and injuries from cuff inflation (**c**, blue arrows)

istics and types, and the interaction between esophageal and airway stents (if a dual stenting procedure is used) is essential [8]. Clinically, tracheoesophageal fistulas (TOFs) can present with symptoms such as coughing during or after fluid intake, dry mouth, neck and chest pain, spontaneous coughing, and sputum-containing food particles. Standard CT scans are very useful for diagnosing TOFs (Fig. 7.5). However, if the fistulous tract is collapsed, standard CT may fail to detect the fistula. In such cases, a CT oral contrast swallow study is often used.

In this study, a diluted non-ionic iodinated contrast agent is recommended. The patient is given a bolus of this contrast agent and instructed to swallow it promptly during the scan. This

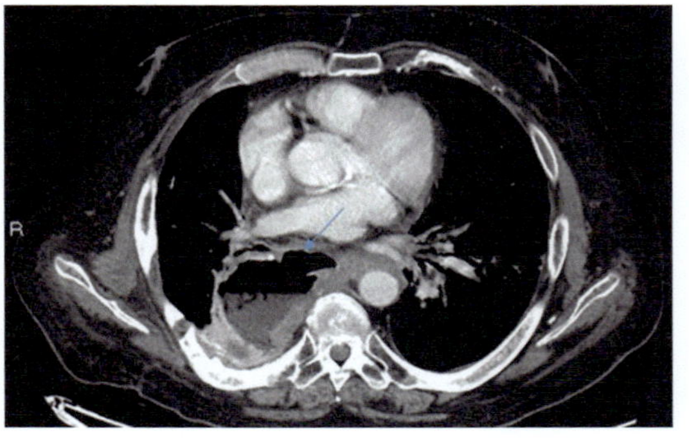

Fig. 7.5 Standard CT examination of a voluminous broncho-esophageal fistula caused by extensive discontinuity of the posterior wall of the esophagus on a neoplastic basis (arrow)

method can accurately visualize the extent of the fistula and any associated complications, such as aspiration.

Spontaneous pneumomediastinum (SPM) is characterized by the presence of free air or gas in the mediastinum without an obvious external cause of injury to the mediastinal structures.

SPM can be triggered by various conditions and activities, including bronchial asthma, diabetic ketoacidosis, intense straining during exercise, inhalation of drugs, and other actions involving the Valsalva maneuver. Typically, SPM is a benign and self-limiting condition that predominantly affects young males [9]. Occasionally, SPM is associated with pneumorrhachis, where air is found in the spinal epidural space. It is very rare for SPM to be accompanied by pneumoperitoneum, with only a few cases reported. Generally, SPM resolves with conservative treatment without the need for invasive interventions [9]. A key finding on CT scans for patients with SPM is the "Macklin effect," which is the presence of air within the interstitial tissues. This appears as linear collections of air adjacent to the bronchovascular sheaths on thoracic CT. The air then dissects into the pulmonary hila and subsequently into the mediastinum. The Macklin effect is also a characteristic sign of alveolar rupture, which can be another cause of pneumomediastinum and is frequently associated with barotrauma, as seen in patients with severe COVID-19 infections (Fig. 7.6). These findings suggest that the virus may induce a vulnerability in the lung parenchyma, potentially triggered by factors such as microvascular thrombosis [10], interstitial inflammation, and disruption of the endothelial barrier. This leads to widespread, COVID-19-specific diffuse alveolar damage, exacerbated by the therapeutic measures, such as mechanical ventilation, that these patients undergo.

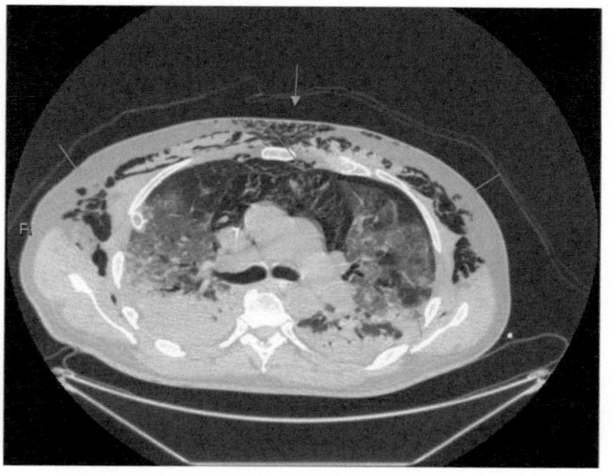

Fig. 7.6 Macklin effect in a patient with COVID-19 infection with pneumomediastinum (orange arrow), subcutaneous emphysema (green arrow), and pulmonary interstitial emphysema (blue arrow) tracking to the mediastinum along the peribronchovascular interstitium

7.3 Pericardial Location

Pneumopericardium is a relatively rare condition compared to isolated pneumomediastinum or pneumothorax. It is characterized by the presence of air within the pericardial cavity [11]. In the adult population, pneumopericardium has frequently been reported following blunt or sharp trauma. Other non-traumatic causes include iatrogenic factors related to invasive procedures such as thoracic surgery, thoracocentesis, endotracheal intubation, or positive-pressure mechanical ventilation. Non-iatrogenic causes may involve underlying infectious processes or a fistulous connection between the pericardium and other air-containing structures, such as the bronchus, gastrointestinal tract, or an abscess. Additionally, there have been cases of spontaneous pneumopericardium occurring in otherwise healthy adults [12, 13]. Clinical manifestations of pneumopericardium can be variable and nonspecific, commonly including chest pain, dys-

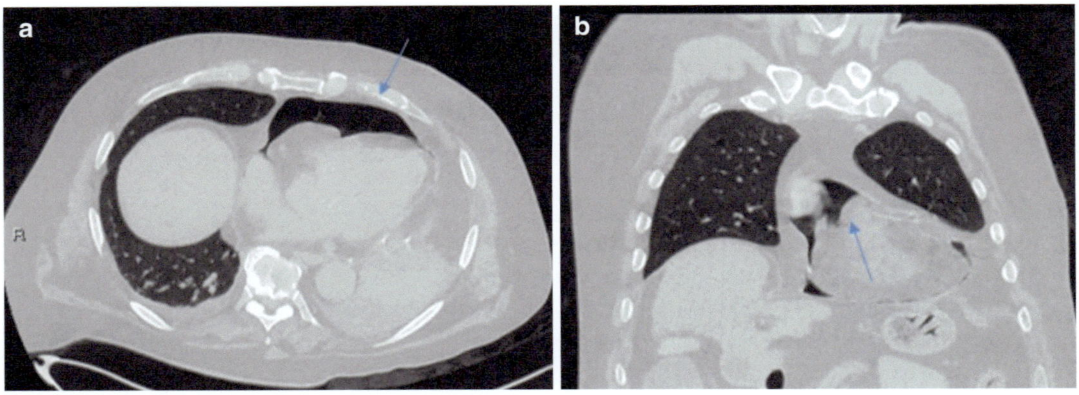

Fig. 7.7 (**a** and **b**) Pneumopericardium (blue arrow) due to complication of drainage placement for pleural effusion

pnea, or palpitations. The symptoms typically correlate with the extent of the pneumopericardium and the underlying cause. In approximately 37% of patients with pneumopericardium, cardiac tamponade may develop, significantly increasing the mortality rate to 58%. Cardiac tamponade occurs when the volume of air in the pericardial cavity is sufficient to obstruct right ventricular filling [13].

The diagnosis of pneumopericardium can be established using conventional chest radiographs, but chest CT is more precise. Chest CT is the preferred method for diagnosing pneumopericardium, especially in complex cases, as it clearly shows the heart being partially or fully surrounded by air (Fig. 7.7) [12]. Although pneumopericardium may resolve spontaneously, acute cardiac tamponade necessitates immediate intervention. In such cases, an emergency pericardiocentesis is required to quickly restore hemodynamic stability, followed by pericardial fenestration or drainage to address the underlying issue [13].

7.4 Pleural Location

The pleural space is the area between the visceral and parietal pleurae. The visceral pleura covers the surface of the lungs and folds back at the root of the lung, known as the pulmonary hilum, to become the parietal pleura, which lines the chest wall and diaphragm [14]. The pleural space typically contains a small amount of fluid, ranging from 1 to 5 mL.

Pneumothorax is a condition characterized by the accumulation of air in one or more areas of the pleural cavity. It can result from the rupture of a bulla, trauma, or iatrogenic causes, such as complications following thoracentesis or positive pressure ventilation [15].

In some cases, it is particularly challenging to differentiate *giant bullous emphysema* from tension pneumothorax due to overlapping presentation symptoms and radiological findings. Landing on the correct diagnosis is imperative to accurately and adequately treat the patient since GBE and tension pneumothorax significantly differ in acuity and overall management, hence the need for a high level of suspicion based on the clinical picture and the use of high-resolution CT [16].

The treatments are vastly different between the two conditions, with GBE consisting mainly of conservative management and tension pneumothorax requiring invasive management. Differentiating between the two conditions is best achieved with HRCT (high resolution computed tomography).

In the case of a large bullous emphysema, as seen in Fig. 7.8, it may be difficult to differentiate it as a large bulla or a pneumothorax, but a careful review of multiple CT images will show that the bulla wall is not parallel to the chest wall and no air is present in the pleura, arguing against a

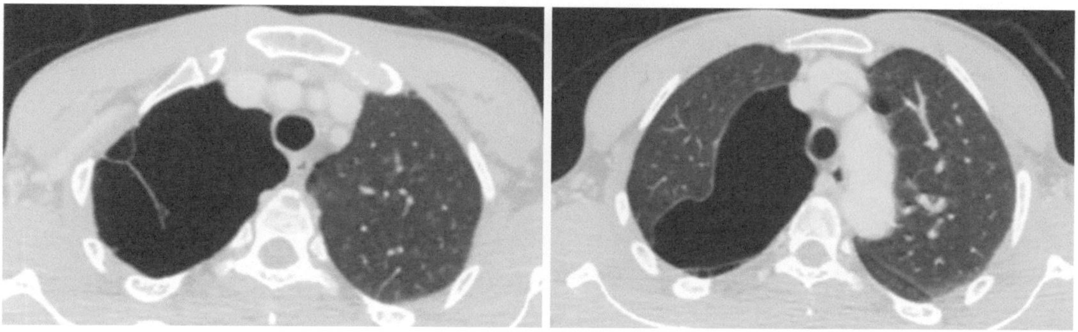

Fig. 7.8 Giant bullos emphysema. Voluminous right apical emphysematous bubble. The absence of a double-wall sign, as illustrate in these images, provides further evidence and increased confidence against the diagnosis of pneumothorax, which can prevent unnecessary chest tube placement

pneumothorax [16]. One of the most valuable signs to distinguish pneumothorax from adjacent giant bullae is the double-wall sign [16]. This sign consists of observing air outlining both sides of the bulla wall parallel to the chest wall. The absence of this sign (Fig. 7.8) provides further evidence and increased confidence against the diagnosis of pneumothorax, which can prevent unnecessary chest tube placement. A further possible but rarer cause of pneumotorax is represented by bronchopleural fistulas. Bronchopleural fistulas are characterized by a direct communication between the pleural space and the bronchial tree or pulmonary parenchyma. These fistulas are typically diagnosed between 1 week and 3 months after lobectomy or pneumonectomy, with the majority being identified between 8 to 12 days post-surgery [17]. They are usually divided as:

Central bronchopleural fistulas occur when the fistula involves the trachea or a lobar bronchus. The primary causes of central bronchopleural fistulas include lung resection, lung transplantation, and trauma to the tracheobronchial tree. The most common cause is the dehiscence of the bronchial stump suture following anatomical resection.

Peripheral bronchopleural fistulas occur when a distal airway, such as segmental bronchi or lung parenchyma, communicates with the pleural space. Possible causes include [17]:

- Necrotizing pneumonia
- Empyema
- Previous radiation therapy
- Ruptured bulla or pulmonary cyst
- Interventional procedures
- Tuberculosis
- Aspergillosis
- Granulomatosis with polyangiitis
- Sarcoidosis

CT imaging allows for the direct visualization of large bronchopleural fistulas. For smaller fistulas, the presence of air bubbles near the bronchial suture or alterations in the pleural air-fluid level can indicate their presence (Fig. 7.9) [17]. CT is regarded as the imaging technique of choice for visualizing and characterizing bronchopleural fistulas [18]. Minimum intensity projection (minIP) reconstructions provide good delineation of the fistulous tract [19].

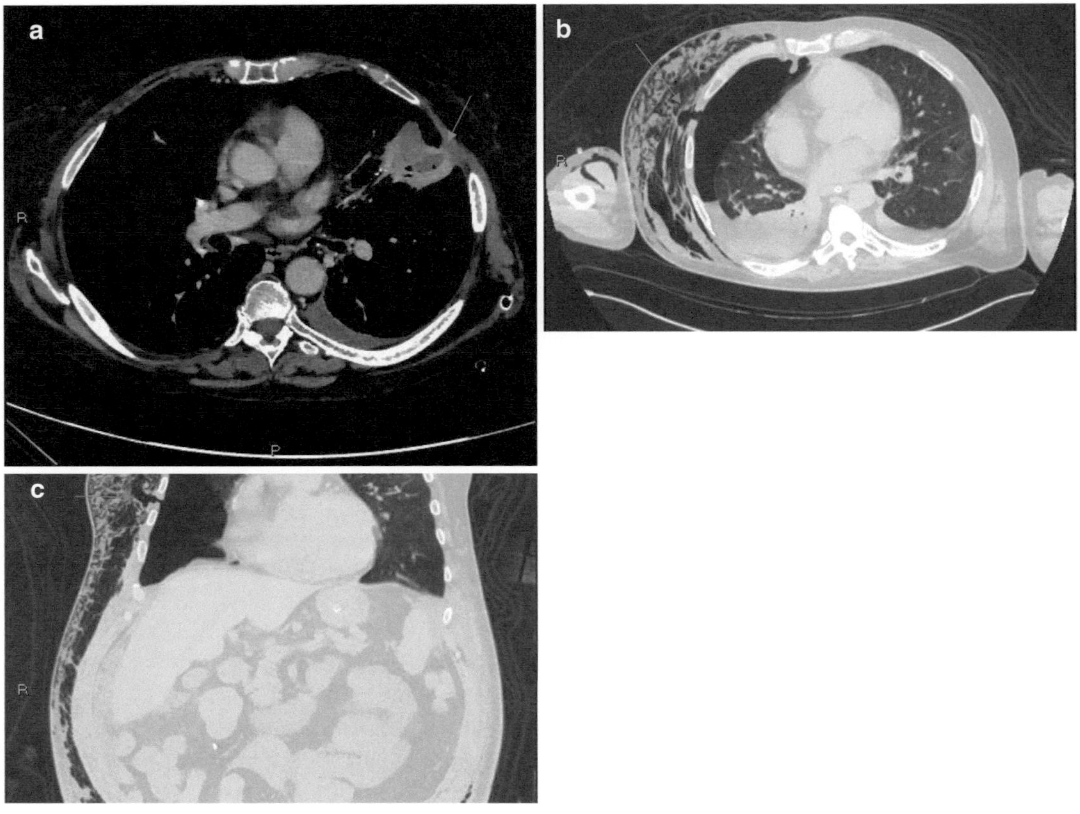

Fig. 7.9 (**a**–**c**) Parenchymal consolidation with a thin tract with the parietal pleural plane (**a**, blue arrow). Subcutaneous emphysema caused by a huge amount of pneumothorax fistulized (**b** and **c** blue arrow) with the right chest wall

CT may show:

- Pneumothorax
- Hydropneumothorax
- Pneumomediastinum
- Underlying lung pathology
- Demonstration of an actual fistulous communication

7.5 Chest Wall Location

Subcutaneous emphysema (SE) refers to the presence of gas in the subcutaneous tissues.

It is commonly used to describe any soft tissue emphysema affecting the body wall or limbs, as the gas can spread into deeper soft tissues and musculature along fascial planes. Subcutaneous emphysema occurs when air accumulates within the subcutaneous fatty tissue, situated superficially to the deep fascia that encloses the skeletal muscle planes [20]. The most common clinical symptom of subcutaneous emphysema is swelling around the neck, often accompanied by chest pain [19]. Crepitus is typically detected during physical examinations of subcutaneous emphysema.

Besides trauma, the most significant causes of subcutaneous emphysema include infectious diseases and iatrogenic complications, such as those resulting from surgical procedures or the insertion of a chest tube [19]. Abnormal air in the body can originate from external or internal sources, such as pneumothorax, pneumomediastinum, pulmonary interstitial emphysema (PIE), or retroperitoneal gas. It can also result from gas-forming microbes, such as those causing necrotizing fasciitis or Fournier gangrene, in these cases, associated CT findings are represented by soft-tissue thickening and swelling, fat stranding, possible presence of air-fluid collections, and enhancement or hyperemia of the fascial planes on contrast-enhanced imaging [20, 21]. Subcutaneous emphysema is readily visible on CT scans, with pockets of gas seen as extremely dark low (air) attenuation areas in the subcutaneous space.

References

1. Varona Porres D, Persiva O, Sánchez AL, Cabanzo L, Pallisa E, Andreu J. Buscando la burbuja: aire torácico extrapulmonar atípico e inusual [Finding the bubble: atypical and unusual extrapulmonary air in the chest]. Radiología. 2021;63(4):358–69. https://doi.org/10.1016/j.rx.2021.02.001.
2. Clements RH, Reddy S, Holzman MD, Sharp KW, Olsen D, Holcomb GW, Richards WO. Incidence and significance of pneumomediastinum after laparoscopic esophageal surgery. Surg Endosc. 2000;14(6):553–5. https://doi.org/10.1007/s004640000164.
3. Iatrogenic TT, Perforation E. J Med Assoc Thail. 2015;98(Suppl 9):S177–83. PMID: 26817229
4. Spapen J, De Regt J, Nieboer K, Verfaillie G, Honoré PM, Spapen H. Boerhaave's syndrome: still a diagnostic and therapeutic challenge in the 21st century. Case Rep Crit Care. 2013;2013:161286. https://doi.org/10.1155/2013/161286.
5. Ghanem N, Altehoefer C, Springer O, Furtwängler A, Kotter E, Schäfer O, Langer M. Radiological findings in Boerhaave's syndrome. Emerg Radiol. 2003;10(1):8–13. https://doi.org/10.1007/s10140-002-0264-1. Epub 2003 Mar 25
6. Ajith Kumar AK, Anjum F. Tracheobronchial tear. In: StatPearls [internet]. Treasure Island (FL): StatPearls Publishing; 2024.
7. Welter S. Repair of tracheobronchial injuries. Thorac Surg Clin. 2014;24(1):41–50. https://doi.org/10.1016/j.thorsurg.2013.10.006.
8. Kim HS, Khemasuwan D, Diaz-Mendoza J, Mehta AC. Management of tracheo-oesophageal fistula in adults. Eur Respir Rev. 2020;29(158):200094. https://doi.org/10.1183/16000617.0094-2020.
9. Al-Mufarrej F, Badar J, Gharagozloo F, Tempesta B, Strother E, Margolis M. Spontaneous pneumomediastinum: diagnostic and therapeutic interventions. J Cardiothorac Surg. 2008;3:59. https://doi.org/10.1186/1749-8090-3-59.
10. De Cobelli F, Palumbo D, Ciceri F, Landoni G, Ruggeri A, Rovere-Querini P, et al. Pulmonary vascular thrombosis in COVID-19 pneumonia. J Cardiothorac Vasc Anesth. 2021;35(12):3631–41. https://doi.org/10.1053/j.jvca.2021.01.011. Epub 2021 Jan 13
11. Brander L, Ramsay D, Dreier D, Peter M, Graeni R. Continuous left hemidiaphragm sign revisited: a case of spontaneous pneumopericardium and literature review. Heart. 2002;88(4):e5. https://doi.org/10.1136/heart.88.4.e5.
12. Iskander S, Amar H, Audrey B, Fabien D. Pneumopericardium: a rare complication of pericardiocentesis. J Cardiovasc Ultrasound. 2016;24(1):55–9. https://doi.org/10.4250/jcu.2016.24.1.55. Epub 2016 Mar 24
13. Uluçam MZ. An extremely rare combination: pneumopericardium, pneumoperitoneum, and subcutanous emphysema-a case report. Cardiol Ther. 2013;2(1):103–10. https://doi.org/10.1007/s40119-012-0008-6.
14. Bilir O, Yavasi O, Ersunan G, Kayayurt K, Giakoup B. Pneumomediastinum associated with pneumopericardium and epidural pneumatosis. Case Rep Emerg Med. 2014;2014:275490. https://doi.org/10.1155/2014/275490.
15. Sakai M, Hiyama T, Kuno H, Mori K, Saida T, Ishiguro T, Takahashi H, Koyama K, Minami M. Thoracic abnormal air collections in patients in the intensive care unit: radiograph findings correlated with CT. Insights Imaging. 2020;11(1):35. https://doi.org/10.1186/s13244-020-0838-z.
16. Ascano MP, Kramer N, Le K. Differentiating Giant bullous emphysema from tension pneumothorax: a case report. Cureus. 2024;16(3):e55988. https://doi.org/10.7759/cureus.55988.
17. Gaur P, Dunne R, Colson Y, Gill R. Bronchopleural fistula and the role of contemporary imaging. J Thorac Cardiovasc Surg. 2014;148(1):341–7. https://doi.org/10.1016/j.jtcvs.2013.11.009.
18. Stern E, Sun H, Haramati L. Peripheral bronchopleural fistulas: CT imaging features. AJR Am J Roentgenol. 1996;167(1):117–20. https://doi.org/10.2214/ajr.167.1.8659354.
19. Adam A, Dixon AK, Schaefer-Prokop C, et al. Grainger & Allison's diagnostic. Radiology. 2020;2. ISBN: 9780702075247
20. Martí de Gracia M, Gutiérrez FG, Martínez M, Dueñas VP. Subcutaneous emphysema: diagnostic clue in the emergency room. Emerg Radiol. 2009;16(5):343–8. https://doi.org/10.1007/s10140-009-0794-x. Epub 2009 Jan 30
21. Aghajanzadeh M, Dehnadi A, Ebrahimi H, Fallah Karkan M, Khajeh Jahromi S, Amir Maafi A, Aghajanzadeh G. Classification and management of subcutaneous emphysema: a 10-year experience. Indian J Surg. 2015;77(Suppl 2):673–7. https://doi.org/10.1007/s12262-013-0975-4.

Chest Compartment Syndrome

8

Carlo Liguori, Luigia Romano,
Maria Giuseppina Scuderi, Maria Elena Porta,
Giuseppe Ruggiero, and Massimo Silva

8.1 Introduction

Blood pressure in the microcirculation determines the adequacy of nutrient blood flow in the capillaries, and this pressure is opposed by both venous and tissue pressures. Compartment syndrome is defined as the inadequate perfusion and oxygenation of organs/tissues within any compartment due to limited blood supply caused by increased pressure within the compartment. Without timely intervention, compartment syndromes cause permanent and irreversible damage to the tissues within the compartment [1]. Without further specification, the term compartment syndrome refers to the extremities (ECS). In the case of other anatomical areas, the specific body compartment must be defined. Indeed, compartment syndrome was first described as an osteofascial phenomenon well-known in the orthopedic and trauma literature [2]. The concept has been expanded to include any body cavity (such as the abdomen and thorax) in which increased tissue pressure reduces capillary perfusion below a level necessary to maintain tissue viability. While abdominal compartment syndrome is a well-recognized clinical entity [3], the thoracic cavity is a significantly less frequent site of compartment syndrome. Keys to the diagnosis and treatment of thoracic compartment syndrome (TCS) include the early recognition of clinical conditions such as increasing airway pressure, falling cardiac output, and worsening acidosis.

C. Liguori (✉)
Diagnostic Imaging Department, ASL NA1 – P.O. San Giovanni Bosco, Naples, Italy

L. Romano · M. G. Scuderi · M. Elena Porta
G. Ruggiero · M. Silva
Department of General and Emergency Radiology, "Antonio Cardarelli" Hospital, Naples, Italy
e-mail: gruggiero1@sirm.org; massimo.silva@aocardarelli.it

8.2 Physiopathology and Classifications of TCS

Compartment walls are made of fascia/connective tissue or bone/connective tissue, which are key determinants of the volume of the compartments. When a closed compartment's pressure increases too much, the microcirculation of the tissues within the compartment is diminished. Two factors are responsible for this condition, either a decrease in a compartment volume or an increase in the contents of a compartment, or sometimes both of these factors act at the same time.

Acute compartment syndrome (ACS) occurs when the interstitial pressure within the compartment exceeds the perfusion pressure at the level of the capillary beds. Elevated intracompartmental pressure (ICP) leads to increased pressure at the venous end of the capillary beds, causing

L. Romano et al. (eds.), *CT of Non-Traumatic Body Emergencies*,
https://doi.org/10.1007/978-3-031-84849-0_8

increased hydrostatic pressure and further increase in ICP, eventually leading to arteriolar compression. Loss of the perfusion pressure gradient results in the onset of ischemia and ultimately leads to cellular anoxia and death. Depending on the organs' normal interstitial pressure and potential for autoregulation, the compartment pressure, which causes organ dysfunction, is between 15 and 25 mmHg. In most compartments, pressures of >30 mmHg critically compromise organ perfusion [4].

More recently, it has been recommended that compartment pressures be interpreted in the context of the difference of diastolic or mean arterial pressure (ΔP = diastolic arterial pressure – compartment pressure) rather than absolute pressures [5]. This approach helps to consider the compartment pressure in the context of the arterial inflow. Once the compartment's perfusion is compromised, a vicious cycle of hypoxia, anaerobic metabolism, edema, further pressure increase, and further decrease of capillary flow takes place. This process is irreversible without intervention [1].

The thoracic cage can also be considered a unique large compartment composed of three sub-compartments: pleura, mediastinum, and pericardium including the heart which can be influenced in its morphology and function by variations in pressure in each of the three surrounding spaces.

Compartment syndrome can be classified as:

- *Primary*: The pathology is within the compartment.
- *Secondary*: No primary pathology or injury within the compartment but pressure increases because of external compression.

According to the above classification TCS can be considered primary in cases of rising pressure after closure of median sternotomy (as first described in an open heart surgery) and secondary in case of pathological conditions, in other thoracic noncardiac structures, determining intrathoracic pressure variations which compromise cardiac function.

8.3 Primary TCS

The condition now known as thoracic compartment syndrome (TCS) was first described in 1975 by Riahi et al. [6] and defined as "*tight mediastinum syndrome*": appearing immediately after approximation of the sternum, it was seen most commonly in patients who had undergone cardiac surgery for valvular disease with an enlarged heart due to compression of the heart by the closed sternum, producing a cardiac tamponade. They treated the "syndrome" with a sternal traction device, after full sternal closure. Thereafter, the TCS has been described in almost 200 reported cases of adult and pediatric patients undergoing cardiac surgical procedures.

In the adult cardiac population, until 1992, the incidence of delayed sternal closure and prolonged open sternotomy ranged from 1.5 to 2.8% [6–9]. In cardiac patients, the main reason for the progressive development of this syndrome, which can be silent for hours, is the increasing airway pressure on the closure of the chest. Sternal closure in these situations may cause additional myocardial compression. Compression of the heart by its surrounding structures can limit the end-diastolic volume of the ventricles and in turn, lead to a decrease in cardiac output. Open chest management has gained acceptance as a technique in the management of hemodynamically unstable patients (myocardial edema, poor hemodynamic indices, primary pulmonary problems, arrhythmias, unsatisfactory hemostasis, and cardiac assist devices) where cardiac compression by sternal closure is not tolerated: compression of the heart by its surrounding structures can limit the end-diastolic volume of the ventricles and in turn lead to decrease in cardiac output.

8.4 Secondary TCS

Computed tomography (CT) is currently accepted as the most valuable imaging modality in evaluating patients with chest trauma or suspected nonvascular, nontraumatic thoracic emergencies [10, 11]. CT provides excellent spatial, contrast, and temporal resolution and allows fast and accurate examination of the mediastinum, heart, pericardium, great vessels, airways, pleural spaces, and pulmonary parenchyma. It is readily available, rapid, noninvasive, easy to perform, and is indicated for patients with chest radiographic findings, indicative of chest pathologies and those with normal chest radiographic findings but strong clinical indications of mediastinal conditions. Intravenous contrast material is routinely used because many patients present with chest pain, and vascular abnormalities are often suspected. The use of oral contrast material is recommended only in patients suspected of having esophageal laceration. Oblique, Coronal and sagittal CT reconstructions are readily available and are useful in mediastinal and great vessel emergencies. In addition, CT provides guidance for draining mediastinal fluid collections and aspirating mediastinal and pericardial air.

Rising peak inspiratory pressure during thoracic wall closure may serve as an early warning that the patient is at risk for TCS. Since the rest of the symptoms (like falling cardiac output and worsening acidosis) are non-specific, clinical suspicion remains a crucial component in the diagnosis of TCS [1].

In most of the cases described in the literature, a marked diminution of the cardiac index is noted. Rising airway pressures on closure of the chest, are the usual marker for the development of this syndrome in the cardiac population. However, the syndrome may not develop for hours and possibly days. The lower cardiac output then leads to increasing acidosis and hypotension, which may be exacerbated by the use of vasoactive agents. The decrease in blood pressure combined with an increased end-diastolic pressure can result in subendocardial ischemia leading to a progressive deterioration of the heart and death.

As well as clinical symptoms, CT imaging is most common based on the depiction of findings suggestive of cardiac compression caused by intrathoracic increased pressure.

The right atrium and ventricle are initially affected by a reduction in right cardiac inflow and right ventricle outflow (stroke volume); secondly, the left cardiac chambers are involved because of a further increase in thoracic pressure, defining the so-called "Beck's triad" (muffled heart sounds, hypotension, and jugular venous distention) in the setting of a cardiac tamponade.

The compression of the heart right chambers causes many highly sensitive but low specificity CT findings, such as:

- Enlargement of the superior vena cava (SVC) with a diameter similar to or greater than the adjacent thoracic aorta.
- Enlargement of the inferior vena cava (IVC) with a diameter greater than that of the adjacent abdominal aorta.
- Periportal lymphedema.
- Reflux of contrast material from the right atrium into the IVC and reflux of contrast material into the azygos vein from SVC.
- Enlargement of hepatic and renal veins [10].

In cases of advanced TCS, when pressure increase affects both right and left chambers configuring a cardiac tamponade-like heart impairment, CT can demonstrate the presence of highly specific features, mainly related to the change of heart shape and silhouette, such as:

Sign of the "flattened heart" (Fig. 8.1), which consists of flattening of the anterior surface of the heart represented by the right ventricle free wall, with a decrease of its anterior-posterior diameter.

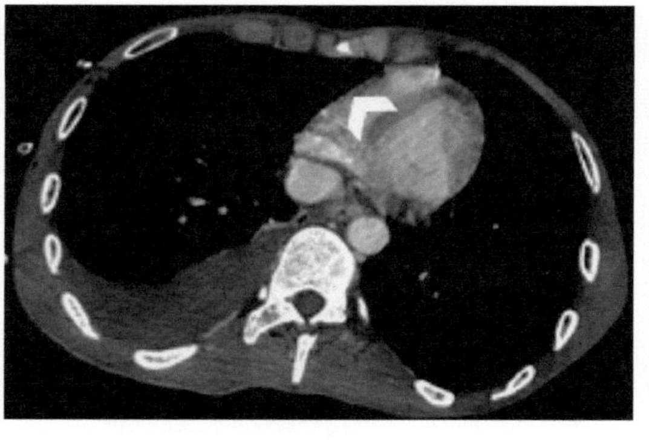

Fig. 8.1 Flattened heart sign (arrow head) consisting in right ventricle normal convex shape loose with reduction of antero-posterior diameter of cardiac chambers

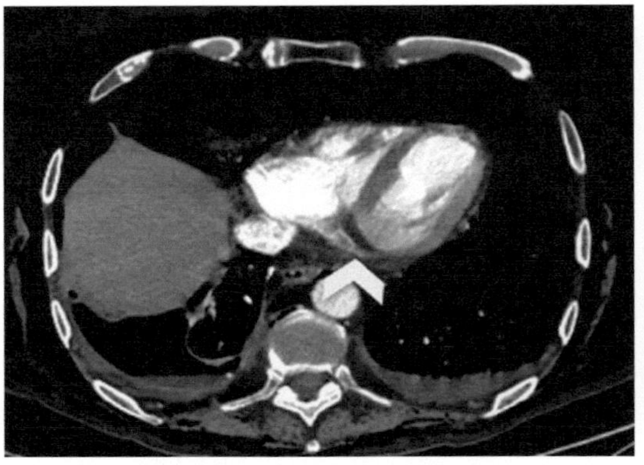

Fig. 8.2 Compression of the coronary sinus (arrow head) consists squeezing of this venous intrapericardial structure at the site of entering the right atrium

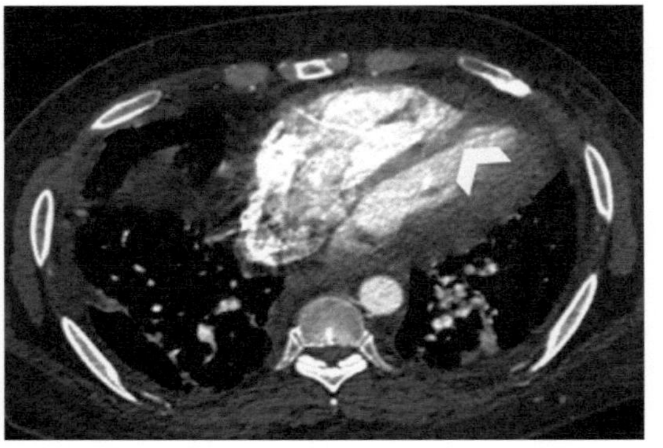

Fig. 8.3 Interventricular septum (IVS) flattening (arrow head) or bowing is an expression of increased pressure on the cardiac chambers with consequent lost of the usual systolic and diastolic convex shape of the left ventricle

It occurs when the increased intrapericardial pressure is sufficient to produce a transient reversal of the transmural right ventricular pressure during diastole, thereby producing a change in the contour of the anterior aspect of the heart with resultant hemodynamic changes [12].

In severe cases, inversion with concave chamber deformity may be seen. Compressive deformity of the cardiac chambers, particularly the thinner and more compliant right-sided chambers, typically manifests at CT as straightening of the right cardiac contour and silhouette.

Compression of the coronary sinus (Fig. 8.2) is a phenomenon similar to the previously described compression of the pulmonary trunk (an entirely intrapericardial vessel) and the short intrathoracic segment of the IVC (which is extrapericardial posteriorly but covered by the pericardium anteriorly).

Angulation or bowing of the interventricular septum (Fig. 8.3) is a finding seen in several thoracic processes that occur with either pressure or volume overload of the right ventricle (such as in constrictive pericarditis or massive pulmonary embolism). This CT finding correlates with the paradoxical motion of the septum [4], which is susceptible to cardiac pressure changes.

8.5 Secondary TCS

TCS is known in the cardiac literature but is still developing in noncardiac/trauma literature. Kaplan et al. [13] described a trauma case where a patient with thoracic and cardiac injuries was treated with delayed sternal closure. The patient experienced multiple episodes of cardiac massage and decompensated in the operating room during attempts to close the thoracic cage. Another trauma-related TCS case was reported by Wandling et al. [14], where the initiation and pathogenesis of TCS were entirely noncardiac following surgical repair of a stab wound injury. TCS may develop secondary to several common thoracic district pathologies involving the mediastinum, pleura, and/or pericardium spaces, as summarized in Table 8.1.

Table 8.1 Secondary causes of TCS

Mediastinum	Pleura	Pericardium
Acute mediastinitis	Tension / pneumothorax	Pericardial effusion
Mediastinal hematoma	Massive hemothorax	Constrictive pericarditis
Tension/Pneumomediastinum		Pericardial haematomas
		Pneumopericardium

8.5.1 Mediastinum

Acute mediastinitis (Fig. 8.4) results from acute inflammation of the connective tissues and fat surrounding the mediastinal structures. It may be classified, based on its cause, as postoperative (the most common), secondary to esophageal perforation, a result of the spread of osteomyelitis from adjacent bone, a direct extension of head and neck infection, or a result of hematogenous spread of infection. Symptoms are nonspecific, including chest pain and fever, necessitating rapid diagnosis. Although chest radiography is the first imaging examination performed to evaluate patients with suspected nonvascular, nontraumatic mediastinal emergencies, the diagnosis of acute mediastinitis and the extent of disease may be determined using CT, the imaging modality of choice in this condition. Common CT findings of acute mediastinitis include increased attenuation of mediastinal fat, free gas bubbles in the mediastinum, and localized fluid collections (Fig. 8.4) [15]. In postoperative complications, *Staphylococcus aureus* is the most common causative microorganism. Sternal dehiscence is frequently associated; the presence of a midsternal diastasis thicker than 3 mm on axial CT images is indicative of dehiscence. In patients with dehiscence, CT findings of acute mediastinitis include air or fluid collections and free air in the mediastinum. The presence of mediastinal gas bubbles and fluid collections on CT images after the 14th postoperative day has sensitivity and specificity approaching 100% for the diagnosis of acute mediastinitis. Additionally, CT may guide diagnostic and therapeutic aspiration of fluid collections [5, 16]. Esophageal perforation may be traumatic (iatrogenic, resulting from surgical, endoscopic, or radiologic procedures, or the ingestion of foreign bodies), neoplastic (esophageal or lung cancers), or spontaneous (Boerhaave syndrome) [17]. CT findings of esophageal rupture include focal esophageal wall thickening, periesophageal fluid collections, free mediastinal air, and oral contrast medium extravasation into the mediastinum and pleural space [4]. In 2010, a study by Shaker et al. [17] reported that early diagnosis and treatment (within 24 hours) are crucial for a successful outcome in patients with esophageal rupture.

Mediastinal hematoma (Fig. 8.5) can be spontaneous or post-traumatic, resulting from a sudden increase in intrathoracic pressure due to coughing, vomiting, or sneezing; a sudden, sustained rise in systemic blood pressure due to malignant hypertension; or hemorrhage into a mediastinal organ or mass (lung, chest wall, aorta) without an underlying bleeding disorder. At unenhanced CT, a hematoma appears as a soft-tissue attenuation mass with areas of high attenuation (>60 HU), indicative of hemorrhage, or as a focal heterogeneous mass and an area of ill-defined soft-tissue thickening in the mediastinum that may extend into the cervical region [5, 18]. A periaortic hematoma typically accompanies thoracic aortic injury and is believed to represent bleeding from small veins in the area or from the vasa vasorum of the aorta itself. CT not only allows direct visualization of periaortic hematoma but also shows the actual aortic injuries, including aortic pseudoaneurysm, changes in aortic contour or diameter, intimal flap, and thrombus, and contrast material extravasation. Multiplanar and volumetric CT reformation are useful in determining the distance of the injury from the aortic arch branches, the length of the injury, the diameter of the aorta above and below the injury, the type of vascular disease, and coexisting anatomic anomalies. Most modern CT scanners are equipped with cardiac gating capability, which permits more accurate evaluation of ascending aortic injury, especially in patients

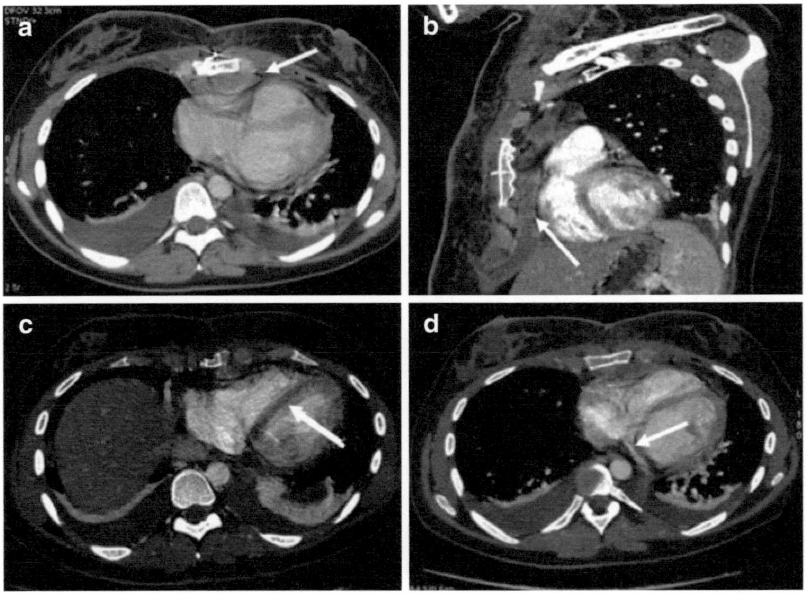

Fig. 8.4 Patient presenting clinical signs of infective mediastinitis after sternal approximation consequent to cardiac revascularization. Fluid dense collection can be seen in the anterior mediastinum (**a**, **b**) (arrows) with signs of thoracic compartment syndrome (TCS) represented by flattening of the right ventricle (arrow) and IVS bowing (**c**) (arrow) associated to coronary sinus squeezing (**d**)

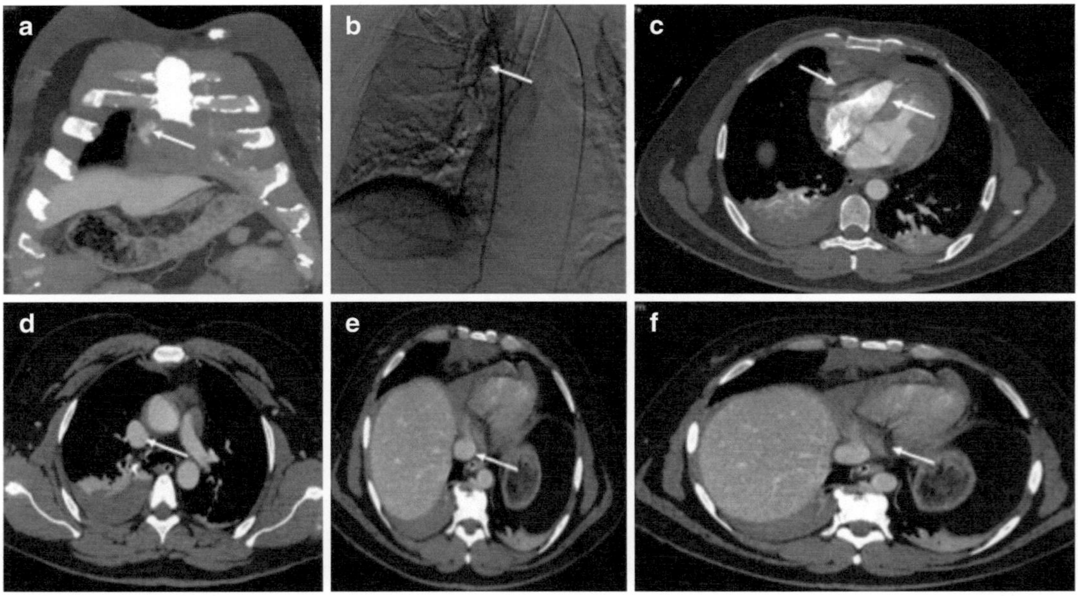

Fig. 8.5 Active bleeding from an internal right mammary artery (arrow) can be appreciated in coronal CT study (**a**), confirmed by Digital Subtraction Angiography IVS bowing (arrow) (**b**). An extensive hematoma in the anterior mediastinum associated with right-sided pleural hematic fluid effusion can be appreciated as well. The victim presented clinical signs of TCS sustained in CT images by IVS bowing (arrow) (**c**), enlargement of Superior Vena Cava (SVC) (arrow) (**d**), enlargement of Inferior Vena Cava (IVC) (arrow) (**e**) and by flattening of right heart, associated to coronary sinus compression (arrow) (**f**)

with tachycardia and marked aortic pulsatile motion. The axial scans are excellent for ruling out ascending aortic injury. The multiplanar and volumetric reformatted images are prepared from an initial non-gated examination [18, 19].

Pneumomediastinum is reported in up to 10% of patients with severe barotrauma due to coughing or asthma; most frequently, the origin remains obscure. It is characterized by the presence of free air around the mediastinal structures. In some cases, pneumomediastinum may result from the extension of cervical or thoracic subcutaneous emphysema, or of a retro-pneumoperitoneum consequent to a hollow viscus rupture. The terminal air spaces of the lung are the most common source of pneumomediastinum. In other cases, it has been attributed to the Macklin effect [20]. Macklin and Macklin [21] first demonstrated that pneumomediastinum can result when air from ruptured alveoli migrates to the mediastinum (a finding confirmed by other investigators). This pathophysiologic process is summed up in three steps: alveolar rupture, air dissection along bronchovascular sheaths, and spreading of this pulmonary interstitial emphysema into the mediastinum. In the presence of a pressure gradient between an alveolus and the interstitium, air ruptures from the alveolus into the perivascular and peribronchial fascial sheath [22]. The Macklin effect is involved in blunt traumatic pneumomediastinum but also in various conditions, such as respiratory distress syndromes, asthma crises, positive-pressure mechanical ventilation, and Valsalva maneuvers. The CT appearance of the Macklin effect is similar to that of pulmonary interstitial emphysema: streaks of air along the bronchovascular bundles may be seen, as well as mediastinal air collections. In less than 2% of patients, pneumomediastinum results from bronchial or tracheal lacerations and is typically parallel to the cartilage rings of the bronchi. Common imaging manifestations of bronchial lacerations are pneumomediastinum and pneumothorax. When there is a complete transection of a bronchus, the lung on the side of the bronchial tear may fall posterolaterally away from the hilum ("fallen lung" sign). The lung falls inferiorly if the patient is upright and posteriorly if the patient is supine, as seen on a CT scan. Tracheal lacerations are usually vertical and longitudinal and located at the junction of the cartilaginous and membranous portions of the trachea. Common findings of tracheal lacerations are cervical subcutaneous emphysema and pneumomediastinum. CT may help identify the site of tracheal laceration in 70%–100% of cases [23].

Tension pneumomediastinum is caused by a substantial increase in intramediastinal pressure resulting from the accumulation of free air. Increased intramediastinal pressure may compress the heart, leading to decreased venous return and compression of the tracheobronchial tree, causing cardiovascular and respiratory collapse. CT is the imaging modality of choice for patients suspected of having tension pneumomediastinum. CT findings include mediastinal free air, flattening of the anterior cardiac contour, compression of the right atrium, uplifting of the heart of the diaphragm, distention of the IVC, compression of the mediastinal vessels, and flattening of the main bronchi [24].

8.5.2 Pleura

Pneumothorax indicates an air collection in the pleural space. It is classified as spontaneous and non-spontaneous.

Spontaneous pneumothorax occurs without any preceding trauma or obvious precipitating causes. Non-spontaneous pneumothorax is classified as traumatic and are subdivided into non-iatrogenic and iatrogenic. Non-iatrogenic pneumothorax can develop following direct or indirect trauma, often to the chest, unrelated to any medical procedure. Iatrogenic pneumothorax results from medical interventions. Whatever the cause or the type of pneumothorax, tension pneumothorax may develop.

Tension pneumothorax (Fig. 8.6) is present when intrapleural pressure exceeds atmospheric pressure throughout expiration [25]. Pneumothorax is a very common traumatic condition that is seen in 15%–40% of all blunt chest trauma patients [17]. Pneumothorax may be caused by ruptured alveoli due to a sudden

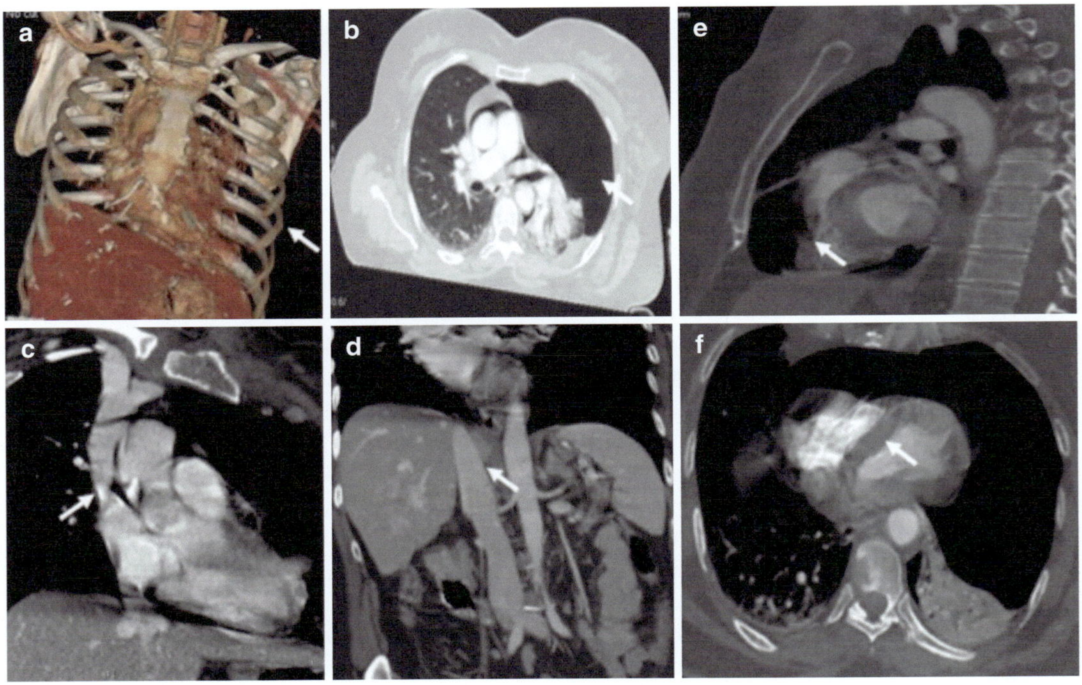

Fig. 8.6 Patient presenting left-sided tension pneumothorax with rib fractures (arrow) (**a**). Pleural space air expansion (arrow) (**b**). Right shifting of mediastinal structures determines compression of cardiac chambers with SVC enlargement (arrow) (**c**) and IVC dilatation (arrow) (**d**). Cardiac silhouette changes are represented by right ventricle convexity inversion (arrow) (**e**) and IVS bowing (arrow) (**f**)

increase in intrathoracic pressure or to blunt crushing force, or deceleration force to the chest, with or without rib fractures. Air in the pleural space accumulates anteriorly and medially in supine patients. As a result, a pneumothorax may be occult on chest radiographs obtained with the patient supine, even though it may be seen on a chest radiograph obtained with the patient upright.

As reported by Wolfman et al. [26] up to 51% of chest trauma patients have an occult pneumothorax, one not seen on an initial chest X-ray but found later with additional imaging. Given the likelihood of progression with mechanical ventilation, early detection with CT is critical, particularly in patients who may require positive pressure ventilation.

With the increased use of CT in trauma patients, pneumothorax is well recognized and do not present any diagnostic difficulty. Mediastinal shift, compromised venous return to the heart, and collapse of the ipsilateral lung maybe present. Tension pneumothorax is a clinical diagnosis (extreme dyspnoea, unilateral chest hyperinflation, cyanosis, and hemodynamic instability); however, it may be suggested at imaging when the following signs are present in addition to the pneumothorax: *(a)* mediastinal shift to the contralateral side, *(b)* flattening or inversion of the ipsilateral hemidiaphragm, and *(c)* hyperexpanded ipsilateral chest. On the other hand, these signs may be seen in a large pneumothorax unaccompanied by hemodynamic compromise. This is probably due to the loss of negative intrapleural pressure on the affected side rather than the presence of positive intrapleural pressure impairing venous return. Nearly 20% of traumatic pneumothorax patients have an accompanying haemothorax.

Massive hemothorax is defined as a hemothorax exceeding 1 liter with clinical signs of shock and hypoperfusion. Blood in the pleural space typically has an attenuation of 35–70 HU. Measurement of pleural fluid attenuation should be routine in the interpretation of chest CT to distinguish simple fluid from acute blood [17].

8.5.3 Pericardium

The pericardial cavity normally contains a small amount of pericardial fluid (15–50 mL) produced by the mesothelial cells that line the serosa. A number of pericardial sinuses and recesses between the reflections of the pericardium serve as a potential space to accommodate a limited amount of additional pericardial fluid, which contributes and increase the pericardial reserve volume [27, 28]. The elevation of the intrapericardial pressure is the result of rapid or slow accumulation of fluid, gas, or tissue within the pericardial cavity. As the pericardial contents initially increase, the pericardial space accommodates the expanding volume of material, without an increase in pressure or compromise of the cardiac chambers until the limit of the pericardial reserve volume is reached. When the limit of pericardial stretch is exceeded, there begins to be compromise of the cardiac chambers, which become smaller for external compression. The rate of accumulation is more significant in establishing cardiac tamponade, than the ultimate size or composition of the pericardial contents [27]. In the acute setting, the pericardium is relatively stiff and noncompliant. Accordingly, acute or rapidly developing pericardial effusions can abruptly increase the intrapericardial pressure and produce cardiac tamponade with as little as 100–200 mL of pericardial fluid, which may result in cardiac dysfunction and death. On the other hand, over time the pericardium can stretch and become more compliant. Therefore, slow or gradual accumulation of pericardial fluid of up to 1000–1500 mL can be tolerated without hemodynamic impairment [17, 29, 30].

Pericardial effusion (Fig. 8.7) originates in the obstruction of venous or lymphatic drainage from the heart. Common causes of pericardial effusion include heart failure, renal insufficiency, infection (bacterial, viral, or tuberculous), neoplasm (carcinoma of lung or breast, lymphoma), and injury (from trauma or myocardial infarction). Echocardiography is considered the primary imaging modality. CT imaging is indicated when loculated or hemorrhagic effusion or pericardial thickening is suspected, or when findings at echocardiography are inconclusive. CT attenuation measurements also enable the initial characterization of pericardial fluid. A fluid collection with attenuation close to that of water is likely to be a simple effusion. Attenuation greater than that of water suggests malignancy, hemopericardium, purulent exudate, or effusion associated with hypothyroidism [29, 31].

Patients with *constrictive pericarditis* frequently present with symptoms of heart failure, such as dyspnea, orthopnea, fatigability, and occasionally may present with liver enlargement and ascites. The most frequent causes of constrictive pericarditis are cardiac surgery and radiation therapy. Clinically, it is difficult to differentiate between constrictive pericarditis and restrictive cardiomyopathy. These two entities are characterized by similar clinical manifestations and similar findings in cardiac catheterization and echocardiography. The diagnosis of constrictive pericarditis is greatly aided by the excellent depiction of the pericardium at CT imaging. Normal pericardial thickness is less than 2 mm [32]; pericardial thickness of 4 mm or more indicates abnormal thickening and when it is accompanied by clinical findings of heart failure, is highly suggestive of constrictive pericarditis. An additional advantage of CT is its high sensitivity in depicting pericardial calcification, which is also associated with constrictive pericarditis. Systemic venous dilatation (particularly in the inferior vena cava), hepatomegaly, and ascites are frequently seen. Tuberculosis (TB) is the most common cause of constrictive pericarditis (Fig. 8.8), with 50% of patients developing constriction despite treatment. Associated findings in TB constrictive pericarditis are pericardial thickening, effusion, lymphadenopathy, and calcifications [32]. The calcifications tend to be thick, irregular, amorphous, and are preferentially located in the atrio-ventricular (AV) grooves. They can be compared with the eggshell calcifications, seen in viral or uremic pericarditis.

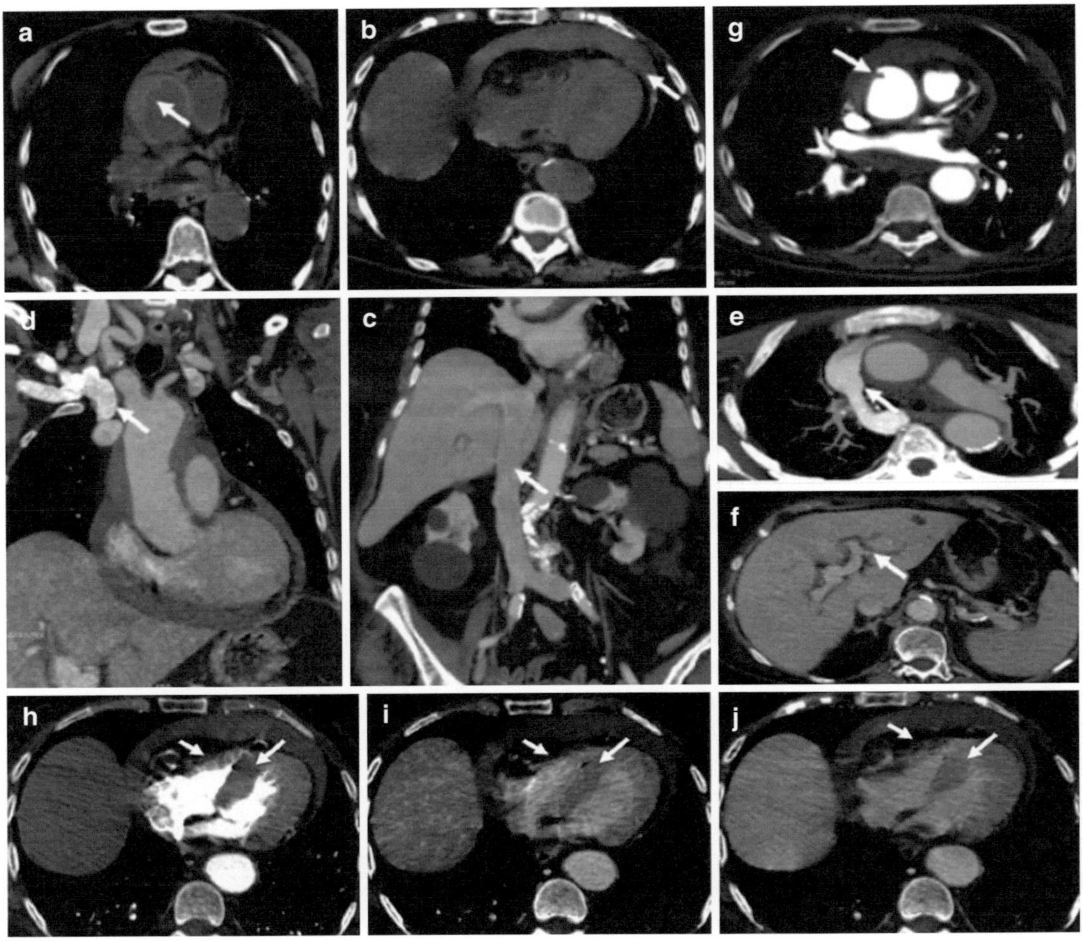

Fig. 8.7 Acute chest pain caused by ascending aorta intimal dissection in an elderly patient under oral anticoagulation therapy. Baseline CT evidences an ascending aortic mural hematoma (arrow) (**a**) accompanied by haemopericardial effusion (arrow) (**b**). In post-contrast scan, TCS clinical signs were present and CT images demonstrate enlargement of the SVC-anonimous right vein (arrow) (**d**) and IVC (arrow) (**c**) with signs of pressure increase in the right chambers: azygos vein contrast media reflux (arrow) (**e**) and hepatic portal spaces edema (arrow) (**f**). There is an intimal flap of the ascending aorta (**g**) associated with mural hematoma. On the cardiac silhouette, right ventricle flattening an IVS bowing can bel clearly appreciated in all three acquisition phases: arterial (arrows) (**h**), venous (arrows) (**i**) and late (arrows) (**j**)

Pericardial thickening may occur in the absence of constrictive pericarditis and may result from inflammation caused by a variety of conditions, including acute pericarditis, uremia, rheumatic heart disease, rheumatoid arthritis, sarcoidosis, and mediastinal irradiation. At contrast-enhanced CT, enhancement of the thickened pericardium indicates inflammation.

Pericardial haematomas may be due to blunt trauma, cardiac surgery, cardiac catheterization, paracentesis, or central line insertion. The blood is of high attenuation initially, which decreases over time. As the hematoma progresses, it organizes and may become fibrotic and calcified. Haematomas do not enhance with IV contrast medium [32]. When diagnosing pericardial fluid

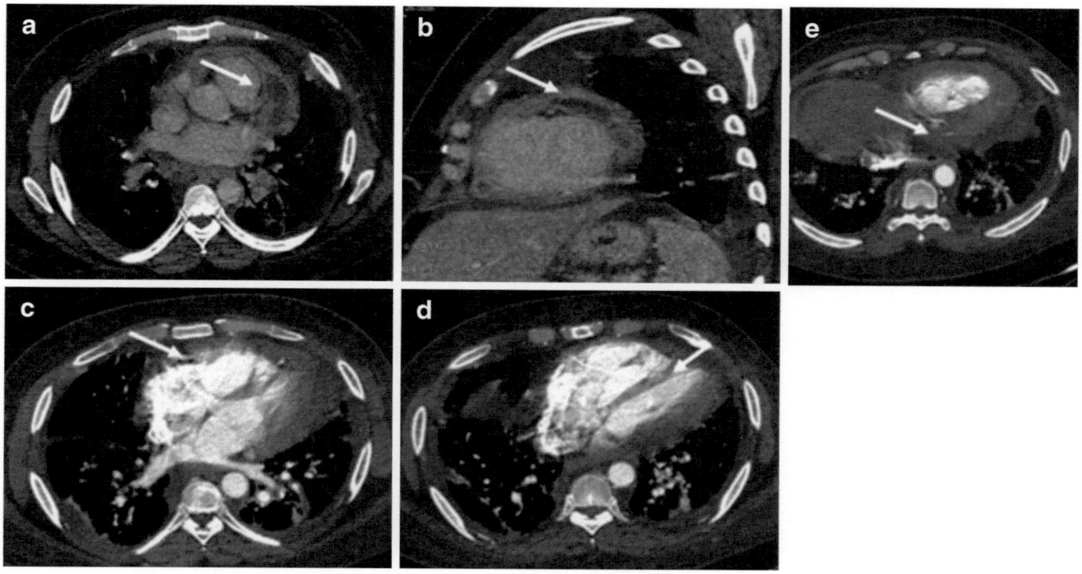

Fig. 8.8 Patient with lung tuberculosis (TB) infection extended to the pericardial sierosa. CT shows inhomogeneous thickening of the pericardium with internal fluid collections (arrows) (**a**, **b**). Pericardial elasticity is compromised with consequential constrictive pericarditis and tamponade-like effect and subsequent TCS. Right ventricle flattening (arrow) (**c**), IVS bowing (arrow) (**d**) and coronary sinus compression (arrow) (**e**) are present

collections, there are many pathologies to consider in order to avoid potential pitfalls. Normal superior pericardial recesses can mimic aortic dissection, intramural aortic hematoma, and enlarged lymph nodes. When considering these differential diagnoses, the Hounsfield attenuation number should be confirmed; for pericardial recesses, this number will be equivalent to that of water and will also be in continuity with the pericardial space. Pericardial effusions should be assessed for size and attenuation on CT. Observed values greater than water suggest that the effusion is caused by blood, malignancy, or infection.

Pneumopericardium (Fig. 8.9) is a well-recognized clinical and radiologic entity. Symptoms are represented by chest pain, dyspnea, cyanosis, hypotension, and tachycardia. Auscultatory findings include a characteristic "mill wheel" murmur [5]. Its causes include trans-sternal surgery and trauma. Trauma is the most common cause of pneumo pericardium and may be blunt or penetrating, iatrogenic (e.g., occurring during or after cardiac surgery), or related to barotrauma secondary to positive pressure ventilation. Nontraumatic causes of pneumopericardium include pericarditis with gas-forming organisms, a direct extension of an inflammatory process from adjacent structures, fistulous communication with air-containing structures (e.g., the stomach, esophagus, airways, and lungs), and extension of a pneumomediastinum into the pericardial cavity.

CT may depict substantial amounts of air in the pericardial cavity with compression and displacement of the heart and associated collapse of the heart chambers, flattening of the anterior border of the heart, and distention of the inferior vena cava. It is an emergent condition and requires immediate pericardial decompression by needle pericardiocentesis and possibly placement of a pericardial drain [33, 34].

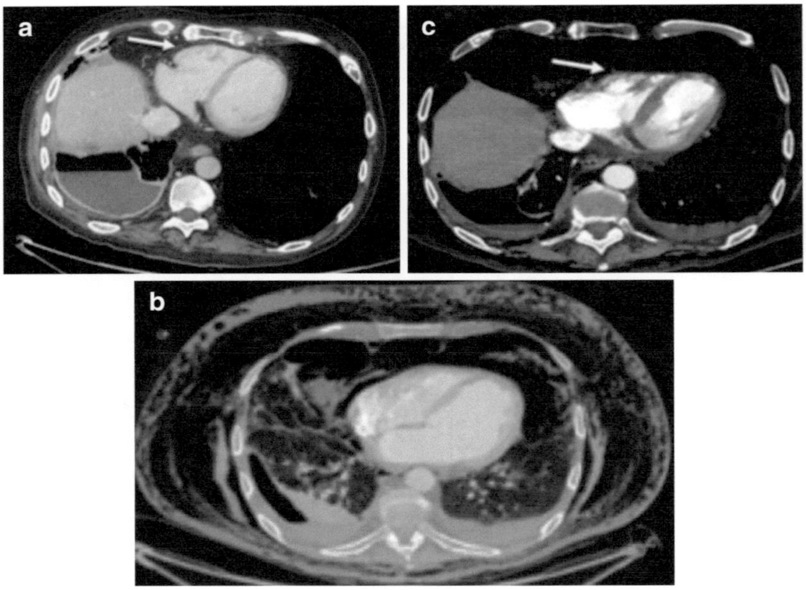

Fig. 8.9 Patient presented with right-sided hydropneumothrax (**a**) and not initially treated by pleural drainage. Same patient after 1 week developed extensive emphysema in cervical and thoracic soft tissues associated with pneumomediastinum and pneumopericardium as well (**b**); TCS clinical signs appeared and CT images show the changing of the right heart and IVS shape (arrow) (**c**) especially if compared to same image 1 week before

References

1. Balogh ZJ, Butcher NE. Compartment syndromes from head to toe. Crit Care Med. 2010;38(9):S445–51. https://doi.org/10.1097/CCM.0b013e3181ec5d09.
2. Haljamae H, Enger E. Human skeletal muscle energy metabolism during and after complete tourniquet ischemia. Ann Surg. 1975;82:9–14. https://doi.org/10.1097/00000658-197507000-00002.
3. Caruso M, Rinaldo C, Iacobellis F, Dell'Aversano Orabona G, et al. Abdominal compartment syndrome: what radiologist needs to know. Radiol Med. 2023;128(12):1447–59. https://doi.org/10.1007/s11547-023-01724-4.
4. Tiwari A, Haq AI, Myint F, Hamilton G. Acute compartment syndromes. Br J Surg. 2002;89(4):397–412. https://doi.org/10.1046/j.0007-1323.2002.02063.x.
5. Cheatham ML, White MW, Sagraves SG, et al. Abdominal perfusion pressure: a superior parameter in the assessment of intra-abdominal hypertension. J Trauma. 2000;49:621–26; discussion, 626–627. https://doi.org/10.1097/00005373-200010000-00008.
6. Riahi M, Tomatis LA, Schlosser RJ, et al. Cardiac compression due to closure of the median sternotomy in open heart surgery. Chest. 1975;67:113–4. https://doi.org/10.1378/chest.67.1.113.
7. Milgater E, Uretzky G, Shimon DV, et al. Delayed sternal closure following cardiac operations. J Cardiovasc Surg. 1986;27:328–31.
8. Mestres CA, Pomar JL, Acosta M, et al. Delayed sterna closure for life-threatening complications in cardiac operations: an update. Ann Thorac Surg. 1991;51:773–6. https://doi.org/10.1016/0003-4975(91)90124-9.
9. Furnary AP, Magovern JA, Simpons KA, et al. Prolonged open sternotomy and delayed sternal closure after cardiac operations. Ann Thorac Surg. 1992;54:233–9. https://doi.org/10.1016/0003-4975(92)91375-j.
10. Liguori C, Tamburrini S, Ferrandino G, et al. Role of CT and MRI in cardiac emergencies. Tomography. 2022;8(3):1386–400. https://doi.org/10.3390/tomography8030112.
11. Valente T, Sica G, Bocchini G, et al. MDCT imaging of non-traumatic thoracic aortic emergencies and its impact on diagnosis and management-A reappraisal. Tomography. 2022;8(1):200–28. https://doi.org/10.3390/tomography8010017.
12. Luyando LH, Calvo J, De Las Heras EG, et al. Tension pericardial collections: sign of 'flattened heart' in CT. Eur J Rad. 1996;23(250):252. https://doi.org/10.1016/s0720-048x(96)00781-4.
13. Kaplan LJ, Trooskin SZ, Santora TA. Thoracic compartment syndrome. J Trauma. 1996;40:291–3. https://doi.org/10.1097/00005373-199602000-00021.
14. Wandling MW, An GC. A case report of thoracic compartment syndrome in the setting of penetrating chest trauma and review of the literature. World J Emerg Surg. 2010;30(5):22. https://doi.org/10.1186/1749-7922-5-22.
15. Garrana SH, Buckley JR, Rosado-de-Christenson ML, et al. Multimodality imaging of focal and diffuse fibrosing mediastinitis. Radiographics. 2019;39:651–67. https://doi.org/10.1148/rg.2019180143.
16. Jolles H, Henry DA, Roberson JP, et al. Mediastinitis following median sternotomy: CT findings. Radiology.

1996;201(2):463–6. https://doi.org/10.1148/radiology.201.2.8888241.
17. Shaheem S, Panikkaveettil H. Aetiology, clinical manifestations, diagnosis, and treatment of oesophageal perforation: a review. Cureus. 2024;16(2):e55041. https://doi.org/10.7759/cureus.55041.eCollection2024Feb.
18. Patel NR, Dick E, Batrick N, Jenkins M, et al. Pearls and pitfalls in imaging of blunt traumatic thoracic aortic injury: a pictorial review. Br J Radiol. 2018;91(1089):201–20. https://doi.org/10.1259/bjr.20180130.
19. Mirvis SE, Shanmuganathan K. Diagnosis of blunt traumatic aortic injury 2007: still a nemesis. Eur J Radiol. 2007;64:27–40. https://doi.org/10.1016/j.ejrad.2007.02.016.
20. Wintermark M, Schnyder P. The Macklin effect: a frequent etiology for pneumomediastinum in severe blunt chest trauma. Chest. 2001;120:543–7. https://doi.org/10.1378/chest.120.2.543.
21. Macklin CC. Transport of air along sheaths of pulmonic blood vessels from alveoli to mediastinum: clinical implications. Arch Intern Med. 1939;64:913–26.
22. Zylak CM, Standen JR, Barnes GR, et al. Pneumomediastinum revisited. Radiographics. 2000;20:1043–57.https://doi.org/10.1148/radiographics.20.4.g00jl131043.
23. Scaglione M, Romano S, Pinto A, et al. Acute tracheobronchial injuries: impact of imaging on diagnosis and management implications. Eur J Radiol. 2006;59:336–43. https://doi.org/10.1016/j.ejrad.2006.04.026.
24. Pinto A, Scaglione M, Scuderi MG, et al. Infections of the neck leading to descending necrotizing mediastinitis: role of multi-detector row computed tomography. Eur J Radiol. 2008;65(3):389–94. https://doi.org/10.1016/j.ejrad.2007.09.024.
25. Baumann MH, Noppen M. Pneumothorax. Respirology. 2004;9(157):164. https://doi.org/10.1111/j.1440-1843.2004.00577.x.
26. Wolfman NT, Myers WS, Glauser SJ, et al. Validity of CT classification on management of occult pneumothorax: a prospective study. AJR. 1998;171:1317–20. https://doi.org/10.2214/ajr.171.5.9798871.
27. Broderick LS, Brooks GN, Kuhlman JE. Anatomic pitfalls of the heart and pericardium. Radiographics. 2005;25:441–53. https://doi.org/10.1148/rg.252045075.
28. Chaturvedi A, Vargas D, Ocazionez D. CT for evaluation of acute pericardial emergencies in the ED. Emerg Radiol. 2018;25(3):321–8. https://doi.org/10.1007/s10140-018-1590-2.
29. Ameli S, Shah PK. Cardiac tamponade: pathophysiology, diagnosis, and management. Cardiol Clin. 1991;9:665–74.
30. Wang ZJ, Reddy GP, Gotway MB, et al. CT and MR imaging of pericardial disease. Radiographics. 2003;23:S167–80. https://doi.org/10.1148/rg.23si035504.
31. Bull RK, Edwards PD, Dixon AK. CT dimensions of the normal pericardium. Br J Radiol. 1998;71:923–5. https://doi.org/10.1259/bjr.71.849.10195005.
32. Troughton RW, Asher CR, Klein AL. Pericarditis. Lancet. 2004;363(9410):717–27. https://doi.org/10.1016/S0140-6736(04)15648-1.
33. Bogaert J, Francone M. Pericardial disease: value of CT and MR imaging. Radiology. 2013;267(2):340–56. https://doi.org/10.1148/radiol.13121059.
34. Su Q, Feng Z, Li T, et al. Tension pneumopericardium leads to cardiac tamponade during hand-assisted ventilation in patients with uremia. J Thorac Cardiovasc Surg. 2008;135(2):432–3. https://doi.org/10.1016/j.jtcvs.2007.10.023.

Part II
Abdomen

9 Clinical Indications to Abdominal CT in Emergency Settings

Mariano Scaglione, Andrea Assenza, Roberto Salis, Stefania Tamburrini, and Salvatore Masala

9.1 Introduction

In the context of acute abdomen (AA), imaging techniques are often required to confirm the diagnosis or when the clinical diagnosis is not straightforward and remains equivocal. Conventional radiography (CR) is still appropriate in a select group of patients with good accuracy in suspected bowel obstruction, perforated viscera, and foreign bodies, while ultrasonography (US) is still the preferred initial modality in pediatric and female/pregnant populations [1]. However, most clinical guidelines indicate that the most appropriate imaging examination depends on the location of the pain, with US being the suggested imaging modality for the right upper quadrant and pelvis and multidetector CT (MDCT) for the remaining quadrants, diffuse abdominal pain, complex clinical scenario, and differential diagnoses.

MDCT is the gold standard imaging technique for evaluating adult patients with acute abdominal pain, providing a rapid and accurate assessment to taper the differential and help in the diagnosis of both surgical and non-surgical causes of pain. According to the ALARA principle, (1) appropriate indication to CT, (2) knowledge of hardware and software modification as well as (3) the choice of the right imaging examination protocol for the right patient and the right time are the crucial points to manage and minimize abdominal and pelvic CT radiation dose, lowing the potential risks of an unnecessary radiation exposure even in the emergency setting.

Therefore, once the decision has been made to perform a CT examination, it is vital to critically examine the significance of each phase in a given CT protocol. Thus, while the non-contrast phase has been abandoned in the vast majority of cases (exception for the search of renal/ureteric stones, free air and ±mesenteric ischemia, pure vascular studies or gastrointestinal bleeding) and double phase CT (arterial and portal venous phases) should be considered just is selected cases (i.e. gastrointestinal bleeding, mesenteric ischemia), porta-venous phase remains the most commonly used single acquisition.

The use of intravenous contrast material is essential in the diagnosis of acute abdomen in the vast majority of cases. Its benefits in CT imaging for acute abdomen include:

Enhancing visualization of vascular structures: including the arteries and veins. This enhance-

M. Scaglione (✉) · A. Assenza · R. Salis · S. Masala
UOC Radiologia Diagnostica, Interventistica e d'Urgenza, Dipartimento di Medicina, Chirurgia e Farmacia, Università degli Studi di Sassari, Sassari, Italy
e-mail: mscaglione@uniss.it; a.assenza@studenti.uniss.it; r.salis15@studenti.uniss.it; samasala@uniss.it

S. Tamburrini
Department of Radiology, Ospedale del Mare-ASL NA1 Centro, Naples, Italy

L. Romano et al. (eds.), *CT of Non-Traumatic Body Emergencies*,
https://doi.org/10.1007/978-3-031-84849-0_9

ment is crucial for identifying abnormalities such as vascular occlusions, aneurysms, or arterial bleeding, which may be contributing to acute abdominal pain.

Improved differentiation of abdominal organs: contrast material aids in distinguishing between different abdominal organs, tissues, and structures. This enhanced tissue contrast facilitates the identification of abnormalities such as inflammation, infection, organ injury, and tumors which may be causing the acute abdomen.

Detection of bowel pathology: the evaluation of the bowel wall, mesenteric vessels, and vascular supply is essential in certain pathologies such as appendicitis/diverticulitis, bowel inflammation, occlusion, mesenteric ischemia, and gastrointestinal bleeding to establish if and when a patient should go to the theatre or to the Interventional Radiology (IR) suite for embolization.

Dynamic imaging: in some cases, acquiring images at different time points after contrast injection, and capturing the arterial and venous phases provides additional information about the perfusion and enhancement patterns of abdominal structures, i.e. bowel pathology which can be helpful in diagnosing certain conditions (bowel occlusion, mesenteric ischemia and ruptured abdominal aneurysms).

Location of pain or tenderness is usually a helpful starting point. The American College of Radiology (ACR) has developed "Appropriateness Criteria" to aid emergency doctors in ordering the most appropriate imaging modality for any specific clinical conditions/query.

9.2 Right Upper Quadrant

Pain in this area can be caused by a wide range of conditions, including:

- Gallstones or inflammation of the gallbladder (cholecystitis), most common,
- Liver conditions such as hepatitis or fatty liver disease,
- Peptic ulcers, gastroenteritis, or constipation,
- Pancreatitis,
- Appendicitis (although this typically causes pain in the lower right quadrant),
- Muscle strain or injury.

Acute cholecystitis is the primary diagnostic consideration in this patient.

The ACR Appropriateness Criteria suggest US as the first imaging modality for patients presenting with right upper quadrant. MDCT of the abdomen in the portal-venous phase can help identify the underlying cause of the right upper quadrant pain by providing detailed images of the liver, gallbladder, pancreas and adjacent hallow viscera. It can be used in equivocal patients and may be used to identify complications of acute cholecystitis, impacted gallstones within the common bile duct, tumors, or other structural issues that may be contributing to the symptoms. Additionally, MDCT is valuable for ruling out certain conditions and guiding further diagnostic and treatment decisions (i.e. magnetic resonance cholangiopancreatography, drainage, and embolization) [2].

9.3 Right Lower Quadrant

The right lower quadrant of the abdomen contains several important structures, including the appendix, cecum, ascending colon, right ovary and fallopian tube (in females), and part of the small intestine. Appendicitis is the primary diagnostic consideration in this patient. In the most common scenario, clinical presentation, physical evaluation, and laboratory tests are usually enough to send the patient with appendicitis to the operating room, without any imaging text. However, it should be emphasized, that uncommon presentation of acute appendicitis are relatively frequent, and pain from acute appendicitis can be referred in any part of the abdomen, therefore clinical examination and imaging studies need to the extended from the right iliac fossa to the whole abdomen. Another important point to remember is that the differential diagnosis of appendicitis includes, intra−/ extra-abdominal and retroperitoneal diseases.

US is often the primary imaging test to confirm the diagnosis of appendicitis, especially in pediatric patient population, and female or pregnant patients. In this context, MRI can be used as the next imaging examination when US is inconclusive [3].

The ACR Appropriateness Criteria suggest MDCT in portal-venous phase as the imaging of choice in non-pregnant adult patients with RLQ pain. The main value of MDCT is to guide through the possible constellation of surgical and non-surgical diagnoses of RLQ pain. As mentioned before, when a CT is planned, it is important to scan the entire abdomen and not only the right iliac fossa. Finally, it is important to take a glance at the lung bases, as pneumonia in the right lower lobe can evoke pain in the RLQ [2].

9.4 Left Upper Quadrant

CT in the portal-venous phase is currently the primary imaging modality for patients with acute left upper quadrant pain, providing detailed images of the organs and structures located in the left upper part of the abdomen. Disorders of the spleen (i.e. splenomegaly and non-traumatic splenic rupture or infarction), pancreatic body and tail (pancreatitis), colonic splenic flexure (i.e. colitis, masses), and left kidney (stones, pyelonephritis) represent a frequent request for MDCT evaluation.

9.5 Left Lower Quadrant

Pain in this area can refer to a wide range of conditions from benign to life-threatening so differential diagnosis must be guided by patient history, physical examination, laboratory tests, and imaging studies which add information to define the best management.

The most common disease in this quadrant is acute diverticulitis, especially in elder patients which is a consequence of an inflammation of a colonic diverticulum.

Other conditions that can cause left lower quadrant (LLQ) pain include colitis, inflammatory bowel disease, bowel obstruction, or hernia, while adnexal pathology, pyelonephritis, and urolithiasis regarding the gynecological and urological systems.

The ACR Appropriateness Criteria recommend MDCT in portal-venous phase of the entire abdomen as the best choice to evaluate LLQ pain. Intravenous contrast material is crucial for detecting bowel wall abnormalities and complications, i.e. an abscess, and for differentiating a simple diverticulitis from a colonic mass. CT is crucial to detect even small extraluminal, intra- and extra-peritoneal air collection which usually indicates a bowel wall perforation implicating a surgical emergency. MDCT is also used for determining the most appropriate management approach in cases of diverticulitis (nonsurgical vs surgical) and to place a percutaneous drainage is cases of large collections/abscesses.

9.6 Flank Pain

Flank pain can be associated with both urinary and extra-urinary causes—such as appendicitis, diverticulitis, gallbladder diseases, chest diseases, and other gastrointestinal conditions with atypical presentation. Patient history, physical evaluation, and laboratory tests are usually enough to differentiate urolithiasis from pyelonephritis. Renal colic is typically associated with urinary tract calculi. It commonly onsets with an acute and intermittent flank pain radiating to the ipsilateral testicle and can be associated with microscopic hematuria, nausea, and vomiting. Conversely, acute pyelonephritis is a severe infection associated with localized pain, fever, leukocytosis, and bacteriuria and with the potential to cause sepsis and shock. In cases of acute onset flank pain/suspicious stone (urolithiasis), the ACR Appropriateness Criteria recommend the use of CT abdomen and pelvis without IV contrast, with ± US/color Doppler frequently used as the initial modality in most European hospitals. An obstruction of the urinary tract can also be related to strictures or tumors. In these cases, a CT urography (CTU), which has largely replaced the traditional intravenous urography in imaging the genitourinary tract, can be considered as further imaging. This imaging technique is used to evaluate the whole urinary system, particularly the upper urinary tract. Standard CTU consists of unenhanced, nephrographic, and pyelographic phases which allows a complete evaluation for the most common urologic causes of hematuria, i.e. calculi, renal masses, and urothelial tumors. After initial unenhanced acquisition, nephrographic phase images are acquired 90–100 seconds after administration of a nonionic contrast agent (80–100 mL of 350 < 400 mg I/mL at 2–4 mL/s). Imaging (2.5- to 5-mm slice thickness) is typically confined to the kidneys during this phase. Nephrographic phase imaging has the highest sensitivity in the detection of renal masses, and correlation with unenhanced images is required to show unequivocal enhancement. Pyelographic phase images are acquired 5–15 minutes after contrast administration to evaluate the urothelium from the kidneys to the bladder [2]. Many institutions are advocating the split-bolus CTU for the evaluation of patients with hematuria and urinary tract diseases because of its lower radiation dose compared with single-bolus three-phase imaging, especially in patients younger than 40 years. Split-bolus CTU uses two sets of image acquisition—an unenhanced phase and synchronous nephrographic-excretory phase. Depending on weight, the patient receives 30–50 mL of IV contrast followed by an additional 50 mL eight minutes later. Images are then acquired 55 seconds following the second dose of IV contrast [4].

9.7 Epigastric Pain

Epigastric pain can be associated with various pathologies including acute gastritis, acute cholecystitis, peptic ulcer disease and perforated ulcer, appendicitis (in atypical scenarios), and pancreatitis. Severe conditions, such as mesenteric ischemia, bowel obstruction, and rupture of an abdominal aneurism can also onset with a localized symptomatology [5]. In this scenario, patient's history, clinical presentation, and laboratory findings are crucial for the differential diagnosis. Acute pancreatitis (AP) is the third most frequent GI cause of hospital admission and can be associated with high morbidity and mortality rates in case of a necrotic condition [6]. According to the Atlanta criteria, the AP diagnosis requires the presence of 2 of the 3 features: acute onset of persistent, severe, epigastric pain often radiating to the back; serum lipase of amylase three times the upper limits of normal; characteristic findings on either MDCT, MRI or US. According to ACR Appropriateness criteria, CT with or without IV contrast in the early phase may not improve clinical outcomes, since widespread necrosis can evolve in few days. It is then crucial to evaluate the grade of severity with furthermore imaging acquisitions, 48–72 hours and five to seven days later from the clinical onset. MDCT protocol with IV contrast provides an overall assessment of the pancreatic parenchyma and complications (Fig. 9.1). Monophasic, portal-venous scan suffices in most cases, while multi-phasic MDCT is recommended in cases of suspicious pancreatic mass causing acute pancreatitis, haemorrhage, arterial pseudoaneurysm and bowel ischemia [6]. However, it should be emphasized that in some cases, elevated serum lipase of amylase can also occur in other potentially life-threatening conditions such as intestinal ischaemia, bowel perforation, etc. Therefore, in the acute setting, keep in mind the differential diagnoses and perform a CT scan (arterial and portal phases) before it is too late.

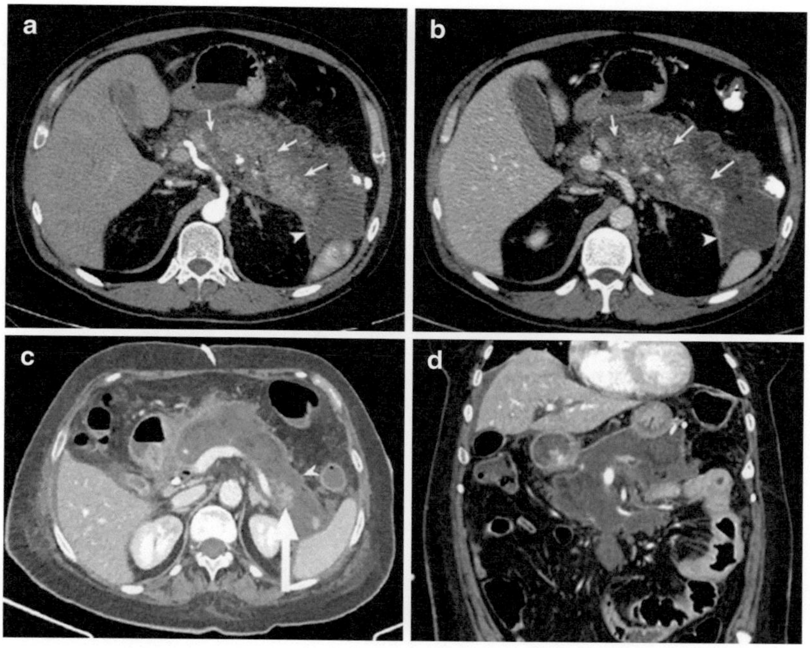

Fig. 9.1 M, 69 yo, acute epigastric pain with back irradiation; LAB: amylase 1500, lipase 800, WBC 8.000, Marshall score 2 for 48H. Contrast-enhanced MDCT in arterial (**a**) and portal (**b**) phase, two contiguous scans, show multiple necrotic foci (arrows) throughout the pancreatic gland in keeping with necrotizing acute pancreatitis with a large acute necrotic collection within the anterior pararenal space (arrowhead). Follow-up CT scan after 7 days (**c**) demonstrates a significant progression of the parenchymal necrosis with a residual enhancing tissue at the pancreatic tail (arrow) and a large necrotic collection within the anterior pararenal space (arrowhead). Coronal reconstruction image (**d**) gives an optimal spatial assessment of the retroperitoneal necrotic collection, with minimal spread around the liver and pelvis

9.8 Non-localized Abdominal Pain

In the case of non-localized pain, clinical evaluation is often not specific and the final diagnosis remains undetermined in about 40/50% even in experienced hands. Common causes include gastrointestinal (GI) perforation, bleeding or inflammation, bowel occlusion (Figs. 9.2 and 9.3) or infarction, pancreatic and hepatobiliary diseases, abscesses, tumors, and even pneumonia. The radiologist's task is often to differentiate non-surgical from surgical causes of pain, indicating the timing for surgery or the need for intervention. The ACR Appropriateness criteria recommend a CT of the abdomen and pelvis with IV contrast (single portal venous phase) as the preferred option. Additional arterial phase (CT-angiography) is strongly recommended in the suspicion of (1) GI bleeding—to exclude or identify the site of bleeding, and to provide "an angiogram", a vascular mapping for selective embolization or the need for surgery—and (2) bowel ischemia to differentiate non-occlusive mesenteric ischemia (common and often missed) from occlusive mesenteric ischemia [2].

CT-Angiography uses a thin-section CT acquisition that is timed to coincide with peak arterial or venous enhancement. The resultant volumetric dataset is interpreted using primary transverse reconstructions as well as multiplanar reformations and 3-D renderings. All elements are essential: (1) timing, (2) reconstructions/reformats, and (3) 3-D renderings. Standard CTs with contrast also include timing issues and recons/reformats. A non-contrast CT scan is often useful to identify pre-existing intra/extraluminal radiopaque items which may interfere with

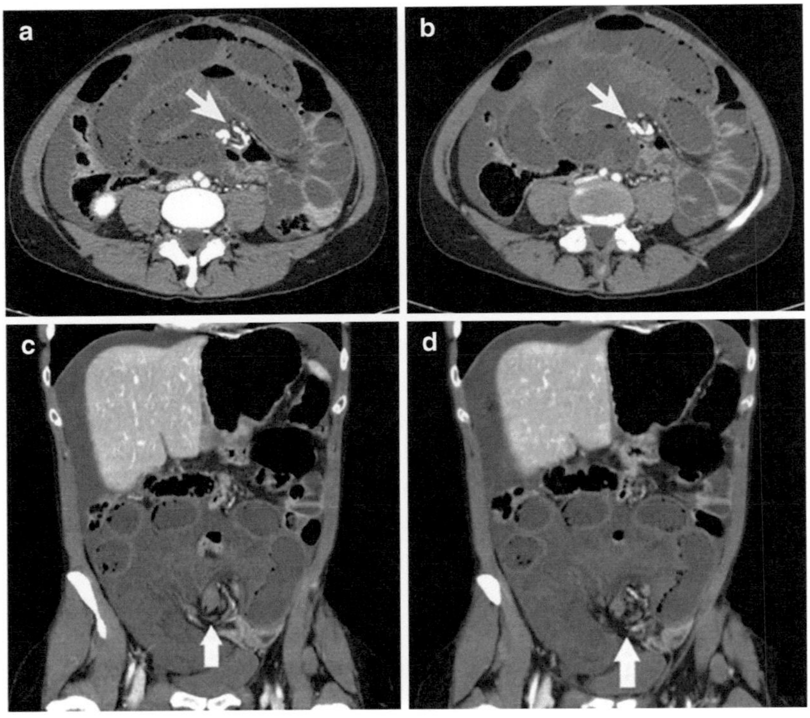

Fig. 9.2 M, 70 yo, presenting with acute abdominal pain and vomiting. Two contiguous axial MDCT scans after IV contrast injection (**a**, **b**) show dilated fluid-filled ilial loops with a decreased enhancement (**a**) and complete swirling appearance of the mesentery around the superior mesenteric artery "whirl sign" (**a**, **b**) (arrows) in keeping with a complicated mesenteric volvulus. Two contiguous MPR images (**c**, **d**) provide an optimal spatial assessment of the small bowel obstruction, mesenteric engorgement, free fluid, and "whirl sign" (arrow). At surgery, a bowel necrosis was found and an ample resection of over 30 cm of small bowel was necessary

the assessment of the pre- and post-contrast status of the bowel wall and mesentery. In cases of suspected bowel perforation, non-contrast CT can be adopted when plain film is inconclusive. However, be aware that evidence of free air in the abdominal cavity may take time to appear even under CT. In such cases, clinical evidence of an ileus, with or without free air/fluid, can be enough to support the clinical suspicion of bowel perforation.

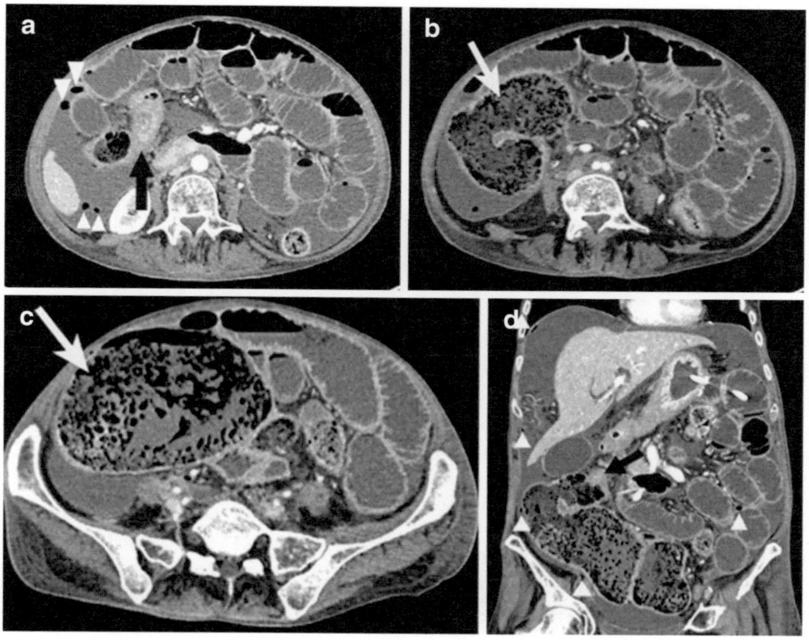

Fig. 9.3 M, 70 yo, presenting with peritonitis and vomiting. Axial contrast-enhanced MDCT scans show a large mass obstructing the hepatic flexure of the colon (**a**, black arrow), dilated small bowel loops with air fluid-levels in the small bowel loops and multiple thin valvulae conniventes, free fluid and locules of free air (**a**, white arrowheads), dilated ascending colon (**b**, arrow) and caecum (**c**, arrow) over 14 cm. Coronal MPR reconstruction image (**d**) gives an optimal overall assessment of the obstructed colonic neoplasm (black arrow), dilated colonic and small bowel loops, free fluid, and gas (white arrowheads). At surgery, a perforated colonic neoplasm with cecal wall necrosis was found

Suspected pathology	Etiology	Clinical symptoms	Major expected CT signs
Acute cholecystitis	Gallstone	Right-upper quadrant pain	Bowel wall thickening, stones, adjacent fat stranding fluid
Appendicitis	Appendicolith	Right-lower quadrant pain	Appendicular wall dilatation/ thickening +/− fat stranding/fluid
Acute diverticulitis	Diverticular disease	Left lower quadrant pain	Diverticula wall thickening, +/− fat stranding, fluid in the pelvis/peritoneal cavity
Renal colic	Urinary tract stone	Flank pain	Urinary tract calculi, hydronephrosis, hydroureter, stranding
Acute pancreatitis	Gallstone/ alcohol abuse	Epigastric/ lumbar pain	(±) Gland enlargement, (+/) necrosis signs, fluid, collections, vessel involvement
Bowel perforation	Parietal inflammation/ foreign body	Sharp and sudden intense abdominal pain	Free air, ± fluid, ileus
Bowel obstruction	Intrinsic and extrinsic cause or intraluminal cause	Increasing cramp-like abdominal pain	Intestinal loops dilatation, U-shaped/C-shaped configuration, transition point, fluid,

(continued)

Suspected pathology	Etiology	Clinical symptoms	Major expected CT signs
Gastrointestinal bleeding	Vascular disease/ ulcer/ inflammation/ neoplasm	Hematemesis/ melena/ coffee-ground vomiting/ hematochezia	Active extravasation within the bowel
Acute mesenteric ischemia	Blood flow sudden interruption	Generalized abdominal pain out of proportion to physical findings	Vessel (± thrombus, ± caliber change); Bowel wall (± thickening/thinning); Peritoneal cavity (± ascites, ± mesenteric engorgement);

References

1. Nelms DW, Kann BR. Imaging modalities for evaluation of intestinal obstruction. .Clin Colon Rectal Surg. 2021;34(4):205–218. https://doi.org/10.1055/s--0041-1729737. Epub 2021 Jun 2. PMID: 34305469; PMCID: PMC8292005.
2. Expert Panel on Gastrointestinal Imaging, Russo GK, Zaheer A, Kamel IR, Porter KK, Archer-Arroyo K, Bashir MR, Cash BD, Fung A, McCrary M, McGuire BM, Shih RD, Stowers J, Thakrar KH, Vij A, Wahab SA, Zukotynski K, Carucci LR. ACR appropriateness criteria® right upper quadrant pain: 2022 update. J Am Coll Radiol. 2023;20(5S):S211–23. https://doi.org/10.1016/j.jacr.2023.02.011.
3. Debnath J, George RA, Ravikumar R. Imaging in acute appendicitis: What, when, and why? Med J Armed Forces India. 2017;73(1):74–9. https://doi.org/10.1016/j.mjafi.2016.02.005. Epub 2016 Mar 29. PMID: 28123249; PMCID: PMC5221358.
4. Wang LJ, Wong YC, Hwang YS, Pang ST, Chuang CK, Chang YH. Split-bolus computed tomography urography (CTU) achieves more than half of radiation dose reduction in females and overweight patients than conventional single-bolus computed tomography urography. Transl Oncol. 2021;14(8):101151. https://doi.org/10.1016/j.tranon.2021.101151. Epub 2021 Jun 8. PMID: 34111709; PMCID: PMC8193142.
5. Expert Panel on Gastrointestinal Imaging, Vij A, Zaheer A, Kamel IR, Porter KK, Arif-Tiwari H, Bashir MR, Fung A, Goldstein A, Herr KD, Kamaya A, Kobi M, Landler MP, Russo GK, Thakrar KH, Turturro MA, Wahab SA, Wardrop RM 3rd, Wright CL, Yang X, Carucci LR. ACR appropriateness criteria® epigastric pain. J Am Coll Radiol. 2021;18(11S):S330–9. https://doi.org/10.1016/j.jacr.2021.08.006.
6. Thoeni RF. Imaging of acute pancreatitis. Radiol Clin North Am. 2015;53(6):1189–208. https://doi.org/10.1016/j.rcl.2015.06.006. Epub 2015 Aug 5.

10 Intra-abdominal Free Air

Antonio Pinto, Daniela Vecchione, Reimy Rodriguez, Maria Rivellini, and Claudia Rossi

10.1 Introduction

Gastrointestinal tract perforations can be determined by several causes, and most of these perforations represent emergency abdominal conditions requiring early recognition and timely surgical treatment [1]. Intra-abdominal free air is the collection of air in the peritoneal cavity (pneumoperitoneum) and/or in the retroperitoneum (pneumoretroperitoneum). Free air can enter the peritoneum in four different ways. Most commonly it involves a peritoneal or retroperitoneal viscus perforation. It may also dissect along mediastinal structures to penetrate the abdomen from the thorax. Iatrogenic or surgical exploration is a third method of entry, and, lastly, the female genital tract provides a fourth pathway of free air entering the peritoneum [2].

Radiographic evidence of free intraperitoneal air was linked to intra-abdominal disease in the early 1900s and continues to be a useful diagnostic tool for perforation of an intra-abdominal viscus [3]. There are four etiologic categories of pneumoperitoneum: iatrogenic, spontaneous, traumatic, and miscellaneous.

About 85% of patients with a ruptured abdominal viscus will present with pneumoperitoneum, most often from a perforated gastric or duodenal ulcer, although perforated colon or small bowel may also present with pneumoperitoneum. Nonsurgical causes of pneumoperitoneum [4–7] are reported in Table 10.1.

Pneumoretroperitoneum is defined by the presence of free air within the retroperitoneal space. The retroperitoneum is the compartmentalized space bounded anteriorly by the posterior parietal peritoneum and posteriorly by the transversalis fascia. It extends from the diaphragm superiorly to the pelvic brim inferiorly [8]. Most often, air is seen surrounding the kidneys and overlying the contour of the iliopsoas muscles. Free air can collect in the retroperitoneal space after perforation of a retroperitoneal bowel segment, or air can spread below the diaphragm from a pneumomediastinum.

It is not uncommon to discover the presence of pneumoperitoneum, pneumoretroperitoneum, pneumomediastinum, pneumothorax, and subcutaneous emphysema in the same patient [9]. Common and uncommon causes of pneumoretroperitoneum [8, 9] are reported in Table 10.2.

Patients with intra-abdominal free air may present with different symptoms, but infrequently are asymptomatic. Symptoms vary in relation to the site of perforation but may include abdominal pain, chest pain, nausea, or vomiting.

A thorough history eliciting the temporal relationship of symptoms and disease progression is critical in order to determine the appropriate

A. Pinto (✉) · D. Vecchione · R. Rodriguez
M. Rivellini · C. Rossi
Department of Support Health Services, Unit of Radiology, CTO Hospital, Azienda Ospedaliera dei Colli, Naples, Italy

L. Romano et al. (eds.), *CT of Non-Traumatic Body Emergencies*,
https://doi.org/10.1007/978-3-031-84849-0_10

Table 10.1 Nonsurgical causes of pneumoperitoneum

Thoracic causes	Cardiopulmonary resuscitation
	Chronic obstructive pulmonary disease/severe coughing
	Median sternotomy
	Mechanical ventilation
	Pneumothorax, tracheal rupture
Abdominal causes	Chronic peritoneal dialysis
	Percutaneous endoscopic gastrostomy
	Pneumatosis cystoides intestinalis
	Scleroderma/Collagen vascular disease
	Spontaneous bacterial peritonitis
Gynecologic causes	Coitus
	Oral-genital insufflation
	Post-partum exercises
	Vaginal instrumentation
Miscellaneous	Amyloidosis
	Cocaine use
	Diving with decompression

From [4], modified

Table 10.2 Common and uncommon causes of pneumoretroperitoneum

Blunt traumatic rupture of the duodenum
Epidural anesthesia
Extension from pneumomediastinum
Extracorporeal shock-wave lithotripsy,
Gas-containing retroperitoneal abscess
Hydrogen peroxide wound irrigation
Necrotizing fasciitis,
Pelvic trauma with perforation of the rectum
Penetrating trauma
Post-diagnostic procedure
Postoperative
Spontaneous colon perforation
Superinfected necrotizing pancreatitis

treatment strategy for all patients with pneumoperitoneum. Patients should be questioned about medical history and pertinent risk factors. The physical examination should focus on the abdomen and the identification of findings that narrow the differential diagnosis. Laboratory tests should be obtained to determine if hematologic or electrolyte abnormalities, or coagulopathy is present that may complicate surgical intervention, and allow the provider to estimate the severity of the illness. Clinical manifestations can include localized abscess formation, inflammatory mass, fistulas, and gastrointestinal hemorrhage. Rare complications secondary to perforation are septicemia, portal pyemia or pyogenic abscess, enterovascular fistulas, and even endocarditis [9]. Even if in the American College of Radiology (ACR) appropriateness criteria [10] the enhanced Computed Tomography of the abdomen and pelvis is considered the most appropriate examination (rating 8) for patients with acute abdominal pain and fever or suspected abdominal abscess, plain radiography remains the most frequently requested examination performed as initial imaging in the assessment of patients who present with acute abdominal pain to the emergency department [11–13].

Multidetector row Computed Tomography (MDCT) is considered the most valuable imaging technique for identifying the presence, the site, and the cause of alimentary tract perforations (Fig. 10.1) [14]. MDCT examination in the emergency setting is performed with the administration of intravenous (iv) contrast medium and includes the thorax if an esophageal perforation is suspected and the entire abdomen, from the dome of the diaphragm to the pubic symphysis. For gastrointestinal tract evaluation, the use of thin sections, high-volume, rapid-bolus scanning technique with state-of-the-art computed tomography (CT) technology is important in differentiating intestinal and abdominal findings. Preliminary unenhanced abdominal CT is relevant in order to detect free air bubbles or fluid collection into the abdominal cavity, hemoperitoneum, and preexisting hyperattenuating material in the bowel wall and lumen such as blood clots, suture materials or retained contrast material. Administration of intravenous contrast medium could be considered essential for all acute intestinal conditions in order to evaluate the bowel wall feature and enhancement, and useful for all differential diagnoses. The range of sensitivity and specificity of MDCT for gastrointestinal perforation is between 80 and 100% [15].

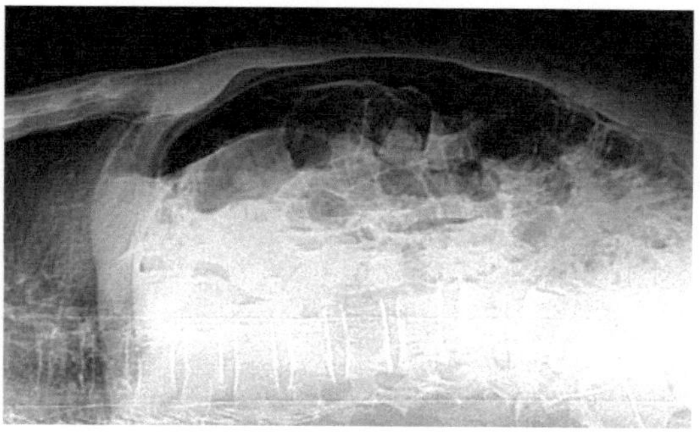

Fig. 10.1 MDCT of the abdomen. Scout view (laterolateral projection). Evidence of free intra-abdominal air

10.2 Intra-abdominal Free Air Due to Esophageal Perforation

The abdominal esophagus is 3 to 4 cm in length and courses to the left of the vertebral column. The esophagus narrows just superior to the gastroesophageal junction and is the site of 12% to 37% of esophageal perforations. Esophageal perforation represents a rare but life-threatening condition. Overall mortality approaches 13.3% but rises significantly after 24 h from symptom onset [16].

The clinical presentation of esophageal perforation mimics other causes of intra-abdominal free air and is dependent on the time of presentation and the level of injury. There needs to be a high index of suspicion for perforation if a patient has an association of chest pain, dysphagia, dyspnea, subcutaneous emphysema, epigastric pain, fever, tachycardia, or tachypnea after any esophageal instrumentation or history of vomiting or retching. The esophageal perforation is more commonly iatrogenic, caused by endoscopic procedures—dilatation for strictures and achalasia [17]—or by surgical complications [18].

CT findings include esophageal wall thickening, mural gas, mural defect(s), cervical or mediastinal fat stranding, free gas/contrast/fluid in the mediastinum, subcutaneous emphysema, pleural effusion, and foreign bodies [19].

The most frequent useful CT findings of esophageal perforation are manifested by extraluminal variable amounts of air, in relationship with elapsed time, and secondly periesophageal fluid collection. CT allows the visualization of very small air or fluid collections, otherwise undetectable, in cases of small tears [20]. Pleural effusions, combined or not with pneumothorax, are also frequently evident. Distal esophageal perforations are usually associated with a left-side pleural effusion or a hydropneumothorax, while a middle perforation is frequently associated with a right-side pleural effusion. In patients with foreign body ingestion, MDCT allows to identification of the size and the correct spatial position of the foreign body, very useful data for removing [21]. In cases of complicated tumours or strictures, an esophago-respiratory fistula, lung abscess, or recurrent aspiration pneumonia may develop. Moreover, lower oesophageal perforations may manifest extraluminal gas that dissects inferiorly into the abdomen and can mimic gastric perforation.

Spontaneous esophageal perforation (Boerhaave syndrome) is caused by incomplete cricopharyngeal relaxation during severe vomiting, resulting in abruptly increased intraluminal pressure with subsequent rupture. Rupture occurs usually at the distal left posterior esophageal wall, accompanied by pneumomediastinum and left pleural effusion [22]. Vomiting, chest pain, and subcutaneous emphysema comprise the Mackler triad which is indicative of this syndrome. Treatment options for esophageal perforation include endoluminal stenting, operative management, and in select cases, nonoperative management.

10.3 Intra-abdominal Free Air Due to Gastric and Duodenal Perforations

Etiologies of pneumoperitoneum from gastric and duodenal sources overlap in many ways. Primary causes include iatrogenic, postoperative, malignant, and benign causes [23]. The most commonly reported cause of gastroduodenal perforation is ulcer disease (Fig. 10.2) linked to both infections with Helicobacter pylori and frequent use of aspirin and other nonsteroidal anti-inflammatory

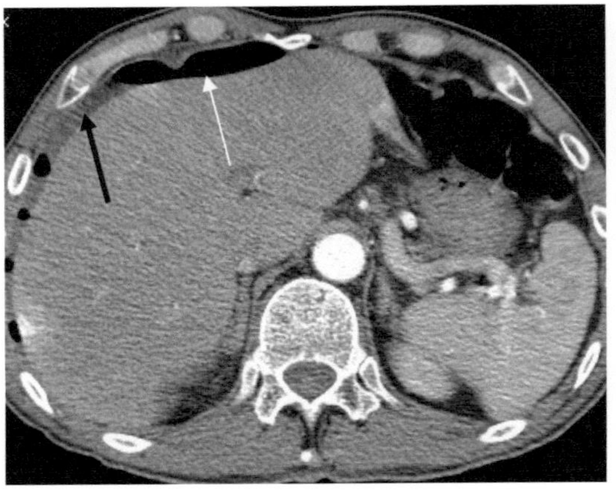

Fig. 10.2 MDCT of the abdomen, axial scan, showing the presence of free air (white arrow) and fluid (black arrow) superficial to the liver. At laparotomy a perforated peptic ulcer was discovered

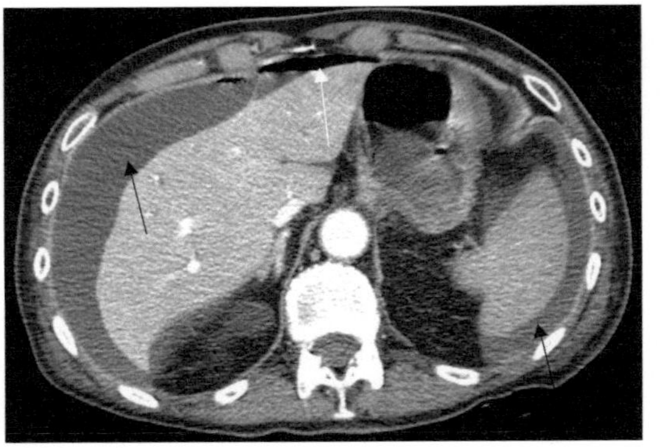

Fig. 10.3 MDCT of the abdomen, axial scan, showing the presence of a small amount of free intraperitoneal air (white arrow). Free fluid in the perihepatic space and in the perisplenic space is also evident (black arrows). At surgery: perforation of the first duodenal portion

drugs [24]. Gastroduodenal perforation connected with a peptic ulcer is usually located at the level of the gastric antrum and duodenal bulb.

The variable location of the ulcer produces different consequences: a deep anterior ulcer may perforate directly into the peritoneal cavity, whereas posterior gastric or duodenal ulcers often determine a confined perforation [24]. Neoplastic causes usually depend on the presence of a tumor that can lead to obstruction or increased endoluminal pressure.

Perforation can also arise from foreign bodies that can be ingested either intentionally or accidentally. Patients with gastroduodenal perforation usually present with signs and symptoms of either local or generalized peritonitis due to the leakage of luminal contents in the peritoneal cavity. Laboratory tests are usually nonspecific, but leukocytosis, metabolic acidosis, and hyperamylasemia may be indicative of the presence of perforation.

The radiologic feature of perforation is the presence of air and/or fluid in the peritoneal cavity (Fig. 10.3), retroperitoneal spaces, mesentery, or ligaments [25]. In some cases, pneumomediastinum or subcutaneous emphysema can also be detected. Direct CT findings of gastroduodenal perforation include extraluminal air (free air) and direct visualization of gastroduodenal tract wall rupture [23, 26]. Indirect CT findings include focal bowel wall thickening (>8 mm in gastroduodenal wall), abnormal bowel wall enhancement, inflammatory changes (abscess and an inflammatory mass adjacent to the bowel), or a fluid collection in the surrounding soft tissues or organs [27].

Air in the lesser sac is commonly due to posterior perforation of the stomach or duodenum. Free air or an air-fluid level crossing the midline and an accentuating falciform ligament (the "falciform ligament sign") and free air confined in the intrahepatic fissure for the ligamentum teres (the "ligamentum teres sign") have been considered to be useful findings in patients with perforation of the duodenal bulb or stomach [28].

Posterior wall peptic ulcers most commonly perforate into the pancreas, resulting in pancreatitis or true abscess formation. Ulcers that perforate into the biliary tree or colon also may lead to fistula [29]. Abscess in the left lobe of the liver or spleen may result from posterior wall penetrating ulcers. Air trapped in the mesenteric folds is seldom seen in gastric perforation.

Gastric perforation associated with malignancy is rare (0.4–6%), occurring particularly with ulcerated masses, e.g. adenocarcinoma, lymphoma, and large gastrointestinal stromal tumours. Irregular wall thickening, submucosal mass, heaped-up ulcer craters, perivisceral soft-tissue extension, peritoneal spread, lymphadenopathy, and distal metastatic disease are highly suggestive of underlying malignancy [30].

Pneumoretroperitoneum is caused by perforation of descending horizontal duodenal tract; extraluminal free air or gas bubbles located only in the retroperitoneal space, in particular in the right anterior pararenal space, have been reported as a reliable CT finding for diagnosing duodenal perforation beyond the bulbar segment, where gas typically outlines the lateral border of the psoas muscle [31].

Anastomotic leaks may be detected at gastroenteric anastomoses. Leaks may also occur at the overseen proximal duodenal stump after Billroth II surgery or after Graham plication of perforated duodenal ulcers. The postoperative contrast examination may show contrast material outside the lumen of the bowel filling a collection or fistula. MDCT is useful for demonstrating the size and location of an abscess cavity or guiding percutaneous drainage of an abscess collection [32]. MDCT is very valuable in the diagnosis of gastroduodenal perforation: the use of three-dimensional reformatting is mandatory to improve the detection of the wall breach when it has not been shown on axial planes.

10.4 Intra-abdominal Free Air Due to Small Intestine Perforations

Perforation of the jejunum or ileum carries an incidence of 1 in 300–350,000 and accounts for 0.4% of cases of acute abdomen [16]. Presentation is nonspecific, consisting of abrupt onset persistent abdominal pain unresponsive to medical therapy which evolves into sepsis and peritonitis if left untreated; nausea and/or vomiting may be present due to intra-abdominal irritation, ileus, or obstruction. Fevers, tachycardia, and hypotension are more concerning features and indicate a more severely ill patient [4]. Whereas gastroduodenal perforation usually results in massive pneumoperitoneum, small bowel perforation accounts for the majority of the cases in which the amount of extraluminal air is too small to be detected by conventional radiography.

Perforation of the mesenteric small bowel can be due to different etiologies: in underdeveloped countries, infection is probably the most common cause, while in industrialized nations, perforation may be due to Crohn's disease, diverticulitis, foreign body, trauma, tumor, mechanical obstruction, primary ischemic event or iatrogenic causes [33–38].

CT findings related to intestinal perforation include the presence of free gas or fluid within the supra- and/or inframesocolic compartments, segmental bowel wall thickening, bowel wall discontinuity, extraluminal oral contrast, mottled extraluminal air bubbles or micropneumoperitoneum, stranding of the mesenteric fat, and abscess formation [34].

Pneumoperitoneum may be absent or too subtle to be detected, as noted in approximately half the cases. For this reason, images should be investigated for indirect findings including bowel wall thickening, mesenteric fluid and stranding, and ancillary findings indicative of the underlying cause such as a mass, an abscess, an incarcerated hernia, or a foreign body [19].

Inflammatory conditions of the small intestines could be considered in evaluating CT examinations of patients with suspected hollow viscus perforations. Crohn's disease and other inflammatory conditions and complications with the presence of abscesses must be accurately noted in location and distribution. A rare condition causing perforations almost localized and covered is represented by small bowel diverticulitis [35], in which wall thickening of the small bowel loop and an adjacent inflammatory mass containing air bubbles could be noted. Small bowel diverticula (Fig. 10.4) are rare and mostly asymptomatic, but they become clinically relevant when complications arise, such as diverticulitis [36].

In the case of evaluation of patients who underwent laparoscopic procedures more frequently such as cholecystectomies, the eventual intestinal perforation due to trocar injury leads to extensive pneumoperitoneum. In fact, small bowel injuries should be suspected when at CT examination a large or an increasing amount of free air is detected following laparoscopic procedures [35].

The small intestine has been reported as the most common site of perforation (59%) in intestinal lymphomas (Fig. 10.5) [38] especially when treated with

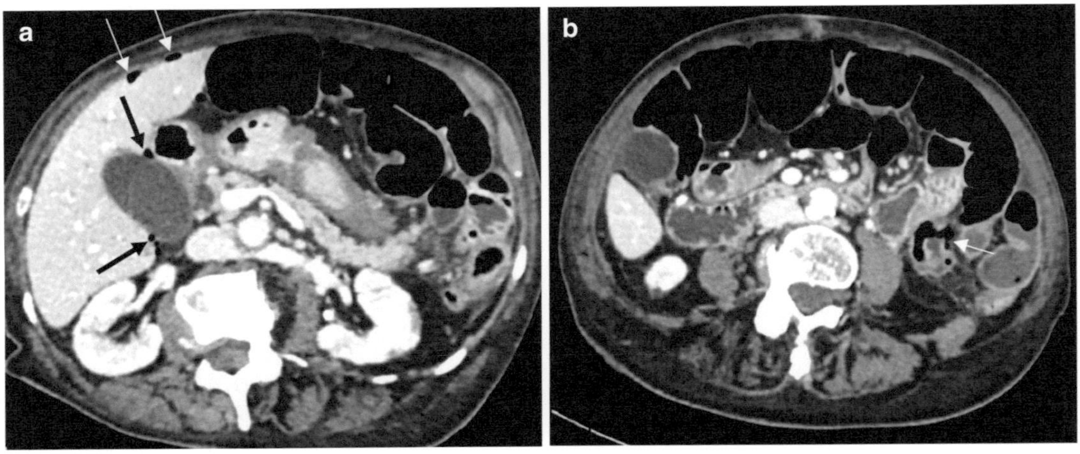

Fig. 10.4 MDCT of the abdomen. Axial scan. Evidence of very small air bubbles in the perihepatic space (white arrows, **a**) and in the pericholecystic space (black arrows, **a**). Evidence of free air in continuity to a jejunal diverticulum (white arrow, **b**). At surgery: perforation of jejunal diverticulum

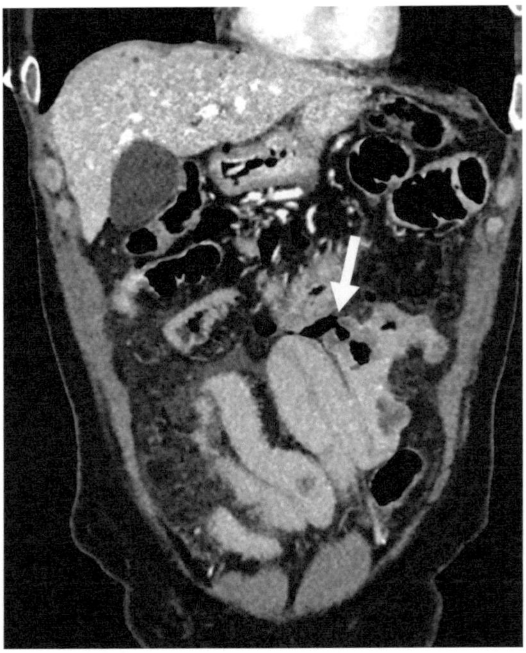

Fig. 10.5 MDCT of the abdomen. Coronal reconstruction. Female patient affected by B-cell lymphoma. Small bowel wall discontinuity with free intramesenteric air (arrow). Fluid and streaky density within the mesentery are also evident

chemotherapy and steroids, in posttransplant lymphoproliferative disorder and following radiation therapy, although adenocarcinomas, gastrointestinal stromal tumours, and metastases can also perforate. When tiny bubbles of free air are embedded in the omentum and mesentery, or if they are located in places such as the anterior peritoneal surface of the liver and among the bowel loops, CT images with the wide window setting can be useful for enhancing the sensitivity to detect this free air [39].

In addition to the presence of gastrointestinal tract perforation, concentrated free air bubbles in close proximity to the bowel wall may help determine the site of perforation because free air bubbles tend to be in the vicinity of the bowel wall from which they arise, and especially when the amount of air is small [1].

10.5 Intra-abdominal Free Air Due to Colorectal Perforation

Colorectal perforation carries the highest complication rate (55%) compared with other gastrointestinal perforation sites. This is related to the bacterial content of the large bowel that evokes bacterial peritonitis.

Nontraumatic colorectal perforation can be caused by inflammatory, neoplastic, or ischemic etiology as well as by iatrogenic injuries and as a postoperative complication [40, 41]. The perforation sites of the large intestine can frequently be correlated with their causes [23]. Malignant neoplasm, diverticulitis (in Western countries), blunt trauma, and ischemia are common causes of perforation on the left side of colonic loops. Inflammatory bowel disease, diverticulitis (in eastern countries), and penetrating trauma tend to be observed on the right side of the colonic loops. The cecum can be perforated in patients with mechanical colonic obstruction. Iatrogenic injuries usually involve the rectum and sigmoid colon [42, 43]: in diagnostic colonoscopy, the rectosigmoid is the most common site of perforation followed by the cecum, while post-polypectomy perforation, in therapeutic colonoscopy, occurs at the site of the excised polyp. A perforated site is typically a large anti-mesenteric tear of the colonic wall if it is caused by the shaft of the endoscope [43]. Patients with colonic or rectal perforation typically develop progressive abdominal pain, which is usually focal initially, but leads to peritonitis if untreated. Signs and symptoms are also dependent on the time of presentation. Patients who present late (days) after perforation are more likely to become systemically ill, whereas patients who present early may have only mild symptoms [44]. Stercoral perforation is related to a localized mucosal ulceration and ischemic pressure necrosis of the bowel wall for vascular occlusion, caused by a stercoraceous mass, most often involving the sigmoid or rectosigmoid. Risk factors include conditions leading to long-standing constipation, often in bedridden patients, such as drug-induced constipation, scleroderma, and an underlying obstructing colonic lesion such as neoplasm or stricture [45]. Direct CT findings of colorectal perforation include extraluminal gas (Fig. 10.6) and oral/rectal contrast, as well as wall discontinuity, faecal material looking like a "dirty" mass (Fig. 10.7) or foreign bodies protruding through the colonic wall or lying free within the abdominal cavity [46–48].

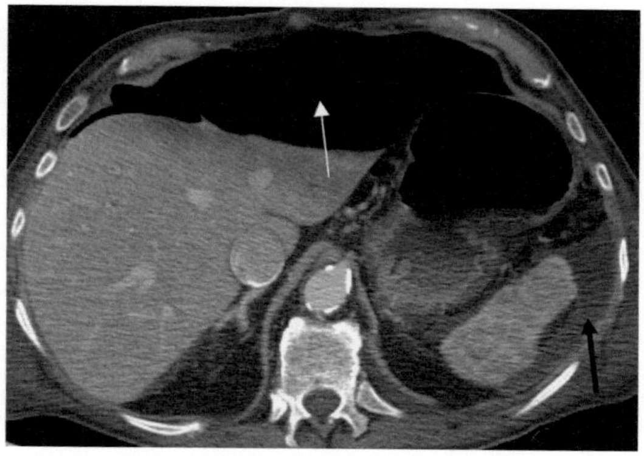

Fig. 10.6 MDCT of the abdomen, axial scan, showing the presence of a large amount of free intraperitoneal air (white arrow). Free fluid in the perisplenic region (black arrow) is also evident. At surgery: perforation of the colon

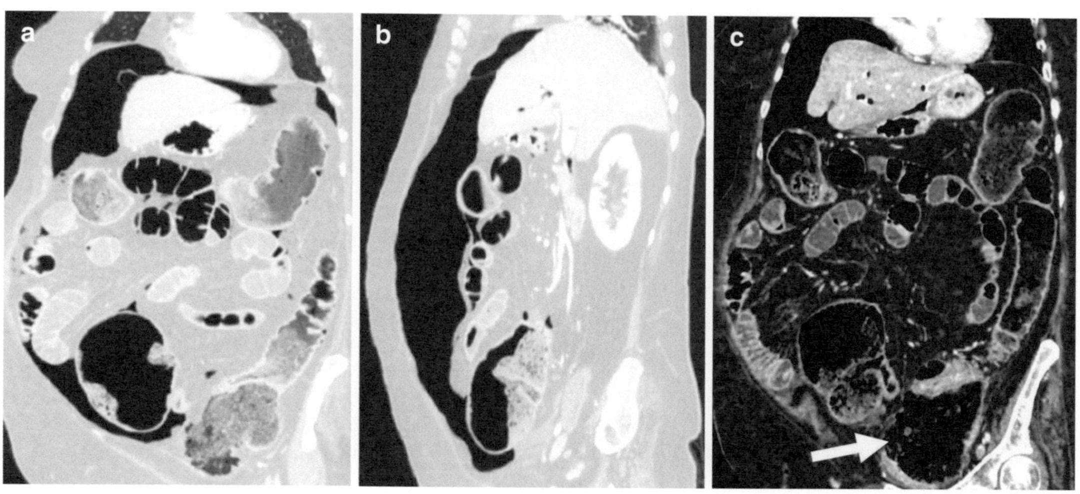

Fig. 10.7 MDCT of the abdomen. MPR reconstructions (coronal reconstruction, **a**; sagittal reconstruction, **b**; coronal reconstruction, **c**). Presence of a large amount of free intra-abdominal air. Faecal material looking like a "dirty" mass is evident in the pelvis (arrow). At surgery: stercoral sigmoid perforation

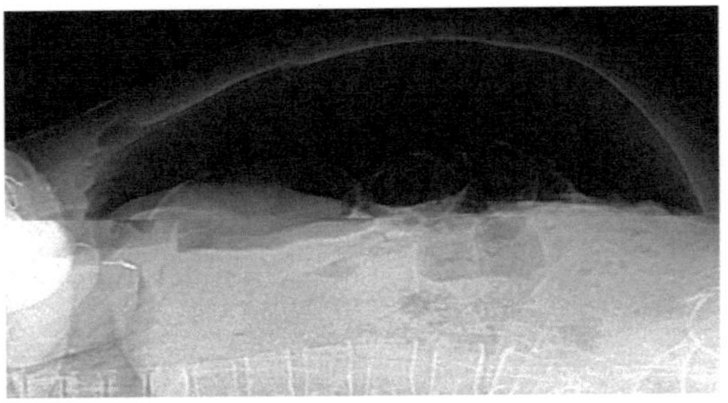

Fig. 10.8 MDCT of the abdomen. Scout view (laterolateral projection). Evidence of massive pneumoperitoneum

Colonic perforation can appear as a massive pneumoperitoneum (Fig. 10.8) with free gas all over the abdomen and pelvis. If free gas is present only in the pelvis, the colon (and not the small bowel) is the usual site of perforation.

Associated CT findings of colorectal perforation include bowel wall thickening, pericolonic fat stranding, free fluid, abnormal wall enhancement, abscess, and the presence of a localized inflammatory mass adjacent to the colon [49, 50].

Perforation of intraperitoneal colon, i.e. of cecum, transverse, sigmoid, and upper 2/3 of the rectum, leads to pneumoperitoneum. Rupture of the retroperitoneal ascending and descending colon results in pneumoretroperitoneum at the right and left anterior pararenal spaces respectively. Posterior rectal perforations can dissect superiorly and cause bilateral pneumoretroperitoneum.

10.6 Conclusion

Gastrointestinal perforations are a frequent cause of acute abdominal symptomatology for patients in the emergency department who requires immediate medical care. The condition is life-threatening. Chances of recovery improve with an early diagnosis and treatment. The diagnosis of alimentary tract perforation on CT examination is generally based on the identification of extraluminal leakage and consequent inflammatory reaction around the perforation site. Extraluminal air is the major specific sign of alimentary tract perforation and MDCT is the most reliable imaging modality for detecting even small amounts of free air.

MDCT allows us to identify the site of gastrointestinal perforations and to determine the most predictive signs in this diagnosis. CT provides superb anatomical detail and diagnostic specificity by directly imaging the intestinal wall, detecting secondary signs of bowel disease within the surrounding mesentery, and depicting even small amounts of extraluminal air or oral contrast leakage into the peritoneal cavity.

References

1. Kim SH, Shin SS, Jeong YY, Heo SH, Kim JW, Kang HK. Gastrointestinal tract perforation: MDCT findings according to the perforation sites. Korean J Radiol. 2009;10(1):63–70. https://doi.org/10.3348/kjr.2009.10.1.63.
2. Winek TG, Mosely HS, Grout G, Luallin D. Pneumoperitoneum and its association with ruptured abdominal viscus. Arch Surg. 1988;123(6):709–12. https://doi.org/10.1001/archsurg.1988.01400300051008.
3. Mularski RA, Ciccolo ML, Rappaport WD. Nonsurgical causes of pneumoperitoneum. West J Med. 1999;170(1):41–6.
4. Tanner TN, Hall BR, Oran J. Pneumoperitoneum. Surg Clin North Am. 2018;98(5):915–32. https://doi.org/10.1016/j.suc.2018.06.004.
5. Williams NM, Watkin DF. Spontaneous pneumoperitoneum and other nonsurgical causes of intraperitoneal free gas. Postgrad Med J. 1997;73(863):531–7. https://doi.org/10.1136/pgmj.73.863.531.
6. Mularski RA, Sippel JM, Osborne ML. Pneumoperitoneum: a review of nonsurgical causes. Crit Care Med. 2000;28(7):2638–44. https://doi.org/10.1097/00003246-200007000-00078.
7. Ustek S, Boran M, Kismet K. Benign pneumoperitoneum after colonoscopy. Case Rep Med. 2010;2010:631036. https://doi.org/10.1155/2010/631036.
8. Goenka AH, Shah SN, Remer EM. Imaging of the retroperitoneum. Radiol Clin North Am. 2012;50(2):333–55, vii. https://doi.org/10.1016/j.rcl.2012.02.004.
9. Welikumbura S, Pham T, Jain A, Williams M, Smart P. Approach to the patient with pneumoretroperitoneum. ANZ J Surg. 2021;91(1–2):206–7. https://doi.org/10.1111/ans.16061.
10. American College of Radiology. ACR appropriateness criteria, 2006. American College of Radiology Web site. http://www.acr.org Expert Panel on Acute Abdominal Pain and Fever or Suspected Abdominal Abscess. Accessed 21 June 2024.

11. Stoker J, van Randen A, Laméris W, Boermeester MA. Imaging patients with acute abdominal pain. Radiology. 2009;253(1):31–46. https://doi.org/10.1148/radiol.2531090302.
12. Grassi R, Romano S, Pinto A, Romano L. Gastroduodenal perforations: conventional plain film, US and CT findings in 166 consecutive patients. Eur J Radiol. 2004;50(1):30–6. https://doi.org/10.1016/j.ejrad.2003.11.012.
13. Smith JE, Hall EJ. The use of plain abdominal x rays in the emergency department. Emerg Med J. 2009;26(3):160–3. https://doi.org/10.1136/emj.2008.059113.
14. Pitiakoudis M, Zezos P, Oikonomou A, Kirmanidis M, Kouklakis G, Simopoulos C. Spontaneous idiopathic pneumoperitoneum presenting as an acute abdomen: a case report. J Med Case Rep. 2011;5:86. https://doi.org/10.1186/1752-1947-5-86.
15. Cadenas Rodríguez L, Martí de Gracia M, Saturio Galán N, Pérez Dueñas V, Salvatierra Arrieta L, Garzón Moll G. Utilidad de la tomografía computarizada multidetector para identificar la localización de las perforaciones gastrointestinales [Use of multidetector computed tomography for locating the site of gastrointestinal tract perforations]. Cir Esp. 2013;91(5):316–23. Spanish. https://doi.org/10.1016/j.ciresp.2012.06.004.
16. Pouli S, Kozana A, Papakitsou I, Daskalogiannaki M, Raissaki M. Gastrointestinal perforation: clinical and MDCT clues for identification of aetiology. Insights Imaging. 2020;11(1):31. https://doi.org/10.1186/s13244-019-0823-6.
17. Merchea A, Cullinane DC, Sawyer MD, Iqbal CW, Baron TH, Wigle D, Sarr MG, Zielinski MD. Esophagogastroduodenoscopy-associated gastrointestinal perforations: a single-center experience. Surgery. 2010;148(4):876–880; discussion 881–882. https://doi.org/10.1016/j.surg.2010.07.010.
18. Sánchez-Pernaute A, Aguirre EP, Talavera P, Valladares LD, de la Serna JP, Mantilla CS, de León AR, Torres A. Laparoscopic approach to esophageal perforation secondary to pneumatic dilation for achalasia. Surg Endosc. 2009;23(5):1106–9. https://doi.org/10.1007/s00464-008-0114-7.
19. Del Gaizo AJ, Lall C, Allen BC, Leyendecker JR. From esophagus to rectum: a comprehensive review of alimentary tract perforations at computed tomography. Abdom Imaging. 2014;39(4):802–23. https://doi.org/10.1007/s00261-014-0110-4.
20. Sdralis EIK, Petousis S, Rashid F, Lorenzi B, Charalabopoulos A. Epidemiology, diagnosis, and management of esophageal perforations: systematic review. Dis Esophagus. 2017;30(8):1–6. https://doi.org/10.1093/dote/dox013.
21. Gagliardi N, Stavolo C, De Gennaro A. Esophageal perforation: assessment with multidetector row computed tomography. In: Romano L, Pinto A, editors. Imaging of alimentary tract perforation, chapter 4. Springer International Publishing Switzerland; 2015. p. 23–7.
22. Liguori C, Gagliardi N, Saturnino PP, Pinto A, Romano L. Multidetector computed tomography of pharyngo-esophageal perforations. Semin Ultrasound CT MR. 2016;37(1):10–5. https://doi.org/10.1053/j.sult.2015.10.005.
23. Ghahremani GG. Radiologic evaluation of suspected gastrointestinal perforations. Radiol Clin North Am. 1993;31(6):1219–34.
24. Lui FY, Davis KA. Gastroduodenal perforation: maximal or minimal intervention? Scand J Surg. 2010;99(2):73–7. https://doi.org/10.1177/145749691009900205.
25. Pinto A, Miele V, Schillirò ML, Nasuto M, Chiaese V, Romano L, Guglielmi G. Spectrum of signs of pneumoperitoneum. Semin Ultrasound CT MR. 2016;37(1):3–9. https://doi.org/10.1053/j.sult.2015.10.00.
26. Faggian A, Berritto D, Iacobellis F, Reginelli A, Cappabianca S, Grassi R. Imaging patients with alimentary tract perforation: literature review. Semin Ultrasound CT MR. 2016;37(1):66–9. https://doi.org/10.1053/j.sult.2015.09.006.
27. Hainaux B, Agneessens E, Bertinotti R, De Maertelaer V, Rubesova E, Capelluto E, Moschopoulos C. Accuracy of MDCT in predicting site of gastrointestinal tract perforation. AJR Am J Roentgenol. 2006;187(5):1179–83. https://doi.org/10.2214/AJR.05.1179.
28. Oguro S, Funabiki T, Hosoda K, Inoue Y, Yamane T, Sato M, Kitano M, Jinzaki M. 64-slice multidetector computed tomography evaluation of gastrointestinal tract perforation site: detectability of direct findings in upper and lower GI tract. Eur Radiol. 2010;20(6):1396–403. https://doi.org/10.1007/s00330-009-1670-5.
29. Chung KT, Shelat VG. Perforated peptic ulcer-an update. World J Gastrointest Surg. 2017;9(1):1–12. https://doi.org/10.4240/wjgs.v9.i1.1.
30. Toprak H, Yilmaz TF, Yurtsever I, Sharifov R, Gültekin MA, Yiğman S, Yildiz Ş. Multidetector CT findings in gastrointestinal tract perforation that can help prediction of perforation site accurately. Clin Radiol. 2019;74(9):736.e1–7. https://doi.org/10.1016/j.crad.2019.06.005.
31. Romano S, Somma C, Sciuto A, Jutidamrongphan W, Pacella D, Esposito F, Puglia M, Mauriello C, Khanungwanitkul K, Pirozzi F. MDCT findings in gastrointestinal perforations and the predictive value according to the site of perforation. Tomography. 2022;8(2):667–87. https://doi.org/10.3390/tomography8020056.
32. Vecchione D, Russo G, Niola R. Role of Multidetector Row Computed Tomography in the diagnosis of gastroduodenal perforation. In: Romano L, Pinto A, editors. Imaging of alimentary tract perforation, chapter 5. Springer International Publishing Switzerland; 2015. p. 29–36.
33. Hines J, Rosenblat J, Duncan DR, Friedman B, Katz DS. Perforation of the mesenteric small bowel: etiologies and CT findings. Emerg Radiol.

2013;20(2):155–61. https://doi.org/10.1007/s10140-012-1095-3.
34. Zissin R, Osadchy A, Gayer G. Abdominal CT findings in small bowel perforation. Br J Radiol. 2009;82(974):162–71. https://doi.org/10.1259/bjr/7877257.
35. Graña L, Pedraja I, Mendez R, Rodríguez R. Jejunoileal diverticulitis with localized perforation: CT and US findings. Eur J Radiol. 2009;71(2):318–23. https://doi.org/10.1016/j.ejrad.2008.04.023.
36. Romano S. Small bowel perforations: imaging findings. In: Romano L, Pinto A, editors. Imaging of alimentary tract perforation, chapter 6. Springer International Publishing Switzerland; 2015. p. 37–44.
37. Reginelli A, Liguori P, Perrotta V, Annunziata G, Pinto A. Computed tomographic detection of toothpick perforation of the jejunum: case report and review of the literature. Radiol Case Rep. 2016;2(1):17–21. https://doi.org/10.2484/rcr.v2i1.52.
38. Katz DS, Scheirey CD, Bordia R, Hines JJ, Javors BR, Scholz FJ. Computed tomography of miscellaneous regional and diffuse small bowel disorders. Radiol Clin North Am. 2013;51(1):45–68. https://doi.org/10.1016/j.rcl.2012.09.004.
39. Lacalamita MC, Moschetta M, Mancini ME, Scardapane A, Angelelli G. Role of CT in the diagnosis of jejunal-ileal perforations. Radiol Med. 2014;119(9):651–7. https://doi.org/10.1007/s11547-013-0375-7.
40. Gong XH, Zhuang ZG, Zhu J, Feng Q, Xu JR, Qian LJ. Differentiation of cancerous and inflammatory colorectal perforations using multi-detector computed tomography. Abdom Radiol (NY). 2017;42(9):2233–42. https://doi.org/10.1007/s00261-017-1134-3.
41. Kothari K, Friedman B, Grimaldi GM, Hines JJ. Nontraumatic large bowel perforation: spectrum of etiologies and CT findings. Abdom Radiol (NY). 2017;42(11):2597–608. https://doi.org/10.1007/s00261-017-1180-x.
42. Araújo AV, Santos C, Contente H, Branco C. Air everywhere: colon perforation after colonoscopy. BMJ Case Rep. 2017;2017:bcr2016219178. https://doi.org/10.1136/bcr-2016-219178. PMID: 28325724.
43. Ponticiello G, Di Nuzzo L, Saturnino PP. Corectal perforation: assessment with MDCT. In: Romano L, Pinto A, editors. Imaging of alimentary tract perforation, chapter 9. Springer International Publishing Switzerland; 2015. p. 61–6.
44. Okamoto T, Ikenoue T, Matsui K, Miyazaki M, Tsuzuku Y, Nishizawa Y, Kubota M. Free air on CT and the risk of peritonitis in peritoneal dialysis patients: a retrospective study. Ren Fail. 2014;36(10):1492–6. https://doi.org/10.3109/0886022X.2014.958953.
45. Heffernan C, Pachter HL, Megibow AJ, Macari M. Stercoral colitis leading to fatal peritonitis: CT findings. AJR Am J Roentgenol. 2005;184(4):1189–93. https://doi.org/10.2214/ajr.184.4.0184118.
46. Saturnino PP, Pinto A, Liguori C, Ponticiello G, Romano L. Role of multidetector computed tomography in the diagnosis of colorectal perforations. Semin Ultrasound CT MR. 2016;37(1):49–53. https://doi.org/10.1053/j.sult.2015.10.007.
47. Singh JP, Steward MJ, Booth TC, Mukhtar H, Murray D. Evolution of imaging for abdominal perforation. Ann R Coll Surg Engl. 2010;92(3):182–8. https://doi.org/10.1308/003588410X12664192075251.
48. Liguori P, Reginelli A, Sparano A, Ruggiero G, Pinto A. Pneumoretroperitoneum associated with "dirty mass": an unusual case of rectal perforation. Radiol Case Rep. 2016;2(1):22–3. https://doi.org/10.2484/rcr.v2i1.51.
49. Ishikawa D, Takehara Y, Takata A, Takamura K, Sato H. Combination of dirty mass volume and APACHE II score predicts mortality in patients with colorectal perforation. World J Emerg Surg. 2021;16(1):17. https://doi.org/10.1186/s13017-021-00359-y.
50. Baş S, Zarbaliyev E. The role of dual-energy computed tomography in locating gastrointestinal tract perforations. Cureus. 2021;13(5):e15265. https://doi.org/10.7759/cureus.15265.

Intraperitoneal Bleeding

11

Claudio Carrubba, Felice D'Antuono,
Dimitri Garifalos, Francesco Giurazza,
and Raffaella Niola

11.1 Introduction

Hemoperitoneum is a common finding in abdominal traumatism [1–3]. Nontraumatic hemoperitoneum is a less frequent situation, requiring prompt diagnosis and treatment. The clinical scenario of abdominal haemorrhage is variable as it may be associated with severe abdominal pain and distention, decreased haematocrit level, or, more rarely, hypovolemic shock [4]. Non traumatic intraperitoneal bleeding may occur spontaneously or may be iatrogenic. Spontaneous haemorrhage has various possible causes, including high-vascularised neoplasms, vascular lesions, spontaneous rupture of spleen, gynaecological conditions. Iatrogenic causes are related to both surgical procedures performed to the peritoneal cavity, and minimally invasive percutaneous or endovascular procedures (Fig. 11.1). In both cases, patients on anticoagulant therapy have a higher risk of developing bleeding.

Supplementary Information The online version contains supplementary material available at https://doi.org/10.1007/978-3-031-84849-0_11.

C. Carrubba · F. D'Antuono · D. Garifalos
F. Giurazza · R. Niola (✉)
Vascular and Interventional Radiology Department, AORN "A. Cardarelli", Naples, Italy
e-mail: claudio.carrubba@aocardarelli.it; felice.dantuono@aocardarelli.it; d.garifalos@studenti.unina.it; francesco.giurazza@aocardarelli.it; raffaella.niola@aocardarelli.it

L. Romano et al. (eds.), *CT of Non-Traumatic Body Emergencies*,
https://doi.org/10.1007/978-3-031-84849-0_11

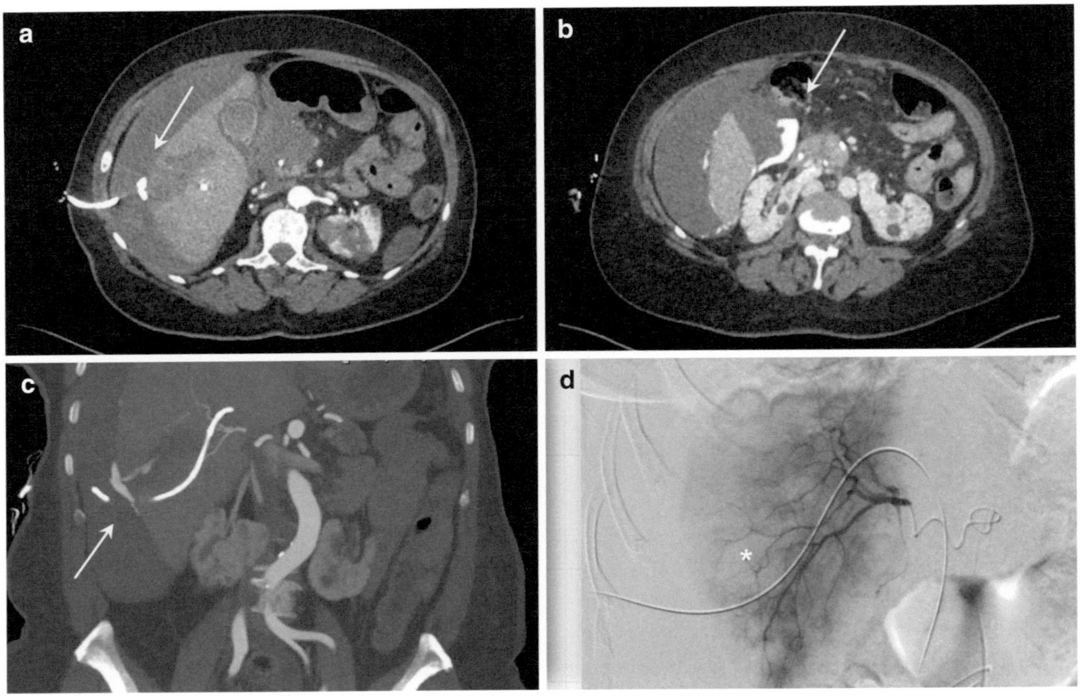

Fig. 11.1 CECT imaging on axial (**a**, **b**) and MIP coronal plans (**c**) of hepatic laceration along with evidence of large subcapsular hepatic hematoma and active extravasation (arrow), caused by the placement of a transhepatic biliary drainage. (**d**) DSA imaging of bleeding embolization (asterisk) performed with PVA particles (300–500 μm)

11.2 Radiology in Abdominal Haemorrhage

The first imaging approach in patients with abdominal symptoms (particularly if lacking unequivocal signs of peritonitis) is generally ultrasonography. On ultrasound, hemoperitoneum may appear iso- or hyperechoic compared to kidney or liver, or even hypo-anechoic, complicating its differentiation from non-bloody ascitic fluid; more commonly, it looks like a collection with heterogeneous echoes, occasionally presenting fluid-fluid levels. The second step (the first in clinically severe patients) is computed tomography (CT), currently the diagnostic gold standard for detecting abdominal bleeding. CT with intravenous contrast medium (IVCM) injection (contrast-enhanced CT; CECT) offers significant advantages in sensitivity, specificity, and comprehensive imaging compared to ultrasound. Additionally, it often identifies the bleeding site and assesses ongoing haemorrhage, determining whether its origin is arterial or venous [5]. Although technical protocols vary significantly between different centres and machines, an exemplary model is provided in Table 11.1.

No universal consensus exists on optimal contrast dosage calculation: some formulas consider body weight, others body surface area, and more complex personalized approaches integrate biometric parameters with heart rate. Additionally, the Italian Society of Medical Radiology (SIRM) emphasizes the importance of the minimal dose compatible with accurate examination to prevent potential contrast-induced nephrotoxicity [6].

11.2.1 Role of Dual Energy CT

In recent years, Dual Energy CT has gained popularity. Utilising X-rays at two different voltages, it takes advantage of different attenuation effects to decompose tissue components within the scan

Table 11.1 CT technical protocol model for a 64 slices machine

CT technical protocol	
Scan and reconstruction parameters	
Scout	AP, LL
Patient positioning	Supine, arms above the head
FOV	Whole abdomen, from diaphragm to pubic symphysis
Scan direction	Craniocaudal
kVp	120 kV
mA	180–230 mA (automatically adjusted)
Pitch	0.984:1
Slice thickness	3 mm
Interval	3 mm
ROI positioning for bolus-tracking	Diaphragmatic aorta (threshold 100–150 HU)
Scan delay	Arterial phase: 10 s Portal/venous phase: 30–35 s after arterial phase Delayed phase (optional): 180–300 s after the injection
Reconstruction slice thickness	1–2 mm
IVCM parameters	
Concentration	High, 350–400 mgI/mL
Volume	90–130 mL
Flow rate	3-4 mL/s

IVCM IntraVenous Contrast Medium; *AP* AnteroPosterior projection; *LL* LateroLateral projection

volume. Special reconstruction software can provide "virtual non-contrast" images by subtracting iodine attenuation effects, reducing artefacts from highly attenuating materials (calcifications, clips, metallic coils), and creating iodine distribution maps. This allows omitting the baseline scan phase, reducing acquisition time, contrast medium dosage, and radiation exposure while maintaining diagnostic accuracy comparable to conventional triphasic CECT protocols [7–9].

11.2.2 Radiological Signs of Hemoperitoneum

CT identification of hemoperitoneum relies on a few but nearly unequivocal radiological signs. The main finding is the presence of intraperitoneal blood, which varies in density over time: initially, on a pre-contrast phase, it shows a density of about 35–40 HU due to high protein content; subsequently, as coagulation occurs, density increases to 60–70 HU, sometimes surrounded by a hypodense halo indicative of peritoneal oedema or clot lysis.

In patients with coagulopathies, the "haematocrit effect" is common, showing a fluid-fluid level within the hematoma due to blood component sedimentation. Blood may migrate within peritoneal spaces and the retroperitoneum over time, generally moving cranio-caudally from the origin site [3, 4]. The higher density hematoma often indicates the bleeding site, termed the "sentinel clot sign." Additionally, identifying hyperdense material within a recent surgical bed, near an aneurysm, or a tumour aids in pinpointing the bleeding source. Mesenteric haemorrhage typically forms a triangular shape (triangle sign) between intestinal loops, which may have thickened walls [1, 2].

11.2.3 Active Bleeding Detection

A crucial role of CT is identifying active bleeding during acquisition, visualized as contrast medium extravasation increasing in volume and changing shape across different phases.

Acquiring a pre-contrast or "baseline" phase allows to identification of haematomas or haemoperitoneum, while also recognizing calcifications/metallic material, or prosthetic elements that might mimic contrast medium extravasation in subsequent phases.

While arterial bleedings are usually apparent in the first post-contrast phase, in patients with large aneurysms or with significantly reduced cardiac output, they may only manifest in the venous phase, leading to misinterpretation and incorrect management of patients that might benefit from prompt endovascular or surgical intervention.

Similarly to contrast extravasation, Pas (pseudoaneurysms) are located within hematomas, but they usually exhibit well-defined margins and stable morpho-volumetry across scan phases, appearing as hypodense on the unenhanced scan, and showing a density comparable to their donor arteries on post-contrast phases; they also require urgent endovascular treatment [10]. Despite CECT being the optimal non-invasive diagnostic tool for bleeding assessment, severe hemodynamic instability (i.e. marked hypotension/shock) or spontaneous bleeding tamponade may prevent contrast medium extravasation detection. In such cases, arteriographic (or endoscopic for suspected gastrointestinal bleeding) examinations are indicated for diagnostic and potentially therapeutic purposes. Similarly, angiography could not detect bleeding showed on CT; in this case, Interventional Radiologist may proceed with an "ex adiuvantibus" embolization of suspicious arterial branches based on CT data.

11.3 Intraperitoneal Bleeding of Hepato-Biliary Origin

Spontaneous hepatic haemorrhage is a rare occurrence, caused by a rupture in the liver tissue without external injury. Patients typically exhibit vague symptoms, most commonly abdominal pain, malaise, and vomiting. Quick diagnosis and treatment are critical, typically involving multiple specialties such as interventional radiology, hepatology, and surgery. The primary cause of nontraumatic liver bleeding is the rupture of highly vascular tumours, both malignant (hepatocarcinoma, angiosarcoma, hemangioendothelioma, hepatoblastoma, rhabdoid sarcoma, and metastases) and benign (hemangioma, adenoma, focal nodular hyperplasia, nodular regenerative hyperplasia, biliary cystadenoma, angiomyolipoma, liver angiosarcomas, and simple cysts) [11]. Hepatocellular carcinoma (HCC) is the most frequent cause of spontaneous haemorrhage, with 10% of cases presenting with bleeding [12, 13]; commonly associated with cirrhosis or chronic liver inflammation. Patients with large or peripherally located tumours, lacking normal overlying tissue, are more prone to rupture [14]. Haemorrhage may result from rupture of parasitic arteries or veins (such as the inferior phrenic), traumatic laceration of a superficial tumour due to minor blunt abdominal trauma, or respiratory movements. Moreover, fast-growing tumours with central necrosis can develop an enlarging central hematoma due to compromised internal neo-vasculature. Imaging findings for such haemorrhages can vary, from minor intrahepatic bleeding to subcapsular haemorrhage and rupture through the hepatic capsule into the peritoneum (leading to subcapsular hematomas, hemoperitoneum, and active peri-tumoral bleeding; Fig. 11.2). Hemoperitoneum related to benign neoplasm is most linked to hepatic adenoma, particularly the inflammatory subtype, being the second highest risk factor for hepatic bleeding [15]. These tumours are frequently found in women of childbearing age with a history of prolonged oral contraceptive use or oestrogen therapy and in men using anabolic steroids [16]. Recognizing a hepatic adenoma is crucial due to the risk of life-threatening haemorrhage. Other potential etiologies include conditions affecting vascular integrity, such as connective tissue disorders (e.g. amyloidosis, systemic lupus erythematosus), polyarteritis nodosa, HELLP syndrome, acute fatty liver of pregnancy, and peliosis hepatis. The main goal of emergency treatment for subcapsular hepatic hematoma is to achieve lasting haemostasis, regardless of the underlying cause. For patients with hypervascular tumours, further definitive oncological intervention should be considered. Treatment typically involves arterial embolization to obtain haemostasis, with hepatectomy reserved for tumour-bearing patients after liver function assessment.

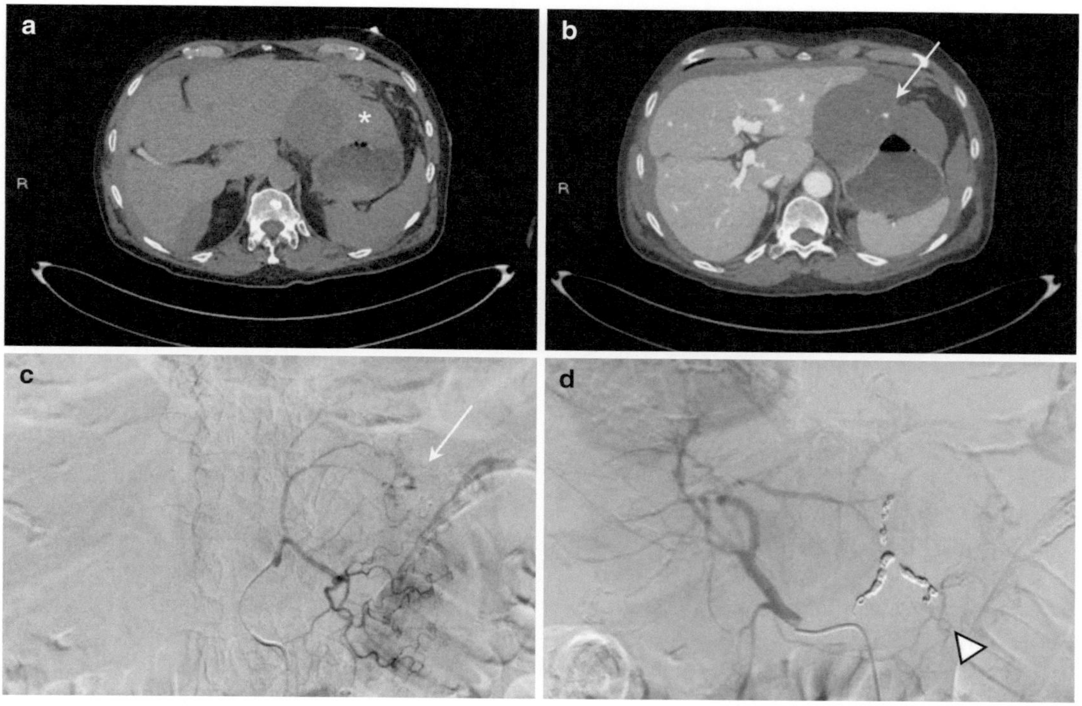

Fig. 11.2 Ruptured HCC. (**a**) Unenhanced CT image shows perihepatic and perisplenic fluid, with an area of slightly higher attenuation (asterisk) indicative of a "sentinel clot" along the left hepatic lobe. (**b**) CECT shows the origin of the bleeding, a breach in an HCC of left hepatic lobe, as well as active extravasation (arrow). (**c**) DSA imaging through a 2.7F microcatheter confirms the findings (**d**) DSA after embolization with coils shows resolution of the bleeding (arrowhead)

11.4 Intraperitoneal Bleeding of Splenic Origin

Non-traumatic Spleen rupture (NTSR) with consequent haemorrhage was first described by Rokitansky in 1861 [17] and is a very rare condition, with a not yet fully understood pathogenesis [18]. NTRS can occur in 1 or 2 phases: single-stage rupture manifests as an acute pattern rapidly progressing to haemorrhagic shock; in the two-stage rupture, a subcapsular hematoma is first formed and the symptomatology is sub-acute combining episodes of epigastric or left hypochondrium pain radiating to the left shoulder (Kehr's sign) [19]. In over 90% of cases, NTSR occurs in patients with an underlying pathological condition causing splenomegaly, typically of viral infectious origin (EBV, CMV), hematologic disorders (leukemias, lymphomas), or neoplastic processes (haemangiomatosis, angiosarcoma, and metastatic tumours) and metabolic disorders (amyloidosis, Gaucher's disease). The most commonly observed symptoms are severe abdominal pain in the left hypochondrium or diffuse throughout the abdomen, peritonitis, and signs of hypotension/shock [20]. CT findings include splenomegaly, heterogeneous enhancement of the organ (sometimes rupture is a late sequela of an infarction), capsular lacerations, hemoperitoneum, intraparenchymal or subcapsular hematoma, and possible active contrast extravasation. In the differential diagnosis of bleeding splenic tumour, the possibility of Peliosis must be kept in mind: this rare condition of unknown cause results in the development of blood-filled cavities in the spleen and, more rarely, the liver, lymph nodes, and bone marrow. These mass-like lesions demonstrate contrast pooling and may also rupture into the peritoneal cavity [21, 22]. Accessory spleens have been reported to occur in 10% to 31% of individuals complications, such as haemorrhage or rupture, are well recognized in the primary spleen, but have only rarely been reported in accessory spleen [23, 24]. Similarly to traumatic spleen injuries, accurate patient management requires grading of the organ damage [25]; indeed, treatment may be conservative, surgical, or transcatheter embolization, depending on the grade of splenic injury and the underlying disease [26].

11.5 Intraperitoneal Bleeding from Visceral Arteries Abnormalities

Non-traumatic abdominal bleeding from visceral arteries, particularly due to aneurysms and pseudoaneurysms, represents an important cause of mortality because they are frequently misdiagnosed and detected only after the rupture has occurred; approximately 25% of visceral artery aneurysms (VAAs) reported in the literature present with rupture [27]. VAA is characterized by a focal dilation exceeding 50% of the expected diameter of the artery, involving all three layers of the vessel; they are rare, with reported incidences ranging from 0.01% to 0.2%, predominantly affecting the splenic artery (60%, Fig. 11.3), followed by the renal artery (22%) and hepatic artery (10%) [28]. Conversely, pseudoaneurysm (PA) results from a contained rupture, lined by adventitia or perivascular tissues rather than all three layers of the artery wall [29]. Spontaneous rupture is a common clinical presentation, particularly in splenic artery aneurysms (3% to 10% incidence), where mortality rates can reach 36% [30]. Pregnancy increases the risk of rupture due to hormonal influences. Superior mesenteric artery aneurysms and pseudoaneurysms, although less prone to rupture, still pose a substantial mortality risk (around 30%), with thrombosis and subsequent intra-abdominal bleeding being more frequent complications [31]. Although Color-Doppler Ultrasound could be useful for early detection, CT angiography remains the gold standard; typical findings include the visualization of a well-defined contrast-filled sac with enhancement similar to the adjacent main artery in both arterial and venous phases, with or without thrombosis, adjacent organ compression, and signs of rupture such as hemoperitoneum, the focal anomaly of the aneurysm walls (blebs) and abrupt change in diameter of the parent vessel [32, 33]. Depending on the extent of thrombosis, the sac may show low attenuation areas, usually in the periphery. Postprocessing with maximum-intensity projection (MIP) and volume rendering (VR) better demonstrates the aneurysm and its origin and improves detection. Furthermore, CTA identifies associated anatomical arterial variations and provides a road map for intervention, generally represented by endovascular techniques, such as coil embolization or stent placement, offering minimally invasive approaches with lower procedural risks compared to traditional surgical repair.

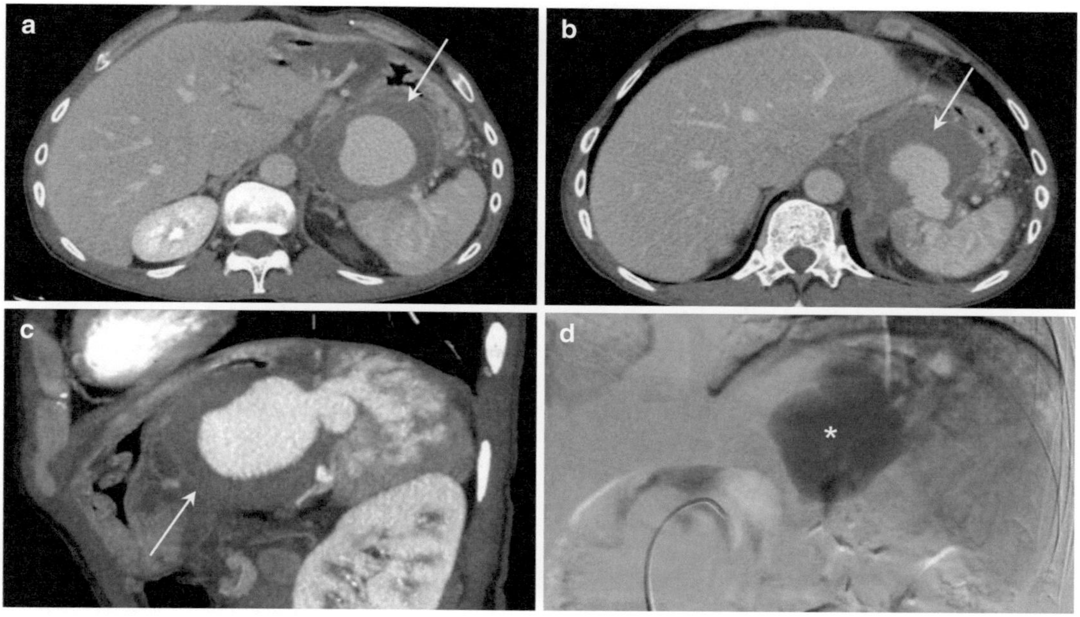

Fig. 11.3 Giant bleeding aneurysm of the splenic artery. CECT imaging in axial (**a**, **b**) and sagittal plans (**c**) show a giant splenic artery aneurysm (arrow), with intraluminal peripheral thrombus (**d**) DSA imaging of the aneurysm (asterisk) through a 5Fr C1 catheter

11.6 Other Causes of Intraperitoneal Bleeding

The most frequent gynaecological causes of hemoperitoneum are ectopic pregnancy (EP) and ruptured ovarian cysts. Other less common causes include endometriosis, which can cause bleeding from endometrial implants, and uterine rupture, often associated with myometrial defects or placenta percreta during labour [34]. EP is a prevalent cause of hemoperitoneum in women of reproductive age; The CT appearance of EP is an extrauterine (most usually adnexal) cystic-like structure with some degree of peripheral enhancement, representing a gestational sac, with or without hemoperitoneum. Haemorrhagic ovarian cysts, particularly corpus luteal cysts, are another common cause of hemoperitoneum; in particular, the increased vascularity of the ovary during the luteal phase may predispose to rupture and bleeding. On CT imaging, a ruptured corpus luteum presents as a shrunken ovarian cyst with a discontinuous, thickened wall. Surrounding hyperattenuating "sentinel clot" may indicate active or recent haemorrhage. Active bleeding may appear as serpiginous or jet-like contrast extravasation adjacent to the cyst, typically observed in the portal phase due to intermittent or venous haemorrhage [35]. The right ovary is more frequently involved due to the protective "cushioning" effect of the sigmoid colon on the contralateral ovary. Peptic ulcer disease is an uncommon but significant cause of intraperitoneal haemorrhage [36]. Abdominal CECT has been effective in visualizing extravasation of contrast material into the gastric lumen, aiding in the diagnosis of active bleeding from gastric ulcers. The use of radiopaque oral contrast material can obscure bleeding sites, emphasizing the importance of appropriate imaging techniques for accurate diagnosis. Pancreatitis-related haemorrhage has a mortality rate exceeding 50%, typically arising from vascular complications as well as pseudoaneurysms or splenic vein thrombosis with segmental portal hypertension, and splenic rupture, often in association with pancreatic pseudocysts [37]. While massive haemorrhage associated with chronic pancreatitis is uncommon, the development of arterial pseudoaneurysms can occur through several mechanisms, such as severe inflammation and enzymatic autodigestion of peripancreatic arteries, or erosion of a pseudocyst into nearby vessels. CT scans may demonstrate features of acute or chronic pancreatitis, bleeding into pancreatic collections or pseudocysts, or vascular complications like pseudoaneurysms and venous thrombosis. Iatrogenic causes of hemoperitoneum related to prior surgery or percutaneous interventions as biopsies or drainages are not infrequent (from 18% to 34% of hemoperitoneum) [38] but generally easy to suspect for the clinical presentation (Hb drop, blood in drainages, abdominal pain) and often of minor entities in cases of percutaneous procedures [39]; CT is essential to identify the site of bleeding and to guide the following treatment.

11.7 The Role of Angiography

Angiographic examination with haemostatic purpose has gained a prominent role in the management of hemodynamically stable patients with active arterial bleeding [40].

Arteriography is a generally well-tolerated procedure, usually performed under local anaesthesia. It is based on the cannulation of a peripheral artery, generally the common femoral artery or the radial artery, via ultrasound-guided puncture and subsequent placement of an introducer sheath (4–5 F) using the Seldinger technique. Under fluoroscopic guidance, through the introducer, a vascular catheter (65–100 cm – 4-5 F) is used to selectively catheterize the suspected vessels. Digital Subtraction Angiogram (DSA) acquisitions are performed during the administration of iodinated contrast medium, preferably via an injector pump, to reduce the operator's exposure to radiation [41]. Angiography systems use some auto-exposure control software to optimize exposure parameters, such as mA, kV, and spectral filtration [42]; operators have a tableside workstation console to dynamically change FOV, framerate (averagely 7,5 fps) or scan protocol.

Acquisitions are made on different projections searching for direct signs of bleeding, such as contrast medium extravasation or pseudoaneurysms, and indirect signs, such as wall irregularities or branch amputations.

It is not always possible to visualize bleeding through a panoramic angiography, especially if it is distal or to a very little extent; in this case, a super-selective catheterization of distal branches by a microcatheter (2.0–2.7 F), with the coaxial technique increases diagnostic sensitivity [43].

Modern angiography systems are equipped with Cone-Beam Computed Tomography (CBCT) technology, based on the rotation of the radiographic tube around the patient; CBCT allows for intraoperative three-dimensional acquisitions, even during the administration of contrast medium [44]. This has been proved to be useful in the endovascular treatment of bleeding, especially in situations where the accuracy of two-dimensional angiographic images is compromised by the presence of hyperdense material (surgical clips, coils, etc.) at the site of interest [45].

Once the bleeding site is identified, interventional radiologists can choose among a large and different number of tools to achieve hemostasis. The choice of the embolic agent is based both on the angiographic findings and the evaluation of the targeted area, as well as on the operator's personal expertise.

References

1. Lubner M, Menias C, Rucker C, Bhalla S, Peterson CM, Wang L, Gratz B. Blood in the belly: CT findings of hemoperitoneum. Radiographics. 2007;27:109–25.
2. Gomez E, Horton K, Fishman EK, Johnson PT. CT of acute abdominopelvic hemorrhage: protocols, pearls, and pitfalls. Abdom Radiol. 2022;47:475–84.
3. Taourel P (ed) CT of the acute abdomen. 2011. https://doi.org/10.1007/978-3-540-89232-8.
4. Furlan A, Fakhran S, Federle MP. Spontaneous abdominal hemorrhage: causes, CT findings, and clinical implications. Am J Roentgenol. 2009;193:1077–87.
5. Ballesta M, Piqueras R, Brugger S, Estellés Lerga P. Non-traumatic spontaneous abdominal haemorrhage. Radiología (English Edition). 2023;65:S73–80.
6. Walgraeve M-S, Pyfferoen L, Van De Moortele K, Zanca F, Bielen D, Casselman JW. Implementation of patient-tailored contrast volumes based on body sur-

face area and heart rate harmonizes contrast enhancement and reduces contrast load in small patients in portal venous phase abdominal CT. Eur J Radiol. 2019;121:108630.
7. Sun H, Hou X-Y, Xue H-D, Li X-G, Jin Z-Y, Qian J-M, Yu J-C, Zhu H-D. Dual-source dual-energy CT angiography with virtual non-enhanced images and iodine map for active gastrointestinal bleeding: image quality, radiation dose and diagnostic performance. Eur J Radiol. 2015;84:884–91.
8. Shaqdan KW, Parakh A, Kambadakone AR, Sahani DV. Role of dual energy CT to improve diagnosis of non-traumatic abdominal vascular emergencies. Abdom Radiol. 2019;44:406–21.
9. Walter SS, Schneeweiß S, Maurer M, Kraus MS, Wichmann JL, Bongers MN, Lescan M, Bamberg F, Othman AE. Virtual non-enhanced dual-energy CT reconstruction may replace true non-enhanced CT scans in the setting of suspected active hemorrhage. Eur J Radiol. 2018;109:218–22.
10. Saad NEA, Saad WEA, Davies MG, Waldman DL, Fultz PJ, Rubens DJ. Pseudoaneurysms and the role of minimally invasive techniques in their management. Radiographics. 2005;25:S173–89.
11. Mortele KJ, Cantisani V, Brown DL, Ros PR. Spontaneous intraperitoneal hemorrhage. Radiol Clin North Am. 2003;41:1183–201.
12. Dewar GA, Griffin SM, Ku KW, Lau WY, Li AKC. Management of bleeding liver tumours in Hong Kong. Br J Surg. 2005;78:463–6.
13. Zhu LX, Wang GS, Fan ST. Spontaneous rupture of hepatocellular carcinoma. Br J Surg. 2005;83:602–7.
14. Kanematsu M, Imaeda T, Yamawaki Y, Seki M, Goto H, Sone Y, Iinuma G, Mochizuki R, Doi H. Rupture of hepatocellular carcinoma: predictive value of CT findings. Am J Roentgenol. 1992;158:1247–50.
15. Molina EG, Schiff ER. Benign solid lesions of the 104. Liver. In: Schiff ER, Sorrell MF, Maddrey WC, editors. Schiff's diseases of the liver. 8th ed. Philadelphia: Lippincott-Raven; 1999. p. 1245–67.
16. Rabe T, Feldmann K, Grunwald K, Runnebaum B. Liver tumours in women on oral contraceptives. Lancet. 1994;344:1568–9.
17. Rokitansky KF, Rokitansky KF. Zwei Fall von spontaner zerreissung der Milz aus der neuesten zeit. Wochenblatt des zeitschift der K.K. Gesselschaft der Aerzte in Wien. 1861;17:42.
18. Aubrey-Bassler FK, Sowers N. 613 cases of splenic rupture without risk factors or previously diagnosed disease: a systematic review. BMC Emerg Med. 2012;12:11.
19. Söyüncü S, Bektaş F, Cete Y. Traditional Kehr's sign: left shoulder pain related to splenic abscess. Ulus Travma Acil Cerrahi Derg. 2012;18:87–8.
20. Mourato Nunes I, Pedroso AI, Carvalho R, Ramos A. Chronic lymphocytic leukaemia and spontaneous rupture of spleen. BMJ Case Reports bcr-2017-221692. 2018.
21. Fujikawa T, Hachiya J, Korenaga T, et al. A case of splenic peliosis. Rinsho Hoshasen. 1986;31:115–58.
22. Tsuda K, Nakamura H, Murakami T, Kozuka T, Yoshii M, Isozaki K, Tsukahara Y, Takami M, Hanada M. Peliosis of the spleen with intraperitoneal hemorrhage. Abdom Imaging. 1993;18:283–5.
23. Halpert B, Györkey F. Lesions observed in accessory spleens of 311 patients. Am J Clin Pathol. 1959;32:165–8.
24. Texeira MB, Hardin WJ. Spontaneous rupture of an accessory spleen. Am Surg. 1974;40:491–3.
25. Ouazzani LCE, Jadib A, Siradji H, Boutachali R, Tabakh H, Siwane A, Touil N, Kacimi O, Chikhaoui N. Spontaneous splenic rupture during infection of cytomegalovirus. A case report. Radiol Case Rep. 2022;17:1741–4.
26. Gayer G, Zandman-Goddard G, Kosych E, Apter S. Spontaneous rupture of the spleen detected on CT as the initial manifestation of infectious mononucleosis. Emerg Radiol. 2003;10:51–2.
27. Rossi M, Krokidis M, Kashef E, Peynircioglu B, Tipaldi MA. CIRSE standards of practice for the endovascular treatment of visceral and renal artery aneurysms and pseudoaneurysms. Cardiovasc Intervent Radiol. 2024;47:26–35.
28. Johal M, Kalaravy M, Ali F, Barve R, Ahmed A, Francis CT, Harky A. Evolving diagnostic and therapeutic options for visceral artery aneurysms. Ann Vasc Surg. 2021;76:488–99.
29. Jia F, Xia G, Zhu Q, Yu S, Hu N, Zhang H. Hepatic artery pseudoaneurysm caused by chronic pancreatitis: case report and literature review. Medicine (Baltimore). 2023;102:e32834.
30. Rinaldi LF, Brioschi C, Marone EM. Endovascular and open surgical treatment of ruptured splenic artery aneurysms: a case report and a systematic literature review. J Clin Med. 2023;12:6085.
31. Kawata A, Imai K, Tamura Y, Kaida T, Mima K, Nakagawa S, Hayashi H, Yamashita Y, Ikeda O, Baba H. Gastrointestinal: superior mesenteric vein aneurysm treated using interventional radiology. J Gastroenterol Hepatol. 2022;37:1209.
32. Saba L, Anzidei M, Lucatelli P, Mallarini G. The multidetector computed tomography angiography (MDCTA) in the diagnosis of splenic artery aneurysm and pseudoaneurysm. Acta Radiol. 2011;52:488–98.
33. Grierson C, Uthappa MC, Uberoi R, Warakaulle D. Multidetector CT appearances of splanchnic arterial pathology. Clin Radiol. 2007;62:717–23.
34. Tonolini M, Foti PV, Costanzo V, Mammino L, Palmucci S, Cianci A, Ettorre GC, Basile A. Cross-sectional imaging of acute gynaecologic disorders: CT and MRI findings with differential diagnosis—part I: corpus luteum and haemorrhagic ovarian cysts, genital causes of haemoperitoneum and adnexal torsion. Insights Imaging. 2019;10:119.
35. Sato F, Uramoto S, Amagai T. Teardrop owl eye appearance in enhanced MDCT for diagnosis of ecto-

pic pregnancy with tubal rupture. Radiology Case Reports. 2023;18:2577–80.
36. Almadi MA, Lu Y, Alali AA, Barkun AN. Peptic ulcer disease. Lancet. 2024;404:68–81.
37. Chagas LA, Albuquerque KS, Soares LE, Machado DC, De Moraes Antunes P, Stern JJ, Dos Santos Romão D, Morais E, Rodrigues da Cunha Fonseca B, Horvat N. Beyond the revised Atlanta classification: a comprehensive review of the imaging assessment of acute pancreatitis and its complications. Abdom Radiol (NY). 2024;50:423. https://doi.org/10.1007/s00261-024-04425-2.
38. Scheinfeld MH, Schwartz C, Jain VR, Goldman IA. Non-traumatic hemoperitoneum in the ED setting: causes, characteristics, prevalence and sex differences. Abdom Radiol. 2021;46:441–8.
39. Atwell TD, Spanbauer JC, McMenomy BP, Stockland AH, Hesley GK, Schleck CD, Harmsen WS, Welch TJ. The timing and presentation of major hemorrhage after 18,947 image-guided percutaneous biopsies. Am J Roentgenol. 2015;205:190–5.
40. Sgalambro F, Giordano AV, Carducci S, et al. The role of interventional radiology in hepatic and renal hemorrhage embolization: single center experience and literature review. Acta Biomedica Atenei Parmensis. 2021;92:e2021405.
41. Rees CR, Duncan BWC. Get the Lead off our backs! Tech Vasc Interv Radiol. 2018;21:7–15.
42. Miraglia R, Maruzzelli L, Cortis K, Tafaro C, Gerasia R, Parisi C, Luca A. Digital subtraction angiography during transjugular intrahepatic portosystemic shunt creation or revision: data on radiation exposure and image quality obtained using a standard and a low-dose acquisition protocol in a flat-panel detector-based system. Abdom Imaging. 2015;40:1808–12.
43. Chatani S, Inoue A, Ohta S, et al. Transcatheter arterial embolization for postoperative bleeding following abdominal surgery. Cardiovasc Intervent Radiol. 2018;41:1346–55.
44. Minami Y, Murakami T, Kitano M, Sakurai T, Nishida N, Kudo M. Cone-beam CT angiography for hepatocellular carcinoma: current status. Dig Dis. 2015;33:759–64.
45. Kamei S, Yamamoto T, Okada H, Kinbara Y, Takahata K, Horikawa Y, Yamada K, Kitajima Y, Hattori T, Suzuki K. Transcatheter arterial embolization using cone-beam computed tomography during angiography and automated vessel detection software for obscure colonic diverticular hemorrhage after unsuccessful endoscopic clipping: a report of two cases. Intervent Radiol. 2021;6:4–8.

Mechanical and Paralitic Ileus 12

Giuseppina Dell'Aversano Orabona,
Francesca Dell'Aversano Orabona, Gaspare Oliva,
Luigi Barbuto, Roberto Ronza,
and Francesca Iacobellis

12.1 Introduction

12.1.1 Physiopathology and Causes

Bowel obstruction is a clinical condition resulting from a mechanical or functional blockage preventing the normal passage of intestinal contents [1, 2]. Obstructions can be *complete* (high-grade), where no material passes, or *incomplete* (low-grade), allowing partial passage of fluids and gas [3]. Intestinal obstruction leads to abdominal distention because of gas and fluid accumulation in the intestine, above the point of transit interruption and lumen contraction [4]. The increased distension determines increased intraluminal pressure with consequent hyper-peristalsis in the first stage, whereas it leads to the opposite effect in the later period. Intraluminal stasis of contents favors bacterial overgrowth in line with the deterioration in peristalsis, leading to an improved passage of these bacteria with their toxins into the blood and lymphatic circulation and a real risk of sepsis in every untreated obstruction. Therefore, if the distension process persists, the resulting increase in intramural pressure within the bowel wall impairs both venous and arterial circulation; this may lead to perforation and necrosis [5]. Approximately 75% of small bowel obstructions (SBO) occur in the small intestine [1]. Adhesions, hernias, and malignancies are the most common causes in Western populations [2]. Large bowel obstructions (LBO) are less frequent, primarily affecting the elderly, with cancer being the leading cause, followed by diverticulitis, volvulus, and adhesions [4].

12.1.2 Clinical Features

Clinical findings for intestinal obstruction lack sensitivity and specificity for definitive diagnosis or identifying complications [2]. Classic symptoms include colicky abdominal pain, vomiting, distension, and absolute constipation. Additionally, unstable vital signs and acidotic blood gases may indicate bowel ischemia. While absolute constipation and abdominal pain are typically predominant in large bowel obstruction (LBO), vomiting tends to occur earlier and more frequently in small bowel obstruction (SBO). Other symptoms vary based on the underlying cause [3].

G. Dell'Aversano Orabona (✉) · G. Oliva
L. Barbuto · R. Ronza · F. Iacobellis
Department of General and Emergency Radiology, "Antonio Cardarelli" Hospital, Naples, Italy
e-mail: giuseppina.dellaversanoorabona@aocardarelli.it; gaspare.oliva@aocardarelli.it; luigi.barbuto@aocardarelli.it; roberto.ronza@aocardarelli.it; francesca.iacobellis@aocardarelli.it

F. Dell'Aversano Orabona
Department of Surgical Science, Anesthesia and Intensive Care, University of Naples "Federico II", Naples, Italy

L. Romano et al. (eds.), *CT of Non-Traumatic Body Emergencies*,
https://doi.org/10.1007/978-3-031-84849-0_12

12.1.3 Imaging

The role of the radiologist is to detect the presence of intestinal obstruction, and define its location, causes, and complications [5]. Plain abdominal radiography continues to be the initial examination in these patients due to its wide availability and relatively low cost, allowing the detection of main bowel obstruction signs as maximally dilated loop measurement (normal lumen diameter: <3 cm in small bowel; <6 cm in the colon; <9 cm in cecum), more than two air-fluids levels, air-fluids levels wider than 2.5 cm, and air-fluids levels differing more than 2 cm in height from one another within the same bowel loop, as well as increased representation of the valvulae conniventes in early stages, or reduced representation in later stages [3]; an additional sign is the paucity of small-bowel gas or the gasless abdomen, due to fluid, rather than gas, filling the dilated small bowel, in the high-grade SBO or in a SBO complicated by a closed-loop obstruction [2]. Nevertheless, radiographs are diagnostic in 50–60% and have been demonstrated to be highly sensitive only for high-grade obstructions. For these reasons, this modality is used as a bridge for further imaging examination needed to assist the therapeutic decision. Standard CT emerged two decades ago as the preeminent imaging modality for preoperative evaluation in bowel obstruction (sensitivity of 90–96%; specificity of 96%; accuracy of 95%), resulting in the best modality for early detection of strangulation and for determining which patients would benefit from conservative management and which patients would benefit from immediate surgical intervention [3].

12.1.4 Treatment and Prognosis

Surgical intervention is necessary for severe obstructions, patients unresponsive to nasogastric decompression, and those with complications like strangulation, vascular compromise, or perforation [2].

Bowel obstruction is a critical emergency. Small bowel obstruction (SBO) is a leading cause of morbidity and mortality, often requiring emergency laparotomy [6]. Large bowel obstruction (LBO) outcomes vary based on underlying cause and comorbidities, but early intervention is crucial. Mortality rates rise significantly with bowel perforation or necrosis (15–30%) [7].

12.2 CT Protocol

There is a consensus on the use of CT for evaluating patients with bowel obstruction. Numerous studies have reported that CT is a valuable tool not only for diagnosing the presence of SBO and LBO, but also for detecting signs of bowel ischemia, identifying the transition point (if present), determining the underlying etiology, and predicting the need for surgical intervention [8]. The CT acquisition typically includes the intravenous administration of iodinated contrast media to assess the bowel wall thickness and enhancement pattern, detect the presence of necrosis, evaluate the enhancement of mesenteric vessels, and identify any concomitant findings [9]. The best phase after intravenous contrast media administration for the study of the intestine is obtained at 60–70 seconds in the portal venous phase; the acquisition volume should include the entire abdomen from the plane just above the diaphragm to a plane just below the symphysis pubis [8]. Oral contrast administration is not recommended in the first instance, since oral contrast does not commonly aid in the diagnosis and may make more difficult the wall enhancement evaluation [9].

12.3 Mechanical Ileus

Only the CT examination may answer the key questions in the emergency setting:

1. *Is obstruction present and at what level?*
2. *What is the cause of the obstruction?*
3. *Is severe or complicated obstruction present?*

Answers to these key questions should represent the radiologist's goal. This information can help guide the surgeon in making critical decisions regarding both operative and nonoperative management, assessing the condition of the bowel loops, and evaluating the risk of complications [1].

12.3.1 First Question: Is the Obstruction Present (and at What Level)?

In the emergency setting, radiologists are called to early detect the presence of a critical condition such as bowel obstruction. There are three main key signs found on CT scan, leading to the correct diagnosis that an obstruction of the bowel is present.

12.3.1.1 Dilatation of Bowel Loops

The first and the major CT finding of bowel occlusion is represented by proximal dilatation of loops with distal decompression [1–3]. CT scans allow precise measurement of the bowel loop caliper by assessing the outer-to-outer diameter on cross-sectional images (Fig. 12.1) [5]. Pathological dilation is defined as >2.5–3 cm for the small bowel, >6 cm for the colon, and >9 cm for the cecum [1–3]. It is important to report the maximum bowel diameter, particularly at the cecum in cases of large bowel obstructions, indeed a cecum diameter >9 cm increases the risk of diastatic perforation [4, 5]. As with X-rays, CT scans reveal air-fluid levels within dilated loops and may show the "string of beads" sign, caused by fluid-filled loops with trapped gas in folds between valvulae conniventes [2]. Confirming bowel obstruction requires demonstrating collapsed loops distal to the obstruction [1, 3].

12.3.1.2 Transition Point

The Transition Zone (TZ) is identified by the point where dilated proximal loops pass into collapsed distal loops, which represents the point of the mechanical or functional obstruction, impeding the normal transit of endoluminal contents. CT cross-sectional imaging accurately identifies the obstruction site by locating the transition zone (TZ) between dilated and nondilated bowel (Fig. 12.2). Starting at the anus and tracing proximally allows for a comprehensive assessment of the large bowel, even in the presence of concurrent small bowel dilation caused by an incompetent ileocecal valve. For higher small bowel obstructions (SBO), tracing antegrade from the stomach aids TZ identification [1, 5, 9]. The presence of the small bowel feces sign, typically found at the TZ, is highly specific for SBO [3]. The most effective tool for detecting the TZ is the

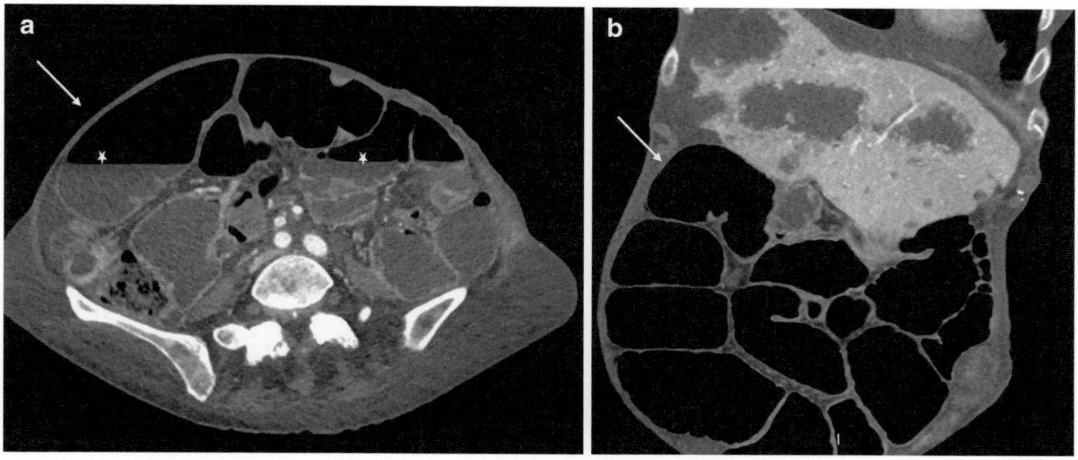

Fig. 12.1 Dilatation of bowel loops. (**a**) Axial and (**b**) coronal CT images in venous phase of a male patient with large bowel obstruction sustained by descendent colon adenocarcinoma with liver metastasis. On CT scans is possible to obtain the precise evaluation of loop dilatation (arrows) measuring from the outer wall to the outer and to identify air-fluid levels (stars) in their context

acquisition technique itself. By acquiring thin-section CT data with near-isotropic voxels, it becomes possible to perform multiplanar and three-dimensional anatomical evaluations, enabling simpler and quicker identification of the transition point [3].

12.3.1.3 Small Bowel Feces Sign

Small bowel feces sign occurs when intraluminal particulate content, gas, and stasis produces a feces-like appearance within the dilated small bowel lumen. This phenomenon is attributed to bacterial overgrowth and partial dehydration of enteric contents caused by stagnant intraluminal flow [3, 9]. The most important finding to remember is that the small feces sign occurs proximal to the obstruction and can localize the exact point of obstruction, so it is considered a good marker for the detection of TZ [5], particularly when associated with distal bowel collapse (Fig. 12.3).

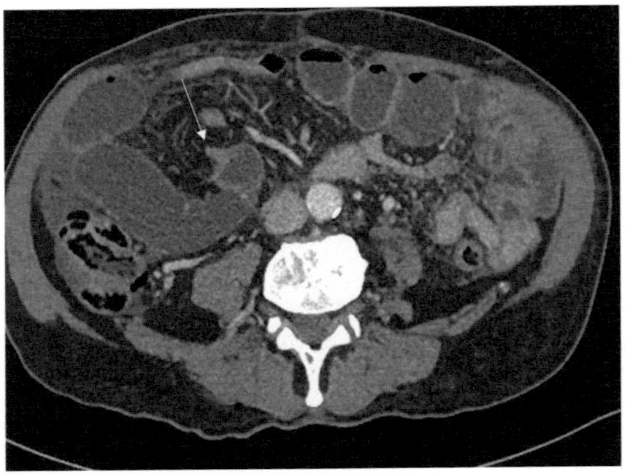

Fig. 12.2 Transition point. Axial CT scan in venous phase of a female patient with small bowel obstruction caused by postoperative adhesive bands. The CT examination shows the point of change in loop's caliper (arrow)

12.3.2 Second Question: What Is the Cause of Obstruction?

Many causes may sustain a bowel obstruction, generally classified as causes of SBO and LBO (Table 12.1) or as *intrinsic* (conditions affecting the loop), *intraluminal* (condition in the lumen), and *extrinsic* causes (condition starting out of the bowel).

Each condition shows specific CT findings that may be used in association with the three main key signs described above, to first detect the presence of bowel obstruction and then to identify the underlying cause.

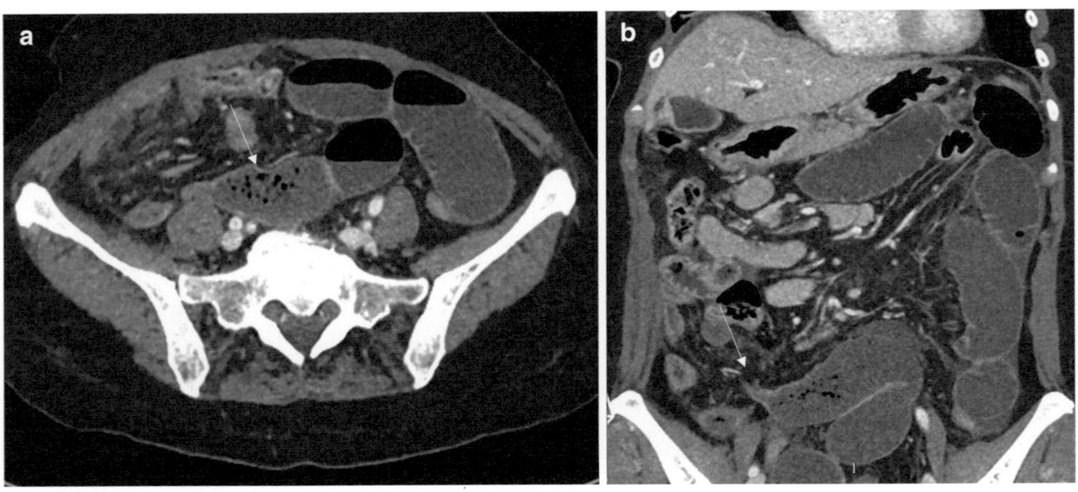

Fig. 12.3 Small Feces Sign. (**a**) Axial CT images in venous phase show the presence of intraluminal particulate contents, gas, and stasis with a feces-like appearance in the dilated small bowel lumen (arrow); (**b**) in the coronal CT view is possible to note how the small feces sign occurs proximal to the obstruction, localizing the exact point of obstruction as potential marker of the transition point (arrow)

Table 12.1 Cause of intestinal obstruction

Small bowel obstruction	Large bowel obstruction
Adhesion	Colorectal cancer
Hernias (external and internal)	Diverticulitis
Neoplasm (extraintestinal and primary)	Volvulus
Crohn's disease	Crohn's disease
Gallstones	Endometriosis
Malrotation	Ischemic strictures
Duplication cyst	Radiation
Diverticulitis	Hernia
Infection	Adhesion
Hematoma	Fecal impaction
Ischemic strictures	Foreign body
Intussusception	
Endometriosis	
Radiation—Foreign body	

The answer to our question (*what is the cause of obstruction?*) is almost always in the transition point [3].

12.3.2.1 Intrinsic Causes

Crohn Disease Up to 80% of patients with CD present with inflammatory behavior, while 5% to 28% have stricturing disease. However, more than 50% of patients with CD develop stricturing or penetrating complications within the first 10 years after diagnosis [10–13]. The bowel obstruction can occur in the small or in the large bowel as a result of the acute presentation of the disease. This is characterized by bowel luminal narrowing secondary to the transmural acute inflammatory process, determining the reduction of loop caliper and mechanical obstruction (Fig. 12.4). It can be also a manifestation of a long-standing disease, which usually results in fibrotic stenosis of affected segments. It is common to recognize the principal CT findings of Crohn's disease at the level of the transition point: the mural hyperenhancement, the fat halo sign as a result of submucosal fat deposition, the bowel wall thickening, the comb sign as a result of engorgement of the vasa recta, the perienteric fat stranding [3, 4].

Neoplasia Primary neoplastic causes of bowel obstructions are possible and less frequent in the small bowel than in the large bowel. Large bowel obstruction is provoked by cancer in about 60% of cases [14]. When a neoplastic intestinal mass presents as a bowel obstruction, it is typically in an advanced state, and appears as asymmetric, irregular mural thickening at the transition point (Fig. 12.5). In this case, it is important to evaluate the presence of lymphadenopathies or distant metastasis. It is important to remember that small bowel involvement by metastatic cancer is more common than involvement by primary neoplasms, frequently in the form of peritoneal carcinomatosis, which is suggested when extrinsic serosal disease involving the small bowel wall is seen in association with a transition point [3, 4].

Volvulus Volvulus and diverticular disease are responsible for other 30% of bowel occlusion [15]. Volvulus is the twisting of the intestine causing obstruction. Twists exceeding 360° typically require surgical intervention. Sigmoid volvulus is more common than cecal volvulus (60–75% vs. 25–33%) with transverse colon and splenic flexure volvulus being rare (1%). A mobile redundant colon on a mesentery and a fixed point about which the colon can twist represents the major predisposing factor leading to a colonic volvulus. Sigmoid volvulus commonly occurs in the elderly, who have an elongated and chronically dilated sigmoid colon [3]. The most sensitive CT findings on cross-sectional images are the presence of a single transition point in the sigmoid and disproportionate enlargement of the sigmoid (Fig. 12.6).

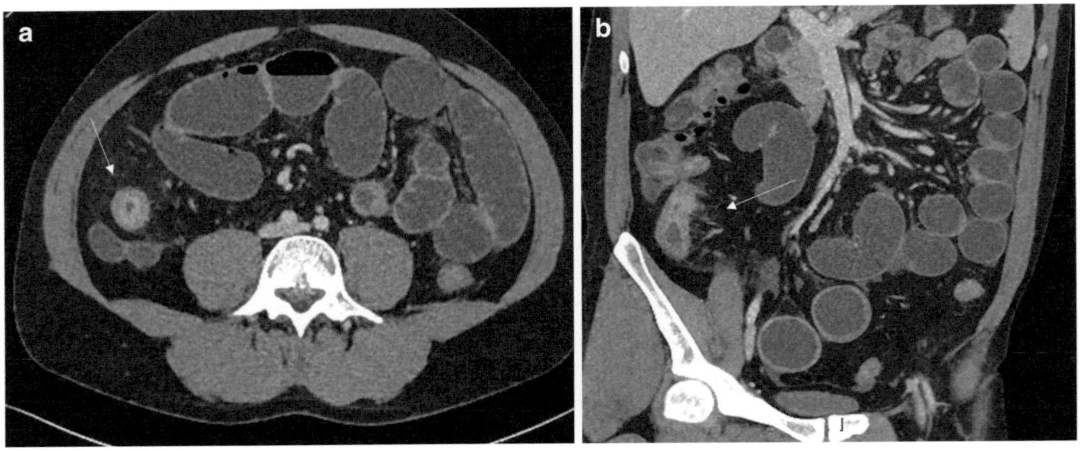

Fig. 12.4 Crohn's disease in a young male patient. (**a**) On axial CT image in the venous phase is possible to identify the bowel luminal narrowing secondary to the transmural inflammatory thickening with mural hyperenhancement (arrow) determining reduction of loop caliper and mechanical obstruction. (**b**) The coronal CT image in the venous phase clearly shows the presence of a comb sign (arrow) as a result of engorgement of the vasa recta and the perienteric fat stranding

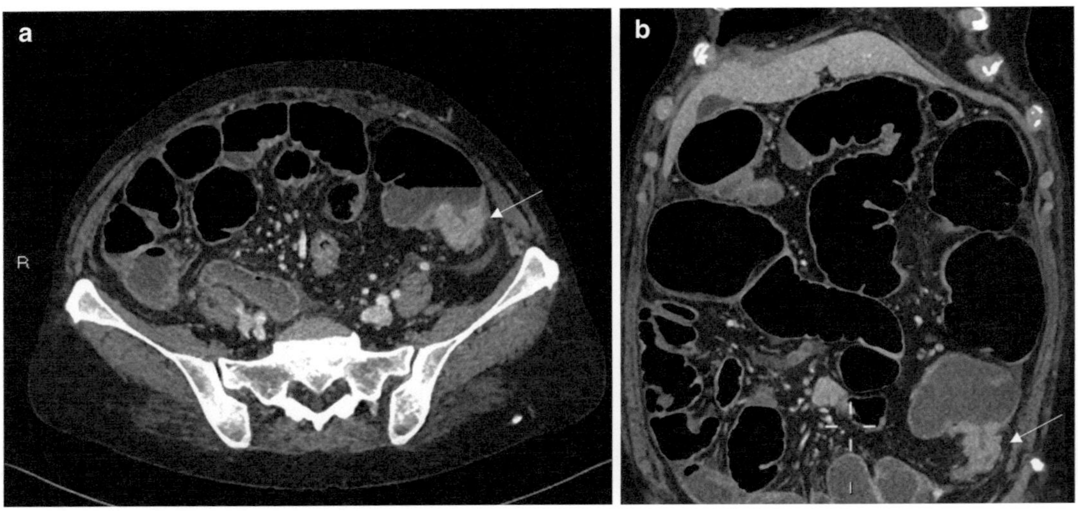

Fig. 12.5 Neoplasm of the large bowel in a 69-year-old female patient. (**a**) The axial and (**b**) coronal CT images in the venous phase show an irregular mural thickening at the transition point, characterized by contrast enhancement and determining a solid neoplastic-based stenosis with contraction of the lumen caliper in the descendent tract of the large bowel

In the sigmoid volvulus, the *coffee bean sign* describes the presence of an air-filled closed loop of the colon, whereas the two side parts of the bean represent the gas-filled segments of the dilated bowel creating an inverted U-shape, whereas the central cleft of the bean represents the double thickness of opposed bowel walls [16]. The *whirl sign*, the appearance of spiraled loops of collapsed bowel with enhancing engorged vessels radiating from the twisted bowel, is often evident at the point of obstruction. Also, a *"beak" sign* can be found at the point of twisting [4].

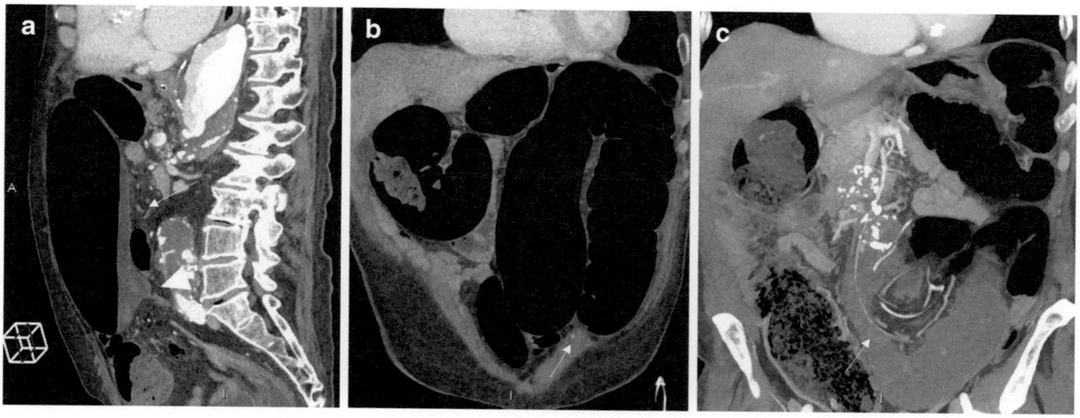

Fig. 12.6 Sigmoid volvulus in elderly male patient. (**a**) The sagittal CT image in the venous phase shows the presence of a transition point in the sigmoid (arrowhead) and disproportionate enlargement of the sigmoid tract of the large bowel (arrow). (**b**) On the coronal CT view in the venous phase is possible to detect the coffee bean sign (arrow) with two side parts of the bean represented by the gas-filled segments of the dilated bowel creating an inverted U-shape and the central cleft of the bean made of the double thickness of opposed bowel walls. (**c**) The MIP reconstruction of the coronal CT image in the venous phase demonstrates the appearance of spiraled and engorged vessels radiating from the twisted bowel (arrow)

Diverticulitis Although less common (10% of all cases of LBO) [15], acute diverticulitis may result in bowel obstruction due to bowel wall edema and pericolonic inflammation. High-grade obstruction is less common in the setting of acute diverticulitis, while, more commonly, obstruction occurs in the setting of multiple episodes of diverticulitis, which causes narrowing and stricture formation. CT findings at the transition point will be characterized by segmental, symmetric bowel wall thickening with hyperemia, which is typically longer in extension than malignant lesions. Pericolonic inflammation and fat stranding are hallmarks of diverticulitis. If the inflammation is severe, intramural and extramural abscesses, as well as perforation with pneumoperitoneum, may be seen. Fluids in the root of the mesentery and vascular engorgement favor the diagnosis of diverticulitis. In contrast, a short segment of colonic wall thickening and the presence of lymph nodes raise the suggestion of a colonic malignancy [4].

Intussusception Intussusception is a relatively rare condition in adults. Intussusceptions secondary to neoplasms, adhesions, or foreign bodies are associated with bowel obstruction, while transient intussusceptions are not associated with this condition. At CT, the presence of a bowel-within-bowel configuration with or without mesenteric fat and mesenteric vessels is pathognomonic for intussusception (Fig. 12.7). A leading mass as the cause of the intussusception can be identified, but this finding should be carefully differentiated from the soft tissue pseudotumor that represents the intussusception itself [3, 17].

Radiation Enteritis Radiation enteritis is a delayed complication of radiation therapy, typically occurring within a year of pelvic irradiation, with an estimated incidence of 1% [18]. Approximately one out of five patients treated by radiation therapy will present clinical signs of radiation enteritis, including obstruction, malabsorption, malnutrition and/or other complications

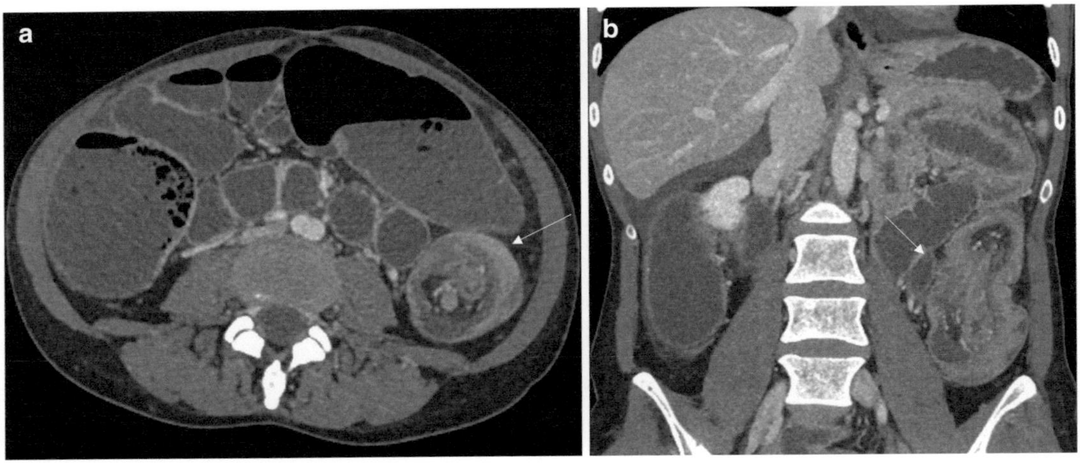

Fig. 12.7 Intussusceptions secondary to large bowel adenocarcinoma in a 47-year-old female patient. (**a**) Axial and (**b**) coronal CT images demonstrate a bowel-within-bowel configuration containing mesenteric fat and vessels. The intussusception is caused by a lead-point mass, seen as irregular mural thickening with contrast enhancement

[19]. It primarily affects the ileum and manifests as bowel obstruction due to adhesive and fibrotic changes in the mesentery. The bowel itself also undergoes changes, including luminal narrowing and dysmotility caused by radiation-induced serositis. CT imaging demonstrates bowel wall thickening, luminal narrowing, angular bowel segments caused by adhesions, and mesenteric retraction. Abnormal enhancement of the thickened bowel wall within the radiation field may also be present.

Infective Enteritis/Enterocolitis Infectious enterocolitis is due to bowel inflammation caused by bacteria, viruses, or parasites. A key radiologic feature of infectious enterocolitis is the typical extended continuous involvement of the bowel produced by the offending organism, classified as duodenitis, small bowel enteritis, proximal or distal, colitis, or proctitis. One of the potentially more serious complications of enteritis is bowel obstruction; however, it remains an extremely rare manifestation of acute bowel infection [20, 21]. Eosinophilic gastrointestinal disease (EGID) is a rare inflammatory disease with unclear etiology that presents with variable degrees of infiltration of eosinophils within the GI tract [22, 23], characterized by intestinal wall thickening and possible features of intestinal obstruction [22]. Bowel obstructions provoked by enteritis/enterocolitis might be partial or total. In some cases, enteritis is discovered because an obstruction is occurring. Partial obstructions might be treated conservatively with bowel decompression (a tube inserted through the nose and suction applied for a few days). Others might need surgery to resolve. The CT examination with contrast media administration is used to identify relevant signs of inflammatory enteritis/enterocolitis (the "comb" sign, enlarged lymph nodes, abscess, fibro-fatty infiltration) and potential complications like bowel obstruction or ischemia [24].

Hematomas Intramural small bowel hematoma may occur secondary to anticoagulant therapy, iatrogenic intervention, or trauma, and can produce bowel obstruction for the luminal narrowing. In these cases, CT will show spontaneously hyperattenuating clot (at unenhanced acquisition) and wall thickening with circumferential, homogeneous, and regular morphology associated with moderate mesenteric infiltration [3].

Vascular Causes Occlusion or stenosis of the mesenteric arterial or venous vascular supply to the bowel usually produces bowel ischemia (described in the dedicated chapter), which causes bowel wall alterations and bowel obstruction due to the impaired persistalsis [3].

12.3.2.2 Extrinsic Causes

Adhesions Across all cases, the most common cause of mechanical intestinal obstruction is believed to be previous abdominal surgeries, accounting for approximately 75% of instances [25]. The main cause of SBO are adhesions, ranging from 50% to 80% of all cases. Almost all of them are postoperative, with a minority secondary to peritonitis. The adhesive bands are not seen at conventional CT; only an abrupt change in the caliber of the bowel is detected without any associated significant inflammation, mass lesion, or bowel wall thickening at the transition point. This finding combined with a history of abdominal surgery usually suggests the diagnosis.

Hernias Hernias are considered the second most common extrinsic cause of SBO, responsible for 10% of cases [3, 26]. Hernias are classified according to the anatomic location of the orifice through which the bowel protrudes, and they are classified as external or internal (less common). An external hernia results from a defect in the abdominal and pelvic wall at sites of congenital weakness or previous surgery (Fig. 12.8a and b). The internal hernia occurs when there is a protrusion of the viscera through the peritoneum or mesentery and into a compartment within the abdominal cavity and the obstruction is based on a closed loop obstruction with two adjacent collapsed loops at the internal hernia orifice (Fig. 12.8c, d, e, f, and g). Diagnosis of an internal hernia is almost always radiologic, whereas external hernias in most cases are obvious at clinical examination [3]. The locations of internal hernias are as follows: right or left paraduodenal (53%), pericecal (13%), foramen of Winslow (8%), transmesenteric and transmesocolic (8%), pelvic and supravesical (6%), sigmoid mesocolon (6%), and transomental (1–4%) [25]. Internal hernias may have three different kinds of hernia orifice: physiologic foramen, unusual peritoneal fossa or recess into the retroperitoneum, and abnormal opening in a mesentery or peritoneal ligament as a result of development defect of fusion. Most mesenteries and peritoneal ligaments consist of two peritoneal layers. Abnormal

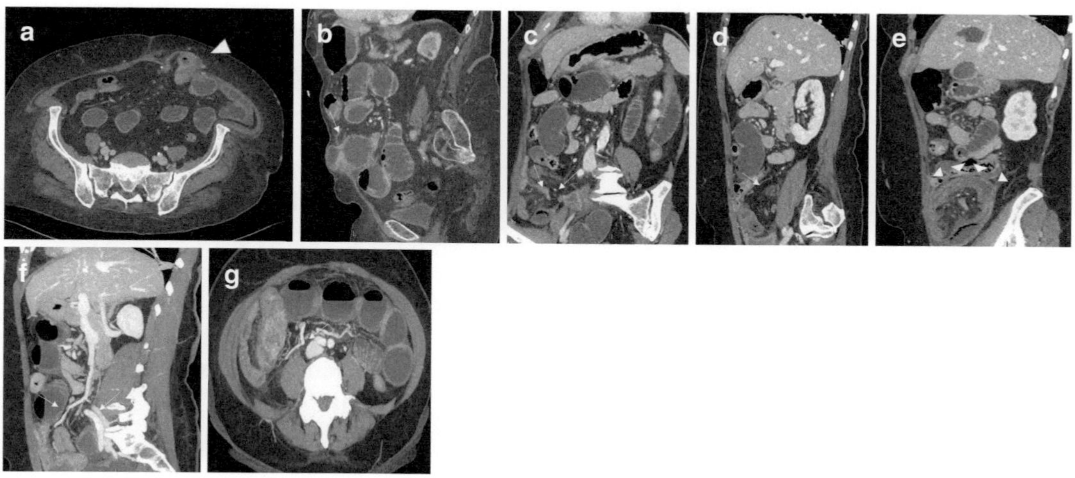

Fig. 12.8 External and internal hernias. (**a**) The axial and (**b**) coronal CT images in the venous phase show the presence of defect in the abdominal left wall with a small bowel loop protrusion (arrowhead) and the exact point of mechanical obstruction (arrow), in a female patient of 72 years old. (**c**) The sagittal CT image of a 56-years old male patient demonstrates the closed loop obstruction with two adjacent collapsed ileal loops at the internal paraceal hernia orifice (arrows) in the right iliac fossa; (**d**) the mesenteric fat and vessels result attracted toward the internal hernia orifice (arrow); (**e**) the external peritoneal layer involving the internal hernia gives a saclike CT appearance (arrowheads); (**f**) on sagittal and (**g**) axial MIP reformatted images is possible to identify the displacement of surrounding structures and key vessels that are unnaturally dislocated by the mass effect (arrows)

openings can arise through both layers (transmesenteric type of internal hernia) or in only one peritoneal layer (intramesenteric type of internal hernia); in the intramesenteric case, the external and intact peritoneal layer involving the herniated loops gives a saclike CT appearance that strongly supports a diagnosis of internal hernia. Unfortunately, this sign is not observed in all types of internal hernias. Definitive diagnosis of internal hernias also requires identification of abnormal displacement of surrounding structures and key vessels that are unnaturally attracted or dislocated by the mass effect of the bowel hernia in a closed space such as the abdominal cavity [27]. Reformatted images are sometimes helpful in assessing the size of the hernial defect, depicting adverse features, and demonstrating hernial anatomy [3].

Endometriosis Endometriosis and other various causes (e.g. carcinomatosis) account for the remaining 10–15% of extrinsic causes of bowel obstructions [28]. The CT findings of intestinal endometriosis can vary based on the size and depth of the endometrial implant, the extent of bleeding from ectopic endometrial tissue, and the degree of surrounding inflammation and fibrosis. Endometrial implants are typically located on the antimesenteric edge of the bowel, and their typical appearance is a solid or cystic nodules, with positive enhancement contiguous with or penetrating the thickened bowel wall. When the endometriotic lesion infiltrates the submucosa, it typically appears as a hypoattenuating layer between the muscularis and the mucosa [3, 29].

12.3.2.3 Intraluminal Causes

The most likely sites of colonic obstruction from intraluminal contents are the rectum (70%) and the sigmoid colon (20%) and the most common cause is *fecal impaction*, occurring primarily in the elderly and debilitated patients or or in patients taking drugs impairing intestinal motility. The CT finding is a large amount of stool located distal to the dilated colon [4].

Gallstone Ileus Gallstone ileus is a rare complication of recurrent cholecystitis, caused by migration of a large gallstone through a biliary-intestinal fistula with subsequent impaction in the bowel and bowel obstruction. The most common site of gallstone impaction is represented by the ileocecal valve. CT pathognomonic findings are the triad of pneumobilia, ectopic gallstone, and bowel obstruction [3].

Bezoar The bowel obstruction secondary to a bezoar is rare with increasing in the last decades owing to the high frequency of gastric outlet surgery that prevents adequate digestion of vegetable fibers, which become impacted, causing obstruction. At CT, a bezoar appears as an intraluminal mass with an ovoid shape and a mottled gas pattern [3].

Distal Intestinal Obstruction Syndrome Distal intestinal obstruction syndrome (DIOS) is a bowel obstruction complication in older children and adults with cystic fibrosis. It results from the impaction of thickened stool due to pancreatic insufficiency and malabsorption. CT findings include small bowel obstruction with characteristic feculent filling defects within the small bowel lumen [3].

Foreign Body Ingestion primarily affects children, mentally impaired individuals, and patients who have undergone endoscopic capsule retention for small bowel evaluation. At CT, the findings consist of bowel obstruction with evidence of a foreign body at the transition point [3].

12.3.3 Third Question: Is Severe or Complicated Obstruction Present?

Based on the pathophysiology evolution of the obstructive process in the bowel, it is possible to identify three different stages of small bowel obstruction: *simple, decompensated, and complicated,* which imply a progressively increasing urgency in the treatment [30, 31].

Simple
The walls of the loops remain of normal thickness, with intensified peristalsis and more prominent valvulae conniventes above the site of obstruction, and no free fluid is seen in the peritoneal cavity.

Decompensated
In this stage, the loop becomes more dilated and the bowel wall is stretched and thin. This causes an impairment in the parietal microcirculation due to the increased endoluminal pressure with transudative loss of fluid into the peritoneal cavity.

Complicated
The persistence of the occlusion leads to vascular impairment of the bowel wall due to progressive congestion with ischemia, necrosis, and perforation [30, 31].

Based on the obstruction mechanism, two different types of bowel obstruction can be identified: simple obstruction and closed-loop obstruction.

12.3.3.1 Simple Obstruction

Simple obstruction of the bowel is considered when the bowel is occluded in one site. The proximal part of the bowel is variably distended, depending on the severity and duration of the process [3, 4].

12.3.3.2 Closed Loop Obstruction

Closed-loop obstructions are diagnosed when a bowel loop of variable length is occluded at two adjacent points along its course. The occlusion can be partial or complete. At CT, axial scans reveal a characteristic fixed radial distribution of several dilated, usually fluid-filled bowel loops with stretched and prominent mesenteric vessels converging toward the point of torsion. The configuration can be U-shaped or C-shaped, depending on the orientation of the closed loop. Because of the presence of contraction of two adjacent bowel segments and the interposed mesentery, a narrow pedicle can be formed, leading to torsion of the loops, and producing a small bowel volvulus. At CT it is possible to recognize a "beak sign" at the site of the torsion, as a fusiform tapering, and occasionally a "whirl sign", as a reflex of rotation of the bowel loops around the fixed point of obstruction [3].

Strangulation is defined as the evolution of a closed-loop obstruction associated with intestinal ischemia. This condition is seen when there is a delay in establishing the correct diagnosis and subsequent surgical treatment. The mortality rate is high [1, 5]. CT findings indicative of strangulation include thickening and spontaneous hyperdensity of the affected bowel wall, a halo or "target sign," pneumatosis intestinalis, and gas in the portal vein. The only specific CT finding is the lack of wall enhancement, asymmetric enhancement, or even delayed enhancement. A recent study reported that increased attenuation of intestinal contents and intestinal walls on non-contrast CT scans may be predictors of bowel necrosis [32]. Localized fluid and hemorrhage in the mesentery can also be seen [3].

12.4 Paralitic Ileus

It is a condition in which there is a functional motor paralysis of the gastro-intestinal tract secondary to neuromuscular failure involving the myenteric (Auerbach's) and submucous (Meissner's) plexus. The intestine fails to transmit peristaltic waves, resulting in a functional obstruction, and allowing fluid and gas to collect in the intestine. It is the small intestine that is predominantly affected, but the colon and stomach could also be involved. The resultant stasis leads to the accumulation of fluid and gas within the bowel with associated distension, vomiting, decrease of bowel sounds, and absolute constipation [33].

Postoperative Ileus In postoperative ileus, motor inhibition is caused by a variety of stimuli, the commonest being tactile stimulation during surgery and peritonitis. Paralytic ileus is commonly seen in postoperative ileus which resolves after 24–48 hours. It might be prolonged if there is hypokalemia, hypoproteinemia, or renal failure; also uremia could produce ileus and peritonitis. Paralitic ileus is sometimes associated with retroperitoneal trauma and hemorrhage, spine or rib fractures, and severe trauma outside the abdomen. Findings on CT include multiple air-fluid levels throughout the abdomen, elevated diaphragm, dilatation of both large and small intestine, and no evidence of mechanical obstruction [33].

Acute Colonic Pseudo-obstruction (ACPO)-Ogilvie Syndrome This syndrome is secondary to interruption of sympathetic innervation of the colon and it is most common in male patients over 60 years of age, already hospitalized with a severe illness. The cecum is routinely distended in ACPO and cecal ischemia and perforation are a major risk if decompression with colonoscopy or surgery is not performed. CT plays a role in the diagnosis of ACPO, allowing to detection of the presence or absence of a transition point [4].

Localized Ileus A localized ileus consists of a localized loop (sentinel loop) of dilated small bowel associated with a local irritation such as acute pancreatitis and other acute intra-abdominal conditions [33].

Generalized Peritonitis Generalized peritonitis is a serious condition resulting from irritation of the peritoneum due to infection or from chemical irritation due to leakage of intestinal contents, such as perforated duodenal ulcer. The peritoneal cavity becomes acutely inflamed with intestinal dilatation and paralytic ileus [33].

12.5 The Essential in the CT Report

The radiologic report should be complete with the most important information for clinicians and surgeons to give them all the necessary for the best management of the patients [32]. The schematic resume here reported may be a useful outline for Radiologists to follow in this not-easy emergency scenario (Table 12.2).

Table 12.2 Findings to report in case of bowel obstruction

What to report		
CT findings		
Loop dilatation (caliper)	Small Bowel (>3 cm)	Large Bowel Colon (>6 cm) Cecum (>9 cm)
Free fluid	Yes	No
Pneumoperitoneum	Yes	No
Wall enhancement	Normal	Ischemia/infarction
Transition point	Present (mechanic ileus)	Absent (paralitic ileus)
Location	Small bowel	Large bowel
Bowel distal to the transition point	Collapsed	Dilated (check if there are further transition point)
Bowel wall thickening at the transition point	Yes	No
Closed loop at the transition point	Yes (check for strangulation)	No

References

1. Nelms DW, Kann BR. Imaging modalities for evaluation of intestinal obstruction. Clin Colon Rectal Surg. 2021;34(4):205–18. https://doi.org/10.1055/s--0041-1729737. Epub 2021 Jun 2. PMID: 34305469; PMCID: PMC8292005.
2. Paulson EK, Thompson WM. Review of small-bowel obstruction: the diagnosis and when to worry. Radiology. 2015;275(2):332–42. https://doi.org/10.1148/radiol.15131519.
3. Silva AC, Pimenta M, Guimarães LS. Small bowel obstruction: what to look for. Radiographics. 2009;29(2):423–39. https://doi.org/10.1148/rg.292085514.
4. Jaffe T, Thompson WM. Large-bowel obstruction in the adult: classic radiographic and CT findings, etiology, and mimics. Radiology. 2015;275(3):651–63. https://doi.org/10.1148/radiol.2015140916.
5. Afzal S, Ahmad F, Farooq F. Role of multi-detector computed tomography in the diagnosis of intestinal obstruction. Cureus. 2023;15(1):e33730. https://doi.org/10.7759/cureus.33730. PMID: 36788830; PMCID: PMC9922381.
6. Jeppesen MH, Tolstrup MB, Kehlet Watt S, Gögenur I. Risk factors affecting morbidity and mortality following emergency laparotomy for small bowel obstruction: a retrospective cohort study. Int J Surg. 2016;28:63–8. https://doi.org/10.1016/j.ijsu.2016.02.059. Epub 2016 Feb 18.
7. Lieske B, Meseeha M. Large bowel obstruction. [Updated 2023 Aug 8]. In: StatPearls [Internet]. Treasure Island (FL): StatPearls Publishing; 2024.
8. Li Z, Zhang L, Liu X, Yuan F, Song B. Diagnostic utility of CT for small bowel obstruction: systematic review and meta-analysis. PLoS One. 2019;14(12):e0226740. https://doi.org/10.1371/journal.pone.0226740. PMID: 31887146; PMCID: PMC6936825.
9. Vercruysse G, Busch R, Dimcheff D, Al-Hawary M, Saad R, Seagull FJ, Somand D, Cherry-Bukowiec J, Wanacata L, Pumiglia L. Evaluation and management of mechanical small bowel obstruction in adults [Internet]. Ann Arbor (MI): Michigan Medicine University of Michigan; 2021.
10. Solberg IC, Vatn MH, Hoie O, et al. Clinical course in Crohn's disease: results of a Norwegian population-based ten-year follow-up study. Clin Gastroenterol Hepatol. 2007;5:1430–8.
11. Henriksen M, Jahnsen J, Lygren I, et al. Clinical course in Crohn's disease: results of a five-year population-based follow-up study (the IBSEN study). Scand J Gastroenterol. 2007;42:602–10.
12. Thia KT, Sandborn WJ, Harmsen WS, et al. Risk factors associated with progression to intestinal complications of Crohn's disease in a population-based cohort. Gastroenterology. 2010;139:1147–55.
13. Gower-Rousseau C, Vasseur F, Fumery M, et al. Epidemiology of inflammatory bowel diseases: new insights from a French population-based registry (EPIMAD). Dig Liver Dis. 2013;45:89–94.
14. Frago R, Ramirez E, Millan M, Kreisler E, del Valle E, Biondo S. Current management of acute malignant large bowel obstruction: a systematic review. Am J Surg. 2014;207(1):127–38.
15. Cappell MS, Batke M. Mechanical obstruction of the small bowel and colon. Med Clin North Am. 2008;92(3):575–97.
16. Stavride E, Plakias C. Coffee bean sign: its meaning and importance. Clin Case Rep. 2020;8(10):2086–7. https://doi.org/10.1002/ccr3.3064. PMID: 33088563; PMCID: PMC7562879.
17. Somma F, Faggian A, Serra N, Gatta G, Iacobellis F, Berritto D, et al. Bowel intussusceptions in adults: the role of imaging. Radiol Med. 2015;120(1):105–17.
18. Miller G, Boman J, Shrier I, Gordon PH. Etiology of small bowel obstruction. Am J Surg. 2000;180(1):33–6. https://doi.org/10.1016/s0002-9610(00)00407-4.
19. Loge L, Florescu C, Alves A, Menahem B. Radiation enteritis: diagnostic and therapeutic issues. J Visc Surg. 2020;157(6):475–85. https://doi.org/10.1016/j.jviscsurg.2020.08.012. Epub 2020 Sep 1.
20. Duffin C, Mirpour S, Catanzano T, Moore C. Radiologic imaging of bowel infections. Semin Ultrasound CT MR. 2020;41(1):33–45. https://doi.org/10.1053/j.sult.2019.10.004. Epub 2019 Oct 14.
21. Sandhu S, Alhankawi D, Prajapati D. *Salmonella typhimurium* as a rare cause of small bowel obstruction. J Community Hosp Intern Med Perspect. 2022;12(4):111–3. https://doi.org/10.55729/2000-9666.1084. PMID: 36262905; PMCID: PMC9533796.
22. Atuiri C, Zhang W, Cronin C. Eosinophilic enteritis causing recurrent small bowel obstruction: a case report. Cureus. 2024;16(2):e54355. https://doi.org/10.7759/cureus.54355. PMID: 38500945; PMCID: PMC10946293.
23. Yun MY, Cho YU, Park IS. Eosinophilic gastroenteritis presenting as small bowel obstruction: a case report and review of the literature. World J Gastroenterol. 2007;13(11):1758–60.
24. Plastaras L, Vuitton L, Badet N, Koch S, Di Martino V, Delabrousse E. Acute colitis: differential diagnosis using multidetector CT. Clin Radiol. 2015;70(3):262–9. ISSN 0009-9260.
25. Menzies D, Ellis H. Intestinal obstruction from adhesions-how big is the problem. Ann R Coll Surg Engl. 1990;72(1):60–3.
26. Takeyama N, Gokan T, Ohgiya Y, Satoh S, Hashizume T, Hataya K, Kushiro H, Nakanishi M, Kusano M, Munechika H. CT of internal hernias. Radiographics. 2005;25(4):997–1015. https://doi.org/10.1148/rg.254045035.
27. Doishita S, Takeshita T, Uchima Y, Kawasaki M, Shimono T, Yamashita A, Sugimoto M, Ninoi T, Shima H, Miki Y. Internal hernias in the era of multidetector CT: correlation of imaging and surgical findings. Radiographics. 2016;36(1):88–106. https://doi.org/10.1148/rg.2016150113. Epub 2015 Nov 20.

28. Catena F, De Simone B, Coccolini F, Di Saverio S, Sartelli M, Ansaloni L. Bowel obstruction: a narrative review for all physicians. World J Emerg Surg. 2019;14:20. https://doi.org/10.1186/s13017-019-0240-7. PMID: 31168315; PMCID: PMC6489175.
29. Gillen N, Kovacs T, Leahy J. Diagnosis and management of small bowel obstruction in the ileum caused by endometriosis: a case report. Case Rep Womens Health. 2023;38:e00522. https://doi.org/10.1016/j.crwh.2023.e00522. PMID: 37440767; PMCID: PMC10334316.
30. Iacobellis F, Laccetti E, Romano F, Altiero M, Scaglione M. Imaging of bowel obstruction and perforation. In: Cova MA, Stacul F, editors. Pain Imaging; 2019. p. 323–46. https://doi.org/10.1007/978-3-319-99822-0_17.
31. Di Mizio R, Scaglione M, editors. Small-bowel obstruction CT features with plain film and US correlations. Springer; 2007.
32. Li BQ, Qi WJ, Yuan M, Wang HY, Chen M, Song ZX, Li Q, Li L, Jiang B, Ma ZL, Xiu DR, Yuan CH. Increased attenuation of intestinal contents at CT indicates bowel necrosis in closed-loop small bowel obstruction. Radiology. 2024;310(2):e231710. https://doi.org/10.1148/radiol.231710.
33. Weledji EP. Perspectives on paralytic ileus. Acute Med Surg. 2020;7(1):e573. https://doi.org/10.1002/ams2.573. PMID: 33024568; PMCID: PMC7533151.

Acute Gastrointestinal Bleeding 13

Marco Di Serafino, Roberto Ronza, Francesca Iacobellis, Luigi Barbuto, Giuseppina Dell'Aversano Orabona, and Gianluca Ponticiello

13.1 Introduction

Acute gastrointestinal bleeding (GIB) is a critical medical condition that necessitates rapid and accurate diagnostic efforts. The annual occurrence of GIB ranges from 20 to 150 instances per 100,000 people, predominantly affecting the upper gastrointestinal (GI) tract [1]. While 80–85% of GIB episodes spontaneously cease, the condition frequently leads to hospital admission and carries substantial risks of morbidity and mortality. These risks are particularly pronounced among older individuals and those with additional health issues. Men are more likely to experience GIB than women, with a ratio of 2:1 [2]. The mortality rate associated with GIB varies from 3.6% to 18% but escalates to 21–40% in situations involving severe bleeding [1, 2]. The most common symptoms include melena, hematemesis, decreasing haemoglobin, and even haemodynamic instability, which necessitates blood pressure stabilization and restoration of intravascular volume [3]. GIB is classified according to whether it originates above or below the ligament of Treitz, thereby distinguishing between upper and lower causes. Upper GIB is more prevalent than lower GIB, occurring about five times more often. The latter originates in the colon in approximately 80% of cases. Upper GIB is divided into variceal and non-variceal categories, with non-variceal further subdivided into non-vascular and vascular origins [1]. Many aetiologies contribute to GIB. The primary reasons for upper GIB are peptic ulcer disease (62%), arteriovenous malformations (10%), gastritis or duodenitis (8%), and oesophageal varices (6%). For lower GIB, the most frequent causes are diverticular disease (40%), colitis and inflammatory bowel disease (21%), neoplasia (14%), coagulopathic haemorrhage (12%), and angiodysplasia, among other conditions. Medications including non-steroidal anti-inflammatory drugs, antiplatelet agents, and anticoagulants, along with anti-angiogenic drugs used in cancer treatment, are recognized as causes of GIB [4]. Anti-vascular endothelial growth factor drugs, notably bevacizumab, have been linked to significant and sometimes life-threatening bleeding in cancer patients, particularly in the rectal area [5]. Determining the location of the bleeding site is crucial for formulating an appropriate management plan [1, 2]. The challenge in identifying the origin of the bleeding stems from its diverse potential causes, the extensive length of the GI tract, and the sporadic nature of the bleeding

M. Di Serafino (✉) · R. Ronza · F. Iacobellis
L. Barbuto · G. Dell'Aversano Orabona
G. Ponticiello
Department of General and Emergency Radiology, "Antonio Cardarelli" Hospital, Naples, Italy
e-mail: marco.diserafino@aocardarelli.it; roberto.ronza@aocardarelli.it; francesca.iacobellis@aocardarelli.it; luigi.barbuto@aocardarelli.it; giuseppinadellaversanoorabona@aocardarelli.it; gianluca.ponticiello@aocardarelli.it

L. Romano et al. (eds.), *CT of Non-Traumatic Body Emergencies*,
https://doi.org/10.1007/978-3-031-84849-0_13

[1–4]. It is imperative not to overlook obscure GIB, which encompasses bleeding types that are less likely to be defined by traditional diagnostic methods such as endoscopy, enteroscopy, and video capsule, than by diagnostic imaging. Both diagnosis and treatment strategies are entirely contingent upon the characteristics of the bleeding and the patient's haemodynamic condition [1]. Therefore, managing patients with GIB necessitates a collaborative effort involving emergency physicians, internal medicine specialists, surgeons, gastroenterologists, and both diagnostic and interventional radiologists. While a significant number of GIB cases can be diagnosed and managed without the need for radiological imaging, this tool remains vital, particularly for patients whose conditions do not improve with endoscopy and/or medical treatments [1–4]. The primary aim of employing diagnostic tools for GIB is to identify the source of the bleeding to enable immediate intervention to manage the haemorrhage if feasible. However, the fact that GIB often presents intermittently or may stop on its own poses a challenge for both diagnosis and treatment [1–4].

13.2 Endoscopy and Diagnostic Imaging

Various methods have been developed to identify the source of acute GIB, such as endoscopy, angiography, nuclear scans using tagged red blood cells, and computed tomography angiography (CTA). Selection of the optimal technique is influenced by factors including the availability of resources; the expertise of the practitioner; the severity, type, and origin of the bleeding; and the overall condition of the patient [1]. Endoscopy demonstrates varying effectiveness in identifying the source of bleeding, with a diagnostic success rate of 48–90%. It frequently struggles to precisely pinpoint the location of ongoing and significant bleeding (1 ml/min). Additionally, its ability to detect bleeding lesions in the colon is compromised when bowel preparation is incomplete [6]. Scintigraphy using tagged red blood cells is highly sensitive and non-invasive, and is capable of identifying slow (0.1 ml/min) venous and arterial bleeds, including those that occur intermittently. This method does not necessitate prior patient preparation, but it is time-intensive, does not pinpoint the precise location of the bleed, and is not accessible 24/7 in many hospitals [1, 7]. Angiography is a costly, invasive, and time-intensive procedure that many hospitals do not offer [1]. CTA is a potentially optimal diagnostic method for acute GIB. It might be able to outperform traditional angiography in identifying GIB, as it is capable of detecting bleeding rates as low as 0.5 ml/min. CTA is quick and widely accessible and provides precise images of the arterial phase. This facilitates the detailed mapping of arterial blood vessels and the identification of contrast medium extravasation into the intestinal lumen, which signifies GIB [1–4]. Furthermore, advancements in isotropic spatial resolution and post-processing techniques for CTA have significantly enhanced its diagnostic capabilities. These improvements enable the detection of very small vascular lesions across multiple orthogonal planes that could be the sources of bleeding. Consequently, in many hospitals, CTA has emerged as the radiological imaging method of choice for haemodynamically stable patients exhibiting symptoms of GIB, particularly in urgent cases. As a leading diagnostic tool, CTA demonstrates exceptional effectiveness in identifying and pinpointing the location of acute GIB, with impressive sensitivity (91%), specificity (99%), accuracy (97.6%), positive predictive value (95%), and negative predictive value (98%) [8]. Its established role in managing lower GIB in stable patients underscores its potential applicability for upper GIB, especially for severe, non-variceal origins or GIB stemming from uncommon or exceedingly rare causes. CTA thereby offers valuable guidance on the timing and approach for treatment [1, 9–11].

13.3 CTA Imaging Approach and Advanced Technologies

Meticulous adherence to the CTA protocol is essential. It is advised to use 100–120 ml of contrast medium with high iodine concentrations at rapid injection speeds (minimum of 4 ml/s). An initial non-contrast computed tomography (CT) scan, followed by an arterial phase scan and possibly one or more delayed phase scans, is often required to identify GIB effectively [1–4]. Obtaining a non-contrast abdominal CT scan is crucial for identifying any pre-existing hyperattenuating materials in the bowel lumen (such as suture material, clips, foreign bodies, orally ingested medications, and coproliths) that could be confused with active bleeding (Fig. 13.1) [1–4]. The arterial phase is crucial for identifying abnormalities in arteries, early venous drainage, vascular clusters, and the primary leakage of contrast medium into the bowel lumen. The arterial phase is obtained using the "bolus tracking" technique, which synchronizes the scanning with the passage of the contrast medium through the aortic arch at the moment it reaches 100 Hounsfield units (HU). This is achieved by setting a region of interest at this specific location. Following the contrast injection, the portal phase is recorded 70–90 s later. This phase plays a key role in monitoring the development of arterial extravasations and pinpointing venous-origin bleeding, potentially revealing slower bleeding locations not detected during the arterial phase (Fig. 13.2) [1–4]. Moreover, the portal phase is valuable in identifying tumours that cause GIB [1–4]. In specific cases, especially in patients with diminished cardiac function or when further exploration of identified pathologies is necessary, it is beneficial to consider late venous phase imaging 5 min post-injection [1]. Images obtained without contrast (baseline phase) should be reconstructed at a thickness of 5 mm and those from the arterial, venous, and late phases at a thickness of 1.25 mm. Post-processing techniques are incredibly beneficial. Techniques such as multiplanar reformatting and maximum intensity projection (MIP) are advantageous for identifying the location of the bleeding section of the bowel and for delineating the mesenteric arteries along with their peripheral branches (Fig. 13.3) [1–4]. During an acute

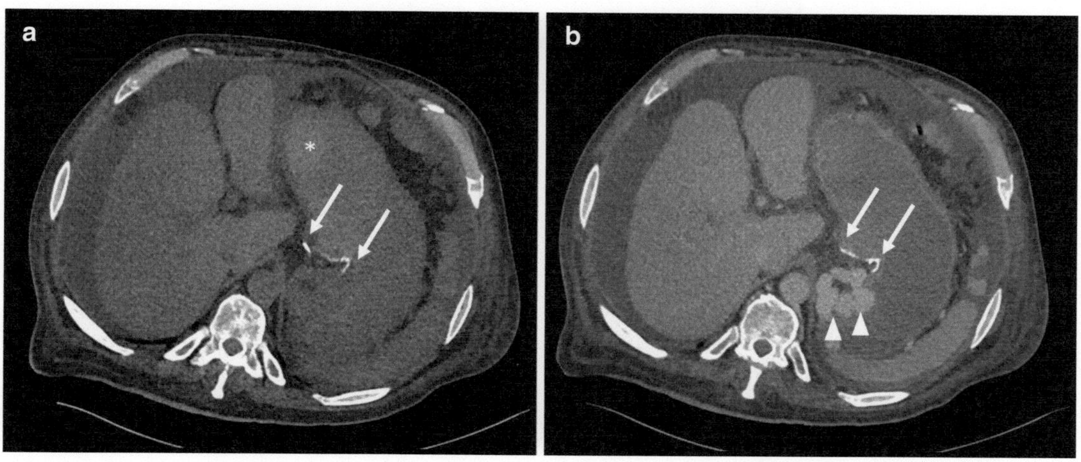

Fig. 13.1 (**a**) Pre-contrast axial CT image showing spontaneous hyperdensity due to metallic clips (white arrows) in a patient with prior gastric bypass, diagnosed with varices and intraluminal "sentinel" blood clots (white asterisk). (**b**) Post-contrast axial CT arterial phase revealing the presence of large gastric varices close to the metallic clips (white arrowheads); no active bleeding was documented during post-contrast CT examination

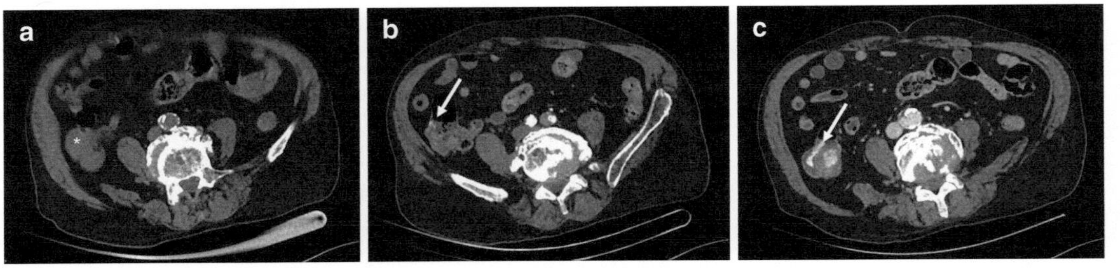

Fig. 13.2 Multiphasic CT examination documenting active intestinal bleeding due to a small caecal mass. Axial non-contrast CT image showed moderate spontaneous hyperdensity within intestinal lumen (**a**). Axial arterial CT image after intravenous contrast media administration (**b**) showed focal intraluminal active blush of iodine contrast media (white arrow), then confirmed in the venous phase as a larger area of incremental hyperdensity (**c**)

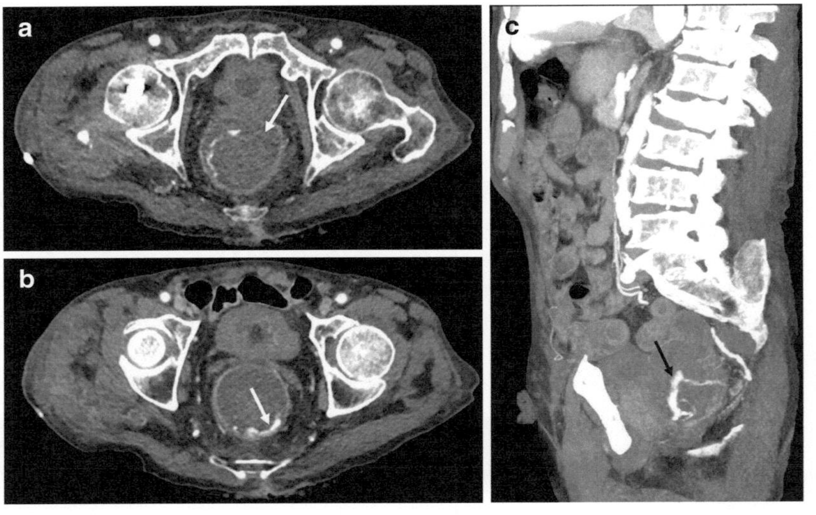

Fig. 13.3 Multiphasic post-contrast CT examination in the arterial (**a**) and venous (**b**) phase of a patient with active hemorrhagic bleeding at the level of the rectum, due to focal angiodysplasia later diagnosed at colonoscopy (white arrows). The MIP post-processing with MPR sagittal reconstruction helped in better defining vascular anatomy, depicting an engorged superior rectal artery (**c**, black arrow)

haemorrhage, a positive oral contrast agent may conceal the leakage of contrast into the bowel lumen, whereas a neutral oral contrast agent could dilute the extravasated contrast, thereby complicating the detection of active bleeding. Consequently, in cases of active bleeding, the administration of oral contrast agents is generally discouraged since they can obscure the source of bleeding [1–4]. In haemodynamically stable patients experiencing occult or intermittent GIB, CT enterography (CTE) with multiphase acquisition is a methodological option. The key distinction between CTE and CTA lies in CTE's utilization of a neutral oral contrast medium (approximately 1.5–2.0 l) to expand the lumen of the small intestine [12]. This expansion enhances the visibility of the mucosal lining and the wall of the small intestine following intravenous (IV) contrast administration, thereby improving the ability to identify lesions on the bowel wall [12]. However, the introduction of oral fluids might dilute any blood present within the lumen [1]. Therefore, while this approach is not suitable during active phases of bleeding, it is beneficial for identifying potential wall lesions in the absence of active bleeding [1]. While the specific protocols for multiphase CTE may differ across radiology departments, the foundational guidelines for administering IV contrast medium are consistent with those outlined for CTA. Consequently, CTE can complement endoscopic methods and CTA in investigating hidden sources of bleeding [1, 13]. Advancements in CT imaging technology have led to the development of dual-energy CTA (DECTA), a method that introduces post-processing techniques leveraging dual-energy technology. DECTA is recognized for its broad range of applications, including its capacity for conducting various analyses and its effectiveness in identifying GI tract diseases [1, 14]. It introduces a virtual non-contrast (VNC) feature, providing an alternative to conventional pre-contrast CT scans in GIB scenarios that could lower radiation exposure by approximately 30% [1, 15]. This feature enables the simulation of a pre-contrast CT scan, facilitating the examination of the presence or absence of iodine in high-density areas without requiring an actual scan. Employing a low-keV virtual monochromatic X-ray image (VMI) not only enhances iodine contrast but also aids in improving the detection of extravasation, leading to highly confident diagnoses. VMIs are generated at energy levels of approximately 40–200 keV, with low-keV images showing increased contrast due to higher contrast medium absorption [14, 15]. Such imaging is even beneficial to patients with reduced renal function or in instances of contrast failure and occasionally produces outcomes akin to traditional contrast-enhanced CT scans. In cases of GIB, VMI usage notably improves bleeding site identification, although it should be noted that low-keV images may increase noise and the visibility of metal artifacts. The clear depiction of vascular structures via low-keV VMI is instrumental in identifying vascular anomalies and assessing arterial anatomy before embolization [14, 15]. Furthermore, low-keV VMI distinctly depicts the vascular structure, thereby enhancing the visibility of vascular anomalies and aiding in the verification of arterial anatomy prior to embolization [15]. Since these analytical images are derived from contrast-enhanced CT scans, the spatial positioning of organs remains completely consistent, thereby enabling image comparisons to be made without the effects of intestinal movement or patient motion influencing the outcomes [15]. An iodine map is an image format in which pixel values reflect iodine density in mg/ml, with contrast agent areas appearing more intense, thereby facilitating an easier distinction between intestinal contents and extravasation [14, 15]. VMIs and iodine maps enhance visibility, especially of extravasation, and maintain consistent organ location for a more assured diagnosis, leading to improved diagnostic reliability and efficiency, especially in ruling out GIB [14, 15]. Techniques that minimize metal density artifacts are also essential, as they diminish distortions from surgical clips, implants, and other foreign bodies [14, 15]. This improves the visibility of contrast material in the vessel lumen and aids in bleeding site identification. The integration of low-energy monochromatic images, iodine maps, and VNC images advances lesion detection and disease characterization within the GI tract (Figs. 13.4 and 13.5) [14, 15]. This offers benefits beyond traditional single-energy CT imaging, especially for conditions involving significant bleeding or the presence of dense material in the bowel. The analytical prowess of DECTA overcomes the limitations of conventional protocols and proves invaluable in radiologically assessing GI haemorrhage [1, 14, 15].

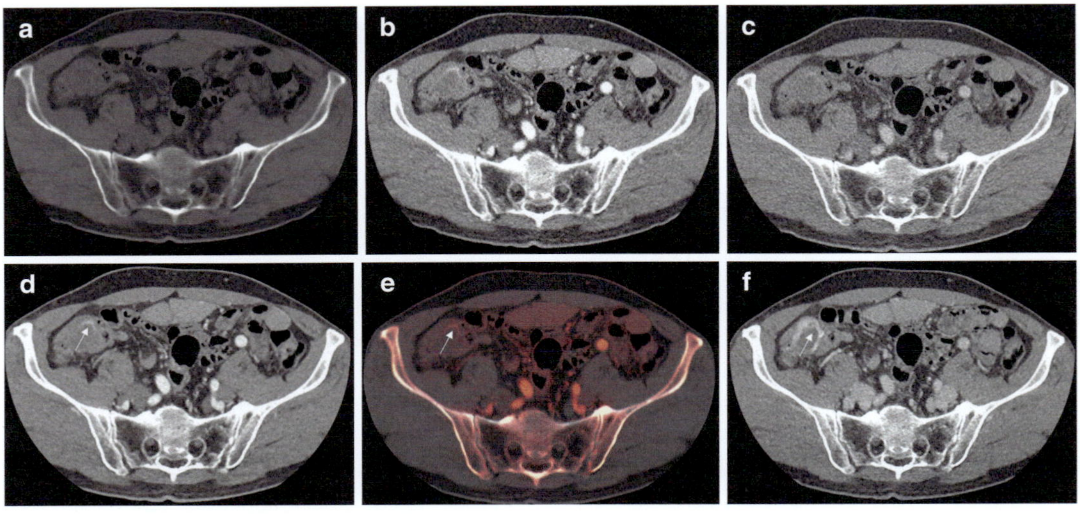

Fig. 13.4 Axial images showing dual energy CT reconstruction in a patient with active intestinal bleeding (white arrows) due to Dieulafoy's lesion of the cecum, including the virtual non-contrast (**a**), the 100kVP source image (**b**), the 140 kVP image (**c**), the mixed 100/140 kVP image (**d**) and the derived iodine color map (**e**). Findings were confirmed in the venous phase (**f**) with the increasing intraluminal bleeding

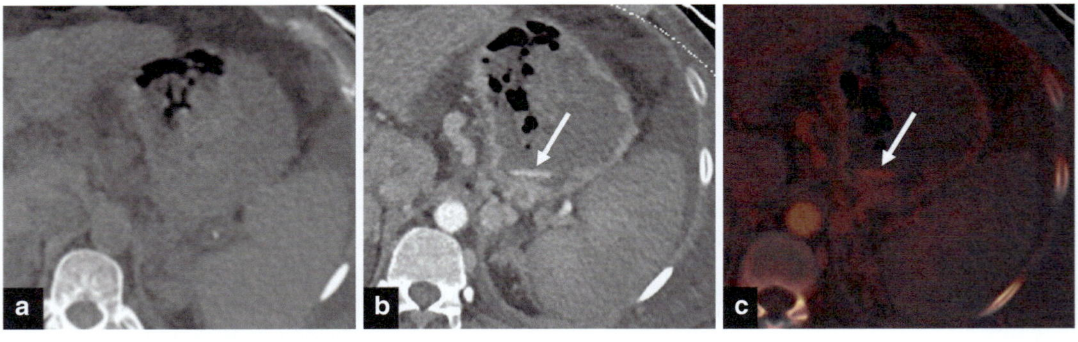

Fig. 13.5 Dual-energy CT examination in a cirrhotic patient diagnosed with gastric variceal bleeding. Virtual non-contrast CT (**a**), arterial phase (**b**) and derived iodine map (**c**) showing active bleeding (white arrows)

13.4 CTA Signs of Bleeding and Common Pitfalls

The most indicative diagnostic sign of CTA for bleeding is the presence of hyper-attenuating contrast medium leaked into the GI lumen. Active bleeding presents as a localized area of high density (90 HU) visible within the GI tract. This may manifest in various shapes, such as linear, jet-like, swirled, ellipsoidal, spot-like, or pooled, and, in some cases, it may occupy the entire bowel lumen, leading to a loop that appears highly attenuated [1–4]. Aside from the specific attenuation values of a haemorrhagic site within the bowel loop lumen, which may not consistently reach the definitive 90 HU threshold if the bleed is thin or diluted, the most effective strategy for identifying and diagnosing GIB involves correlating observations from the arterial phase with those from the basal and venous phases [1–4]. The key diagnostic indicator is the variation in the appearance of the extravasated contrast medium across these phases, from arterial to venous. This conclusively confirms active bleeding, particularly when no hyper-attenuating material is observed in the region of the lumen during the initial basal phase [1–4]. Additionally, it is important to note that, in cases of low-flow bleeding, arterial-origin contrast extravasation might become visible only during the venous phase (Fig. 13.6) [1]. Meanwhile, in patients who had recent bleeding but are not actively bleeding during the CTA, a hyperdense clot may be observed within the intestinal lumen (Fig. 13.7) [1–4]. This is referred to as a "sentinel" clot and serves as a marker for the location of prior active bleeding. Active arterial leakage of contrast media can be distinguished from clotted blood through CT attenuation values [1–4]. On a CTA scan, the attenuation values for active arterial extravasation vary from 90 to 274 HU, with an average of 155 HU, while clotted blood exhibits attenuation values ranging from 28 to 82 HU, with a mean of 54 HU. Additional, less prominent CTA indicators comprise highly attenuated fat surrounding the bowel, thickening of the intestinal wall, polyps, tumours, and enlarged blood vessels [1–4, 16]. The location of contrast medium leakage seen in CTA images matches precisely with the bleeding site identified through angiography. CTA demonstrates a sensitivity of 90.9% and a specificity of 99% for detecting

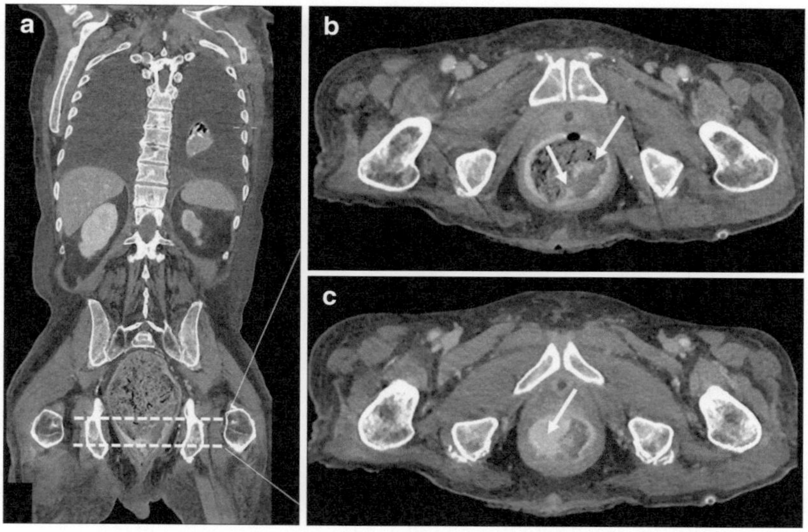

Fig. 13.6 Venous phase post-contrast CT examination of stercoral inflammatory colitis in a bedbound elderly patient. Coronal image (**a**) with axial reconstruction at two different relevant levels (**b**–**c**) showed the different blood dispositions (white arrows) in active bleeding, impacted by the presence of feces within the rectal lumen

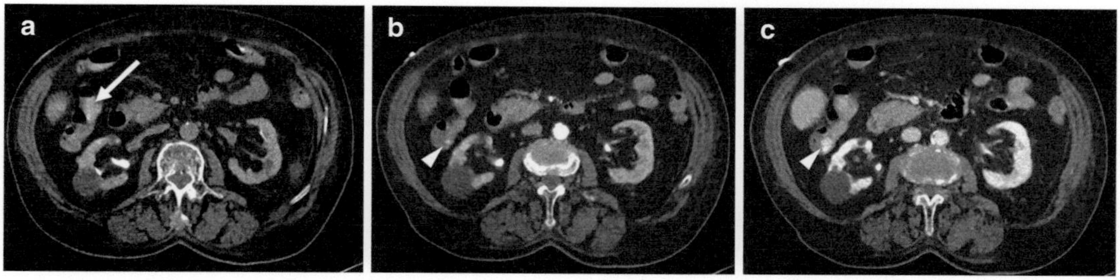

Fig. 13.7 Non-contrast CT scan in a patient with rectorrhagia referred to a tertiary care center from a peripheral hospital, showing sentinel blood clot sign in the ascending colon (**a**, white arrow), visible as an area of higher attenuation close to the anatomic site of hemorrhage (then diagnosed as intestinal angiodysplasia at colonoscopy). Arterial (**b**) and venous (**c**) phases at post-contrast CT examination confirmed the site of active bleeding close to the sentinel clot sign (white arrowheads)

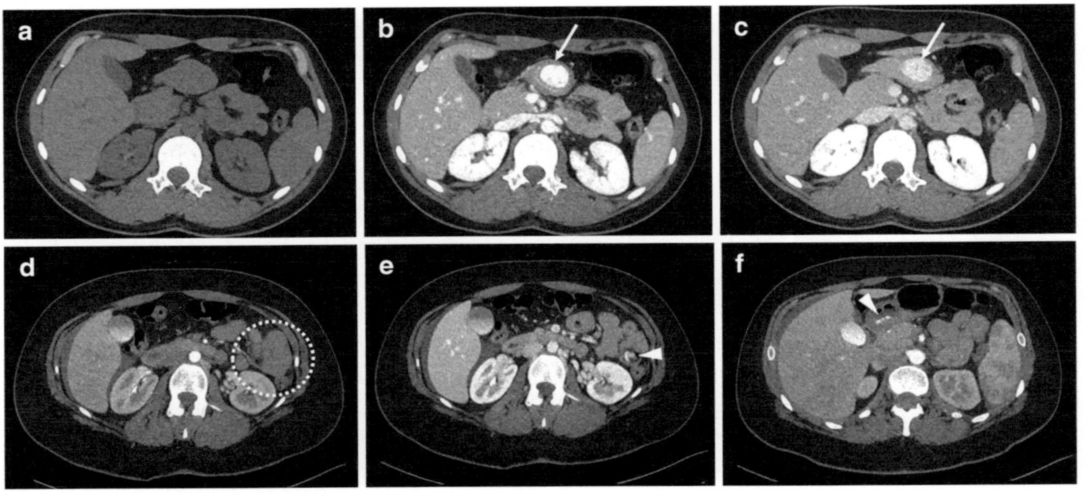

Fig. 13.8 Possible intestinal bleeding mimics. Upper row: Multiphasic CT examination with axial pre-contrast (**a**), arterial (**b**) and venous (**c**) phase, documenting a vividly enhancing gastric lesion (white arrows) that could mimic active bleeding; the lesion finally resulted in pathology in a hypervascular tumor of the gastric wall (glomus tumor of the stomach). Bottom row: Multiphasic CT examination showing spontaneous intraluminal hyperdensity in the jejunum in the venous phase (**e**, white arrowheads), not visible at the same level in the arterial phase (**d**, dotted line); revising arterial phase acquisitions (**f**), the same hyperdensity was seen in the gastric antrum, thus suggesting migrated ingested foreign bodies (white arrowheads)

acute GIB, along with 100% accuracy in identifying the exact location of the acute GIB [1–4, 16]. Post-processing analysis, particularly the detailed review of MIP reconstructions, is crucial in all GIB cases [1–4, 16, 17]. Such analysis can uncover subtle bleeding not evident in the original images or more clearly delineate vascular anomalies, thereby offering a level of anatomical detail akin to angiographic studies [1, 16]. Understanding the typical diagnostic errors when analysing CTA for GIB is crucial. Cone-beam artifacts can create misleading signals of high-density material in the bowel lumen, though DECTA post-processing methods can mitigate these issues to some extent [1–4, 18]. Additionally, it is important to recognize the various incidental findings that may emerge during a CTA scan. Finally, special attention should be given to early indicators of hypovolemic shock in severe bleeding scenarios, collectively referred to as the "CT hypoperfusion complex" [19]. Several conditions must be considered in the differential diagnosis, including the presence of pre-existing high-density materials within the bowel lumen (such as metallic clips, sutures, foreign objects, drugs, or residual contrast agent), hypervascular GI tumours (including stromal tumours, carcinoid tumours, and adenocarcinomas), intraluminal hypervascular metastases (from melanoma, breast cancer, or renal cell carcinoma), solid masses that do not exhibit morphological changes during arterial/portal phase imaging, intestinal trauma, intestinal ischemia, gastric and duodenal ulcers, and colonic angiodysplasia (Fig. 13.8) [1, 20]. Furthermore, a true diverticulum, the most common congenital abnormality of the GI tract, should also be considered. This is typically found in the distal ileum, around 60–100 cm from the ileocecal valve, and warrants attention in the differential diagnosis process [1, 20].

13.5 Conclusions

GIB frequently leads to hospital admission and often necessitates the involvement of specialized centres and a collaborative approach that encompasses emergency physicians, internal medicine experts, surgeons, gastroenterologists, and both diagnostic and interventional radiologists. Although many GIB cases spontaneously improve or can be managed with medical and endoscopic treatments, imaging plays a crucial role, particularly when endoscopy is inconclusive. Within the range of imaging options, CTA stands out as the premier method for a prompt and precise diagnosis of GIB. CTA offers high sensitivity and effectiveness in informing the appropriate therapeutic approach. Furthermore, dual-energy acquisition methods enhance contrast resolution, thereby enabling the detection of bleeding sites with reduced contrast medium and radiation doses for the patient. Radiologists must be knowledgeable about the correct applications of CTA, DECTA, and other diagnostic imaging techniques for patients experiencing acute GIB. Understanding the typical imaging results and potential errors is crucial for accurately diagnosing and treating these patients.

References

1. Di Serafino M, Iacobellis F, Schillirò ML, Dell'Aversano Orabona G, Martino A, Bennato R, Borzelli A, Oliva G, D'Errico C, Pezzullo F, Barbuto L, Ronza R, Ponticiello G, Corvino F, Giurazza F, Lombardi G, Niola R, Romano L. The role of CT-angiography in the acute gastrointestinal bleeding: a pictorial essay of active and obscure findings. Tomography. 2022;8(5):2369–402. https://doi.org/10.3390/tomography8050198.
2. Guglielmo FF, Wells ML, Bruining DH, Strate LL, Huete Á, Gupta A, Soto JA, Allen BC, Anderson MA, Brook OR, Gee MS, Grand DJ, Gunn ML, Khandelwal A, Park SH, Ramalingam V, Sokhandon F, Yoo DC, Fidler JL. Gastrointestinal bleeding at CT angiography and CT enterography: imaging atlas and glossary of terms. Radiographics. 2021;41(6):1632–56. https://doi.org/10.1148/rg.2021210043.
3. DiGregorio AM, Alvey H. Gastrointestinal Bleeding. 2023 Jun 5. In: StatPearls [Internet]. Treasure Island (FL): StatPearls Publishing; 2024.
4. Wortman JR, Landman W, Fulwadhva UP, Viscomi SG, Sodickson AD. CT angiography for acute gastrointestinal bleeding: what the radiologist needs to know. Br J Radiol. 2017;90(1075):20170076. https://doi.org/10.1259/bjr.20170076. Epub 2017 Apr 26. PMID: 28362508; PMCID: PMC5594987
5. Zhu X, Tian X, Yu C, Hong J, Fang J, Chen H. Increased risk of hemorrhage in metastatic colorectal cancer patients treated with bevacizumab: an updated meta-analysis of 12 randomized controlled trials. Medicine (Baltimore). 2016;95(34):e4232. https://doi.org/10.1097/MD.0000000000004232. PMID: 27559943; PMCID: PMC5400309.
6. Kim BS, Li BT, Engel A, Samra JS, Clarke S, Norton ID, Li AE. Diagnosis of gastrointestinal bleeding: a practical guide for clinicians. World J Gastrointest Pathophysiol. 2014;5(4):467–78. https://doi.org/10.4291/wjgp.v5.i4.467. PMID: 25400991; PMCID: PMC4231512.
7. Grady E. Gastrointestinal bleeding scintigraphy in the early 21st century. J Nucl Med. 2016;57(2):252–9. https://doi.org/10.2967/jnumed.115.157289. Epub 2015 Dec 17
8. Wu LM, Xu JR, Yin Y, Qu XH. Usefulness of CT angiography in diagnosing acute gastrointestinal bleeding: a meta-analysis. World J Gastroenterol. 2010;16(31):3957–63. https://doi.org/10.3748/wjg.v16.i31.3957. PMID: 20712058; PMCID: PMC2923771.
9. Di Serafino M, Martino A, Manguso F, Ronza R, Zito FP, Giurazza F, Pignata L, Orsini L, Niola R, Romano L, Lombardi G. Value of multidetector computed tomography angiography in severe non-variceal upper gastrointestinal bleeding: a retrospective study in a referral bleeding unit. Abdom Radiol (NY). 2024; https://doi.org/10.1007/s00261-024-04208-9. Epub ahead of print.
10. Martino A, Amitrano L, Guardascione M, Di Serafino M, Bennato R, Martino R, de Leone A, Orsini L, Romano L, Lombardi G. The role of computed tomography for the prediction of esophageal variceal bleeding: current status and future perspectives. World J Gastrointest Endosc. 2023;15(12):681–9. https://doi.org/10.4253/wjge.v15.i12.681. PMID: 38187916; PMCID: PMC10768040.
11. Martino A, Di Serafino M, Orsini L, Giurazza F, Fiorentino R, Crolla E, Campione S, Molino C, Romano L, Lombardi G. Rare causes of acute non-variceal upper gastrointestinal bleeding: a comprehensive review. World J Gastroenterol. 2023;29(27):4222–35. https://doi.org/10.3748/wjg.v29.i27.4222. PMID: 37545636; PMCID: PMC10401659.
12. Deepak P, Pundi KN, Bruining DH, Fidler JL, Barlow JM, Hansel SL, Harmsen WS, Wells ML, Fletcher JG. Multiphase computed tomographic enterography: diagnostic yield and efficacy in patients with suspected small bowel bleeding. Mayo Clin Proc Innov Qual Outcomes. 2019;3(4):438–47. https://doi.org/10.1016/j.mayocpiqo.2019.09.001. PMID: 31993562; PMCID: PMC6978607.
13. Unno M, Hashimoto S, Shimizu K, Onoda H, Tanabe M, Shirasawa T, Goto A, Hamabe K, Okamoto T, Nishikawa J, Ito K, Sakaida I. Combined use of computed tomography enterography/enteroclysis and capsule endoscopy improves the accuracy of diagnosis of small bowel bleeding. Intern Med. 2021;60(16):2545–55. https://doi.org/10.2169/internalmedicine.6785-20. Epub 2021 Aug 15. PMID: 34393155; PMCID: PMC8429301.

14. Trabzonlu TA, Mozaffary A, Kim D, Yaghmai V. Dual-energy CT evaluation of gastrointestinal bleeding. Abdom Radiol (NY). 2020;45(1):1–14. https://doi.org/10.1007/s00261-019-02226-6.
15. Okamura-Kawasaki M, Uesugi Y, Yabusaki S. Dual-energy CT for gastrointestinal bleeding. BJR Open. 2023;5(1):20220054. https://doi.org/10.1259/bjro.20220054. PMID: 37035764; PMCID: PMC10077409.
16. Artigas JM, Martí M, Soto JA, Esteban H, Pinilla I, Guillén E. Multidetector CT angiography for acute gastrointestinal bleeding: technique and findings. Radiographics. 2013;33:1453–70.
17. Di Serafino M, Severino R, Laviani F, Maroscia D. Three-dimensional computed tomography rendering of pedunculated colon polyp: new "clapper-bell" sign pedunculated polyp at 3D computed tomography. Radiol Case Rep. 2016;11(4):292–5. https://doi.org/10.1016/j.radcr.2016.07.005. PMID: 27920846; PMCID: PMC5128358.
18. Stuber T, Hoffmann MH, Stuber G, Klass O, Feuerlein S, Aschoff AJ. Pitfalls in detection of acute gastrointestinal bleeding with multi-detector row helical CT. Abdom Imaging. 2009;34(4):476–82. https://doi.org/10.1007/s00261-008-9437-z.
19. Di Serafino M, Viscardi D, Iacobellis F, Giugliano L, Barbuto L, Oliva G, Ronza R, Borzelli A, Raucci A, Pezzullo F, De Cristofaro MG, Romano L. Computed tomography imaging of septic shock. Beyond the cause: the "CT hypoperfusion complex". A pictorial essay. Insights Imaging. 2021;12(1):70. https://doi.org/10.1186/s13244-021-01006-5. PMID: 34089401; PMCID: PMC8178660
20. Scaglione M, et al., editors. Emergency radiology of the abdomen, medical radiology. Diagnostic imaging. Berlin Heidelberg: Springer-Verlag; 2012. https://doi.org/10.1007/978-3-540-88256-5.

Part III

Bowel Inflammations and Infections

14 Enteritis and Colitis

Armando Perrella, Nunzia Di Meglio, Giulio Bagnacci, Francesco Giuseppe Mazzei, and Maria Antonietta Mazzei

14.1 Introduction

Enteritis and colitis are heterogeneous diseases with many causes, from inflammatory to infectious and ischaemic, so their differential diagnosis is broad. Each case has a substantially different management strategy, which makes appropriate radiological identification crucial. From an imaging perspective, the findings are relatively nonspecific, necessitating an overall assessment of all signs present to formulate a hypothesis regarding the underlying disease process. The majority of patients in this setting present with generalized abdominal pain, and the integration of clinical information (e.g. alvus alteration, comorbidities, drug therapy) and blood tests (e.g. white blood cell count, C-reactive protein and lactates values) is an important tool to support the radiological diagnosis. Although a definitive diagnosis often depends on endoscopic biopsy results, stool culture findings, or other clinical features, it is the radiologist's responsibility to assist in guiding the diagnosis. The gold-standard imaging modality in suspected enteritis and colitis is contrast-enhanced computed tomography (CECT). Particularly in the acute phase and in the emergency setting, CT can provide crucial information to guide diagnosis, identify major complications, and suggest appropriate therapeutic management. Nevertheless, preliminary investigations should be conducted prior to CT, particularly X-ray, which is effective in identifying significant differential diagnoses, such as bowel obstruction, or in detecting complications, such as the presence of toxic megacolon or pneumoperitoneum, which indicates bowel perforation. Ultrasonography (US) indications for acute enteritis and colitis are limited to cases involving young/paediatric patients, where the limitation of radiation exposure should be mandatory. In these cases, the use of CT is recommended in cases of nondiagnostic US and in cases where there is a discrepancy between the clinical symptoms and negative imaging findings observed in the US examination [1]. In contrast, magnetic resonance imaging (MRI), has only limited indications for the emergency phase study of intestinal loops. MRI can play a role in the diagnosis and monitoring of the therapeutic response in Crohn's disease (CD) and ischemic colitis [2]. With regard to the methodology of performing the CT scan, it should be noted that pre-contrastographic scan-

A. Perrella · N. Di Meglio · G. Bagnacci
M. A. Mazzei (✉)
Department of Medical, Surgical and Neuro Sciences, University of Siena, Diagnostic Imaging Unit, Azienda Ospedaliera Universitaria Senese, Siena, Italy
e-mail: armando.perrella@unisi.it; giulio.bagnacci@unisi.it; mariaantonietta.mazzei@unisi.it

F. G. Mazzei
Emergency Diagnostic Unit, Azienda Ospedaliera Universitaria Senese, Siena, Italy

L. Romano et al. (eds.), *CT of Non-Traumatic Body Emergencies*,
https://doi.org/10.1007/978-3-031-84849-0_14

ning is not mandatory. However, it does allow for the detection of ancillary findings, such as spontaneous hyperdensity of the bowel walls or their lumen, which may be suggestive of haemorrhagic necrosis. The optimal evaluation of bowel wall enhancement is conducted in the enteric phase (45–50 seconds after the intravenous contrast media injection begins) and/or the portal venous phase (60–70 seconds after the intravenous contrast media injection begins). Dual-energy CT (DECT) is a technique that enhances contrast resolution while simultaneously reducing the volume of contrast medium required. The enhanced contrast resolution of DECT is achieved through the use of iodine decomposition maps (which provide a quantitative and qualitative assessment of iodine distribution) and virtual monoenergetic reconstructions at low energies (approximately 40–55 keV). This enables a more accurate assessment of intestinal mucosal and wall enhancement patterns and a more confident differential diagnosis of conditions lacking enhancement, such as intestinal ischemia. Furthermore, DECT is especially advantageous for elderly patients with multiple comorbidities and low estimated glomerular filtration rates. There is no evidence to support the use of oral contrast, which may even mask the mucosal enhancement pattern: it is often poorly tolerated by patients with nausea and abdominal pain. Following intravenous administration of contrast medium, the findings are extremely variable, ranging from parietal thickening of the loops, which may be diffuse, segmental (10–30 cm), or focal (<10 cm), to bowel distention. In the post-contrastographic phase, different patterns of intestinal wall enhancement can be identified, which may suggest various diagnoses (Table 14.1). This chapter will concentrate on the principal CT characteristics of infectious enterocolitis and primary and secondary forms of inflammatory enterocolitis.

Table 14.1 The main CT signs found in the various forms of enteritis and colitis

CT findings	Description	Differential diagnosis	Imaging pattern
Bowel wall or intraluminal hyperdensity	Spontaneous hyperdensity of the intestinal wall or its luminal content due to haemorrhagic necrosis phenomena. This sign is detectable in the CT scan without contrast medium	Bowel ischemia Trauma or Spontaneous Hematoma	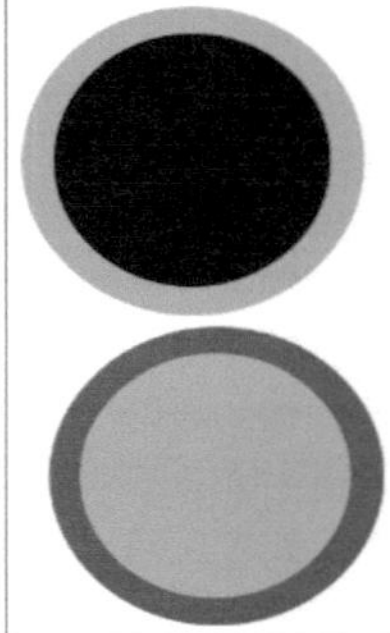
Bowel wall hyperenhancement	Marked enhancement of the intestinal mucosa due to vasodilation phenomena	Acute IBD Infectious diseases Reperfusion after bowel ischemia	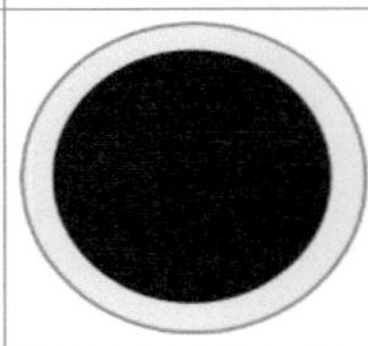
Bowel wall hypoenhancement	Reduced vascularisation of the walls of the bowel loops—diffuse or in comparison with other bowel loops	Intestinal ischemia	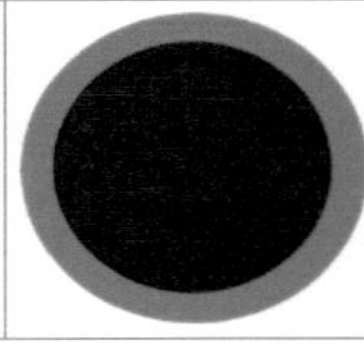

(continued)

Table 14.1 (continued)

CT findings	Description	Differential diagnosis	Imaging pattern
Target or halo sign with edematous submucosa	Target appearance of the bowel wall due to enhancing mucosa and muscularis mucosa with edemigenous thickening of the submucosa tonaca in between	Infectious diseases Acute IBD Intestinal ischemia (venous or non-occlusive) Reperfusion after bowel ischemia Portal hypertension	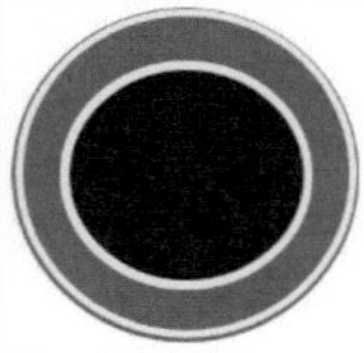
Target sign with fat metaplasia submucosa	Target appearance of the bowel wall due to fat metaplasia of submucosa tonaca. This sign is due to a chronic inflammatory process	Chronic IBD or Celiac disease (especially duodenum or proximal jejunum) Obesity Chemotherapy	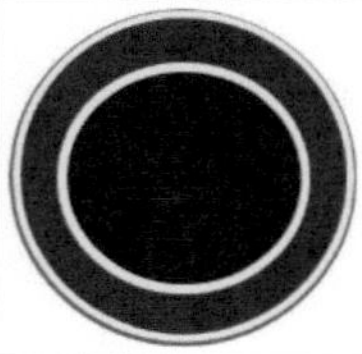
Ascites		Infectious diseases Acute IBD Intestinal ischemia	–
Mesenteric edema/ fat stranding		Infectious diseases Acute IBD Intestinal ischemia (venous type and reperfusion phase)	–
Mesenteric lymphadenopathies		Infectious enteritis Acute IBD	–

IBD Inflammatory Bowel Disease

14.2 Infective Enteritis and Colitis

Infectious enterocolitis is a condition characterized by bowel inflammation, which may be caused by bacteria, viruses, or parasites. In such cases, the CT findings are non-specific and a key element in the differential diagnosis is the topographical distribution of the loops involved, which allows one to suggest the possible aetiological agent. Duodenitis is most commonly associated with Helicobacter pylori infection, which is a differential diagnosis with peptic ulcers and non-steroidal anti-inflammatory drug (NSAID) induced inflammation [3]. Duodenitis is characterized by the presence of parietal thickening with submucosal edema and periduodenal fat stranding, and a duodenal fold thickness of greater than 4 mm, which may be accompanied by erosions. The thickening of the duodenal folds may sometimes appear nodular, especially when the viscera is distended, due to hyperplasia of Brunner's glands [4]. In the case of small bowel infections, parasitic enteritis, which is caused by parasitic protozoa and helminths, including Giardia and Strongyloides species, most often involves the proximal small bowel. In contrast, bacteria such as non-typhoidal Salmonella, Shigella, and Yersinia species typically affect the distal small bowel. The role of imaging in small bowel enteritis is constrained by the poorly characterizing findings: intestinal loops are thickened and edematous, with moderately thickened and smooth folds caused by infiltration of the lamina propria and submucosa by macrophages packed with acid-fast organisms [5]. Lymphadenomegaly and ascites may be present in disseminated infection (Fig. 14.1). Furthermore, the scarcity of imaging findings that are useful in the differential diagnosis is attributable to the fact that a considerable proportion of patients with acute enteritis do not undergo radiological and endoscopic investigations, but are treated with empirical supportive therapy [4]. In helminthiasis, the presence of larvae and worms within the intestinal lumen may also be identified through CT examinations. Anisakis larvae, for instance, have been observed

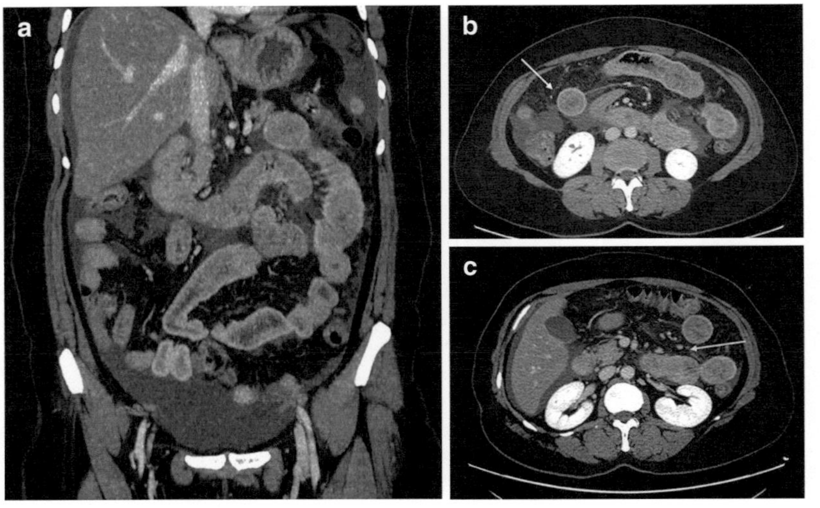

Fig. 14.1 CT image of infectious salmonella enteritis: (**a**, **b**) bowel loops are thickened and edematous (target appearance, white arrow) with mucosal hyperenhancement. Ascites (**a**, **b**) and lymphadenopathy (white arrow in **c**) are also present

within the stomach and colon, manifesting as thin, elongated structures. Additionally, the adult worms Ascaris lumbricoides have the capacity to reach lengths of up to 40 cm, which can result in complications such as bowel obstruction, volvulus, and intussusception. The Mycobacterium avium-intracellular (MAI) complex may be an additional aetiological agent leading to enteritis associated with chronic diarrhea, abdominal pain, malabsorption, weight loss, lymphadenopathy, and hepato-splenomegaly in immunocompromised patients. MAI complex infection more commonly involves the jejunum, causing wall thickening which may be nodular, often associated with large and hypoattenuating mesenteric and retroperitoneal lymphadenopathies. It can be indistinguishable from a giardiasis or Cryptosporidium infection. Neutropenic enteritis or typhlitis is a potentially fatal infection of the distal ileum, cecum, and proximal ascending colon in severely neutropenic patients caused by enteric pathogens. CT of the abdomen usually reveals thickening of an ileal loop with mural stratification, resulting from low-attenuation submucosal edema and inflammation, as well as cecal inflammation. Tuberculosis, typhlitis, and amebiasis most frequently affect the distal ileum and cecum. Due to the distribution of intestinal lymphatics, intestinal tuberculosis mainly impacts the ileocecal region. A comprehensive autopsy series revealed the disease involved the distal ileum in 90% of cases, the cecum in 75%, the ascending colon in 51%, and skip lesions were also observed and it often occurs in patients without radiographic evidence of pulmonary disease [6]. Intestinal tuberculosis is characterized by diffuse circumferential thickening of the terminal ileum, occasionally accompanied by a fibrotic stenotic valve and the medial wall of the cecum. This condition is often associated with large lymphadenopathy, which can sometimes be necrotic. It may also be associated with peritoneal involvement with peritoneal and mesenteric nodules, fibrotic adhesions, and variable amounts of hyperattenuating ascites due to protein and cellular debris. In the colon, Yersinia and Salmonella species frequently infect the ascending portion, whereas Shigella species infect the descending colon. Pancolitis can be seen in Clostridium Difficile, Cytomegalovirus, and Escherichia Coli infections (Fig. 14.2). Acute colitis often presents with acute abdominal pain, and a CT scan is performed as a general overview before the exact etiology of the picture is defined. In this scenario, where laboratory and clinical correlations are often poor, the differential diagnosis with other diseases, in particular ischaemic colitis, is particularly complex. However, three features would seem most likely to be associated with infectious colitis: (1) the "empty colon" sign, i.e. the complete absence of gas, fluid, and faeces in the colic lumen; (2) the absence of

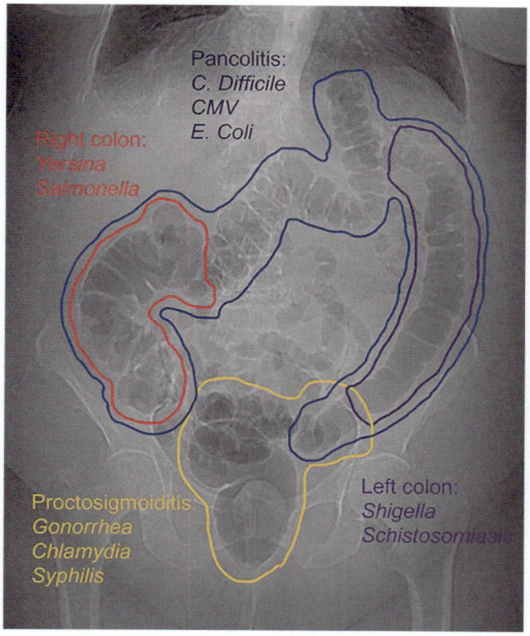

Fig. 14.2 Distribution of the main forms of infectious colitis according to the aetiological agent

enlarged lymph nodes, which are more frequently associated with inflammatory bowel disease (IBD) as well as simultaneous small bowel involvement; (3) the continuous involvement of the colic tract, which differs from the segmental involvement of ischaemic colitis [4, 7]. Although in 10% of cases, there may be diffuse ischaemia, ischaemic colitis usually affects the watershed areas (splenic flexure or rectosigmoid junction), which have reduced vascular compensation, or specific vascular territories (i.e. superior or inferior mesenteric artery) [7]. Some types of colitis are characterized by distinctive CT findings, such as pancolitis caused by Clostridium difficile. Clostridioides difficile colitis, also known as pseudomembranous colitis, is a common cause of antibiotic-associated infectious colitis in hospitalized patients with multiple comorbidities. It is clinically characterized by diarrhea, fever, abdominal pain, and distension and, if undiagnosed and untreated, it continues to have a high mortality rate due to fulminant colitis, toxic megacolon, and subsequently perforation. Characteristic CT findings include involvement of the whole colon, including the rectum (although up to 40% of cases may involve only the right colon), with marked oedematous wall thickening involving mucosa and submucosa, irregular mucosal outline and presence of the thumbprint and accordion signs. The thumbprinting sign results from regular edematous thickening of the colonic folds, which project into the aerated colonic lumen, while the accordion sign derives from the contrast between the hypervascular mucosa, the submucosal oedematous thickening of the haustral folds and the formation of pseudomembranes on the luminal surface of the colon (Fig. 14.3). Additionally, since it is primarily a mucosal/submucosal infectious process, it is not frequently associated with fat stranding, while free fluid may be present (in up to 40% of cases). Pseudomembranous colitis produces one of the most severe degrees of colonic wall thickening among all types of colitis. In addition to pseudomembranous colitis, Clostridium difficile can cause an isolated form of acute enteritis in immunocompromised patients: in this case, it is associated with non-specific CT findings (distended, fluid-filled small bowel loops, ascites, and mesenteric fat stranding). Proctosigmoiditis could be caused by sexually transmitted infections, including gonococcal or chlamydia infection, and syphilis. On CT examination, they are characterized by edematous wall thickening of the sigmoid colon and rectum with loss of haustration and sometimes ulcerations and/or fistulas. The main differential diagnoses include ischemic proctitis or post-radiation proctitis.The main diagnostic challenge in infectious enterocolitis is the differentiation between ischaemic colitis and IBD, using imaging alone. The differential diagnosis of intestinal ischemia may be straightforward in cases of occlusive forms, where the presence of arterial or venous thrombosis, intestinal pneumatosis, or the presence of air in the porto-mesenteric venous system can be identified. However, the diagnosis is more complex in non-occlusive ischaemic forms with signs of reperfusion (oedematous thickening of the intestinal wall on CT). As previously stated, these are distinguished by segmental involvement of the intestinal loops, with a greater prevalence in the watershed regions (splenic flexure or rectosig-

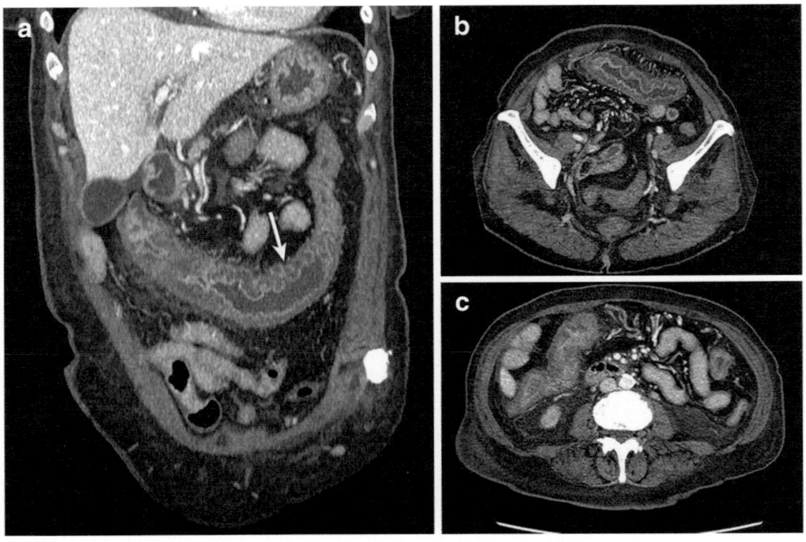

Fig. 14.3 Pseudomembranous colitis. The whole colon is involved in the infectious process, with marked edematous thickening of the submucosal tonaca, mucosal hyperenhancement, and irregular mucosal outline (arrow) (**a**). The thumbprint (**b**) and the accordion sign (**c**) are also visible

moid junction). Additionally, there is an absence of lymphadenopathies and the presence of extraintestinal findings, including splenic and renal parenchymal ischaemia and atherosclerosis of the mesenteric vessels.

14.3 Inflammatory Enterocolitis

Inflammatory enterocolitis can be primary (IBD, vasculitis) or secondary (i.e. drug-induced disorders, radiation therapy enterocolitis, graft versus host disease).

14.3.1 Inflammatory Bowel Diseases (IBD)

IBD refers to a group of chronic remitting and relapsing diseases characterized by a gastrointestinal inflammatory process that may be associated with multisystemic and extraintestinal manifestation; ulcerative colitis (UC) and Crohn's disease (CD) are the most common types of IBD and they differ in histopathological, topographical, and imaging features (Table 14.2).

CD can affect simultaneously any part of the gastrointestinal tract, from the mouth to the anus, but the small bowel and the terminal ileum is the most common location (70–80% of cases) [4]. It is not rare to encounter patients with disease involving only the colon or anorectal area in the emergency setting (up to 30% of cases). The CD is characterized by a chronic and relapsing transmural inflammation, initially limited to the mucosa with lymphoid hyperplasia and neutrophilic cryptitis, which may progress to involve the entire intestinal wall and mesentery, leading to a fibrostenotic phase and a penetrating disease responsible for complications such as fistula, abscess, and free perforation. There is increasing evidence of an association between stricture formation and penetrating bowel disease; in fact, fistulae usually form in the mid or proximal aspect of the stricture, whereas in the absence of stricture, penetrating disease is very unlikely [8]. CT has a pivotal role in the diagnosis of the disease and the detection of complications, which are a major cause of morbidity in CD. The signs of small bowel inflammation on CECT include the following: (1) bowel wall thickening greater than or equal to 3 mm; (2) mural edema and peri-

Table 14.2 Main CT differences in Crohn's disease and ulcerative colitis

CT features	Crohn's disease	Ulcerative colitis
Location	Can affect any part of the GI tract, from mouth to anus	Restricted to the colon and rectum
Distribution	Patchy, with "skip lesions" (areas of normal tissue between affected areas)	Continuous inflammation starting from the rectum
Bowel wall thickening	Often significant and asymmetric (greater than 1 cm; approx. 11–13 mm)	Usually mild to moderate and symmetric/concentric (approximately 8 mm)
Mucosal enhancement	Patchy mucosal enhancement	Diffuse mucosal enhancement
Colon wall appearance	"Cobblestone" appearance due to deep ulcerations and transmural inflammation	Uniform, shallow ulcerations
Ileocecal valve involvement	Frequently involved, often thickened and narrowed	Rarely involved
Strictures	Common, especially in the small intestine	Less common
Fistulas	Common, can be entero-enteric, entero-cutaneous, etc	Rare
Abscesses	Can be present, especially if there are fistulas	Rare
Mesenteric fat wrapping	Often present (also called "creeping fat")	Not typically seen
Lymphadenopathy	Frequently observed	Less common
Perianal disease	Common, including abscesses and fistulas	Rare
Inflammatory pseudopolyps	Rare	Common

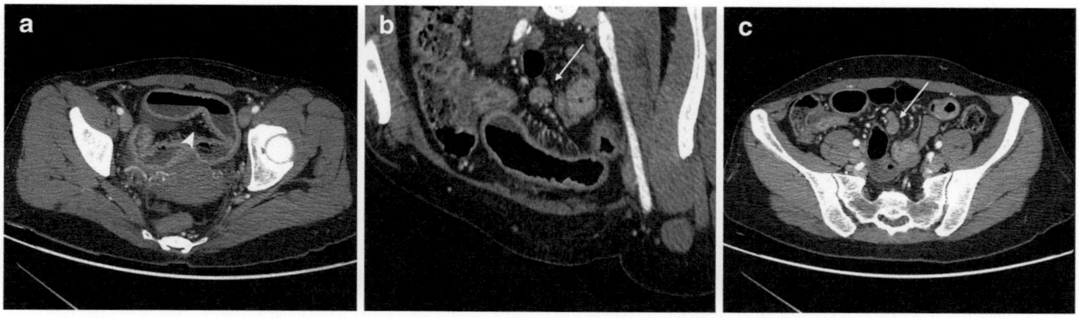

Fig. 14.4 Involvement of the terminal ileum in Crohn's Disease: there is a thickening of the bowel wall with hyperenhancement, fat stranding (arrowhead) (**a**) and lymphadenopathy (white arrows in **b** and **c**). In the coronal reconstruction (**b**), the comb sign is visible

enteric fat stranding; (3) segmental mural hyperenhancement; and ulcerations (Fig. 14.4). Wall thickness should be evaluated and measured in a bowel segment that is adequately distended by fluid or enteric contrast material and should be subdivided as mild (3–5 mm) moderate (>5–9 mm), or severe (≥10 mm). Bowel wall thickening greater than 15 mm is atypical for CD and neoplasia should be excluded. Segmental mural hyperenhancement may be asymmetric, stratified, or homogeneous and is visible in a noncontracted segment of the small bowel. The asymmetric/eccentric mural hyperenhancement is a specific imaging finding for small bowel CD and often involves the mesenteric border of a small bowel loop more than the antimesenteric border. Stratified mural hyperenhancement is defined as hyperenhancement of both the inner and outer (trilaminate) or only the inner (bilaminar) of the bowel wall; it could be associated with a combination of submucosal edema, intramural fat deposition, or fibrosis, and inflammatory infiltration. Homogeneous symmetric mural hyperenhancement, which is rare, is transmural hyperenhancement that uniformly involves the entire bowel wall and can have many other causes besides CD, including fibrosis, infiltration, ischaemia, collagen deposition, or shock bowel [9, 10].

Other characteristic CT signs of CD are the engorged and enlarged vasa recta that supply and drain an inflamed bowel loop, defined as comb sign, and the hypertrophy of the mesenteric fat adjacent to diseased bowel segments (fibrofatty proliferation or creeping fat sign), which displaces surrounding structures and bowel loops. Also, lymphadenopathies and submucosal fat deposition (fat halo sign) often occur [11].

Strictures, fissures, fistulas, and abscess formations are frequent complications in CD, secondary to transmural inflammation as opposed to UC, and they are considered hallmark features. Sinuses and fissures are blind-ending inflammatory tracts that penetrate through the full thickness of the bowel wall. Fistulae, which may be enteroenteric, enterovesical, enterocutaneous, perianal, and colovaginal, can be classified as simple or complex: a complex fistula is defined as the presence of more than one fistulous tract and can result in an asterisk-shaped or cloverleaf appearance. Abscess is a fluid collection with rim enhancement well-defined wall, with or without internal gas bubbles and/or air-fluid level, and it may be confined to the bowel wall or pericolic and mesenteric fat, or may involve adjacent structures, such as the psoas muscle and retroperitoneum, bladder, and perirectal/perianal region. Perianal or rectal fistulae are another common finding in colonic or rectal disease; when possible, perianal fistulas should be reported using Park's or St James' classification system. Up to one-third of patients develop stricture within 10 years of the diagnosis: a stricture is defined as a bowel segment with luminal narrowing and unequivocal dilation (i.e. $\geq$3 cm) of the upstream bowel segment; conversely, luminal narrowing is defined as luminal diameter reduction of at least 50% compared with that of a normal adjacent bowel loop. A stricture can be present with or without active inflammation; when it is present, the location and length of the stricture and imaging findings of concurrent inflammation or upstream dilation should be reported. A bowel stricture may be present without upstream dilation (<3 cm); for example, a fistula could decompress the upstream small bowel segment or if there are two or more strictures close, in which case the distal stricture may not have associated upstream dilation. However, strictures with active inflammation in the ileum, especially at the terminal loops, can be a common cause of bowel obstruction (upstream dilatation >4 cm), hence the indication for CT. Thrombosis of the mesenteric vein can occur in CD, usually adjacent to an inflamed loop, and it can be acute (distended vein) or chronic (interrupted or narrowed vein).

UC is typically confined to the colon and is characterized by a diffuse, symmetric, and continuous distribution starting from the rectum. Bowel wall thickness is concentric with a mean value lower than CD due to confined mucosal and submucosal inflammation (Fig. 14.5). The haustral folds undergo two major changes: early on in the disease, they may be edematous and thickened, and in chronic disease, they may become blunted or completely effaced (ahaustral) with foreshortening of the colon [8]. CT is often insensitive to UC early mucosal disease. Some CT findings are the inflamed and thickened bowel, with a target appearance due to concentric rings of varying attenuation (i.e. mural stratification) [12]. Strictures are also common due to marked muscolaris mucosae hypertrophy and are not all malignant. When most of the mucosa has been lost, islands of mucosa remain giving it a pseudopolyp appearance, whereas in areas of mucosal denudation, abnormal thinning of the bowel may also be evident (Fig. 14.6). In chronic cases, the colon loses the normal haustral marking with a luminal narrowing, bowel shortening, and smooth-walled and cylindrical appearance (lead pipe sign). Another chronic feature is represented

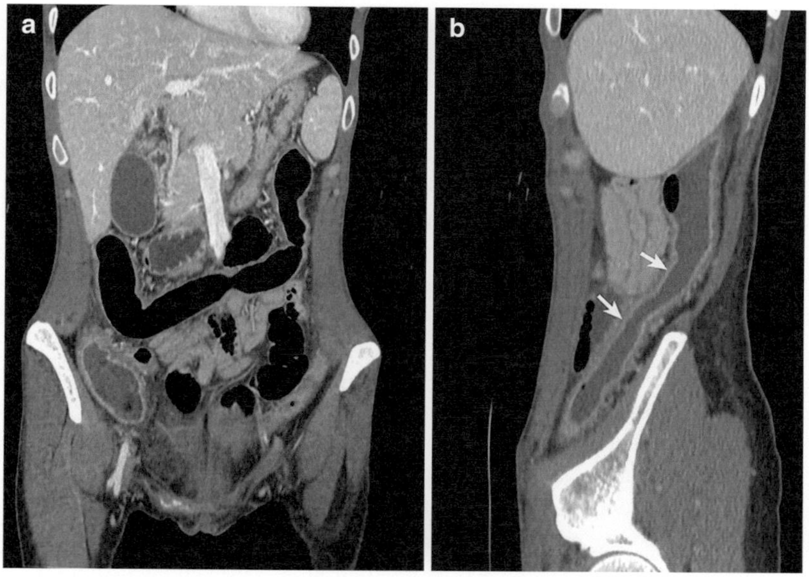

Fig. 14.5 Example of ulcerative rectocolitis with diffuse, symmetrical, and continuous distribution from the rectum (**a**). The colon has lost its normal haustral markings (**b**) with luminal narrowing, bowel shortening, and a smooth cylindrical appearance (lead pipe sign arrows)

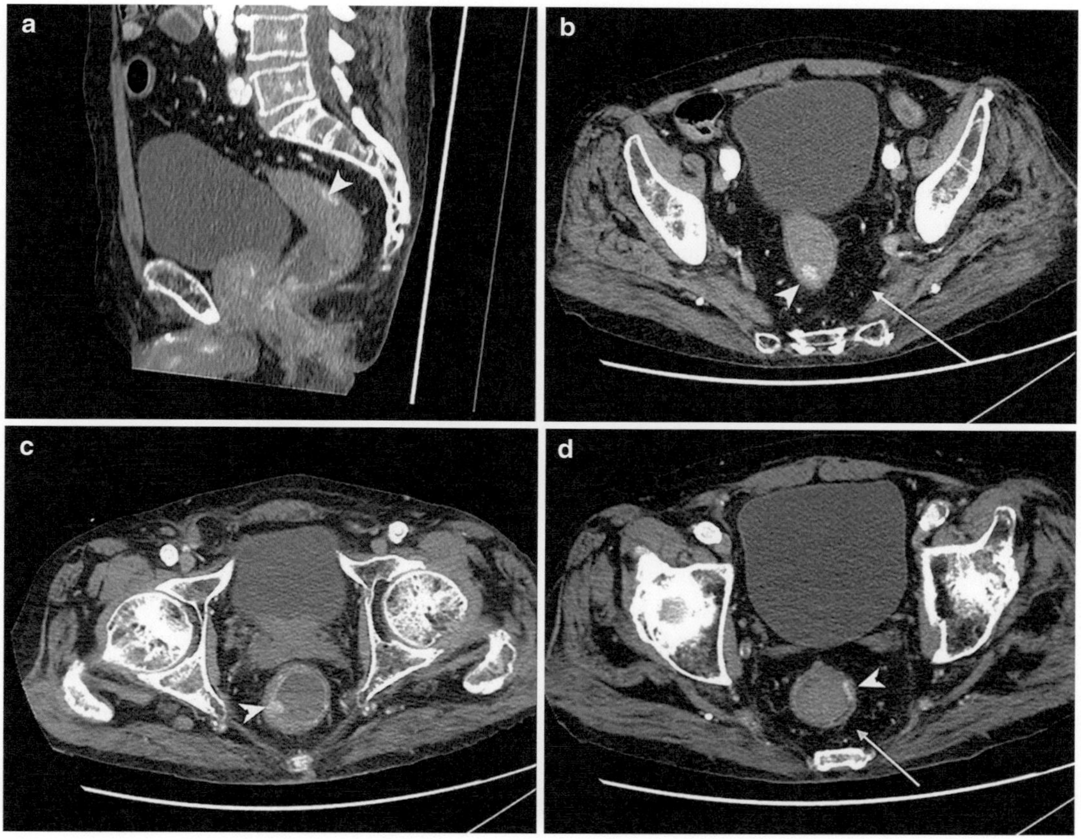

Fig. 14.6 Involvement of the rectum and sigmoid colon in ulcerative colitis (**a**) with fibrofatty proliferation (arrow, **b**), fat halo sign (arrow, **d**) and multiple hypervascular mucosal pseudopolyps (arrowheads, **a**–**d**)

by submucosal fat deposition, particularly in the rectum (fat halo sign), derived from the chronic inflammatory process. Extramural fat deposition (fibrofatty proliferation) is also common in the perirectal space, with presacral space widening. Complications in UC are toxic megacolon and colorectal carcinoma. Toxic megacolon is a potentially lethal complication of UC that results from the extension of the mucosal inflammation into the colonic smooth-muscle layer with the destruction of ganglion cells. As a result, the bowel becomes aperistaltic and begins to dilate. It is characterized by total or segmental nonobstructive colonic dilatation (>6 cm) with systemic toxicity. Colorectal carcinoma could be suspected when there is a focal loss of mural stratification with an excessive mural thickness or sessile lesions: in these cases, endoscopic evaluation is required [13].

14.3.2 Inflammatory Enterocolitis

Abdominal manifestations of rheumatologic disease may result from primary involvement with Systemic lupus erythematosus (SLE), Scleroderma, Henoch-Schonlein purpura, or complications of therapy. Serositis and intestinal vasculitis can present with severe abdominal pain and may masquerade as an acute surgical abdomen. Lupus enterocolitis presents as chronic ulcerations in the bowel wall or as acute ischemic enteritis that results from mesenteric vasculitis or vascular occlusion associated with the antiphospholipid syndrome. The jejunum (80%) and ileum (85%) are common sites of involvement. Radiological diagnosis is based on CECT findings of bowel wall edema (>3 mm) with "halo-sign" or "target sign", increased attenuation of mesenteric fat with fat-stranding and engorgement of mesenteric vessels with "coombs sign" [14]. Scleroderma is a complex multisystem connective tissue disorder, affecting the gastrointestinal tract through dysmotility, muscular atrophy, and fibrosis, which reflected the imaging features. The esophagus is the second most frequently involved organ after the skin, but the involvement of the proximal small bowel (duodenum and jejunum) and distal large bowel (anorectal) are also common. Diagnosis is based on CECT; often we can see dilated fluid-filled esophagus (up to 6 cm in caliber), dilatation of duodenum and jejunum with a transition to non-dilated distal small bowel and wall thickening of the jejunum with tightened jejunal folds which can remember the hide-bound sign. This radiologic finding is the radiographic representation of the smooth muscle atrophy and fibrosis that occurs as a result of foreshortening of the small bowel in scleroderma; "faeces-sign" could be present. In the large bowel, the atrophy of the smooth muscle in the colonic wall causes dilatation and loss of haustral pattern leading to "wide-mouth" diverticula that can become ulcerated, infected, or even perforate from fecal impaction; colonic hypomotility can cause delayed gut transit time and subsequently, constipation with potentiated bacterial overgrowth which can ultimately lead to malabsorptive diarrhea. The absence of surrounding inflammatory fat stranding is important to differentiate from acute infectious or inflammatory causes of bowel wall thickening; pneumatosis cystoid intestinalis, characterized by clusters of gas within the bowel wall, is a possible intestinal complication of scleroderma for stasis of luminal contents that can facilitate bacterial overgrowth [15]. Henoch-Schonlein purpura is a small vessel vasculitis mediated by type III hypersensitivity with deposition of IgA immune complex in the walls of vessels. On CT imaging, bowel involvement is seen as multifocal symmetric, circumferential wall thickening with target appearance and mural stratification, presence of skip areas, with involvement of unusual sites like stomach, duodenum, and rectum; associated findings include free intraperitoneal fluid, ileus of the affected loop, vascular engorgement in the adjoining mesentery and non-specific lymphadenopathy (Fig. 14.7) [16, 17].

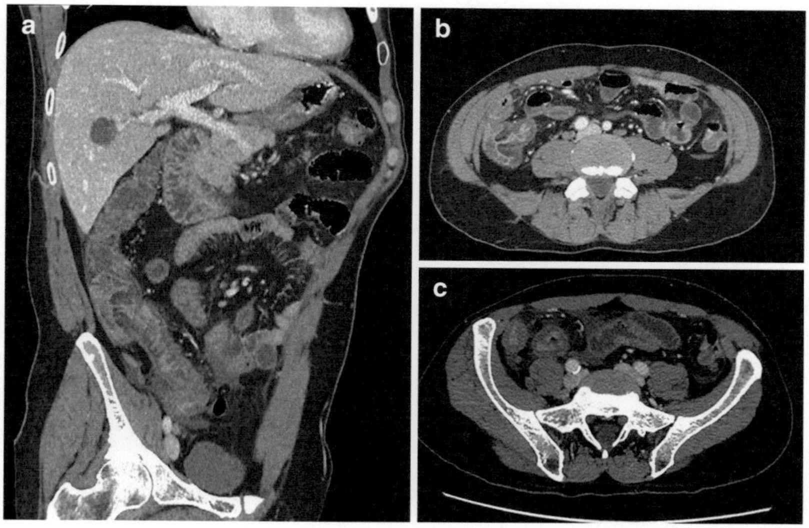

Fig. 14.7 Case of terminal ileal enteritis and right colitis of vasculitic origin in a patient with Henoch-Schonlein purpura. Significant symmetric and concentric thickening of the bowel wall is present with target appearance (**a**, **b**); involvement of the ileocecal valve, swollen and edematous (**b**), and fat stranding adjacent to the intestinal loops are also visible (**c**)

14.3.3 Drug-Induced Disorders and Radiation Therapy Enterocolitis

A number of drugs have been observed to induce a range of abnormalities in the small intestine and colon. Anticoagulants, such as warfarin, have been associated with an increased risk of gastrointestinal bleeding or intramural hematomas, which may be identified as an increased bowel wall density on unenhanced CT scans. Narcotics and anticholinergic drugs can cause small bowel hypomotility. Chemotherapy drugs, particularly antimetabolites such as 5-fluorouracil, have the potential to cause mucosal damage within the first 3 days of treatment, leading to symptoms such as nausea, vomiting, and diarrhea, with marked wall thickening of the distal ileum with smooth, thickened, or effaced ileal folds on CT imaging. A diagnosis is typically suggested based on a clinical history of recent chemotherapy. Additionally, oral molecular-targeted agents such as Tyrosine Kinase Inhibitors (erlotinib, sorafenib, sunitinib, and imatinib) have been associated with enterocolitis related to the oral administration route. Enteritis and colitis have rarely been reported in immune checkpoint inhibitors (ICI) therapies, with a median time to onset of gastritis estimated to be approximately 4–9 months following the initiation of therapy [18]. On CT imaging, enteritis is characterized by diffuse wall thickening of the small bowel with mucosal hyperenhancement, distension of the lumen with fluid, and adjacent fat stranding (Fig. 14.8) [19, 20]. With regard to colonic involvement, two different types of extent have been described: (i) focal/segmental colitis (focal for a few centimeters and segmental for 10–30 cm), which is seen in a bowel segment with pre-existing diverticulosis and is characterized by short segment bowel wall thickening with mural stratification, such as a "target" or "halo" appearance, mucosal hyperenhancement and pericolic fat stranding; (ii) diffuse colitis (>30 cm), which is characterized by the mucosal hyperenhancement, vessel engorgement, bowel wall thickening, fat stranding and fluid stagnation in the lumen. The degree of bowel wall thickness was graded as mild (4–8 mm), moderate (8–12 mm), and severe (>12 mm), which is modified from the criteria described by Bharucha et al. [21, 22]. Ulcers, focal inflammation, and stenosis can be induced by NSAIDs, but they are very difficult or impossible to detect on CT. NSAID-induced webs or diaphragms may be seen as 2- to 5-mm wide ringlike strictures encircling the small bowel [23]. ACE inhibitors can cause gastrointestinal angioedema, characterized by circumferential

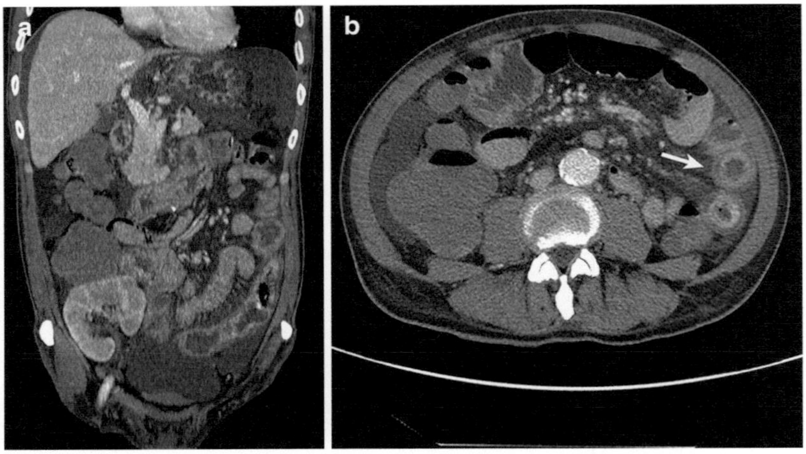

Fig. 14.8 Acute enteritis following treatment with checkpoint inhibitors: diffuse oedematous thickening (target appearance, arrow) of the jejunum and ileum with the presence of ascites (**a**) and mesenteric fat stranding (**b**)

bowel wall thickening (approximately 4–9 mm) with target appearance, mesenteric edema due to engorged vasa rectae, and ascites on CT [24, 25]. A review by Benson et al. highlights ascites as a key feature in distinguishing ACE inhibitor-induced visceral angioedema from infectious enteritis [26]. Radiation therapy may lead to enterocolitis, presenting as bowel wall thickening and submucosal edema, with risks increased by high doses and concurrent chemotherapy.

Radiation-induced enterocolitis is a deterministic effect, which results from the toxic effects of radiation therapy on the wall and vasculature of the small and large intestines. About 5–15% of patients treated with radiotherapy (usually >4500 cGy) develop chronic radiation enteropathy. Some risk factors could increase the occurrence of this complication of treatment: high radiation dose, metabolic syndrome (atherosclerosis, hypertension, and diabetes mellitus), and treatment combination with chemotherapy. In pelvic radiotherapy, enteritis of the small bowel typically involves the more fixed terminal ileum and manifests as bowel wall thickening and submucosal edema at CT examination. CT may also show bowel luminal narrowing or small bowel obstruction or fistulas between the bowel (especially the colon) and the bladder or vagina, as further complications of treatment.

14.3.4 Graft-Versus-Host Disease

Acute graft-versus-host disease (GVHD) is a frequent and serious complication after allogenic hematopoietic stem cell transplant which involves multiple organ systems but is most commonly seen in the gastrointestinal tract. It occurs in about 30% to 50% of patients and develops in 3 to 11 weeks. Acute GVHD gastrointestinal tract usually occurs with abdominal pain, anorexia, diarrhea, vomiting, and gastrointestinal bleeding and is often complicated by sovra-infection by cytomegalovirus, adenovirus, and Clostridium difficile infection [27]. It is crucial to combine radiological findings with clinical history, including the timing of the transplant, laboratory values, and any stool studies and dermatologic findings. CT may reveal a diffusely thickened small bowel wall with mucosal hyperenhancement, extensive submucosal edema of the ileum and jejunum with mural stratification and target sign, mesenteric congestion, thickening of the bowel wall with engorgement of the vasa recta adjacent and bowel dilatation. In advanced cases, there could be present pneumatosis. Often there is gastric wall thickening and some extraintestinal findings in the abdomen: ascites, periportal edema, biliary abnormalities, and thoracic manifestations. The main differential diagnosis in these patients may include neutropenic enterocolitis (most commonly involves the cecum and ascending colon and occasionally involves the ileum in contradistinction to GVH) and infectious enterocolitis (e.g. pseudomembranous colitis and CMV). Viral infection often is segmental rather than diffuse involvement and CMV colitis has a similar appearance to typhlitis, predominantly affecting the terminal ileum, cecum, and right colon. Chronic GVHD develops 3 to 13 months after transplantation and is characterized by strictures or stenosis related to fibrosis of the lamina propria and submucosa with subsequent bacterial overgrowth, mostly in the upper to a mid-third of the esophagus.

References

1. Mazzei MA, Guerrini S, Cioffi Squitieri N, Cagini L, Macarini L, Coppolino F, Giganti M, Volterrani L. The role of US examination in the management of acute abdomen. Crit Ultrasound J. 2013;5 Suppl 1(Suppl 1):S6. https://doi.org/10.1186/2036-7902-5-S1-S6.
2. Mazzei MA, Guerrini S, Cioffi Squitieri N, Imbriaco G, Chieca R, Civitelli S, Savelli V, Mazzei FG, Volterrani L. Magnetic resonance imaging: is there a role in clinical management for acute ischemic colitis? World J Gastroenterol. 2013;19(8):1256–63. https://doi.org/10.3748/wjg.v19.i8.1256.
3. Juanpere S, Valls L, Serra I, Osorio M, Gelabert A, Maroto A, Pedraza S. Imaging of non-neoplastic duodenal diseases. A pictorial review with emphasis on MDCT. Insights Imaging. 2018;9(2):121–35. https://doi.org/10.1007/s13244-018-0593-6.
4. Duffin C, Mirpour S, Catanzano T, Moore C. Radiologic imaging of bowel infections. Semin Ultrasound CT MR. 2020;41(1):33–45. https://doi.org/10.1053/j.sult.2019.10.004.
5. Frager DH, Frager JD, Brandt LJ, Wolf EL, Rand LG, Klein RS, Beneventano TC. Gastrointestinal complications of AIDS: radiologic features. Radiology. 1986;158(3):597–603. https://doi.org/10.1148/radiology.158.3.3003792.
6. Rubesin SE. Inflammatory disorders of the small bowel other than Crohn's disease. In: Gastrointestinal Radiology, 2-Volume Set (Fourth Edition); 2015.
7. Balthazar EJ, Yen BC, Gordon RB. Ischemic colitis: CT evaluation of 54 cases. Radiology. 1999;211(2):381–8. https://doi.org/10.1148/radiology.211.2.r99ma28381.
8. Maddu KK, Mittal P, Arepalli CD, Shuaib W, Tewari A, Khosa F. Colorectal emergencies and related complications: a comprehensive imaging review—noninfectious and noninflammatory emergencies of colon. AJR Am J Roentgenol. 2014;203(6):1217–29. https://doi.org/10.2214/AJR.13.12323.
9. Guglielmo FF, Anupindi SA, Fletcher JG, Al-Hawary MM, Dillman JR, Grand DJ, Bruining DH, Chatterji M, Darge K, Fidler JL, Gandhi NS, Gee MS, Grajo JR, Huang C, Jaffe TA, Park SH, Rimola J, Soto JA, Taouli B, Taylor SA, Baker ME. Small bowel Crohn disease at CT and MR enterography: imaging atlas and glossary of terms. Radiographics. 2020;40(2):354–75. https://doi.org/10.1148/rg.2020190091.
10. Bruining DH, Zimmermann EM, Loftus EV Jr, Sandborn WJ, Sauer CG, Strong SA, Society of Abdominal Radiology Crohn's Disease-Focused Panel. Consensus recommendations for evaluation, interpretation, and utilization of computed tomography and magnetic resonance enterography in patients with small bowel Crohn's disease. Radiology. 2018;286(3):776–99. https://doi.org/10.1148/radiol.2018171737.
11. Bruining DH, Zimmermann EM, Loftus EV Jr, Sandborn WJ, Sauer CG, Strong SA, Society of Abdominal Radiology Crohn's Disease-Focused Panel. Consensus recommendations for evaluation, interpretation, and utilization of computed tomography and magnetic resonance enterography in patients with small bowel Crohn's disease. Gastroenterology. 2018;154(4):1172–94. https://doi.org/10.1053/j.gastro.2017.11.274.
12. Deepak P, Bruining DH. Radiographical evaluation of ulcerative colitis. Gastroenterol Rep (Oxf). 2014;2(3):169–77. https://doi.org/10.1093/gastro/gou026.
13. Gore RM, Balthazar EJ, Ghahremani GG, Miller FH. CT features of ulcerative colitis and Crohn's disease. AJR Am J Roentgenol. 1996;167(1):3–15. https://doi.org/10.2214/ajr.167.1.8659415.
14. Kirby JM, Jhaveri KS, Maizlin ZV, Midia M, Haider E, Khalili K. Abdominal manifestations of systemic lupus erythematosus: spectrum of imaging findings. Can Assoc Radiol J. 2009;60(3):121–32. https://doi.org/10.1016/j.carj.2009.06.001.
15. Delaney FT, Fenlon HM, Buckley B, Welaratne I, Cronin CG. Multimodality imaging of the gastrointestinal manifestations of scleroderma. Clin Radiol. 2021;76(9):640–9. https://doi.org/10.1016/j.crad.2021.04.014.
16. Prathiba Rajalakshmi P, Srinivasan K. Gastrointestinal manifestations of Henoch-Schonlein purpura: a report of two cases. World J Radiol. 2015;7(3):66–9. https://doi.org/10.4329/wjr.v7.i3.66.
17. Sampat HN, McAllister BP, Gaines DD, Ostrov B. Terminal ileitis as a feature of Henoch-Schönlein purpura masquerading as Crohn disease in adults. J Clin Rheumatol. 2016;22(2):82–5. https://doi.org/10.1097/RHU.0000000000000361.
18. Nishimura Y, Yasuda M, Ocho K, Iwamuro M, Yamasaki O, Tanaka T, Otsuka F. Severe gastritis after administration of nivolumab and ipilimumab. Case Rep Oncol. 2018;11(2):549–56. https://doi.org/10.1159/000491862.

19. Messmer M, Upreti S, Tarabishy Y, Mazumder N, Chowdhury R, Yarchoan M, Holdhoff M. Ipilimumab-induced enteritis without colitis: a new challenge. Case Rep Oncol. 2016;9(3):705–13. https://doi.org/10.1159/000452403.
20. Guerrini S, Bagnacci G, Perrella A, Meglio ND, Sica C, Mazzei MA. Dual energy CT in oncology: benefits for both patients and radiologists from an emerging quantitative and functional diagnostic technique. Semin Ultrasound CT MR. 2023;44(3):205–13. https://doi.org/10.1053/j.sult.2023.03.006.
21. Bharucha AE, Tremaine WJ, Johnson CD, Batts KP. Ischemic proctosigmoiditis. Am J Gastroenterol. 1996;91(11):2305–9.
22. Kim KW, Ramaiya NH, Krajewski KM, Shinagare AB, Howard SA, Jagannathan JP, Ibrahim N. Ipilimumab-associated colitis: CT findings. AJR Am J Roentgenol. 2013;200(5):W468–74. https://doi.org/10.2214/AJR.12.9751.
23. Levi S, de Lacey G, Price AB, Gumpel MJ, Levi AJ, Bjarnason I. "Diaphragm-like" strictures of the small bowel in patients treated with non-steroidal anti-inflammatory drugs. Br J Radiol. 1990;63(747):186–9. https://doi.org/10.1259/0007-1285-63-747-186.
24. Turcu AF, White JA, Kulaga ME, Skluth M, Gruss CB. Calcium channel blocker-associated small bowel angioedema. J Clin Gastroenterol. 2009;43(4):338–41. https://doi.org/10.1097/MCG.0b013e31815cf6b9.
25. Vallurupalli K, Coakley KJ. MDCT features of angiotensin-converting enzyme inhibitor-induced visceral angioedema. AJR Am J Roentgenol. 2011;196(4):W405–11. https://doi.org/10.2214/AJR.10.4856.
26. Benson BC, Smith C, Laczek JT. Angiotensin converting enzyme inhibitor-induced gastrointestinal angioedema: a case series and literature review. J Clin Gastroenterol. 2013;47(10):844–9. https://doi.org/10.1097/MCG.0b013e318299c69d.
27. Jones B, Kramer SS, Saral R, Beschorner WE, Yolken RH, Townsend TR, Yeager AM, Lake A, Tutschka P, Santos GW. Gastrointestinal inflammation after bone marrow transplantation: graft-versus-host disease or opportunistic infection? AJR Am J Roentgenol. 1988;150(2):277–81. https://doi.org/10.2214/ajr.150.2.277.

15 Appendicitis

Gaspare Oliva, Stefania Daniele,
Giuseppina Dell'Aversano Orabona,
Giuliana Giacobbe, Luigi Barbuto,
and Luigia Romano

15.1 Introduction

In Europe and United States, acute appendicitis is the most common cause of acute abdominal pain requiring surgery. More than 5% of the population develops appendicitis at some point in their lives, typically during adolescence and between the ages of 20 and 30, though it can occur at any age. Other conditions affecting the appendix include carcinoids, carcinoma, villous adenomas, and diverticula [1–3]. The appendix can also be affected by Crohn's disease or ulcerative colitis with pancolitis (inflammatory bowel disease).

15.2 Clinical Approach

15.2.1 Etiology of Appendicitis

Appendicitis is generally thought to be caused by the obstruction of the appendiceal lumen, typically due to lymphoid hyperplasia, but sometimes due to the presence of a fecalith, foreign body, tumor, or even parasites. The obstruction leads to distention, excessive bacterial growth, ischemia, and inflammation. If untreated, this can result in necrosis, gangrene, and perforation of the appendix. If the perforation is contained by the omentum, an appendiceal abscess can develop.

G. Oliva (✉) · S. Daniele · G. Dell'Aversano Orabona
G. Giacobbe · L. Barbuto · L. Romano
Department of General and Emergency Radiology, "Antonio Cardarelli" Hospital, Naples, Italy
e-mail: gaspare.oliva@aocardarelli.it; stefania.daniele@aocardarelli.it; giuseppina.dellaversanoorabona@aocardarelli.it; giuliana.giacobbe@aocardarelli.it; luigi.barbuto@aocardarelli.it; luigia.romano@aocardarelli.it

L. Romano et al. (eds.), *CT of Non-Traumatic Body Emergencies*,
https://doi.org/10.1007/978-3-031-84849-0_15

15.2.2 Symptoms and Signs of Appendicitis

There are many variations in the symptoms of appendicitis in more than 50% of patients (Tables 15.1 and 15.2). The pain may not be localized, especially in infants and children. Tenderness may be diffuse or, in rare cases, absent. Bowel movements are usually less frequent or absent; if diarrhea is present, a retrocecal appendix should be suspected. Red or white blood cells may be present in the urine.

Atypical symptoms are common in elderly patients and pregnant women; in particular, the pain is less severe and local tenderness less pronounced.

15.2.3 Diagnosis of Appendicitis

- Clinical evaluation
- Ultrasound especially in young patients with localized abdominal pain
- Abdominal CT scan

When the classic symptoms of appendicitis are present, the diagnosis is clinical. In these patients, delaying appendectomy to perform imaging studies only increases the likelihood of perforation and consequent complications. In patients with atypical or equivocal findings, imaging should be performed without delay. Contrast-enhanced CT has reasonable accuracy in diagnosing appendicitis and can also reveal other causes of acute abdomen [4]. Graded compression ultrasound can usually be performed quickly and does not use radiation (a particularly important consideration in children and young patients) [5], but it can be limited by the presence of intestinal gas and is less useful for identifying nonappendiceal causes of pain. Appendicitis remains primarily a clinical diagnosis. Selective and judicious use of imaging studies can reduce the rate of negative laparotomies.

In this regard, it is worth mentioning the opportunity offered by the diagnostic score proposed by Alvarado, based on the clinical laboratory approach. The Alvarado score (also known as the MANTRELS score) is a clinical decision rule and predictor of the likelihood of acute appendicitis (Table 15.3) [6, 7].

The score can be useful for decision-making when evaluating nonspecific imaging or ambiguous ultrasound findings. It is more effective at ruling out appendicitis with a score of less than 5 than at confirming appendicitis with a score greater than 7.

Table 15.1 Symptoms of appendicitis

Classic symptoms of acute appendicitis:
Epigastric or periumbilical pain followed by brief nausea, vomiting, and anorexia
After a few hours, the pain shifts to the lower right abdominal quadrant and increases with coughing and movement

Table 15.2 Clinical signs of appendicitis

Direct and rebound tenderness in the lower right quadrant, localized at McBurney's point (junction of the middle and outer thirds of the line connecting the navel with the anterior superior iliac spine)
Pain in the lower right quadrant with palpation of the lower left quadrant (Rovsing's sign)
Increased pain caused by passive extension of the right hip joint, which tenses the iliopsoas muscle (psoas sign)
Pain produced by passive internal rotation of the flexed thigh (obturator sign)
A low-grade fever is common

Table 15.3 The Alvarado score

Criteria
Migration of pain to the right lower quadrant (+1 point)
Anorexia (+1 point)
Nausea or vomiting (+1 point)
Tenderness in the right lower quadrant (+2 points)
Rebound tenderness (+1 point)
Elevated temperature (> 37.3 °C or 99.1 °F) (+1 point)
Leukocytosis >10,000 (+2 points)
Shift (of leukocytes) to the left (+1 point)
Score total
5–6 points: possible acute appendicitis
7–8 points: probable acute appendicitis
9–10 points: very probable acute appendicitis

15.3 Anomaly of Position

The vermiform appendix is unique among human organs in that it does not have a fixed anatomical position. Its location can change as the proximal part of the large intestine lengthens, ultimately displacing the appendix into the right iliac fossa. During this displacement, the appendix can assume various positions as shown in Fig. 15.1.

We have to remind also the possible herniation involving the Appendix:

- Amyand hernia: This is the herniation of the appendix into an inguinal hernia. It occurs in less than 1% of inguinal hernias, with appendicitis found in 0.13% of these cases. It is most common in male patients [8].
- De Garengeot hernia: This is the herniation of the appendix into the femoral canal. It is even rarer than Amyand hernia and is most common in female patients.

Although these are rare occurrences, it is important to remember the possible agenesis of the appendix, either partial or complete, as well as the possible duplication of the appendix, also partial or complete. With particular reference to possible appendiceal duplication, it is important to remember that with the term "alimentary tract duplication" we mean a group of congenital anomalies that are characterized by the presence of a well-developed smooth muscle layer and epithelial lining ("the gut signature" described by various authors in the literature), and their connection to a part of the gastrointestinal tract.

15.4 CT Study Protocol

There is ongoing debate about the best CT protocol for evaluating patients with signs and symptoms of acute appendicitis, including the use of intravenous and oral contrast agents. At our institution, in the emergency setting, we routinely use only intravenous contrast material and perform trifasic study protocol, with dual-energy acquisition during the venous phase; indeed dual-energy CT has emerged as a promising tool with various clinical applications in abdominal imaging already demonstrated [9]. By characterizing materials based on their differential attenuation at two different energy levels, dual-energy CT can help determine the composition of internal body constituents. This technology allows for the selective identification of iodine, enabling the assessment of an organ's enhancement pattern, including the detection of hyperenhancement in inflammatory processes or ischemic changes due to vascular compromise. Additionally, quantification of iodine uptake with contrast-enhanced dual-energy CT has been suggested as a useful method for differentiating between inflammatory and neoplastic conditions [10]. In addition to monoenergetic imaging, iodine mapping can detect areas of hyperenhancement within the intestinal wall. One imaging feature of acute appendicitis is mural enhancement due to hyperemia, which can be subtle in the early stages of the illness. Clinical experience at our institution suggests that dual-energy CT can be useful for evaluating acute appendicitis, just using iodine overlay maps that improve physicians diagnostic confidence (Fig. 15.2). Similarly, iodine quantification techniques can identify complications such as early ischemic or gangrenous changes and perforation, indicated by discontinuity in the enhancement of the appendiceal wall, a finding often subtle or undetectable with conventional single-energy CT.

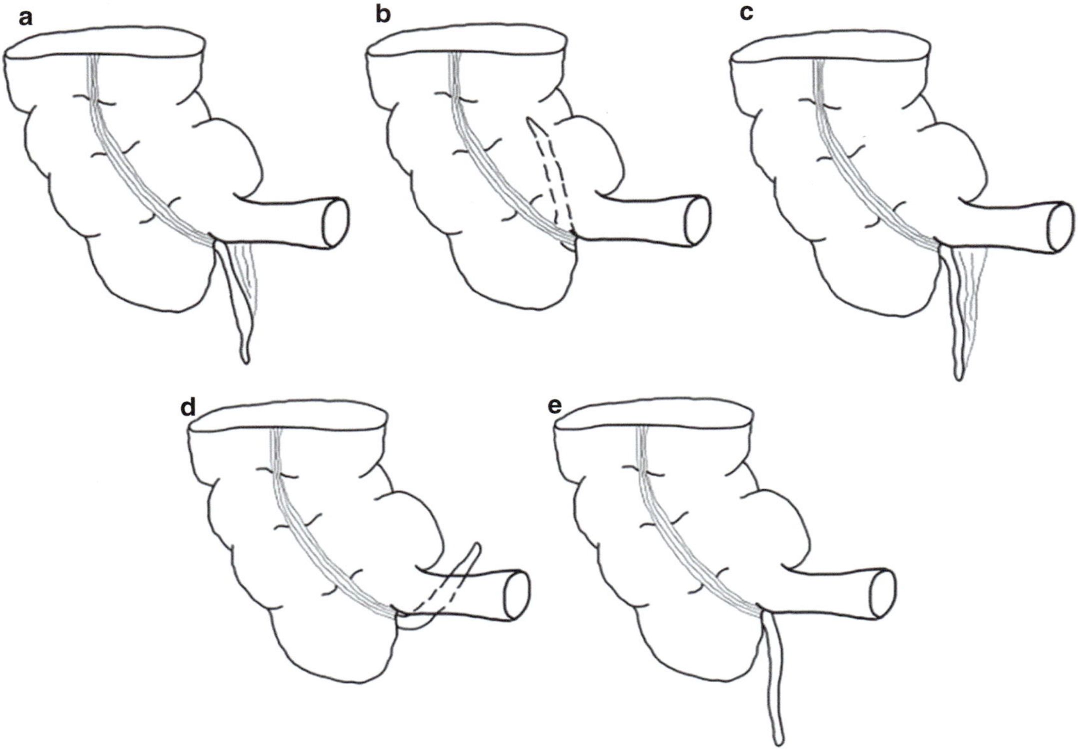

Fig. 15.1 Position variations: (**a**) Normal position. (**b**) Retrocecal appendix. (**c**) Pelvic appendix. (**d**) Mesocolic appendix. (**e**) Funnel-shaped appendix

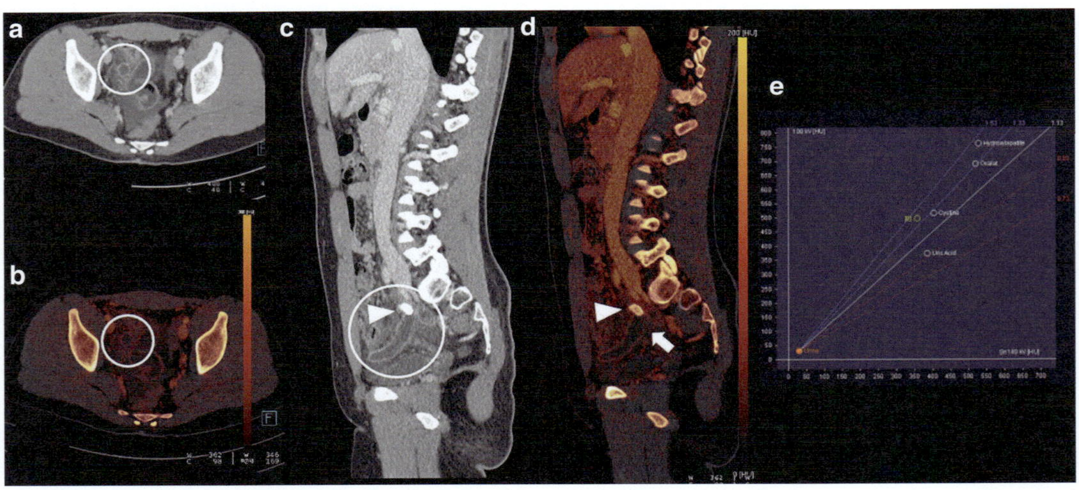

Fig. 15.2 DECT scan in patient with appendicitis. In (**a**) is possible to recognize the flogistic hyperemic thickening of the walls, especially in the apex (circle) much more evident in the iodine mapping (**b**); in MPR sagittal plane (**c**) is well shown the whole course of the appendix (circle) and evidence of large appendicolith at the base (arrowhead in **c** and **d**). Additionally, the iodine map (**d**) allows us to identify with better diagnostic accuracy the parietal perfusion defect of the cecal appendix in the posterior wall (arrow), due to tensive ischemia. In (**e**) picture is shown the possible analysis of the composition of the appendicolith obtainable in post-processing thanks to the DE acquisition

The use of oral contrast agents would involve a wait of approximately 60–90 minutes from administration before the diagnostic acquisition. Therefore, this practice is not well suited for managing critically ill patients in an emergency scenario, although it can be utilized when the patient is stable or in an elective setting when it is effective for distinguishing conditions that are part of the differential diagnosis for acute appendicitis, such as Meckel's diverticulum and tubo-ovarian diseases. By the way, the selected protocol should meet the needs of the referring clinicians and be suitable for the specific patient, though this ideal can be challenging to achieve in emergency settings. Dose reduction strategies should be implemented to minimize the patient's radiation exposure while maintaining the image quality necessary for a high level of diagnostic accuracy.

The use of multiplanar reconstructions (MPR) may help in the identification of the appendix [11].

15.5 Key CT Findings

It is possible to categorize CT findings of acute appendicitis into changes in the appendix, cecum, and periappendiceal region [12].

15.5.1 Appendiceal Changes

A key indicator of acute appendicitis on CT is appendiceal thickening. Many authors, drawing from sonography literature, define appendiceal thickening on CT as an outer-wall-to-outer-wall transverse diameter greater than 6 mm [13]. However, sonographic measurements often involve graded compression of the right lower quadrant (RLQ), potentially altering the diameter, whereas CT images do not use compression. Thus, applying sonographic standards to CT may not be accurate. Some authors suggest a threshold of greater than 7 mm for CT-defined thickening. Even so, this threshold may not be ideal. Research by Brown et al. indicates that a normal appendix can measure over 6 mm in 42% of asymptomatic outpatient adults, with an upper normal limit of 10 mm. Consequently, an appendiceal diameter between 6 and 10 mm is considered indeterminate. Due to the significant overlap between normal and abnormal appendices, relying on a single-diameter threshold is overly simplistic. Instead, the appendiceal diameter should be interpreted alongside clinical and other CT findings. Additional appendiceal indicators include wall thickening (≥3 mm), wall hyperenhancement, mural stratification, appendicolith(s), and intramural gas. Appendicoliths are found in one-third of appendicitis cases. While they are associated with appendicitis, they are not diagnostic on their own due to low specificity, as they can also appear in asymptomatic individuals. However, their presence can be prognostically significant, as they increase the likelihood of appendiceal perforation (Fig. 15.3).

15.5.2 Cecal Changes

Key CT findings in the cecum, particularly the apex, include apical thickening, the arrowhead sign, and the cecal bar sign. While diffuse cecal thickening is possible, it is less specific for appendicitis. The arrowhead sign is characterized by focal cecal wall thickening around the appendiceal orifice, where enteric contrast material in the cecum forms a triangular shape pointing to the abnormal appendix [14]. The cecal bar sign involves inflammatory soft tissue at the base of the appendix, separating it from the contrast-filled cecum. These signs are best visualized in patients with a distended cecum from enteric contrast, particularly after oral contrast administration (Fig. 15.4).

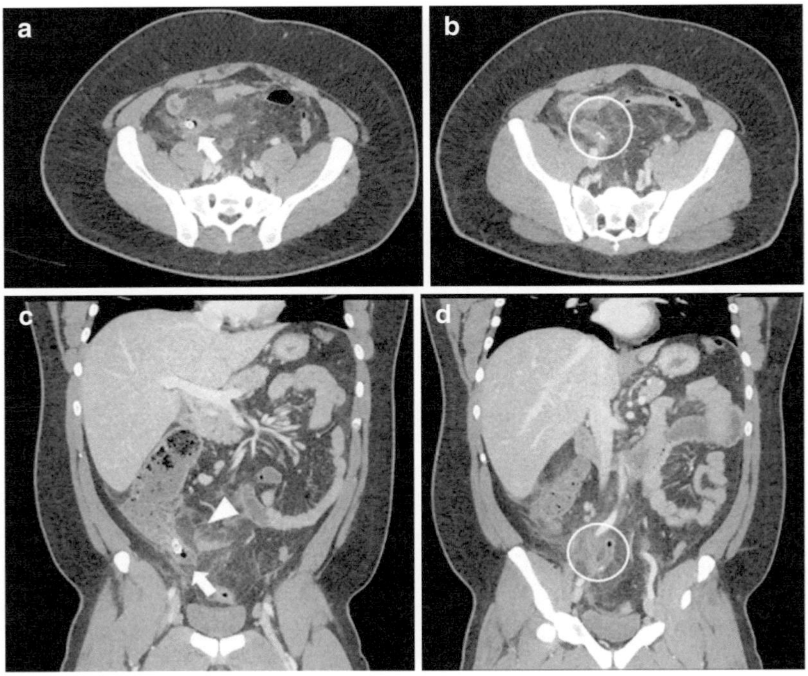

Fig. 15.3 Phlegmonous appendicitis with thickening and hyperemia of the walls and evidence of multiple appendicoliths (**a**, **b**), the largest at the base (arrow in **a**). Additionally, air and fluid are visible within the lumen throughout the appendix (circle in **b** and **d**). There are diffuse signs of reactive hypertrophy of the perivisceral fat (arrowhead in **c**)

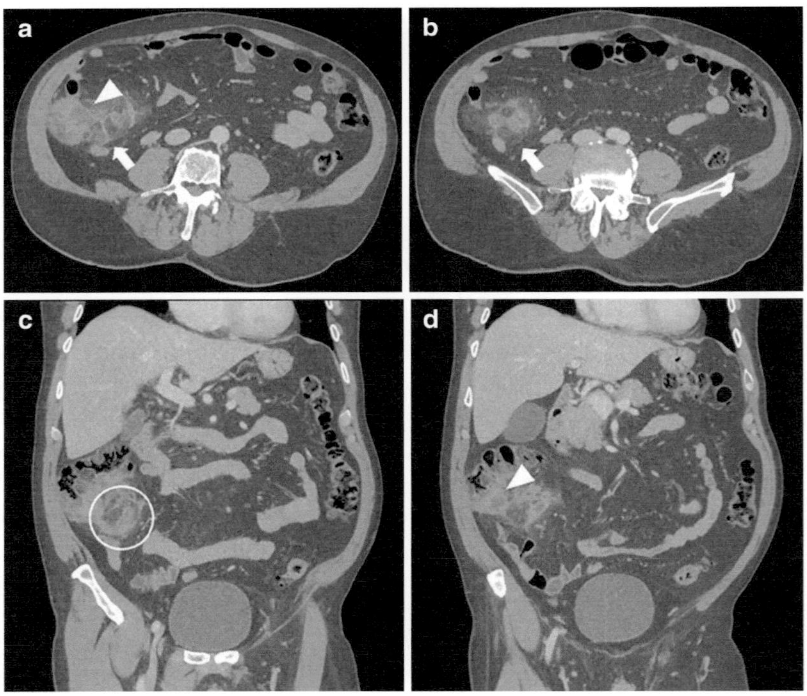

Fig. 15.4 Phlegmonous appendicitis with pericecal involvement—the cecal appendix (circle in **c**) exhibits thickened and hyperemic walls with widespread signs of hypertrophy in the periappendiceal fat (arrow in **a** and **b**). The predominant signs are cecal involvement, including intramural abscess collections within the cecum (arrowhead in **a** and **d**)

15.5.3 Inflammatory Changes in the RLQ

Periappendiceal inflammation includes fat stranding around the appendix, thickening of the lateral conal fascia and mesoappendix, extraluminal fluid, phlegmon, abscess formation, mild enlargement of ileocecal lymph nodes, and inflammatory thickening of nearby structures. Depending on the appendix's location, secondary inflammation may affect the ascending colon, terminal ileum, sigmoid colon, and urinary bladder. However, periappendiceal signs are not specific to appendicitis as they can occur in various other RLQ disorders. Moreover, the sensitivity of these signs may be decreasing as CT scans are being performed earlier in the course of acute appendicitis, reducing the prevalence and severity of periappendiceal fat stranding and other inflammatory changes on CT (Fig. 15.5).

15.5.4 Atypical Pattern of Appendicitis

Careful examination of the entire appendix, from its origin to its most distal portion, is crucial during imaging to avoid missing a diagnosis of focal/segmental or tip appendicitis [15, 16]. It is important to note that the normal appendiceal tip has a bulbous shape and is typically wider in diameter than the rest of the appendix (Fig. 15.4).

Inflammation of the remaining appendix after an appendectomy is called stump appendicitis. Surgical removal of the inflamed appendiceal stump, known as repeat or completion appendectomy, is typically recommended [17] (Figs. 15.6 and 15.7).

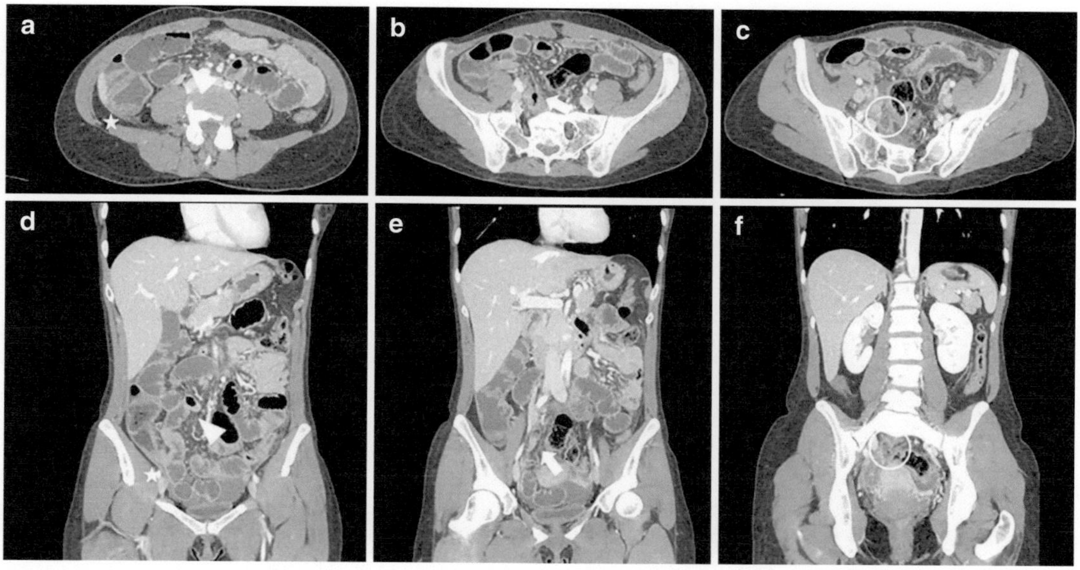

Fig. 15.5 Acute appendicitis with associated small bowel obstruction. In **a** and **d**, there is fluid distension of the small intestine (arrowhead) and fluid imbibition with reactive thickening of the lateroconal fascia in the right iliac fossa (star). In **b** and **e** the cecal appendix is of increased caliber with thickened and hyperemic walls, its lumen is distended by air and enteric material (arrow). In **c** and **f** the apex of the appendix shows enteric material within the lumen and focal wall discontinuity due to perforative complication (circle)

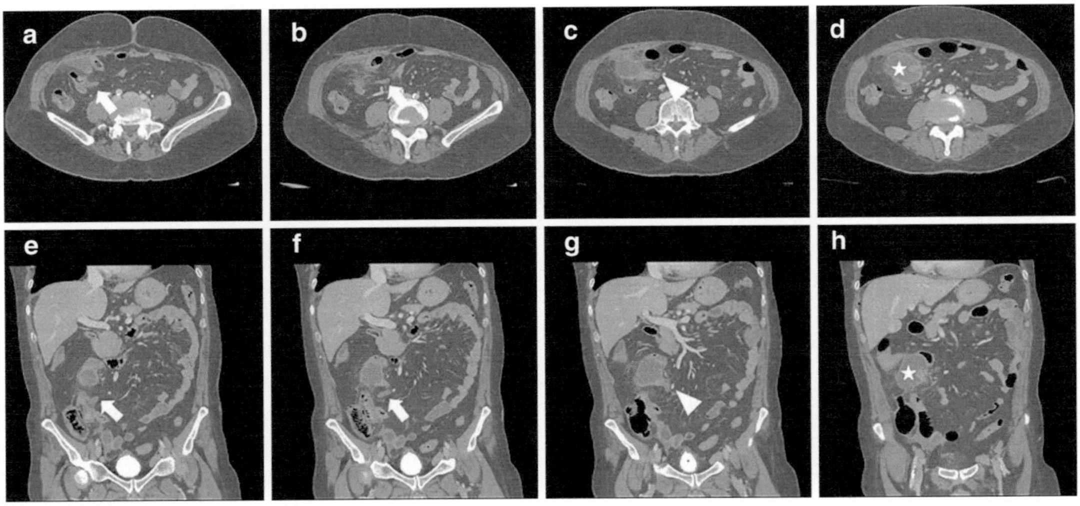

Fig. 15.6 Tip appendicitis . In picture **a** and **e**, the appendix's normal emergence is visible. In picture **b** and **f**, the proximal and middle parts of the appendix show regular caliber and thickness. Picture **c** and **g** reveal tip appendicitis (arrowhead), accompanied by a near abscess collection extending toward the anterior abdominal wall. In images **d** and **h**, an appendicolith is seen inside the fluid collection (star), indicating a perforation at the apex of the appendix

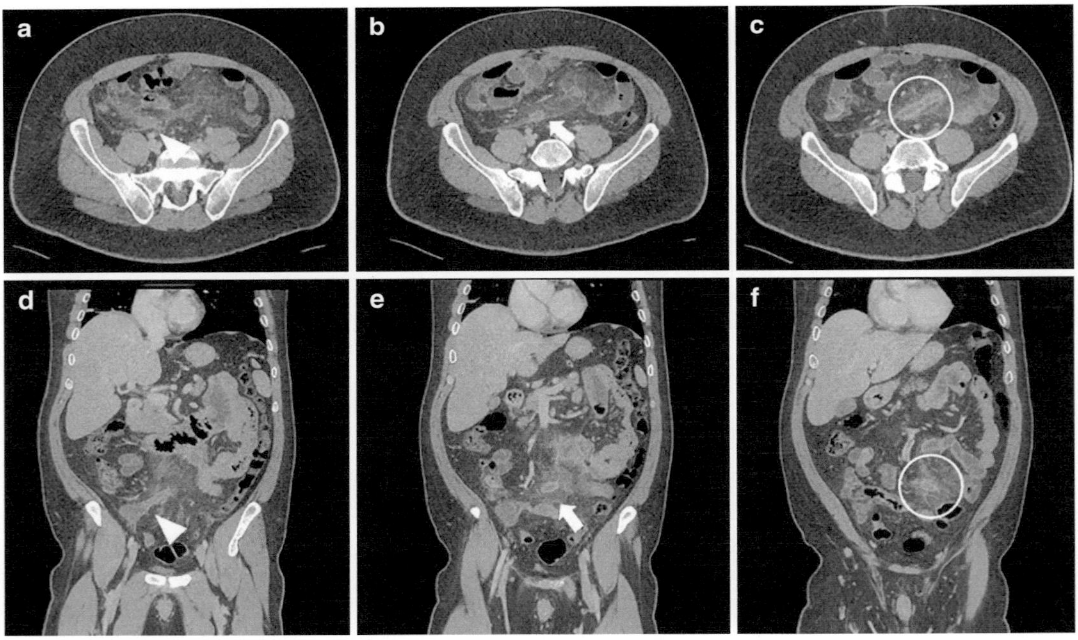

Fig. 15.7 Anomaly in the position and course of the cecal appendix, particularly long: phlegmonous appendicitis with emergence indicated by the arrowhead in **a** and **d**, course of the viscera in the hypogastric region, arrow in **b** and **e**, and with apex on the left side with widespread reactive hypertrophy of the neighboring fat, circle in **c** and **f**

15.6 Major Complications

Complications from acute appendicitis are often a result of delayed diagnosis or treatment, leading to the progression of inflammation and infection. Common complications include perforation, periappendiceal abscess, peritonitis, bowel obstruction, and septic involvement of mesenteric vessels. The use of CT imaging is crucial in identifying these complications early and improving patient outcomes. The table below (Table 15.4), adapted from a recent meta-analysis [18], summarizes the pooled sensitivity and specificity measures for various CT features associated with complicated appendicitis.

15.6.1 Perforation

If appendicitis progresses, parts of the appendiceal wall can become ischemic or necrotic, leading to perforation. On CT, perforation is suggested by periappendiceal inflammation, although this is a nonspecific finding. Interestingly, the presence of appendicoliths on CT increases the likelihood of perforation, possibly because appendicoliths accelerate the rate of perforation. Therefore, the presence of one or more appendicoliths along with periappendiceal inflammation is nearly diagnostic of perforation and defects in the enhancement of appendiceal wall may be appreciated when perforation occurs. In a retrospective study, Horrow et al. demonstrated that specifically looking for five CT findings—extraluminal air, extraluminal appendicolith, abscess, phlegmon, and a defect in the enhancing appendiceal wall—provides excellent sensitivity (95%) and specificity (95%) for detecting perforation in patients with known appendicitis who underwent preoperative CT [19].

15.6.2 Periappendiceal Abscess

An abscess is the most common complication of a perforated appendix [20]. It remains localized if periappendiceal fibrinous adhesions develop before the rupture. CT imaging typically reveals a loculated, rim-enhancing fluid collection that may exert a mass effect on nearby bowel loops. For large abscesses (>4 cm), the recommended

Table 15.4 Pooled sensitivity and specificity, of individual CT features [18]

CT feature	Pooled sensitivity (%)	Pooled specificity (%)
Extraluminal appendicolith	14	100
Abscess	69	91
Extraluminal air	34	99
Appendiceal wall enhancement defect	59	99
Periappendiceal fat stranding	94	95
Ileus	29	95
Periappendiceal fluid collection	42	81
Periappendiceal fat stranding	94	95
Ileus	29	95
Periappendiceal fluid collection	42	81
Ascites	24	81
Intraluminal air	23	74
Intraluminal appendicolith	24	84
Appendiceal dilatation	94	52
Cecal wall thickening or abnormal	48	82
Lymph node enlargement	58	53
Relatively increased appendiceal enhancement	87	16

treatment is percutaneous drainage followed by a delayed appendectomy.

15.6.3 Peritonitis

Bacterial peritonitis is a serious complication resulting from an early rupture of the appendix before the formation of inflammatory adhesions. This condition is more common in young children due to the rapid progression to perforation. CT and sonography show interloop fluid and free fluid tracking along the peritoneal reflections, often far from the appendix. Common locations include the pelvis, paracolic gutters, and the subhepatic, subphrenic, and hepatorenal spaces. Fluid in the lesser sac suggests other diagnoses, such as pancreatitis or a perforated peptic ulcer. Contrast-enhanced CT helps differentiate bacterial peritonitis from ascites by revealing enhancement and thickening of peritoneal reflections, inflammatory changes in the mesentery and omentum, engorgement of regional mesenteric vessels, and hyperemic changes in adjacent bowel segments.

15.6.4 Bowel Obstruction

In rare cases, acute appendicitis can cause mechanical bowel obstruction, likely due to the entrapment of the distal ileum in a periappendiceal inflammatory mass. More commonly, small-bowel obstruction occurs as a late complication of appendectomy, caused by postoperative fibrous adhesions in the peritoneal cavity.

15.6.5 Septic Seeding of Mesenteric Vessels

Appendicitis can lead to complications such as pylephlebitis, pylethrombosis, or hepatic abscesses due to an ascending infection along the draining mesenteric-portal venous system. Occasionally, patients with cryptogenic portal hypertension resulting from pylethrombosis have a recent or remote history of appendicitis.

15.6.6 Gangrenous Appendicitis

Gangrenous appendicitis occurs due to intramural and arterial thrombosis. CT findings include pneumatosis (air within the appendiceal wall), a shaggy appearance of the appendiceal wall, and patchy areas of mural nonperfusion.

15.6.7 Fistula

A fistula can form from a perforated appendix to adjacent organs such as the bowel, bladder, vagina, uterus, or skin. This complication, known as fistulation, is a rare outcome of perforated appendicitis [21] (Fig. 15.8).

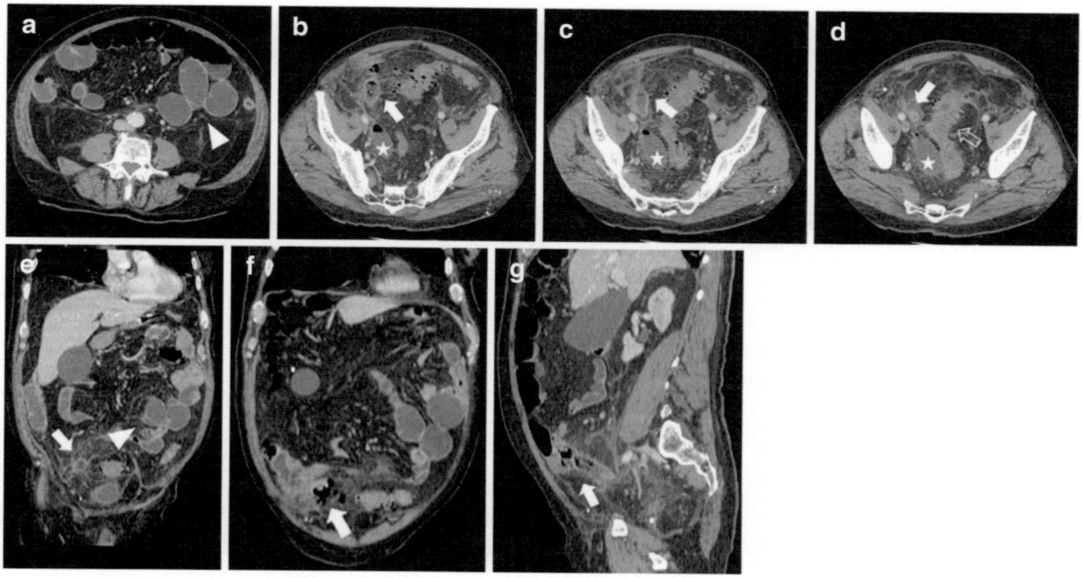

Fig. 15.8 Complicated appendicitis. The cecal appendix is distended by enteric/fecaloid material (arrow in pictures **b**–**g**), perforated at the base with evidence of multiple abscess collections containing fluid and air in the mesentery and pelvis (star). There is also diffuse thickening of the sigmoid wall, with multiple diverticular protrusions associated with hypertrophy of the perivisceral adipose tissue due to reactive sigmoiditis (empty arrow in **d**) and small bowel obstruction (arrowhead in **a**)

15.7 Differential Diagnosis

Several alternative conditions can clinically and radiologically mimic appendicitis or secondary involve the appendix. Accurate diagnosis is crucial because many of these conditions are self-limiting and can be effectively managed with conservative treatment. In the following table (Table 15.5), we summarize many pathologies that can mimic the clinical symptoms of acute appendicitis. Notably, conditions such as cecal/colic diverticulitis and Crohn's disease are among the most common causes of secondary or reactive appendicitis [3].

Table 15.5 Differential diagnosis of appendicitis

Differential diagnosis of appendicitis
Acute mesenteric adenitis
Acute gastroenteritis
Pelvic inflammatory disease
Urinary tract infection
Ureteral stone
Ruptured Graafian follicle
Epiploic appendagitis
Endometriosis
Ovarian torsion
Ruptured ectopic pregnancy
Meckel's diverticulum
Bowel intussusception
Crohn's disease
Yersiniosis
Perforated peptic ulcer
Henoch-Schònlein purpura

15.8 Conclusion

CT study is a precise and effective method for diagnosing acute appendicitis. Although the optimal CT technique for evaluating patients with suspected acute appendicitis is still under discussion, it is now proven that CT with intravenous contrast agent, is highly accurate. Good knowledge of CT findings is crucial for correctly diagnosing acute appendicitis, distinguishing it from other conditions, and identifying complications. However, CT has some disadvantages, including exposure to ionizing radiation, potential adverse reactions to IV contrast material, partially limited evaluation of acute gynecologic disorders, and possibly inadequate visualization of the appendix in thin individuals. Therefore, ultrasound remains an important tool and is often preferred as the initial imaging modality particularly in children, adolescents, thin young adults and women of reproductive age, with potential gynecologic causes of pain in RLQ.

References

1. Kwon LM, Lee K, Kim M-J, Lee IJ, Kim GC. Acute ileal diverticulitis: computed tomography and ultrasound findings. Diagnostics. 2023;13:1408. https://doi.org/10.3390/diagnostics13081408.
2. Lee KH, Lee HS, Park SH, Bajpai V, Choi YS, Kang S-B, et al. Appendiceal diverticulitis. J Comput Assist Tomogr. 2007;31:763–9. https://doi.org/10.1097/RCT.0b013e3180340991.
3. Levine CD, Aizenstein O, Wachsberg RH. Pitfalls in the CT diagnosis of appendicitis. Br J Radiol. 2004;77:792–9. https://doi.org/10.1259/BJR/95663370.
4. Brillantino A, Iacobellis F, Brusciano L, Abu-Omar A, Muto G, Amadu AM, et al. Accuracy of computed tomography in staging acute appendicitis and its impact on surgical outcome and strategy: a multi-center retrospective case-control study. Radiol Med. 2023;128:415–25. https://doi.org/10.1007/S11547-023-01619-4.
5. Dirks K, Calabrese E, Dietrich CF, Gilja OH, Hausken T, Higginson A, et al. EFSUMB position paper: recommendations for gastrointestinal ultrasound (GIUS) in acute appendicitis and diverticulitis. Ultraschall Med. 2019;40:163–75. https://doi.org/10.1055/A-0824-6952.
6. Alvarado A. A practical score for the early diagnosis of acute appendicitis. Ann Emerg Med. 1986;15:557–64. https://doi.org/10.1016/S0196-0644(86)80993-3.
7. Alfredo A. Improved Alvarado Score (MANTRELS) for the early diagnosis of acute appendicitis. Int J Surg Res Pract. 2019;6:6. https://doi.org/10.23937/2378-3397/1410098.
8. Constantine S. Computed tomography appearances of Amyand hernia. J Comput Assist Tomogr. 2009;33:359–62. https://doi.org/10.1097/RCT.0B013E3181837FD9.
9. Abu-Omar A, Murray N, Ali IT, Khosa F, Barrett S, Sheikh A, et al. Utility of dual-energy computed tomography in clinical conundra. Diagnostics (Basel). 2024;14:775. https://doi.org/10.3390/DIAGNOSTICS14070775.
10. Murray N, Darras KE, Walstra FE, Mohammed MF, McLaughlin PD, Nicolaou S. Dual-energy CT in evaluation of the acute abdomen. Radiographics. 2019;39:264–86. https://doi.org/10.1148/RG.2019180087.
11. Paulson EK, Harris JP, Jaffe TA, Haugan PA, Nelson RC. Acute appendicitis: added diagnostic value of coronal reformations from isotropic voxels at multidetector row CT. Radiology. 2005;235:879–85. https://doi.org/10.1148/RADIOL.2353041231.
12. Leite NP, Pereira JM, Cunha R, Pinto P, Sirlin C. CT evaluation of appendicitis and its complications: imaging techniques and key diagnostic findings. AJR Am J Roentgenol. 2005;185:406–17. https://doi.org/10.2214/AJR.185.2.01850406.
13. Moteki T, Horikoshi H. New CT criterion for acute appendicitis: maximum depth of intraluminal appendiceal fluid. Am J Roentgenol. 2007;188:1313–9. https://doi.org/10.2214/AJR.06.1180/ASSET/IMAGES/06_1180_05B.JPEG.
14. Rao PM, Wittenberg J, McDowell RK, Rhea JT, Novelline RA. Appendicitis: use of arrowhead sign for diagnosis at CT. Radiology. 1997;202:363–6. https://doi.org/10.1148/RADIOLOGY.202.2.9015058.
15. Shademan A, Tappouni RFR. Pitfalls in CT diagnosis of appendicitis: pictorial essay. J Med Imaging Radiat Oncol. 2013;57:329–36. https://doi.org/10.1111/J.1754-9485.2012.02451.X.
16. Chin CM, Lim KL. Appendicitis: atypical and challenging CT appearances: resident and fellow education feature. Radiographics. 2015;35:123–4. https://doi.org/10.1148/rg.351140122.
17. Kanona H, Al Samaraee A, Nice C, Bhattacharya V. Stump appendicitis: a review. Int J Surg. 2012;10:425–8. https://doi.org/10.1016/J.IJSU.2012.07.007.
18. Kim HY, Park JH, Lee YJ, Lee SS, Jeon JJ, Lee KH. Systematic review and meta-analysis of CT features for differentiating complicated and uncomplicated appendicitis. Radiology. 2017;287:104–15. https://doi.org/10.1148/RADIOL.2017171260.

19. Iacobellis F, Iadevito I, Romano F, Altiero M, Bhattacharjee B, Scaglione M. Perforated appendicitis: assessment with multidetector computed tomography. Semin Ultrasound CT MR. 2016;37:31–6. https://doi.org/10.1053/J.SULT.2015.10.002.
20. Horrow MM, White DS, Horrow JC. Differentiation of perforated from nonperforated appendicitis at CT1. Radiology. 2003;227:46–51. https://doi.org/10.1148/RADIOL.2272020223.
21. See TC, Watson CJE, Arends MJ, Ng CS. Atypical appendicitis: the impact of CT and its management. J Med Imaging Radiat Oncol. 2008;52:140–7. https://doi.org/10.1111/J.1440-1673.2008.01932.X.

Diverticulitis

16

Costanza Camillo, Maria Giuseppina Scuderi,
Roberto Ronza, Maria Laura Schillirò,
Marco Di Serafino, and Francesca Iacobellis

16.1 Introduction

Acute colonic diverticulitis (ACD) is defined as an episode of acute lower abdominal pain caused by diverticular inflammation; it's a complication of colonic diverticulosis and one of the presentations of diverticular disease [1]. Acute diverticulitis represents the second most common cause of acute abdomen in the Western world and is considered an abdominal emergency.

The etiopathogenesis of diverticular disease is multifactorial and still highly debated; advanced age, combined with lifestyle factors and a genetic predisposition, especially contribute to its development; Table 16.1 summarizes the main etiopathogenic factors that can contribute to the development of diverticular disease [2].

Diverticula are small pouches that develop at weak spots in the intestinal wall, usually where blood vessels penetrate the circular muscle layers. Acute diverticulitis occurs when these diverticula become inflamed and then perforate. Initially, the opening of a diverticulum is blocked by fecal matter and undigested food particles (such as seeds), which increases internal pressure and leads to inflammation. This can escalate to a small or large perforation of the diverticulum, allowing bacteria to escape and infect the surrounding pericolic tissue, resulting in localized inflammatory response around the diverticulum. The sigmoid colon, due to its high intraluminal pressure and narrow diameter, is the most frequent location for the formation of diverticula [3].

C. Camillo (✉) · M. G. Scuderi · R. Ronza
M. L. Schillirò · M. Di Serafino · F. Iacobellis
Department of General and Emergency Radiology, "Antonio Cardarelli" Hospital, Naples, Italy
e-mail: costanza.camillo@aocardarelli.it; maria.scuderi@aocardarelli.it; roberto.ronza@aocardarelli.it; marialaura.schilliro@aocardarelli.it; marco.diserafino@aocardarelli.it; francesca.iacobellis@aocardarelli.it

L. Romano et al. (eds.), *CT of Non-Traumatic Body Emergencies*,
https://doi.org/10.1007/978-3-031-84849-0_16

Table 16.1 Etiopathogenic factors

Age	Incidence increases with age due to the progressive weakening of the colonic wall
Low-fiber diet	A low-fiber diet causes increased intraluminal pressure, contributing to the formation of diverticula
Sedentary lifestyle	Lack of physical activity can impair intestinal motility and increase the risk of diverticulosis
Obesity	High body mass index is associated with increased intestinal pressure and risk of diverticulosis
Genetic predisposition	A family history of diverticulosis can increase susceptibility to the condition
Chronic constipation	Chronic constipation leads to persistent straining and increased pressure in the colon, facilitating the formation of diverticula
Inflammation and intestinal stress	Chronic inflammation and intestinal stress can contribute to the weakening of the colonic wall and the formation of diverticula
Drugs	Medications such as non-steroidal anti-inflammatory drugs and steroids may influence the risk of diverticulosis

CT of the abdomen and pelvis with intravenous contrast is universally recognized as the best useful imaging method for diagnosing and assessing diverticular inflammation [4].

16.2 CT Findings

The clinical presentation of a patient experiencing an episode of acute diverticulitis generally includes pain in the lower abdominal quadrants, especially on the left side, radiating to the inguinal and lumbosacral regions, fever, and increased inflammatory markers. In the rarer cases where complications have already developed, the patient may present with irritative urinary symptoms, pneumaturia, and fecaluria (in the case of fistulas), obstinate constipation, and subocclusive intestinal symptoms (in the case of stenosing forms).

In the clinical suspicion of acute diverticulitis, especially in younger patients presenting with localized acute abdominal pain, the diagnostic workflow can begin performing an abdominal—pelvic ultrasound (US); typical US findings include the presence of diverticular outpouchings, along with intestinal wall thickening, pericolic fluid, that may be organized into a well-defined collection, and increased echogenicity of the surrounding fat tissue. CE-CT is the imaging modality of choice, allowing for confirmation of the diagnosis and alternatively providing differential diagnoses, classifying the patient to determine the indication for conservative or surgical treatment, or planning the surgical and/or interventional radiology therapeutic pathway [4, 5]. The acquisition volume should extend at least from the diaphragm to the pubic symphysis; the study protocol necessarily includes a pre-contrast phase. Diagnostic completion with the administration of rectal contrast is indicated in cases of acute diverticulitis complicated by fistulas between the colon and adjacent pelvic organs and in the evaluation of post-surgical complications [6, 7].

On CE-CT, diverticula appear as saccular air-filled outpouchings of the colonic wall. In pre-contrast acquisitions, they can appear spontaneously hyperdense due to fecal residues. CT findings of uncomplicated acute diverticulitis can be classified into "intestinal" and "extraintestinal" signs. The primary intestinal finding to evaluate is wall thickening: if the colonic segment is contracted, a wall thickness of up to 8 mm is considered normal; when the colonic wall is distended, segmental thickening is defined as a wall thickness (maximum distance between the sierosa and the mucosal profile) of 4 mm or more, measured relative to the longitudinal axis of the viscus [8]. The maximum value of colonic

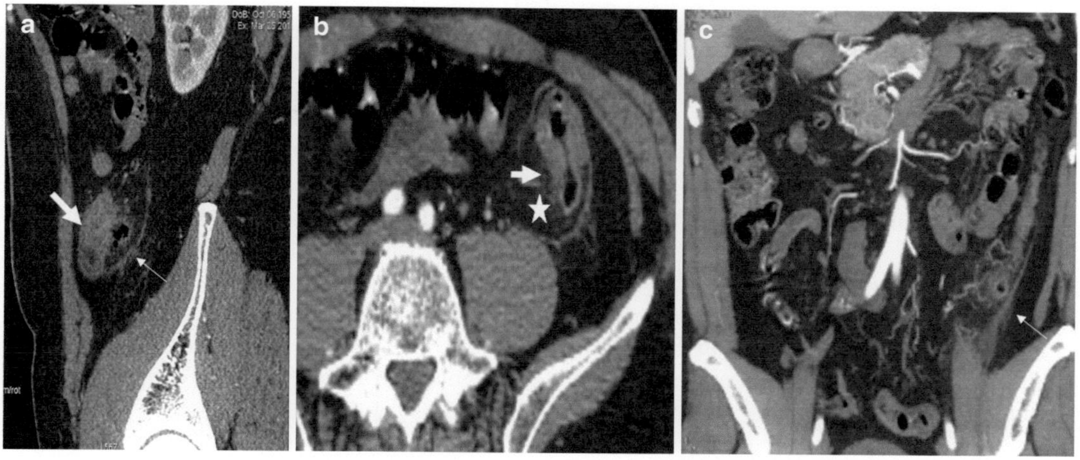

Fig. 16.1 Sagittal (**a**), axial (**b**), and coronal (**c**) CE- CT images (**a–c** arterial phase), show left colonic wall thickening (**a**, **b** short arrow) and fat stranding (**b**, star). Also, thickening and fluid collection of the left latero-conal fascia (**a**, **c** thin arrow) are typical CT findings of uncomplicated diverticulitis

wall thickening in patients with ACD, can predict the probability of recurrent diverticulitis and may be useful in determining which patients might benefit from elective partial colectomy. Secondly, on CE-CT, the length of the involved colonic segment should be assessed, expressed in millimeters or as a percentage of the segment involved relative to the entire colon, as well as the "diverticular density." The latter is defined as the number of diverticula distributed along the colon. Dickerson et al. proposed a severity scale that classifies diverticula based on the distance between them: few (more than 5 cm apart), mild (1–5 cm apart), moderate (less than 1 cm apart), and severe (no distance between them) [9].

Extraintestinal CT findings in ACD refer to "mesenteric findings" and "vascular findings". Increased density of pericolic fat, so-called "fat stranding", often disproportionate considering mural thickening, associated with pericolic fluid collection is typical mesenteric findings. The most severe progression of pericolic fat stranding is the formation of a phlegmon: an inflammatory mass, oval or round in shape, not defined by enhancing walls, and located adjacent to the thickened segment of the colon (Fig. 16.2). The presence of fluid at the root of the mesentery (known as the "comma sign") and the thickening of the lateroconal fascia are additional characteristic CT findings (Fig. 16.1) [4].

Congestion of the mesenteric vessels adjacent to the colonic segment affected by the acute inflammatory process can be clearly appreciated on CE-CT and is known as the "centripede sign". Hematogenous dissemination of the inflammatory process from the mesenteric veins draining the affected colonic site is the basis for the development of ascending septic thrombophlebitis. On CE- CT, this is diagnosed by the presence of small, multiple filling defects in the porto-mesenteric venous system, which may have heterogeneous content due to the presence of intraluminal gas with a purulent significance, accompanied by circumferential thickening of the perivascular adipose tissue. Rarely, thrombophlebitis can be complicated by the formation of distant abscesses, especially in the liver, pulmonary thromboembolism, or septic emboli [10].

16.3 CT Spectrum of Complications

Identifying complications of acute diverticulitis is essential for its management and therapy; CT has high sensitivity and specificity. The CT findings of complications are:

- *Intestinal perforation*: The presence of free air near the inflamed intestinal segment, identified as small air bubbles or an air collection, is the result of inflammatory damage and subsequent wall necrosis. Free air can have a "pericolonic" distribution when located within 5 cm of the inflamed intestine or, in more severe cases, spread into the peritoneum and retroperitoneum. CT, especially with the appropriate window setting, has excellent contrast resolution to detect even the smallest air bubbles (Fig. 16.2) [11].
- *Abscess*: A collection defined by a fluid component, sometimes fluid-air, with thick, hypervascularized walls. It can have an "intramural," pericolonic, or "distant" distribution. Larger abscesses (>4 cm) may benefit from percutaneous drainage treatment (Fig. 16.3) [12]. The development of abscess collections near adjacent organs leads to contiguous involvement, such as the formation of a tubo-ovarian abscess near a sigmoid diverticulitis (Fig. 16.4). Alternatively, hematogenous dissemination from the highly inflamed colonic mucosa can lead to distant organ involvement (liver, lung, brain, and spinal cord).
- *Fistula*: An abnormal communication between two adjacent organs or tissues. It can complicate an existing abscess collection or be the predisposing cause of abscess formation, such as a myometrial abscess complicating a colo-uterine fistula. Only a small percentage of

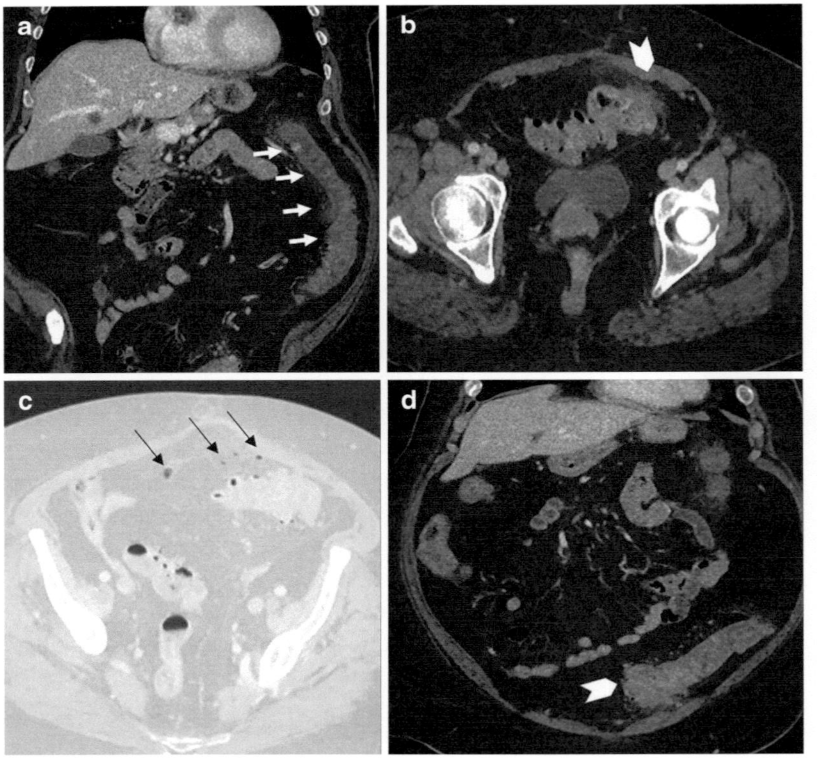

Fig. 16.2 Coronal (**a**, **d**), axial (**b**, **c**) CE-CT images (**a**, **d** arterial phase; **b**, **c** venous phase), show a long inflamed segment of the descending colon (**a**, white arrows), with peri- diverticular inflammation and, adjacent to the colonic walls, an oval-shaped inflammatory mass without enhancing-walls, defined as a peridiverticular phlegmon (**b**, **d** arrowhead). Lung window axial CT image (**c**) allows the identification of very small bubbles of free air, indicating diverticulitis complicated by micro-perforation (**c**, black arrows)

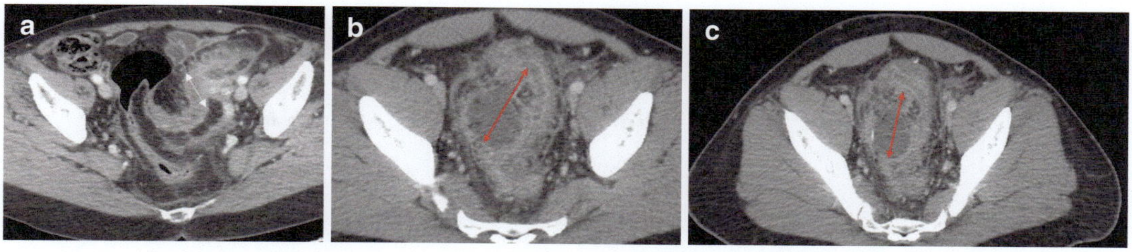

Fig. 16.3 Axial (**a**, **b**, **c**) CE- CT images (**a**–**c** venous phase), show acute colonic diverticulitis complicated with abscesses located near the sigmoid colon, with diameter <4 cm in figure **a** (white arrow) and >4 cm in figures **b** and **c** (red arrows)

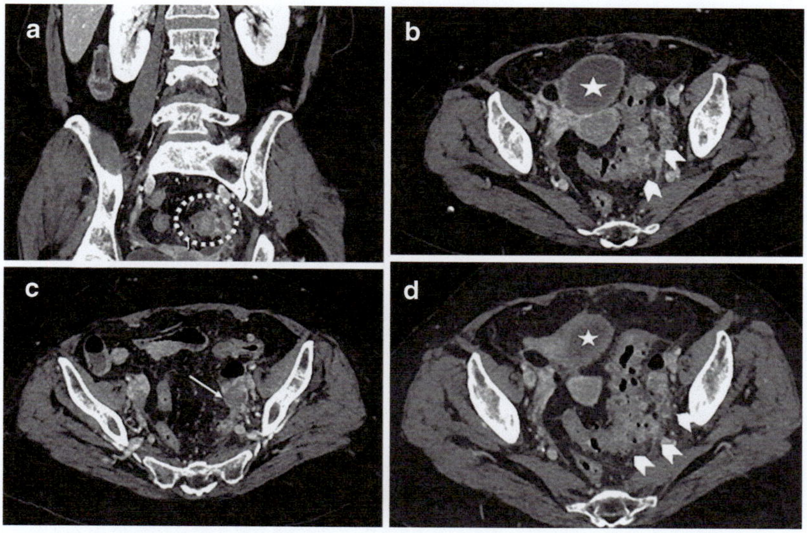

Fig. 16.4 Coronal (**a**) and axial (**b**, **c**, **d**) CE- CT images (**a**–**d** venous phase), show a scenario of sigmoid diverticulitis complicated by diverticular perforation with fistulization into the left iliac space (**b**, **d**, arrowheads), and the presence of a fluid-gas collection in that area, involving the ipsilateral ovary (**c**, thin arrow), increased in volume and with a heterogeneous structure due to inflammatory-abscess involvement (**a**, dottered circles); further diverticular perforation more caudally with adjacent fluid-air level (**b**, **d** white stars)

acute diverticulitis cases are complicated by fistula formation (Fig. 16.5). The most frequent types, in order of prevalence, are colo-vesical, colo-cutaneous, colo-vaginal, colo-enteric, and colo-uterine. A colo-vesical fistula can be suspected on CE-CT by the presence of free air within the bladder lumen along with heterogeneous wall thickening (Fig. 16.6) [13].

- *Bleeding*: Often associated with conditions of chronic diverticulitis; the rationale lies in the presence of vessels at the point of weakness through which the mucosa protrudes. On pre-contrast CT scans, spontaneously hyperdense content may suggest the presence of intraluminal blood. The densitometric increase in subsequent post-contrast study phases indicates active contrast extravasation and thus active bleeding (Fig. 16.7).
- *Peritonitis*: This is the most severe complication of acute diverticulitis, posing a life-threatening risk. The etiological cause is the perforation of the colonic viscus; thus, it can be purulent when caused by a pericolonic abscess or fecal when a non-inflamed diverticulum perforates. Suspicious CT findings

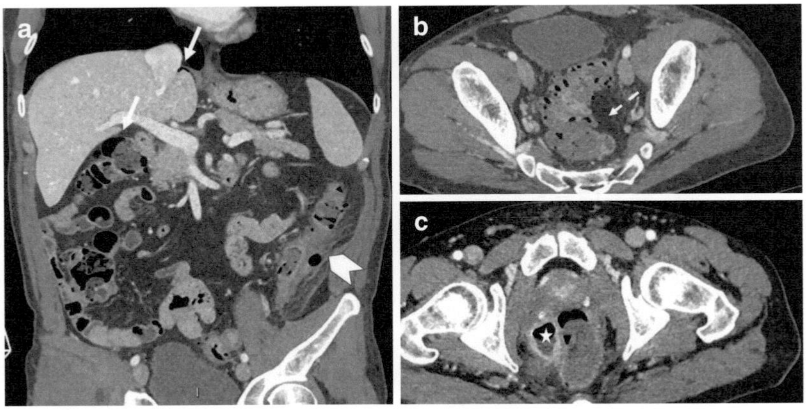

Fig. 16.5 Coronal (**a**) contrast-enhanced CT image (venous phase), shows perforation with free air bubbles, located in the right subdiaphragmatic area and in the supramesocolic area (**a**, arrows), and a segmental inflammatory thickening of the descending colon with signs of perivisceritis and air pockets adjacent to the colonic walls (**a**, arrowhead). In the same patient, axial (**b**, **c**) contrast–enhanced CT images (arterial phase) show further wall thickening at the distal sigmoid colon (**b**, dotted arrow), where there is a fistulous tract with the rectal wall feeding an abscess collection distributed in the right pararectal space (**c**, star)

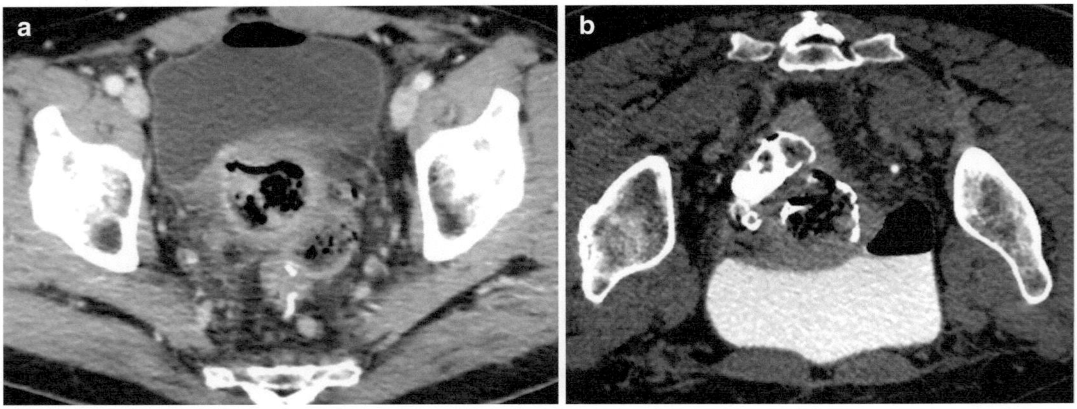

Fig. 16.6 Axial CT image in the venous phase (**a**) shows a case of colonic diverticulitis complicated by the presence of free air in the bladder (**a**, short arrow), a finding suggestive of a colo-vesical fistula. This diagnostic hypothesis is confirmed after the administration of contrast medium via the transrectal route (**b**), which, with the patient in the prone position, reveals bladder opacification

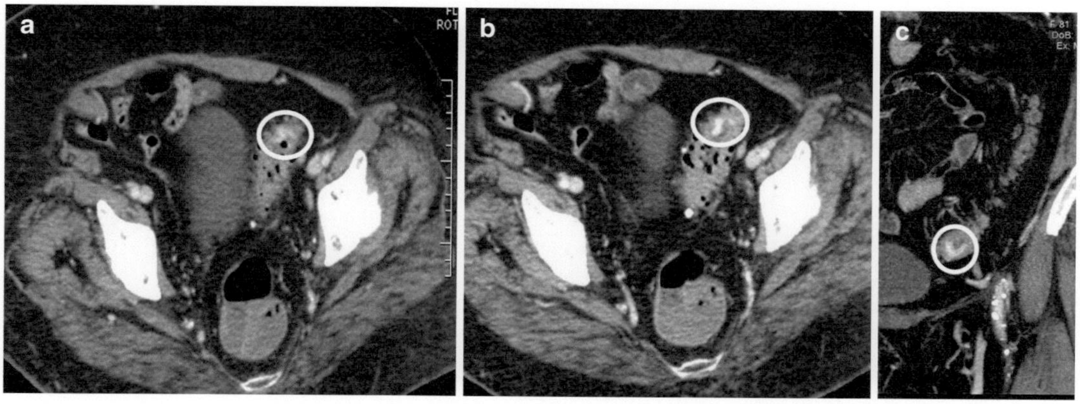

Fig. 16.7 Axial (**a**, **b**) and sagittal (**c**) contrast-enhanced arterial (**a**), portal (**b**), and delayed (**c**) CT phases, show active arterial contrast extravasation within a diverticulum in the left colonic segment; this is more apparent in the later phases of the study (circle, **b**, **c**), which is a typical finding of active bleeding

include the presence of free fluid in the peritoneal recesses, often with fluid or particulate content, thickening, and hyperemia of the peritoneal layers, along with CT signs of perforation.

16.4 Staging

The historically most validated and used classification for acute diverticulitis (ACD) is that of Hinchey, proposed in 1978 and based on clinical and surgical findings (Table 16.2) [14]. With the advent of multi-slice CT and the establishment of a conservative surgical approach, numerous modifications and integrations have been made to it; in particular, Kaiser et al. introduced a classification specifically integrated with CT findings, which included stage 0, represented by mild diverticulitis; stage Ia represented by wall thickening associated with pericolonic reaction, and stage Ib, which involves the presence of a pericolonic or mesocolic abscess (Table 16.2). In 2015, a new classification based on radiological findings was introduced and incorporated into the WSES guidelines for managing Acute Colonic Diverticulitis [12]. This classification categorizes ACD into two groups: complicated and uncomplicated. Uncomplicated ACD is characterized solely by thickening of the diverticular wall, accompanied by increased density of the pericolic fat. Complicated acute diverticulitis is categorized into four stages, determined by the extent of the infectious process, as detailed in Table 16.2. For each stage, appropriate treatment recommendations are provided. Conservative treatment is suggested for stages Ia and Ib, while percutaneous drainage is recommended for abscesses larger than 4 cm (stage IIa). Surgical intervention is advised for stages IIb, III, and IV. Specifically, for stable patients in stages IIb and III, surgical resection with anastomosis is recommended, while Hartman's resection is advised for unstable patients in stages IIb and III or those in stage IV [12].

Regardless of the classification chosen, both intestinal and extraintestinal findings, as well as the presence of complications, must be included in the CT report in order to guide patient management.

Table 16.2 Classifications for ACD

STAGE	Hinchey classification	Modified Hinchey Classification by Kaiser et al.	WSES classification
0		Mild clinical diverticulitis	Uncomplicated diverticulitis
I	Pericolic abscess or phlegmon		Complicated diverticulitis
Ia		Confined pericolic inflammation/ phlegmon	Pericolic air bubbles or little pericolic fluid without abscess
Ib		Pericolonic/mesocolic abscess	Abscess <4 cm
II	Pelvic, distant intraabdominal, or retroperitoneal abscess	Pelvic, distant intraabdominal, or retroperitoneal abscess	
IIa			Abscess >4 cm
IIb			Distant air (>5 cm from inflamed bowel segment)
III	Generalized purulent peritonitis	Generalized purulent peritonitis	Diffuse fluid without distant free air
IV	Generalized fecal peritonitis	Generalized fecal peritonitis	Diffuse fluid with distant free air (persistent hole in the colon)

16.5 Differential Diagnosis

The CT diagnosis of acute diverticulitis is based on the detection of diverticula associated with signs of perivisceral inflammation [15]. However, the clinical symptoms can sometimes be atypical, necessitating a differential diagnosis.

The main differential diagnoses for acute diverticulitis include acute appendicitis, particularly when the ascending colon is involved and there is localized right flank abdominal pain. In such cases, multiplanar CT reconstructions allow for the easy identification of the anatomical structure involved, even in subtler cases where the inflamed appendix, originating from an ectopic cecum in the pelvis, might reach a non-inflamed diverticulum of the sigmoid colon. In omental infarction, the involvement of mesenteric adipose tissue is more prominent compared to colonic wall thickening [16]. Epiploic appendicitis is characterized by an adipose density mass located adjacent to the colonic wall, with a marked peripheral hypervascularization rim. The finding of a colo-vesical fistula is also typical of Crohn's disease: a distinguishing CT sign that can aid in the differential diagnosis is the postero-lateral localization relative to the bladder walls in complicated acute diverticulitis, whereas it is generally located on the right antero-lateral bladder side in the case of a Crohn's disease complication.

The most important differential diagnosis concerns colorectal adenocarcinoma, which becomes necessary in cases presenting with perforation. CT elements suggestive of oncological pathology include greater wall thickening of a "short" colonic segment (<5 cm), disproportionate to the pericolic inflammation, the interruption of the normal enhancement pattern of the colon, and the presence of mesenteric and pericolic lymphadenopathy (Fig. 16.8) [17].

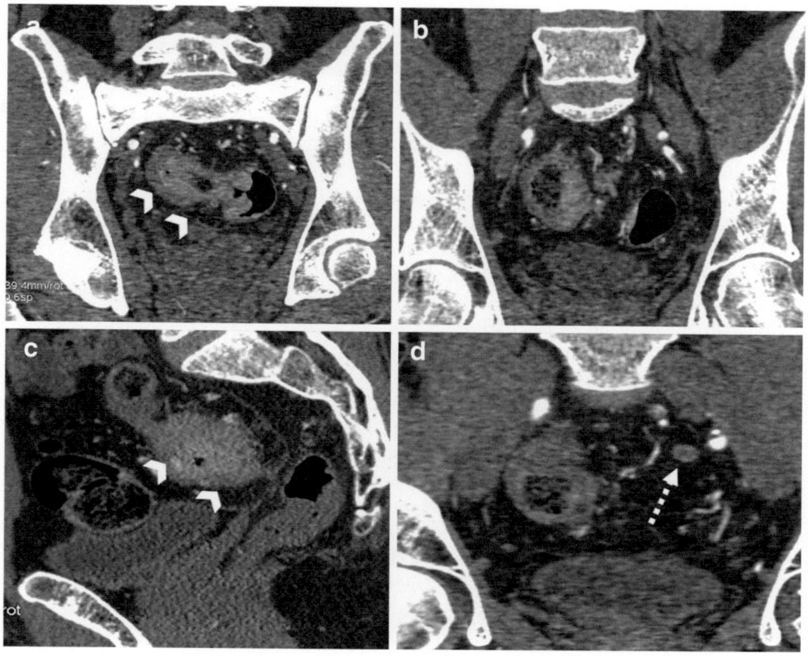

Fig. 16.8 Coronal (**a**, **b**, **d**) and sagittal (**c**) CE-CT images during the arterial phase, show stenosing colonic wall thickening (**a**, **c** arrowheads) corresponding to a sigmoid adenocarcinoma associated with malignant lymphadenopathy (**d**, dotted arrow)

References

1. Hong MK, Skandarajah AR, Hayes IP. Diverticulosis, diverticular disease and diverticulitis – definitions and differences. J Stomal Therapy Australia. 2015;35:8.
2. Stollman N, Raskin JB. Diverticular disease of the colon. Lancet. 2004;363(9409):631–9. https://doi.org/10.1016/S0140-6736(04)15597-9. PMID: 14987890.
3. Strate LL, Morris AM. Epidemiology, pathophysiology, and treatment of diverticulitis. Gastroenterology. 2019;156(5):1282–1298.e1. https://doi.org/10.1053/j.gastro.2018.12.033. Epub 2019 Jan 17. PMID: 30660732; PMCID: PMC6716971.
4. Minordi LM, Larosa L, Berte G, Pecere S, Manfredi R. CT of the acute colonic diverticulitis: a pictorial essay. Diagn Interv Radiol. 2020;26(6):546–51. https://doi.org/10.5152/dir.2020.19645. PMID: 33180020; PMCID: PMC7664754.
5. Destigter KK, Keating DP. Imaging update: acute colonic diverticulitis. Clin Colon Rectal Surg. 2009;22(3):147–55. https://doi.org/10.1055/s--0029-1236158. PMID: 20676257; PMCID: PMC2780264.
6. Sugi MD, Sun DC, Menias CO, Prabhu V, Choi HH. Acute diverticulitis: key features for guiding clinical management. Eur J Radiol. 2020;128:109026. https://doi.org/10.1016/j.ejrad.2020.109026. Epub 2020 Apr 30. PMID: 32422553.
7. Expert Panel on Gastrointestinal Imaging, Galgano SJ, McNamara MM, Peterson CM, Kim DH, Fowler KJ, Camacho MA, Cash BD, Chang KJ, Feig BW, Gage KL, Garcia EM, Kambadakone AR, Levy AD, Liu PS, Marin D, Moreno C, Pietryga JA, Smith MP, Weinstein S, Carucci LR. ACR appropriateness criteria® left lower quadrant pain-suspected diverticulitis. J Am Coll Radiol. 2019;16(5S):S141–9. https://doi.org/10.1016/j.jacr.2019.02.015. PMID: 31054740.
8. Fernandes T, Oliveira MI, Castro R, Araújo B, Viamonte B, Cunha R. Bowel wall thickening at CT: simplifying the diagnosis. Insights Imaging. 2014;5(2):195–208. https://doi.org/10.1007/s13244-013-0308-y. Epub 2014 Jan 10. PMID: 24407923; PMCID: PMC3999365.
9. Dickerson EC, Chong ST, Ellis JH, Watcharotone K, Nan B, Davenport MS, Al-Hawary M, Mazza MB, Rizk R, Morris AM, Cohan RH. Recurrence of colonic diverticulitis: identifying predictive CT findings-retrospective cohort study. Radiology. 2017;285(3):850–8. https://doi.org/10.1148/radiol.2017161374. Epub 2017 Aug 24. PMID: 28837412.
10. Perez-Cruet MJ, Grable E, Drapkin MS, Jablons DM, Cano G. Pylephlebitis associated with diverticulitis. South Med J. 1993;86(5):578–80. https://doi.org/10.1097/00007611-199305000-00020. PMID: 8488411.
11. Sessa B, Galluzzo M, Ianniello S, Pinto A, Trinci M, Miele V. Acute perforated diverticulitis: assessment with multidetector computed tomography. Semin Ultrasound CT MR. 2016;37(1):37–48. https://doi.org/10.1053/j.sult.2015.10.003. Epub 2015 Oct 9. PMID: 26827737.
12. Sartelli M, Weber DG, Kluger Y, Ansaloni L, Coccolini F, Abu-Zidan F, Augustin G, Ben-Ishay O, Biffl

WL, Bouliaris K, Catena R, Ceresoli M, Chiara O, Chiarugi M, Coimbra R, Cortese F, Cui Y, Damaskos D, De' Angelis GL, Delibegovic S, Demetrashvili Z, De Simone B, Di Marzo F, Di Saverio S, Duane TM, Faro MP, Fraga GP, Gkiokas G, Gomes CA, Hardcastle TC, Hecker A, Karamarkovic A, Kashuk J, Khokha V, Kirkpatrick AW, Kok KYY, Inaba K, Isik A, Labricciosa FM, Latifi R, Leppäniemi A, Litvin A, Mazuski JE, Maier RV, Marwah S, McFarlane M, Moore EE, Moore FA, Negoi I, Pagani L, Rasa K, Rubio-Perez I, Sakakushev B, Sato N, Sganga G, Siquini W, Tarasconi A, Tolonen M, Ulrych J, Zachariah SK, Catena F. 2020 update of the WSES guidelines for the management of acute colonic diverticulitis in the emergency setting. World J Emerg Surg. 2020;15(1):32. https://doi.org/10.1186/s13017-020-00313-4. PMID: 32381121; PMCID: PMC7206757.
13. Woods RJ, Lavery IC, Fazio VW, Jagelman DG, Weakley FL. Internal fistulas in diverticular disease. Dis Colon Rectum. 1988;31(8):591–6. https://doi.org/10.1007/BF02556792. PMID: 3402284.
14. Hinchey EJ, Schaal PG, Richards GK. Treatment of perforated diverticular disease of the colon. Adv Surg. 1978;12:85–109. PMID: 735943.
15. Pereira JM, Sirlin CB, Pinto PS, Jeffrey RB, Stella DL, Casola G. Disproportionate fat stranding: a helpful CT sign in patients with acute abdominal pain. Radiographics. 2004;24(3):703–15. https://doi.org/10.1148/rg.243035084. PMID: 15143223.
16. Tonerini M, Calcagni F, Lorenzi S, Scalise P, Grigolini A, Bemi P. Omental infarction and its mimics: imaging features of acute abdominal conditions presenting with fat stranding greater than the degree of bowel wall thickening. Emerg Radiol. 2015;22(4):431–6. https://doi.org/10.1007/s10140-015-1302-0. Epub 2015 Mar 1. PMID: 25725796.
17. Lips LM, Cremers PT, Pickhardt PJ, Cremers SE, Janssen-Heijnen ML, de Witte MT, Simons PC. Sigmoid cancer versus chronic diverticular disease: differentiating features at CT colonography. Radiology. 2015;275(1):127–35. https://doi.org/10.1148/radiol.14132829. Epub 2014 Nov 26. PMID: 25426771.

Acute Mesenteric Ischemia and Infarction

17

Francesca Iacobellis, Costanza Camillo, Martina Caruso, Giuseppina Dell'Aversano Orabona, Antonio Brillantino, and Luigia Romano

17.1 Introduction

Intestinal ischemia is a pathological condition that derives from an inadequate blood supply to the gastrointestinal tract, which can be acute or chronic, resulting in ischemic or necrotic alterations, depending on the severity and timing of occurrence. When acute in manifestation, it occurs a cascade of events, rapidly evolving, with the release of inflammatory products into the circulation, and bacterial translocation in the peritoneal cavity and in the systemic circulation, which if not stopped leads the patient to death due to multi-organ failure [1, 2].

Acute mesenteric ischemia (AMI) has a reported incidence of 0.63–12.9 per 100,000 people per year; there are less specific data for chronic mesenteric ischemia (CMI), for whom is assumed an incidence of up to 3 per 100,000 inhabitants per year [3]. The diagnosis is difficult, so, maintaining a high index of suspicion and treating it early, may help in reducing the mortality rates that are high, ranging between 50% and 80% [4, 5]. The incidence of AMI increases exponentially with age, particularly in patients aged 75 years or older [5].

Imaging plays a fundamental role because clinical symptoms are rather subtle in their onset and unspecific, so, severe abdominal pain out of proportion to physical examination findings should be assumed to be AMI until disproven, and enhanced computed tomography (CT) should be performed without delay in any patient with suspicion for AMI [5]. Other symptoms may include nausea, vomiting, diarrhea, and hematochezia. Biohumoral alterations are not sufficiently accurate to conclusively identify the presence or absence of ischemic or necrotic bowel, although elevated l-lactate, leukocytosis, and D-dimer may help in some cases [5–7].

17.2 Etiology

AMI can arise from various etiologies primitively involving the mesenteric vessels, including embolic or thrombotic occlusion of mesenteric arteries, nonocclusive mesenteric ischemia (due to low flow states), or mesenteric venous thrombosis. Furthermore, there are conditions in which bowel ischemia arises from secondary vessel

F. Iacobellis (✉) · C. Camillo · M. Caruso
G. Dell'Aversano Orabona · L. Romano
Department of General and Emergency Radiology, "Antonio Cardarelli" Hospital, Naples, Italy
e-mail: francesca.iacobellis@aocardarelli.it; costanza.camillo@aocardarelli.it; martina.caruso@aocardarelli.it; giuseppinadellaversanoorabona@aocardarelli.it

A. Brillantino
Department of Surgery, "A. Cardarelli" Hospital, Naples, Italy
e-mail: antonio.brillantino@aocardarelli.it

L. Romano et al. (eds.), *CT of Non-Traumatic Body Emergencies*,
https://doi.org/10.1007/978-3-031-84849-0_17

involvement, as it occurs in strangulated hernias, bowel and mesenteric traumas, and in neoplasms compressing or infiltrating mesenteric vessels [8].

Particularly, arterial mesenteric ischemia accounts for the majority of cases (60–85%) and mainly manifests in men with cardiovascular risk factors in the fifth decade, patients with stenosis of the superior mesenteric artery (20–35%), young patients with vasculitis (5%), patients who take cocaine, hemodialyzed patients, patients with COVID-19 [5].

Fairly frequent is the nonocclusive mesenteric ischemia (NOMI) occurring in approximately 20–30% of cases of AMI, usually as a consequence of artery vasoconstriction associated with low splanchnic blood flow, as in patients who have suffered myocardial infarctions, in patients with heart failure, or with extensive bleeding or in complex patients admitted to intensive care. These etiologies are increasing because of an increased number of critically ill patients and the improvement of intensive care [5, 9]. This type of intestinal ischemic damage represents one of the most difficult diagnostic challenges in the field of intestinal ischemia, due to the variability of manifestation of the CT imaging findings.

Venous Mesenteric Ischemia occurs in a minority of cases (5–15%) and mainly affects women in the fourth decade, patients with prothrombotic states (myeloproliferative disorders, mutation of the prothrombin gene or antiphospholipid antibody syndrome, neoplasms or intestinal infectious-inflammatory states, COVID-19), cirrhotic patients [5].

17.3 Diagnostic Approach and Imaging Modalities

The early hallmark of mesenteric ischemia is severe pain with minimal physical findings, eventually associated with mild tachycardia. When necrosis develops, signs of peritonitis appear. Patients may have blood in the stool due to the progression of bowel wall ischemia. A sudden onset of pain suggests but is not diagnostic of an arterial embolism, whereas a more gradual onset is typical of venous thrombosis. Patients with a history of postprandial abdominal discomfort (which suggests intestinal angina) may have arterial thrombosis or arterial compression phenomena, such as Dunbar syndrome or superior mesenteric artery syndrome [10].

Each patient suspected of having AMI needs to perform enhanced CT as soon as possible, as it represents the diagnostic gold standard and gives all the elements useful to plan the treatment [5], however, in cases where the onset of symptoms is subtle, diagnostic approach may vary depending on patient's clinical presentation, and so, in some cases, it may happen that it starts with abdominal ultrasound and abdominal X-ray whose findings depend on the etiology and phase of the ischemia and, anyway, cannot give a definitive and complete diagnosis.

Doppler ultrasound examination of the celiac and mesenteric vessels may have a role in elective settings in selected patients [11, 12] as well as MRI, whose role can be considered in the follow-up of patients with ischemic colitis [13, 14].

17.4 CT Imaging Findings

The CT protocol to be adopted is a complete, multi-phase protocol, as described in the dedicated chapter, this is because to obtain a complete understanding of the pathology, findings of arterial and venous vessels, mesentery, intestinal walls, and abdominal cavity must be explored, as well as a differential diagnosis must be carried out and any incidental findings must be reported comprehensively.

In the setting of mesenteric ischemia, the precontrast phase is useful for identifying the spontaneous hyperdensity of the bowel (i.e. when hemorrhagic necrosis occurs) and for comparison purposes with the subsequent post-contrast phases to evaluate the bowel wall enhancement.

The arterial phase is important to obtain an adequate depiction of the arterial vascular tree and detect arterial vascular findings such as atheromatous plaques, thrombotic occlusion, and arterial dissection, to evaluate the arterial vessels patency and to evaluate the arterial bowel wall enhancement.

The venous phase is indispensable for the evaluation of the venous vessels patency and to study of the enhancement of the bowel wall [1].

Dual-energy CT may improve the early detection of bowel ischemia by increasing the conspicuity of hypoenhancing bowel segments on low–kiloelectron volt and iodine material density images (Fig. 17.1) [15].

The late phase is actually optional, it may be helpful in patients in whom the contrast dynamics are suboptimal in the two previous phases of the study and for differential diagnostic purposes.

The role of post-processing is very important: having thin layer acquisitions available to be able to reconstruct them to obtain good multiplanar reconstruction (MPR) and good maximum intensity projection (MIP).

CT imaging findings vary depending on the etiology as well as on the conditions of the patient's mesenteric circulation which, thanks to the anatomical structure in anastomotic arcades, allows blood flow compensation to be obtained, within certain limits, in the event of a sectorial deficit, this has influence on the extent and entity of the ischemic damage and, consequently, on the related CT findings [8] (Table 17.1).

To systematize the findings and consequently simplify understanding, dedicated animal models examined macroscopically, with imaging methods and with histology have been developed [13, 16–19].

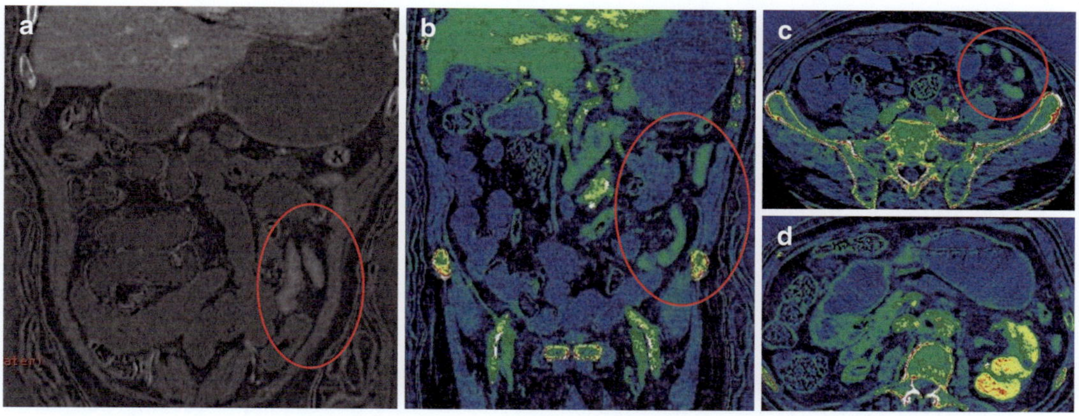

Fig. 17.1 Seventy-three-year-old male with acute abdominal pain. Note that dual-energy CT acquisitions in the venous phase (**a**, greyscale, **b–d** color coded iodine perfusion maps) improve the detection of ischemic bowel segments by increasing the conspicuity of hypoenhancing bowel segments. Note in the figures the normally perfused bowel (**a–c** circle, green depicted) compared with other non-perfused segments (blue depicted)

Table 17.1 Imaging of mesenteric ischemia: CT findings

	Arterial ischemia/ infarction	Reperfusion after arterial ischemia	Nonocclusive mesenteric ischemia	Venous ischemia/ infarction
Vascular findings	Complete or partial thrombotic arterial occlusions	Restoration of post-obstructive arterial flow	Normally patent or variably atheromatous vessels	Thrombotic or mechanical venous occlusion
Bowel wall findings	Thin walls ("paper thin") with reduced or absent enhancement	Walls thickened due to congestion with marked enhancement	Alternation of loops with thin walls (ischemic phase) and loops with thickened walls (reperfusion phase) depending on the presence of compensatory mechanisms	Thickened walls with stratified appearance and increased post-contrastographic enhancement
Mesentery findings	Thin peripheral arterial branches	Congested mesentery	Thin peripheral arterial branches	Congested mesentery
Peritoneal cavity findings	Fluid, serum-blood or air in relation to the evolution of visceral damage	Serum-blood or air in relation to the evolution of visceral damage	Fluid, serum-blood or air in relation to the evolution of visceral damage Altered perfusion of abdominal parenchymatous organs	Serum-blood or air in relation to the evolution of visceral damage

17.5 Notes on Intestinal Vascular Anatomy

The arterial vascular supply to the intestine (20% of cardiac output) is guaranteed by:

- Celiac trunk: gastroduodenal artery which supplies the distal portion of the cardias, the stomach, the I and II duodenum
- Superior mesenteric artery: guarantees arterial supply from the III-IV duodenum to the transverse colon
- Inferior mesenteric artery: supplies from the splenic flexure to the superior rectum.

Furthermore, there is a large anastomotic network between the various arterial vascular branches, which physiologically guarantees adequate perfusion to each intestinal segment and ensures that when a vascular occlusion occurs, there are others that can compensate, unless they are not compromised by widespread atheromasia or previous surgical alterations.

Considering the existence of these phenomena is critical to understanding imaging findings.

Intestinal venous drainage is ensured by the superior mesenteric vein for the entire small intestine and the ascending and transverse colon, and by the inferior mesenteric vein for the descending colon up to the superior rectum. The venous drainage of the middle and lower rectum is ensured by the middle and inferior rectal veins which flow into the inferior vena cava.

17.5.1 Arterial Mesenteric Ischemia

In the arterial mesenteric ischemia, vessel findings (Fig. 17.2) may vary from compression/infiltration of the mesenteric arteries to thrombotic plaque obstructing the lumen or unstable aortic or mesenteric plaque causing peripheral embolism. In this last case, the occlusion of distal arterial vessels goes beyond the resolving power of CT, therefore in these cases, the diagnosis will derive from the presence of unstable plaques or embolic phenomena and from the findings of the bowel wall and abdominal cavity.

Actually, bowel wall findings are the most important to make the diagnosis, and the decreased wall enhancement is the main feature related to bowel ischemia [20]. The extension of the involved bowel depends on the level of arterial vessel obstruction and on the capability to restore the blood flow downstream of the obstructed vessel.

In the early stage of ischemia, in the context of the mesentery, the arterial vessels become less

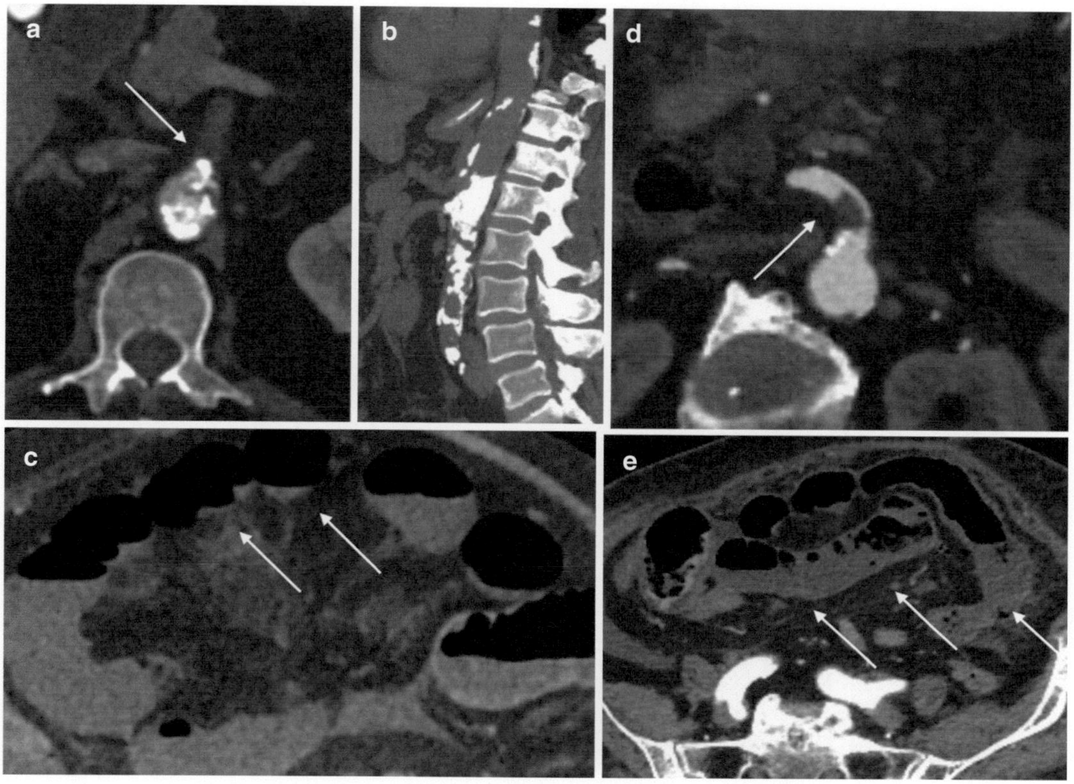

Fig. 17.2 Vessel findings. (**a**) complete thrombotic occlusion of the superior mesenteric artery (**a**, arrow) in the presence of diffuse calcifications of the abdominal aorta (**b**), causing acute arterial mesenteric ischemia (**c**). Note in **c** the paralitic ileus of the bowel loops, with thinned hypoperfused walls. (**d**) Atheromasic, non-calcified plaque partially occupying the lumen of the superior mesenteric artery and causing distal embolism with signs of bowel ischemia (**e**). Note in **e** the presence of paralitic ileus with thinned walls, without wall enhancement (**e**, arrow)

noticeable and of reduced caliber and the bowel reacts with spastic reflex ileus with reduced bowel wall enhancement (Fig. 17.3) [18], if the ischemia persists, the spastic reflex ileus gives way to the hypotonic reflex ileus and, then, to the paralitic ileus in which the bowel become dilated, with thinned and hypoperfused wall and with gas–fluid mixed stasis in the lumen (Fig. 17.4). When these findings occur, ischemia is usually already in an advanced stage, peritoneal fluid is usually present and becomes progressively more dense due to translocation phenomena in the peritoneum. In very late stages of necrosis, bowel wall pneumatosis and gas in mesenteric venous vessels appear (Fig. 17.5) [18].

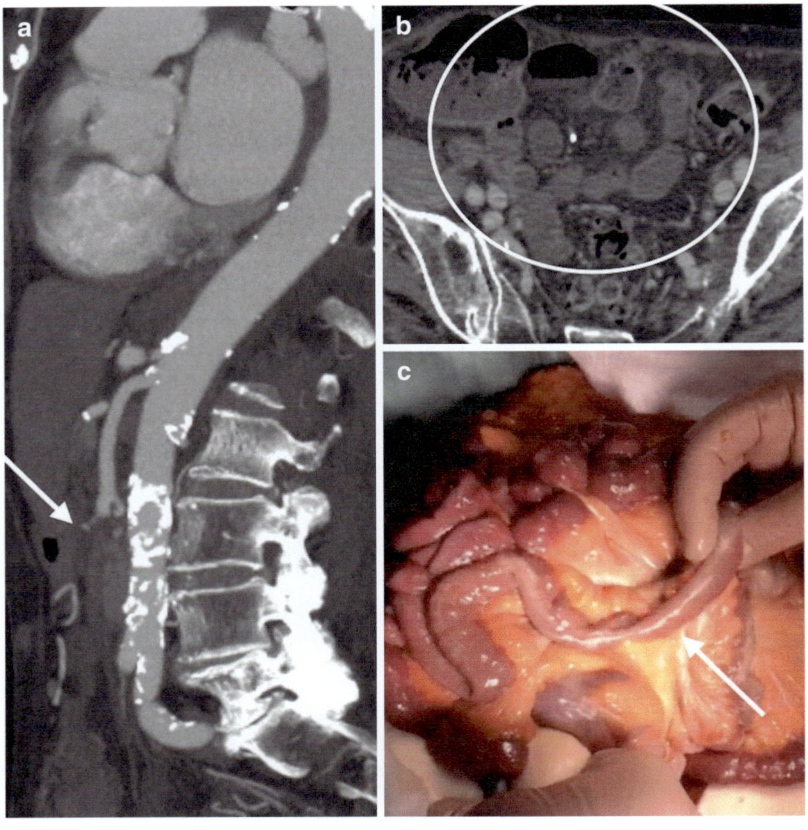

Fig. 17.3 Seventy-four male patient with early occlusive arterial ischemia. Note the complete thrombotic occlusion of the superior mesenteric artery (**a**, arterial phase, sagittal plane, arrow) causing reduced perfusion of the small bowel loops (**b**, white circle) presenting in spastic reflex ileus (**c**, arrow), without free peritoneal fluid. (Authors would like to thank Dr. Francesco Scardi, Department of Emergency Surgery of the "A. Cardarelli" Hospital, directed by Dr. Maurizio Castriconi, for the intraoperative picture (**c**))

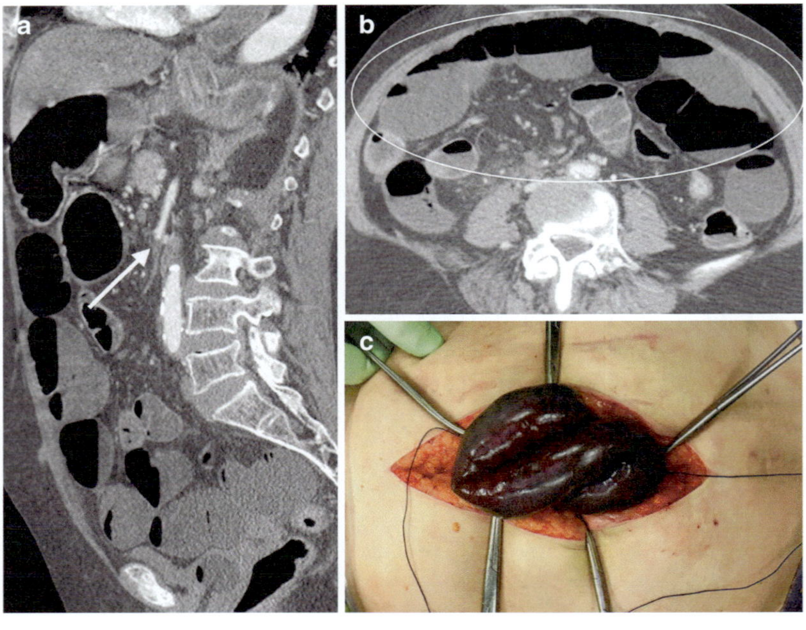

Fig. 17.4 Seventy-four female patient with abdominal pain, hypotension, bloody diarrhea following chemotherapy. Note the complete thrombotic occlusion of the superior mesenteric artery (**a**, arterial phase, sagittal plane, arrow) causing reduced perfusion of the small bowel wall (**b**, circle), diffusely dilated in paralitic ileus, with thinned wall. Intraoperative findings (**c**) confirmed the extensive, advanced small bowel ischemia

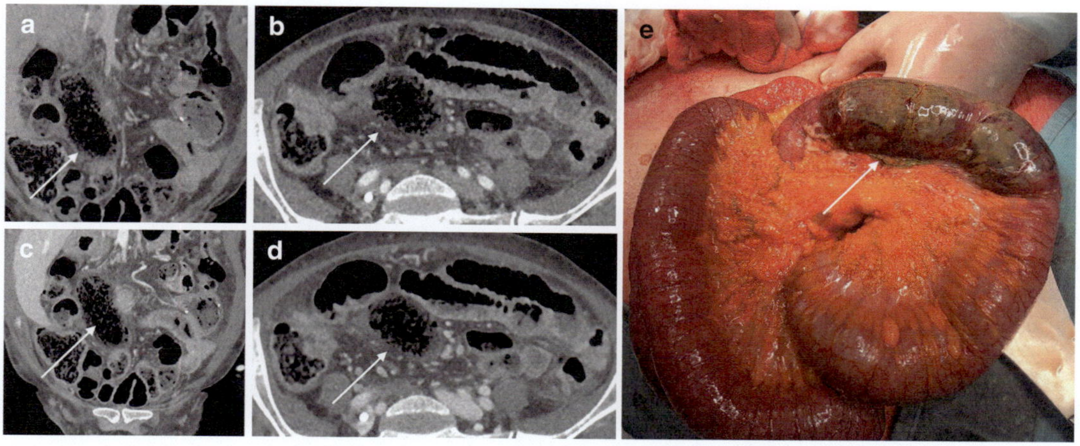

Fig. 17.5 Fifty-six year-old female patient with acute abdomen (**a**, **b** arterial phase, **c**, **d** venous phase, **e**, intraoperative finding). Note the necrotic small bowel segment (**a**–**d** arrow) with extremely thinned and unenhanced wall and intramural pneumatosis. CT findings were confirmed at surgery and the patient underwent small bowel resection. (Authors would like to thank Dr. Antonio Brillantino, Department of Emergency Surgery of the "A. Cardarelli" Hospital, directed by Dr. Maurizio Castriconi, for the intraoperative picture (**c**))

17.5.2 When Reperfusion Occurs: Ischemia-Reperfusion Phenomena

If blood reperfusion occurs, due to therapy or to collateral arterial vessels, the possibility of restoring the bowel wall depends on the time lapsed from ischemia. Indeed in ischemia-reperfusion phenomena, the arriving blood supplies a territory variably damaged by the ischemic phase and what began as a "dry ischemia-infarction", with a thin wall and bloodless mesentery, now takes on the appearance of a hemorrhagic infarct, due to the endothelial damage suffered in the ischemic phase which promotes blood transudation and inflammation with edema when the flow is restored [17]. This a result of oxidative stress following reperfusion that increases reactive oxygen species and local inflammation leading to cell death [20]. So, when reperfusion occurs the bowel wall becomes thickened, variably stratified with hypoattenuating oedema of the submucosa and hyperenhancement of the mucosa (Fig. 17.6) [17]. Furthermore, fat stranding may coexist in the adjacent mesentery, showing dilated draining veins and free fluid with variable density, depending on the entity of the wall damage [17, 20].

17.5.3 Ischemic Colitis

Ischemic colitis can be considered, usually, as a sub-entity of arterial AMI reflecting a localized colon ischemia-reperfusion injury [20]. Indeed, ischemic colitis is mostly caused by transient splanchnic hemodynamic variations which impede blood flow in the inferior mesenteric artery, or inferior mesenteric artery spasm [20]. The cause is actually rarely identified and at CT examination inferior mesenteric artery results are usually patent. It can be intended as a localized colon ischemia-reperfusion injury as, in the majority of cases, the superior mesenteric artery and the compensatory circle determined by the anastomotic vascular arches which supply the territories of the inferior mesenteric artery from the superior mesenteric artery, are patent. This guarantees that in the presence of a defect in the arterial vascular supply in the inferior mesenteric artery, there may be reperfusion from the superior mesenteric arterial vascular district and so the injured colon will show findings related to ischemia followed by reperfusion, with thickened wall with submucosal hypodensity due to edema and mucosal hyperenhancement and pericolic fat stranding. IC is usually segmental, with a sharp

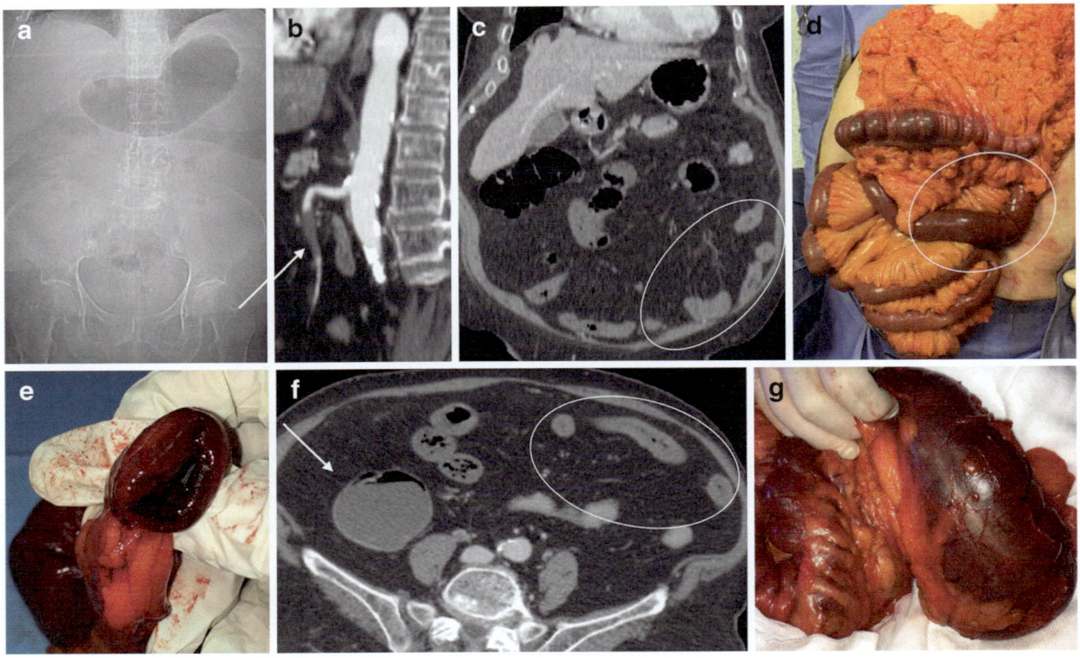

Fig. 17.6 Seventy-nine year-old female patient with acute abdomen (**a**, CT scout, **b** arterial phase sagittal view, **c**, venous phase coronal view, **d**, **e** intraoperative findings, **f**, venous phase axial view, **g** intraoperative findings). Note at the CT scout (**a**) the reduced representation of intestinal meteorism associated with reflex gastrectasia, in **b** is seen the segmental obstruction of the superior mesenteric artery lumen (**b**, arrow) with downstream opacification, causing mixed ischemic-reperfusion phenomena. Indeed, in **c** is seen thickening of some small bowel loops (**c**, **f** circle) due to reperfusion damage, appearing dark at the following surgical exploration (**d**, circle) with intramural blood extravasation (**e**). Furthermore there are findings of advanced ischemia, without reperfusion, involving the cecum (**f**, arrow) that appear with thinned, hypoperfused wall and brownish at the surgical exploration

definition between the involved and uninvolved colon, even if, rarely, may affect the whole colon (Fig. 17.7).

The condition is usually transient and gradually there is a progressive restoration [13, 21, 22].

However, in vasculopathic patients and in all cases in which no circulation compensation occurs, the deficit in the blood supply from the inferior mesenteric artery leads to progressive ischemia of the colonic wall up to parietal necrosis, similar to what was previously explained regarding arterial ischemia not followed by reperfusion (Fig. 17.8) [14, 23, 24].

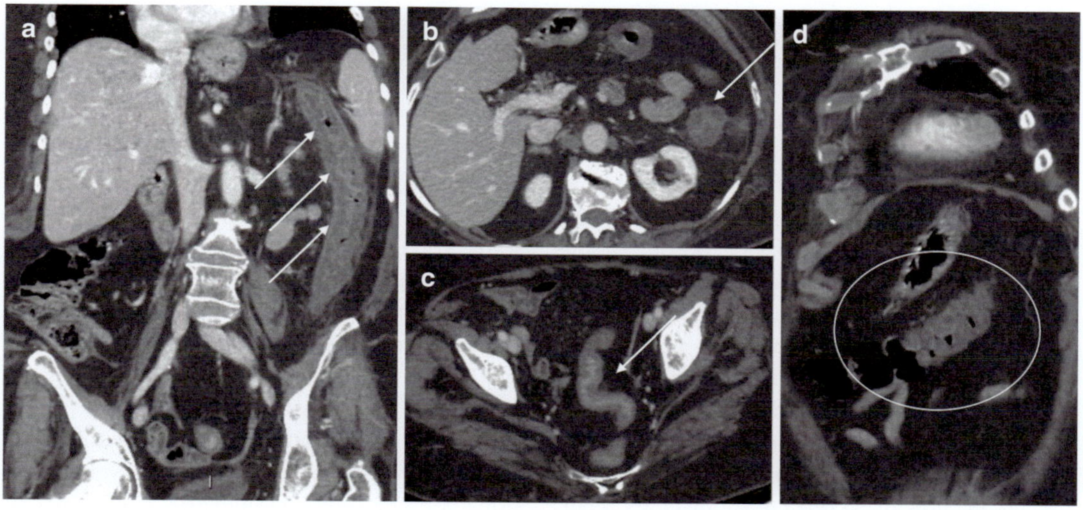

Fig. 17.7 Fifty year-old female with acute abdominal pain and rectorrhagia. Note the thickening of the colon with mucosal hyperemia, submucosal edema and pericolic free fluid (**a–c** arrows), with clear demarcation of the affected segment from the unaffected ones (**d**). There are no signs of active bleeding, the rectorrhagia is caused by the mucosal ischemic-reperfusion damage. (From: Iacobellis et al. [14], licensed under CC-BY 4.0)

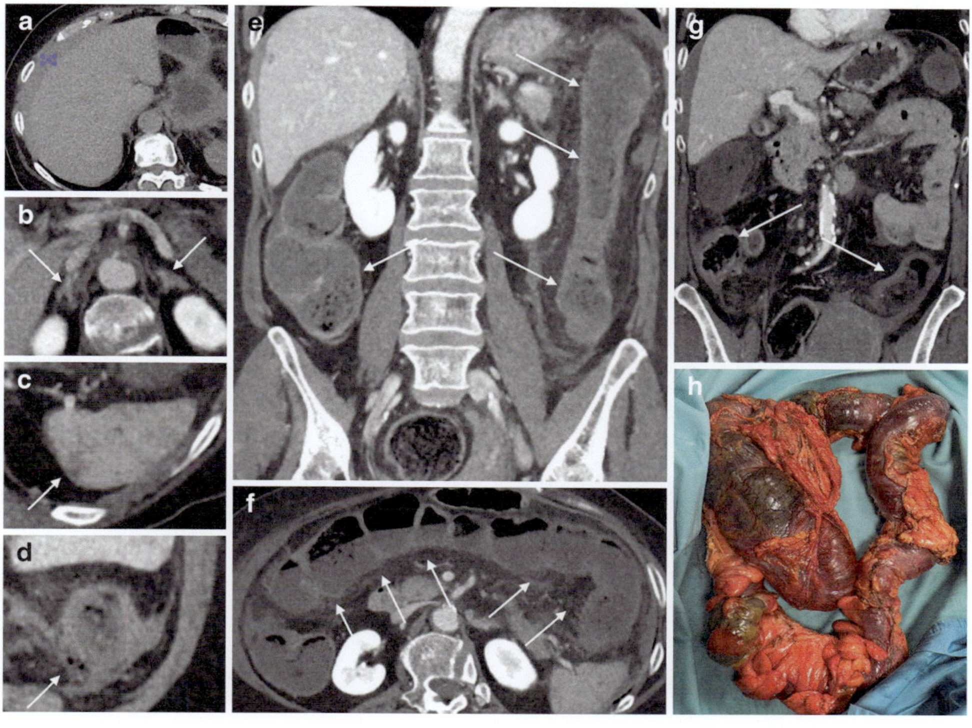

Fig. 17.8 Seventy year-old female patient with acute abdominal pain and syncope. Note the presence of spontaneously hyperdense peritoneal free fluid 66 HU (**a**, circle), hyperdensity of the adrenal cortex (**b**, arrows), inhomogeous enhancement of the spleen (**c**, portal phase, arrow), diffuse slight colonic wall thickening (**e–g**, arrows) with inhomogeneous enhancement and focal wall defect at the descending segment (**d**, arrow) consistent with extensive colonic ischemia due to ineffective colonic reperfusion, with focal ischemic perforation, in a setting of splanchnic hypoperfusion. Intraoperative finding (**h**) confirmed the extensive colonic ischemia and led to colectomy. (Authors would like to thank Dr. Michele Lanza, Department of Emergency Surgery of the "A. Cardarelli" Hospital, directed by Dr. Maurizio Castriconi, for the intraoperative picture (**c**))

17.6 Nonocclusive Mesenteric Ischemia

Nonocclusive mesenteric ischemia (NOMI) usually occurs in critically ill patients with low-flow states or with altered regulation of the splanchnic circulation and is related to impaired arterial mesenteric flow due to hypoperfusion. In this form of mesenteric ischemia, the vessel finding is given by thinned vessels, often diffusely atheromatous, with a poorly appreciable lumen of the distal branches. The bowel wall findings vary depending on the degree and extent of the intestinal ischemic injury and the therapies administered or the attempts at circulation compensation. Indeed, in cases of NOMI not followed by reperfusion, the bowel wall findings are the same as described for arterial mesenteric ischemia, whereas when reperfusion occurs there will be findings similar to what has already been described for the ischemia phenomena followed by reperfusion. In these last cases, frequently encountered is the inhomogeneity of post-contrastographic enhancement of the bowel walls, some of them may have thin walls (ischemic hypoperfusion phase) and others may be thickened (reperfusion phase), with variable wall enhancement. However, additional findings that can help in the diagnosis are those affecting the abdominal parenchymatous organs, in fact in NOMI the circulation deficit involves the entire splanchnic district so more or less severe perfusion alterations will be found affecting the parenchymas (Fig. 17.9) [8, 9, 20, 24].

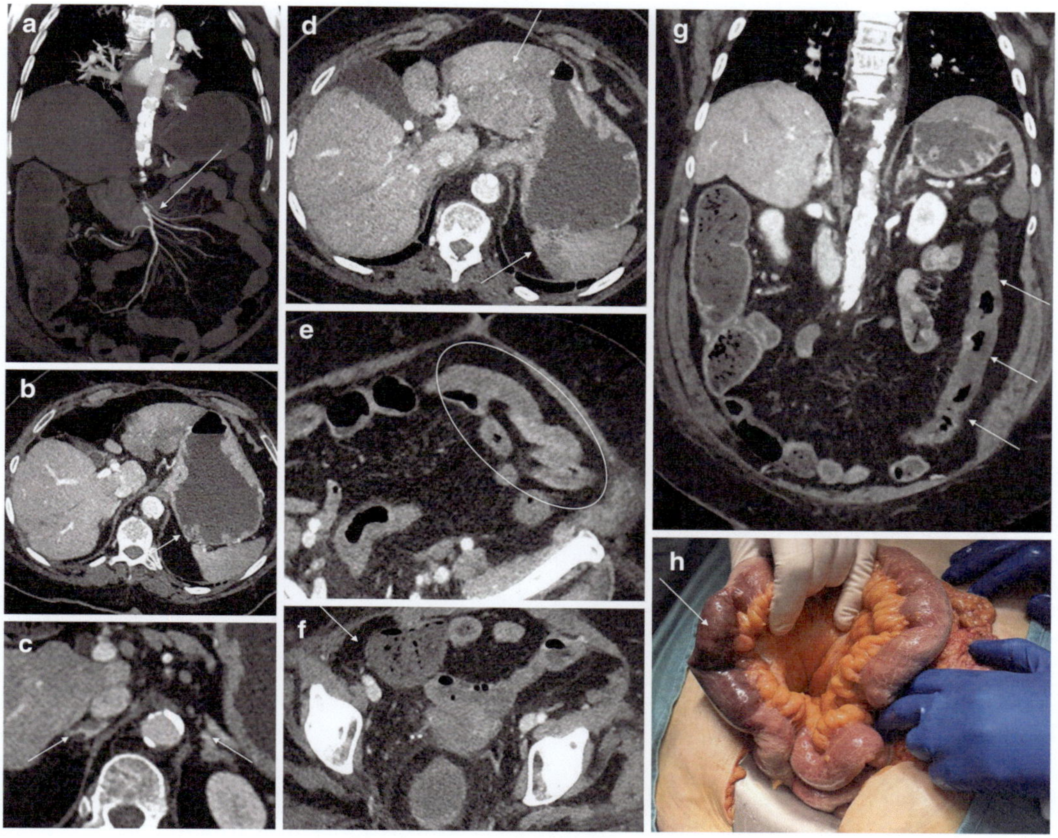

Fig. 17.9 Seventy-five year-old female patient with cardiac failure. Note the reduced caliper of the superior mesenteric artery and its branches (**a**, arterial phase, MIP reconstruction, arrow), the gastrectasia (**b**, arrow), bilateral hyperdensity of the adrenal cortex (**c**, arrows), inhomogeous enhancement of the liver and spleen (**d**, portal phase, arrow), inhomogeneous enhancement of the small bowel wall (**e**, portal phase, circle) due to ischemia-reperfusion phenomena, the presence of a small bowel segment in advanced stage of ischemia with thinned and unenhanced wall in the right iliac fossa (**f**, arrow) and inhomogeneous thickening of the colonic wall (**g**, arrows). Surgical exploration confirmed the splanchnic hypoperfusion with segmental advanced ischemia of a small bowel segment (**h**, arrow). (Authors would like to thank Colleagues of the Department of Emergency Surgery of the "A. Cardarelli" Hospital, directed by Dr. Maurizio Castriconi, for the intraoperative picture (**c**))

17.7 Venous Mesenteric Ischemia

In case of obstructive compromise of the venous vascular side, the vessel finding is represented by venous luminal obstruction of various etiologies (e.g. thrombotic, adhesions, infiltrative), whereas the bowel wall findings depend on the entity of congestion of the upstream territory, therefore, wall thickening with an increased post-contrastographic enhancement of the bowel wall, with a variably stratified appearance will be detected. The mesentery will appear congested, with increased vessel representation and with a variable amount of fat stranding and free fluid, depending on the entity of the damage. The lack of outflow of catabolites and vascular congestion cause, however, an ischemic damage and in the late phases, the absence of wall enhancement and pneumatosis may be observed (Fig. 17.10) [8, 17, 20, 24].

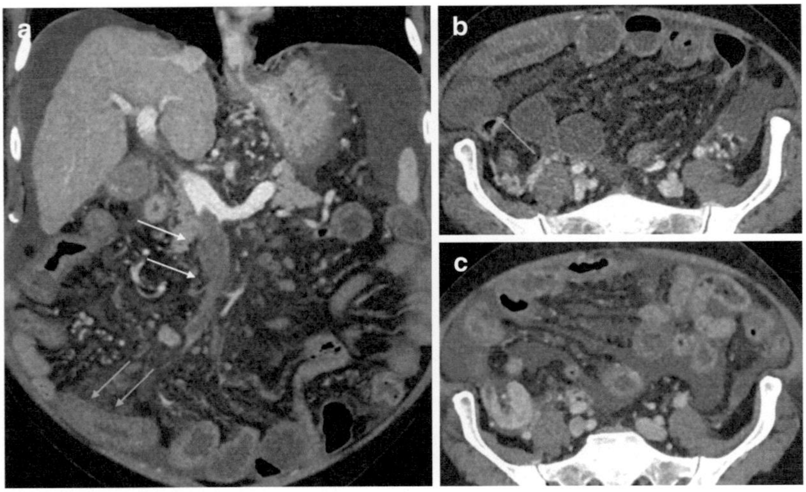

Fig. 17.10 Fifty-seven year-old male patient with cirrhosis and thrombotic occlusion of the superior mesenteric vein (**a**, portal phase, coronal view, white arrows) occupying the whole venous lumen and causing venous mesenteric ischemia (**a**, green arrows). The ischemic small bowel loop shows a thickened wall (**a**, green arrow) with reduced enhancement (**b**, green arrows). Patient underwent medical therapy with anticoagulant drugs and some days later showed a restoration of the bowel tone and wall enhancement (**c**)

17.8 Differential Diagnoses

The main pathological conditions that enter into the differential diagnosis with mesenteric ischemia are infectious, inflammatory enteritis and colitis, graft-versus-host disease, actinic enteritis, and chronic inflammatory intestinal disease. The anamnesis, the distribution of the damage, and the imaging appearance of the alterations of the loop, as well as the clinical-laboratory and endoscopic examinations, can guide the differential diagnosis, although this sometimes remains actually complex to be made.

Among the CT findings of acute mesenteric ischemia it should be considered that:

Luminal dilatation can be found in mechanic and paralytic ileus.

Bowel wall thickening with stratified appearance is a fairly frequent finding in bowel pathologies, indeed it can be found in infectious enteritis, acute stage of Crohn's disease, and acute radiation enteritis [25, 26].

Intestinal wall pneumatosis, although usually considered a sign of necrotic damage to the bowel wall, may be also associated with several non-surgical benign conditions such as cystic pneumatosis (Fig. 17.11), connective tissue disease, emphysema, asthma, and in these cases patients are usually asymptomatic with normal bowel wall thickness and enhancement pattern and absence of porto-mesenteric gas. Intestinal wall pneumatosis can also be found in non ischemic bowel conditions such as sepsis, or luminal overdistension (Fig. 17.11) [27].

The clinical history and symptoms, the pattern of bowel involvement (segmental with skip areas in Crohn's disease), the opacification of the vessel lumen, and, mainly, the bowel wall enhancement, help in differentiating these entities from bowel ischemia/infarction [28, 29].

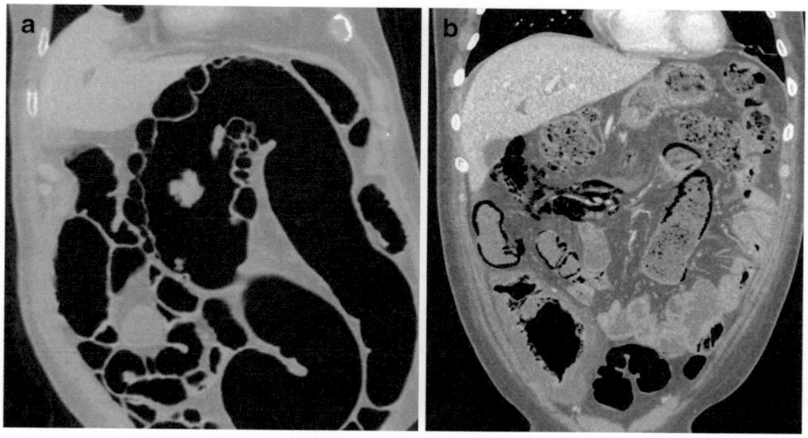

Fig. 17.11 Two different cases of non-surgical pneumatosis: (**a**) cystic pneumatosis, (**b**) septic pneumatosis. In the first case any therapy is needed, in the second case medical therapy is necessary

17.9 The Emergency Radiologist Role: Treatment Implications

Radiologists play a critical role in guiding therapeutic decisions by accurately characterizing the extent and severity of mesenteric ischemia through imaging. Indeed, early diagnosis is essential to prevent bowel necrosis and associated morbidity and mortality. Treatment strategies vary based on patient conditions and the underlying etiology and severity of AMI. If there are signs of advanced ischemia/necrosis, the approach is surgical, if the intestinal involvement is not so extensive as to not allow any possible resection. When there are signs of early or moderated ischemia, in arterial occlusions, urgent revascularization via endovascular or surgical techniques can be attempted. In NOMI it is important the optimize systemic perfusion and supportive measures, whereas, in mesenteric venous thrombosis, anticoagulation therapy can be first attempted. Ischemic colitis, being usually an ischemia-reperfusion phenomenon, needs supportive medical treatment. Obviously, in cases where the ischemic damage is secondary to other causes (infiltrative, compressive, traumatic) the treatment will be aimed at the primary cause [5].

17.10 Vascular Compression Syndromes

We believe it is necessary to mention some clinical conditions, usually not included among the causes of acute mesenteric ischemia, as they are not strictly at risk of causing rapidly evolving intestinal ischemia, but which can cause recurrent acute abdominal pain, in usually young patients, and base their pathophysiology on mixed, partly ischemic, mechanisms.

We refer to celiac artery compression syndrome (also known as median arcuate ligament syndrome, Dunbar syndrome, or celiac axis syndrome) and superior mesenteric artery compression disorder.

These syndromes are commonly seen in young and otherwise healthy individuals. They can present with a wide array of vague abdominal symptoms, such as abdominal pain, nausea, vomiting, weight loss, and in severe cases, acute abdominal hemorrhage, arterial ischemia, embolism, or venous stasis and thrombosis [11, 30]. This diversity of symptoms makes diagnosing these conditions particularly challenging in clinical practice.

Dunbar syndrome presents as a condition where the proximal celiac trunk experiences external compression due to the median arcuate ligament being abnormally positioned lower than usual. The pathophysiology of Dunbar syndrome is still a subject of debate. Two primary theories have emerged to elucidate its symptoms: one pertaining to vascular factors and the other to neurogenic factors. The vascular theory suggests that compression of the mesenteric vasculature leads to mesenteric ischemia, resulting in symptoms such as abdominal angina. Conversely, the neurogenic theory proposes that splanchnic vasoconstriction occurs due to stimulation of the celiac ganglion and the celiac plexus [30]. Patients usually present with relapse postprandial symptoms including pain, nausea, vomiting, diarrhea, and unexplained weight loss. CT helps in the diagnosis allowing three-dimensional visualization of compressed celiac artery and can show changes like post stenotic dilatation. Celiac artery compression can be better noted during expiration, adopting MPR in the sagittal views, with eventually associated collaterals developed due to the compression, usually from the superior mesenteric artery (Fig. 17.12) [31]. Usually, no significant alterations in the stomach or small bowel wall enhancement are detected since compression of the celiac trunk occurs as a transitory event.

Superior mesenteric artery compression is an infrequent vascular compression disorder (Fig. 17.13). It occurs when the superior mesenteric artery (SMA) undergoes acute angulation, compressing the third part of the duodenum and causing luminal obstruction. Patients may present acutely with signs and symptoms of duodenal obstruction or with long-standing vague abdominal symptoms, early satiety and anorexia, or recurrent episodes of abdominal pain, associated with vomiting. Symptoms depend on the course of the superior mesenteric artery, with a short angle with the aorta of 9–35° (normal value 38–56°), and a reduction in the distance between the aorta and the superior mesenteric artery of 2–8 mm (normal value 10–28 mm). This arterial course may cause compression of the duodenum, of the left renal vein, or, also, of mesenteric

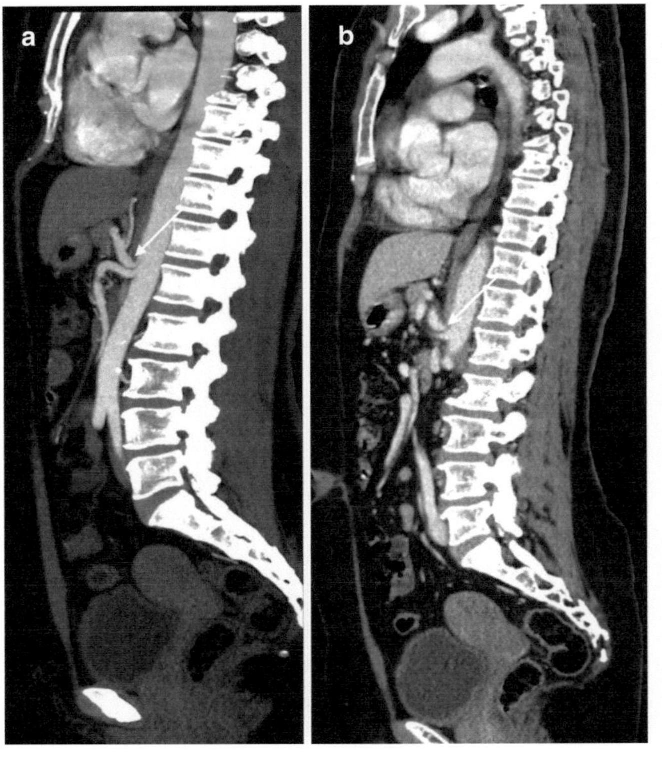

Fig. 17.12 A case of Dunbar syndrome: young patient complaining of persistent abdominal pain. Note in both images (**a**, arterial phases, **b**, venous phase, sagittal plane, arrows) the compression of the celiac trunk

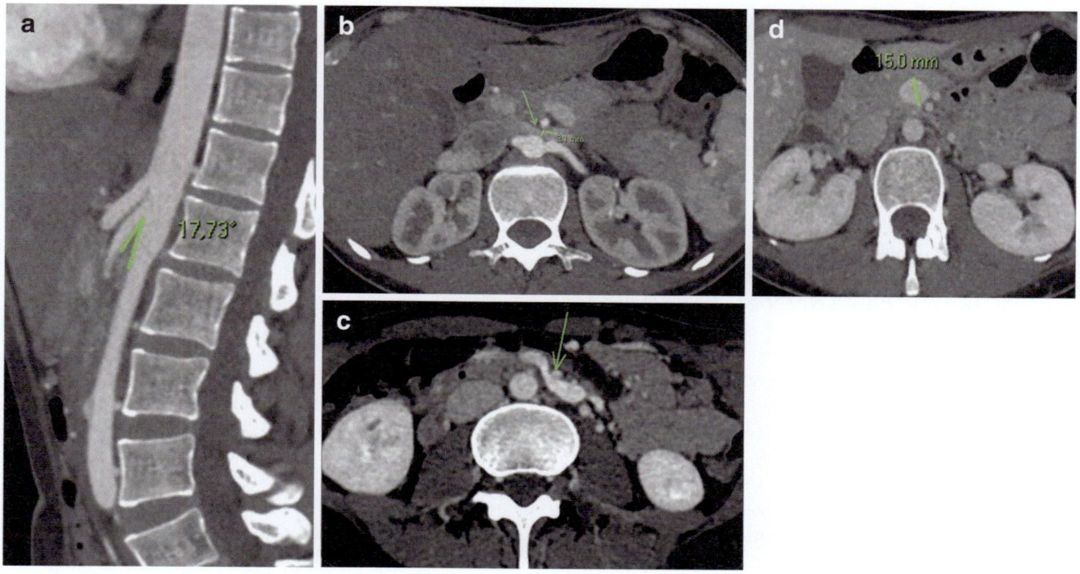

Fig. 17.13 Twenty-four-year-old female patient complaining of persistent abdominal pain in left flank. There is a reduced aorto-mesenteric angle (**a**) causing compression of the left renal vein (**b**, arrow) and of a venous mesenteric vessel (**c**, arrow) causing venous mesenteric dilation upstream (**d**, arrow)

venous vessels, being responsible in this last case of late postprandial symptoms due to mesenteric venous congestion. This form often causes anorexia and weight loss, establishing a vicious circle that causes a further worsening of symptoms, given that the presence of a well-represented fat pad between the superior mesenteric artery and the aorta can reduce the acuteness of the emergency angle of the superior mesenteric artery.

The treatment of these syndromes may vary being usually surgical in Dunbar Syndrome, and both conservative or surgical in the superior mesenteric artery syndrome, depending on the compressed anatomical structure and the degree of compression [30].

17.11 Conclusion

AMI and bowel infarction represent severe and time-sensitive conditions requiring prompt radiological evaluation for accurate diagnosis and intervention. Radiologists are pivotal in identifying characteristic imaging features that aid in timely management decisions. Familiarity with imaging modalities, typical findings, and differential diagnoses is essential for optimizing patient care and outcomes in cases of AMI.

References

1. Copin P, Zins M, Nuzzo A, Purcell Y, Beranger-Gibert S, Maggiori L, Corcos O, Vilgrain V, Ronot M. Acute mesenteric ischemia: a critical role for the radiologist. Diagn Interv Imaging. 2018;99(3):123–34. https://doi.org/10.1016/j.diii.2018.01.004
2. Peoc'h K, Nuzzo A, Guedj K, Paugam C, Corcos O. Diagnosis biomarkers in acute intestinal ischemic injury: so close, yet so far. Clin Chem Lab Med. 2018;56(3):373–85. https://doi.org/10.1515/cclm-2017-0291
3. Oehler H, Eichler K, Derwich W, Schnitzbauer AA, Schreckenbach T. Epidemiologie und Diagnostik der mesenterialen Ischämie [Epidemiology and diagnostics of mesenteric ischemia]. Chirurgie (Heidelb). 2024;95(5):347–52. German. https://doi.org/10.1007/s00104-023-02021-6.
4. Monita MM, Gonzalez L. Acute Mesenteric Ischemia. [Updated 2023 June 26]. In: StatPearls [Internet]. Treasure Island (FL): StatPearls Publishing; 2024. Available from: https://www.ncbi.nlm.nih.gov/books/NBK431068/ accessed on April 22, 2024.
5. Bala M, Catena F, Kashuk J, et al. Acute mesenteric ischemia: updated guidelines of the World Society of

Emergency Surgery. World J Emerg Surg. 2022;17:54. https://doi.org/10.1186/s13017-022-00443-x.

6. Brillantino A, Iacobellis F, Renzi A, Nasti R, Saldamarco L, Grillo M, Romano L, Castriconi M, Cittadini A, De Palma M, Scaglione M, Di Martino N, Grassi R, Paladino F. Diagnostic value of arterial blood gas lactate concentration in the different forms of mesenteric ischemia. Eur J Trauma Emerg Surg. 2018;44(2):265–72. https://doi.org/10.1007/s00068-017-0805-7. Epub 2017 June 13. PMID: 28612169.
7. Blauw JTM, Metz FM, Nuzzo A, van Etten-Jamaludin FS, Brusse-Keiser M, Boermeester MA, Peppelenbosch M, Geelkerken RH, Dutch Mesenteric Ischaemia Study group. The diagnostic value of biomarkers in acute mesenteric ischaemia is insufficiently substantiated: a systematic review. Eur J Vasc Endovasc Surg. 2024;67(4):554–69. https://doi.org/10.1016/j.ejvs.2023.08.059. Epub 2023 Aug 26. PMID: 37640253.
8. Theodore S, Xia T, Saillant N. Intestinal Ischemia – etiology and foundational concepts. NEJM Evid. 2024;3(3):EVIDra2300266. https://doi.org/10.1056/EVIDra2300266.
9. Di Serafino M, Viscardi D, Iacobellis F, Giugliano L, Barbuto L, Oliva G, Ronza R, Borzelli A, Raucci A, Pezzullo F, De Cristofaro MG, Romano L. Computed tomography imaging of septic shock. Beyond the cause: the "CT hypoperfusion complex". A pictorial essay. Insights. Imaging. 2021;12(1):70. https://doi.org/10.1186/s13244-021-01006-5.
10. Acute Mesenteric Ischemia By Parswa Ansari, MD, Hofstra Northwell-Lenox Hill Hospital, New York. Reviewed/Revised Apr 2023 https://www.msdmanuals.com/professional/gastrointestinal-disorders/acute-abdomen-and-surgical-gastroenterology/acute-mesenteric-ischemia. Accessed on April 29/2024.
11. Acampora C, Di Serafino M, Iacobellis F, Trovato P, Barbuto L, Sangiuliano N, Costigliola L, Romano L. Insight into Dunbar syndrome: color-Doppler ultrasound findings and literature review. J Ultrasound. 2021;24(3):317–21. https://doi.org/10.1007/s40477-019-00422-0.
12. Reginelli A, Genovese E, Cappabianca S, Iacobellis F, Berritto D, Fonio P, Coppolino F, Grassi R. Intestinal Ischemia: US-CT findings correlations. Crit Ultrasound J. 2013;5 Suppl 1(Suppl 1):S7. https://doi.org/10.1186/2036-7902-5-S1-S7.
13. Iacobellis F, Berritto D, Somma F, Cavaliere C, Corona M, Cozzolino S, Fulciniti F, Cappabianca S, Rotondo A, Grassi R. Magnetic resonance imaging: a new tool for diagnosis of acute ischemic colitis? World J Gastroenterol. 2012;18(13):1496–501. https://doi.org/10.3748/wjg.v18.i13.1496.
14. Iacobellis F, Narese D, Berritto D, Brillantino A, Di Serafino M, Guerrini S, Grassi R, Scaglione M, Mazzei MA, Romano L. Large bowel Ischemia/Infarction: how to recognize it and make differential diagnosis? A review. Diagnostics (Basel). 2021;11(6):998. https://doi.org/10.3390/diagnostics11060998.
15. Potretzke TA, Brace CL, Lubner MG, Sampson LA, Willey BJ, Lee FT Jr. Early small-bowel ischemia: dual-energy CT improves conspicuity compared with conventional CT in a swine model. Radiology. 2015;275(1):119–26. https://doi.org/10.1148/radiol.14140875.
16. Berritto D, Somma F, Landi N, Cavaliere C, Corona M, Russo S, Fulciniti F, Cappabianca S, Rotondo A, Grassi R. Seven-Tesla micro-MRI in early detection of acute arterial ischaemia: evolution of findings in an in vivo rat model. Radiol Med. 2011;116(6):829–41. English, Italian. https://doi.org/10.1007/s11547-011-0676-7.
17. Somma F, Berritto D, Iacobellis F, Landi N, Cavaliere C, Corona M, Russo S, Di Mizio R, Rotondo A, Grassi R. 7T μMRI of mesenteric venous ischemia in a rat model: timing of the appearance of findings. Magn Reson Imaging. 2013;31(3):408–13. https://doi.org/10.1016/j.mri.2012.08.003.
18. Berritto D, Iacobellis F, Somma F, Corona M, Faggian A, Iacomino A, Feragalli B, Saba L, La Porta M, Grassi R. 7T mMR in the assessment of acute arterial mesenteric ischemia in a rat model. J Biol Regul Homeost Agents. 2013;27(3):771–9.
19. Saba L, Berritto D, Iacobellis F, Scaglione M, Castaldo S, Cozzolino S, Mazzei MA, Di Mizio V, Grassi R. Acute arterial mesenteric ischemia and reperfusion: macroscopic and MRI findings, preliminary report. World J Gastroenterol. 2013;19(40):6825–33. https://doi.org/10.3748/wjg.v19.i40.6825.
20. Garzelli L, Ben Abdallah I, Nuzzo A, Zappa M, Corcos O, Dioguardi Burgio M, Cazals-Hatem D, Rautou PE, Vilgrain V, Calame P, Ronot M. Insights into acute mesenteric ischaemia: an up-to-date, evidence-based review from a mesenteric stroke centre unit. Br J Radiol. 2023;96(1151):20230232. https://doi.org/10.1259/bjr.20230232.
21. Berritto D, Iacobellis F, Mazzei MA, Volterrani L, Guglielmi G, Brunese L, Grassi R. MDCT in ischaemic colitis: how to define the aetiology and acute, subacute and chronic phase of damage in the emergency setting. Br J Radiol. 2016;89(1061):20150821. https://doi.org/10.1259/bjr.20150821.
22. Iacobellis F, Berritto D, Fleischmann D, Gagliardi G, Brillantino A, Mazzei MA, Grassi R. CT findings in acute, subacute, and chronic ischemic colitis: suggestions for diagnosis. Biomed Res Int. 2014;2014:895248. https://doi.org/10.1155/2014/895248.
23. Di Grezia G, Gatta G, Rella R, Iacobellis F, Berritto D, Musto LA, Grassi R. MDCT in acute ischaemic left colitis: a pictorial essay. Radiol Med. 2019;124(2):103–8. https://doi.org/10.1007/s11547-018-0947-7.
24. Reginelli A, Iacobellis F, Berritto D, Gagliardi G, Di Grezia G, Rossi M, Fonio P, Grassi R. Mesenteric ischemia: the importance of differential diagnosis for the surgeon. BMC Surg. 2013;13 Suppl 2(Suppl 2):S51. https://doi.org/10.1186/1471-2482-13-S2-S51.

25. Fernandes T, Oliveira MI, Castro R, Araújo B, Viamonte B, Cunha R. Bowel wall thickening at CT: simplifying the diagnosis. Insights Imaging. 2014;5(2):195–208. https://doi.org/10.1007/s13244-013-0308-y.
26. Marín-Díez E, Crespo Del Pozo J. Diagnostic approach to small-bowel wall thickening: Beyond Crohn's disease and cancer. Radiologia (Engl Ed). 2021;63(6):519–30. https://doi.org/10.1016/j.rxeng.2020.11.008.
27. Lassandro F, Mangoni de Santo Stefano ML, Porto AM, Grassi R, Scaglione M, Rotondo A. Intestinal pneumatosis in adults: diagnostic and prognostic value. Emerg Radiol. 2010;17(5):361–5. https://doi.org/10.1007/s10140-010-0868-9.
28. Sinha D, Kale S, Kundaragi NG, Sharma S. Mesenteric ischemia: a radiologic perspective. Abdom Radiol (NY). 2022;47(5):1514–28. https://doi.org/10.1007/s00261-020-02867-y.
29. Olson MC, Bach CR, Wells ML, Andrews JC, Khandelwal A, Welle CL, Fidler JL. Imaging of Bowel Ischemia: an update, from the AJR special series on emergency radiology. AJR Am J Roentgenol. 2023;220(2):173–85. https://doi.org/10.2214/AJR.22.28140. Epub 2022 Aug 10. PMID: 35946859.
30. Gozzo C, Giambelluca D, Cannella R, Caruana G, Jukna A, Picone D, Midiri M, Salvaggio G. CT imaging findings of abdominopelvic vascular compression syndromes: what the radiologist needs to know. Insights Imaging. 2020;11(1):48. https://doi.org/10.1186/s13244-020-00852-z.
31. Iqbal S, Chaudhary M. Median arcuate ligament syndrome (Dunbar syndrome). Cardiovasc Diagn Ther. 2021;11(5):1172–6. https://doi.org/10.21037/cdt-20-846.

18 Abdominal Compartment Syndrome

Martina Caruso, Chiara Rinaldo,
Giuliana Giacobbe, Maria Laura Schillirò,
Gianluca Ponticiello, and Francesca Iacobellis

18.1 Introduction

Compartment syndrome is a pathological condition characterized by increased pressure within a closed anatomical space, which compromises perfusion and reduces the functionality of the organs and tissues within that space. While it is well-known in the extremities, usually as complication of traumatic injuries, it is less recognized in the abdomen. Although the harmful effects of increased intra-abdominal pressure (IAP) were first documented more than 100 years ago, with a focus on understanding how abdominal pressure impacts renal blood flow and cardiac return, the term "abdominal compartment syndrome" (ACS) was introduced in 1989 by Fietsam et al. to describe the pathological condition occurred in a patient undergoing repair of ruptured abdominal aortic aneurysm [1]. In 2004, the World Society of Abdominal Compartment Syndrome (WSACS), composed of European, Australian, and North American surgical, trauma, and critical care specialists, published expert definitions, clinical practice guidelines, and research recommendations for intra-abdominal hypertension (IAH) and ACS [1]. WSACS defines IAH as a persistent increase of IAP above 12 mmHg, whereas normal abdominal pressure is less than 8 mmHg. Acute increased intra-abdominal volume (such as hemoperitoneum or ascites) or decreased abdominal wall compliance can lead to IAH. This, in turn, can decrease venous return, resulting in low cardiac output, impaired renal function, oliguria, and decreased respiratory compliance, leading to hypoxemia. These conditions can cause multiple organ failure. ACS is defined by a sustained IAP greater than 20 mmHg accompanied by new organ dysfunction and/or failure [2]. The direct measurement of IAP requires placement of an intraperitoneal catheter connected to an external pressure transducer or saline manometer, but this method is invasive. For that, in clinical practice, the indirect measurement through urinary bladder pressure is preferred. Since this method is not always feasible, alternative diagnostic tools should be considered, such as computed tomography (CT) [3]. The presence of certain CT findings in critically ill patients, for instance, round belly signs, elevation of the diaphragm, and narrowing of inferior vena cava, can raise suspicion of ACS, and abdominal CT can help identify possible causes [2, 4].

M. Caruso (✉) · C. Rinaldo · G. Giacobbe
M. L. Schillirò · G. Ponticiello · F. Iacobellis
Department of General and Emergency Radiology, "Antonio Cardarelli" Hospital, Naples, Italy
e-mail: martina.caruso@aocardarelli.it; chiara.rinaldo@aocardarelli.it; giuliana.giacobbe@aocardarelli.it; marialaura.schilliro@aocardarelli.it; gianluca.ponticiello@aocardarelli.it; francesca.iacobellis@aocardarelli.it

L. Romano et al. (eds.), *CT of Non-Traumatic Body Emergencies*,
https://doi.org/10.1007/978-3-031-84849-0_18

18.2 Pathophysiology and Risk Factors

The abdomen is an enclosed anatomical space. Consequently, any increase in intra-abdominal volume and/or any decrease in the abdominal compliance, which relies on the elasticity of the abdominal wall and the diaphragm's elastic recoil, may lead to a rise in IAP. Obesity, rectus sheath hematoma, and burns with abdominal eschars may reduce abdominal wall compliance, while gastric distention, mechanical and paralytic ileus, and massive hemoperitoneum may increase the intra-abdominal volume, representing risk factors for the development of IAH/ACS.

IAH and ACS are categorized as primary, secondary, or recurrent based on duration and etiology. Primary ACS, also known as "surgical" ACS, is characterized by IAH of relatively short duration, linked to injuries or diseases that involve the abdominopelvic region, such as high-grade traumatic parenchymal injuries, liver transplantation, endovascular repair of ruptured abdominal aortic aneurysm, hemorrhagic pancreatitis, and massive ascites or hemoperitoneum [5–11]. In detail, ACS develops in 5–20% of patients with severe abdominal trauma, 30% of those post-liver transplantation, and 10% of severe acute pancreatitis cases [12–15]. Primary ACS often needs surgical or radiologic intervention [16]. Secondary ACS, also known as "medical" ACS, arises from extra-abdominal conditions, such as sepsis, major burns, large-volume intravenous resuscitation, or massive transfusion in case of shock [17, 18]. Finally, recurrent ACS refers to the return of ACS symptoms after an earlier episode of primary or secondary ACS has been resolved. Recent studies indicate that primary IAH accounts for 46% of cases [8].

As mentioned above, progressively increasing IAP significantly affects various organ systems, creating a vicious cycle in IAH and ACS, which further deteriorates systemic conditions and can lead to multi-organ failure.

First, rising IAP increases intrathoracic pressure due to the upward displacement of the diaphragm. As a result, increased intrathoracic pressure directly compresses the heart, aorta, and lung parenchyma [19]. The reduced cardiac compliance and ventricular contractility determine a decrease in cardiac output. The compression of the aorta leads to an increase in systemic vascular resistance. Finally, the increased intrathoracic pressure causes basilar lung parenchyma atelectasis, therefore a reduction of total lung capacity, functional residual volumes, and a ventilation-perfusion mismatch [19]. As a consequence, tachypnea, hypercapnia, and hypoxia occur. IAH-induced atelectasis has been demonstrated to increase the rate of pulmonary infections [1]. Renal dysfunction is a significant complication in patients with ACS, resulting from a multifactorial pathophysiological process. Direct mechanical pressure on the kidneys and renal vasculature reduces renal blood flow and the glomerular filtration rate, while also interfering with venous drainage. This triggers the activation of the renin-angiotensin-aldosterone system, which increases systemic vascular resistance and further impairs cardiac output [20]. Renal dysfunction in ACS can manifest as oliguria, potentially progressing to anuria. In detail, oliguria can occur at an IAP of 15 mmHg, while anuria of 30 mmHg [21]. Even though the heart, lungs, and kidneys are the organs most affected by IAH, almost every other organ system, such as the gut, liver, and central nervous system, is impacted. The increased IAP may reduce mesenteric blood flow, decrease mucosal vascularization, and may compress thin-walled mesenteric veins, resulting in venous hypertension and intestinal edema. Visceral swelling contributes to an increase in IAP, perpetuating a vicious cycle that leads to worsening malperfusion bowel ischemia, decreased intramucosal pH, feeding intolerance, and systemic metabolic acidosis [22].

Reduced hepatic arterial and portal venous flow impairs hepatic cell function and liver perfusion, leading to decreased lactate clearance and altered mitochondrial function [1]. IAH results in elevation of intracranial pressure by decreased lumbar and cerebral venous blood flow and increased cerebral arterial blood flow secondary to increased $PaCO2$ [23]. Lastly, the direct compression of the inferior vena cava reduces venous return, resulting in peripheral edema and a higher risk of deep venous thrombosis [24].

18.3 Clinical Diagnosis

ACS should always be suspected in patients with tensely distended abdomen and organ dysfunction or failure, often represented by hypotension, oliguria/anuria, respiratory failure, and alteration of the sensorium. The abdomen distention may be missed in overweight or pregnant patients, or patients with burns to the abdominal wall. However, most patients with ACS are critically ill and recovered inside and outside the intensive care units, different pathological conditions may co-exist, so other reasons, such as sepsis and acute respiratory distress syndrome, may act as confounding factors [25, 26]. As mentioned above, IAP may be directly measured by positioning an intraperitoneal catheter connected to an external pressure transducer. Since this method is invasive, in clinical practice, the indirect measurement through urinary bladder pressure with the patient in the supine position is preferred. Unfortunately, this technique is not always reliable or feasible, such as in the presence of pelvic hematomas and/or fractures, neurological bladder, pelvic packing, or bladder injuries. Therefore, in such clinical conditions, the imaging role is more relevant in raising the suspicion of IAH/ACS as well as in patients outside the ICUs, in whom the measurement of bladder pressure is not usually performed.

18.4 CT Findings of IAH and ACS

In patients with IAH/ACS imaging is useful to assess the underlying cause and guide the most appropriate treatment, surgical and/or medical, since the diagnosis is clinical. However, the measurement of IAP is not routinely performed in ICUs and especially outside the ICUs, where critical conditions leading to IAH or ACS may also occur and be underestimated. In these latter situations the role of imaging becomes very important, because, through suggestive imaging findings, the suspicion of IAH or ACS in critically ill patients should be raised and will be confirmed or not by measuring the IAP. Identifying patients with IAH or ACS at earlier stages could potentially improve their outcomes [27].

Abdominal CT examination should be conducted with the injection of an intravenous contrast agent followed by a multiphasic acquisition; arterial and portal-venous phases are mandatory, while the late phase is optional. At least one CT scan should include the chest, usually the venous phase, but if specific chest diseases are present or suspicious, a pulmonary and/or arterial chest acquisition should be considered [28–35]. This CT protocol allows a comprehensive evaluation of vessels, abdominal parenchyma, and bowel [36–38].

The CT features suggestive of IAH/ACS are several, but their specificity is low and their diagnostic performance remains unclear since only very few retrospective and prospective studies have been conducted on small populations [2, 4, 39–42]. However, the coexistence of several CT signs in critically ill patients may increase the specificity for diagnosing or ruling out IAH/ACS [2].

18.4.1 Round Belly Sign

On axial CT scan the morphology of the normal abdomen is oval, in case of distention it becomes round. So, round belly sign (RBS) refers to the round morphology of a tense and distended abdomen of patients with IAH/ACS on an axial CT scan. To objectify the degree of distention it is necessary to calculate the abdomen ratio (AR): the ratio of anteroposterior to transverse abdomen diameter measured on axial CT scan at the level where the left renal vein crosses the aorta, excluding the subcutaneous fat (Fig. 18.1) [39]. The reported normal value of AR is ≤ 0.80, however, there is no consensus about the diagnostic accuracy of the RBS in the IAH/ACS as well as the AR value to differentiate patients with and without IAH/ACS. According to Pickhardt et al., who first described this imaging sign, the AR cutoff value of 0.80 may differentiate patients with

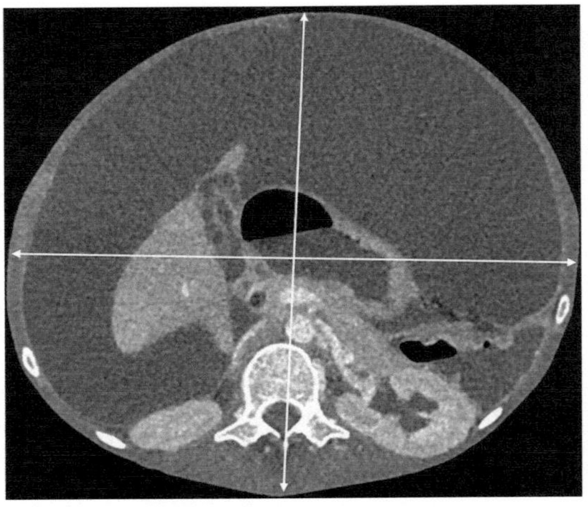

Fig. 18.1 Contrast-enhanced CT exam, axial plane, venous phase. Positive round belly sign [ratio of antero-posterior to transverse abdomen diameter (AR) >0.8] in a patient with massive neoplastic ascites and proven ACS. Anteroposterior abdomen diameter = 25.7 cm; Transverse abdomen diameter = 30 cm; AR = 0.86

and without ACS with a sensitivity of 100% and a specificity of 94% [39]. These results were not confirmed by Bouveresse et al., who achieved a sensitivity of 24% and specificity of 100% with an AR threshold >0.8, and a sensitivity of 95% and specificity of 50% with an AR threshold >0.65 to discriminate high-risk critically patients with and without IAH [2]. On the other hand, Patel et al. observed an AR of less than 0.7 in 20 of 21 patients with ACS, and Bo-Kyung et al. did not notice a significant difference in AR between ACS patients and control subjects (0.83 ± 0.10 vs 0.81 ± 0.05) [43, 44]. Furthermore, the RBS was not demonstrated as an independent predictor of ACS in critically ill patients with IAH [40]. Therefore, since any severe abdominal disease may cause significant abdominal distention and the pathogenesis of IAH and ACS involves the acute pathologic elevation of the IAP, the RBS cannot be considered a specific imaging finding of these conditions. It should only raise suspicion in clinicians when seen in an appropriate clinical setting, and additional imaging findings should be sought [2]. For instance, in patients with acute pancreatitis, the presence of RBS combined with moderate to severe ascites and more than 50% pancreatic necrosis may indicate the presence of IAH (Fig. 18.2) [41].

18.4.2 Peritoneal-to-Abdominal Height Ratio

In addition to AR, Bouveresse et al. suggested measuring the peritoneal-to-abdominal height ratio (PAR) along the midline and excluding subcutaneous fat. PAR is calculated as the ratio of antero-posterior peritoneal compartment diameter (distance from the linea alba to the posterior aspect of the duodenum) and antero-posterior abdomen diameter (distance from the linea alba to the posterior fascia (Fig. 18.3) [2]. The Authors observed that a PAR threshold of ≥0.52 may discriminate high-risk critical patients with and without IAH with a sensitivity of 57% and a specificity of 85% (AUC: 0.826), making reliable the diagnosis of IAH with a PPV of 80% [2]. Furthermore, the authors demonstrated that among several evaluated CT signs, both the increase of the PAR and of the AR are significantly associated with the presence of IAH [2].

18.4.3 Bowel Wall Thickness Enhancement

The wall thickness of the small and/or large bowel on post-contrast CT scans is defined as a thickness greater than 3 and 5 mm for the small and large bowel, respectively. This CT sign is potentially linked to IAH (Fig. 18.4) and could be caused by venous congestion and related ischemia [18, 43]. Al-Bahrani et al. conducted a multivariate regression analysis based on CT findings suspicious of ACS, such as RBS, narrowing of

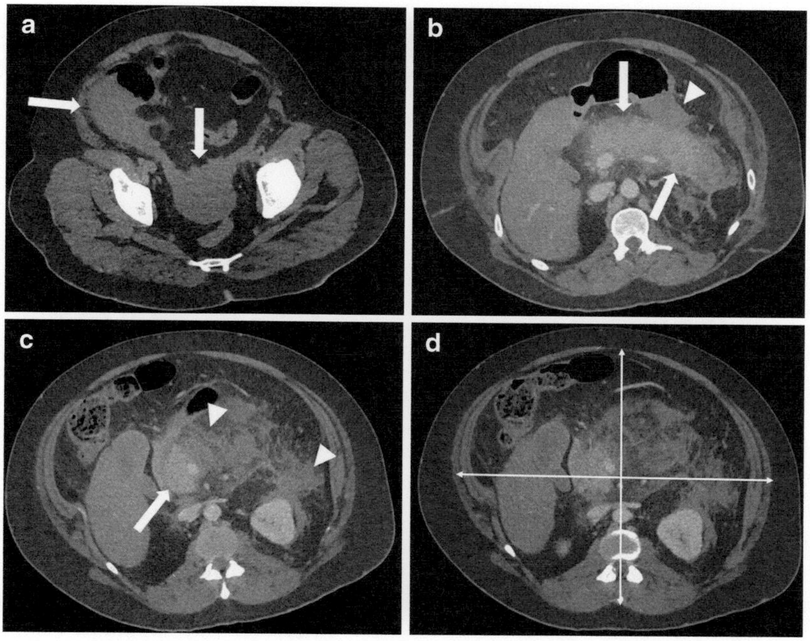

Fig. 18.2 Male patient, 41 years old, with acute necrotizing and hemorrhagic pancreatitis. (**a**) Pre-contrast CT scan, axial plane. Moderate amount of hemoperitoneum in the pelvis and right iliac fossa (white arrows). (**b** and **c**) Post-contrast CT scan, venous phase, axial plane. Pancreas appears markedly swollen with heterogeneous enhancement (white arrows). This is accompanied by peripancreatic and perigastric fluid accumulation, which seems to be forming acute necrotic collections (arrowheads). (**d**) Post-contrast CT scan, venous phase, axial plane. Positive round belly sign with an AR of 0.86 (Anteroposterior abdomen diameter = 28.4 cm; Transverse abdomen diameter = 33 cm)

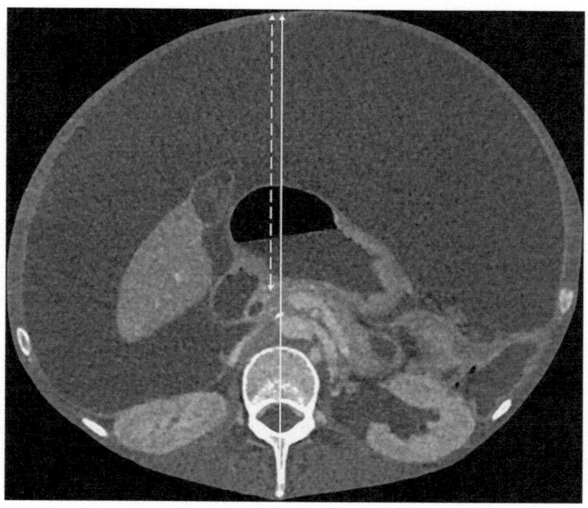

Fig. 18.3 Contrast-enhanced CT exam, axial plane, venous phase. Peritoneal-to-abdominal height ratio [ratio of anteroposterior peritoneal compartment diameter and anteroposterior abdomen diameter (PAR), n.v. <0.52] in the same patient of Fig. 18.1 with massive neoplastic ascites and proven ACS. Anteroposterior peritoneal compartment diameter (dashed arrow) = 15.3 cm; anteroposterior abdomen diameter (continuous arrow) = 25.6 cm; PAR = 0.60

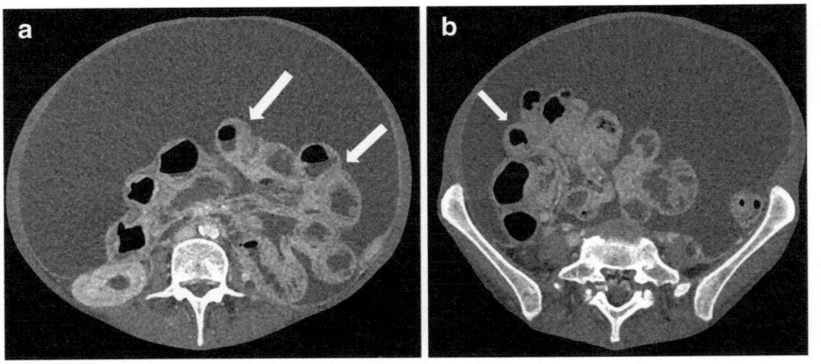

Fig. 18.4 Contrast-enhanced CT exam, axial plane, venous phase. (**a** and **b**) Two different slices of the same patients with massive ascites and positive round belly signs. The small bowel wall was thickened and with increased enhancement (white arrows)

upper intra-hepatic inferior vena cava, direct renal compression or displacement, contour deformity of solid abdominal viscera, and elevation of the diaphragm. Among these features, the bowel wall thickening was the only independent predictor of ACS with a sensitivity of 44.4% and specificity of 84.6% [40].

On a pre-contrast CT scan the bowel wall appears thickened and hyperdense. The wall enhancement may be stratified in the early stage of IAH, while it becomes progressively inhomogeneous and decreases in later stages. If the underlying condition is not resolved, the congestion can lead to ischemia and eventually infarction of the intestinal wall [35, 38, 45, 46].

18.4.4 Elevation of the Diaphragm

Elevation of the diaphragm, one of the most common CT findings in patients with clinically proven ACS, is defined as dome of the diaphragm reaching the tenth thoracic vertebral body or above (Fig. 18.5) [15].

18.4.5 Narrowing of Inferior Vena Cava

A slit-like appearance (<3 mm) of the inferior vena cava on two or three contiguous CT slices as well as flattened renal veins (Fig. 18.6) may be observed in patients with IAH or ACS. However, this sign is also present in case of hypovolemic shock, associated with increased bowel enhancement. Therefore, the clinical setting should be considered for differential diagnosis [2, 43, 44].

18.4.6 Mosaic Liver Perfusion Sign

Hepatic venous congestion hinders liver perfusion, therefore heterogeneous contrast enhancement of the liver parenchyma in the arterial and portal venous phases may be observed due to the presence of hypodense areas (mosaic liver perfusion sign) [2]. In the late CT phase, the parenchymal enhancement generally becomes more uniform [2].

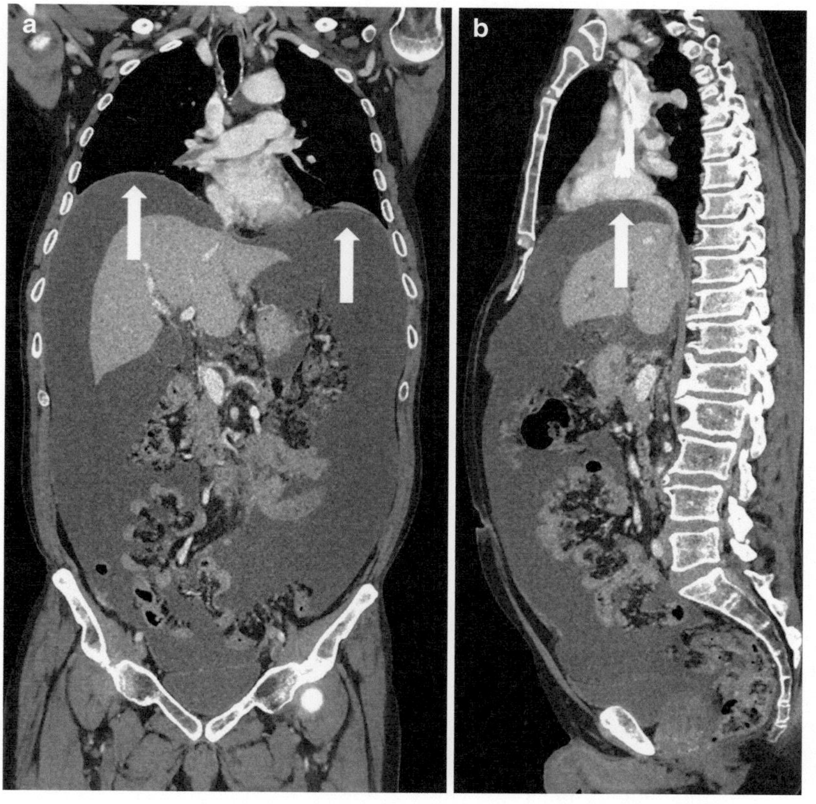

Fig. 18.5 Contrast-enhanced CT exam, coronal (**a**) and sagittal (**b**) MPR reconstruction. Elevation of the diaphragm (white arrows), with the dome reaching the level of the eighth thoracic vertebral body, in a patient with peritoneal carcinomatosis and massive neoplastic ascites

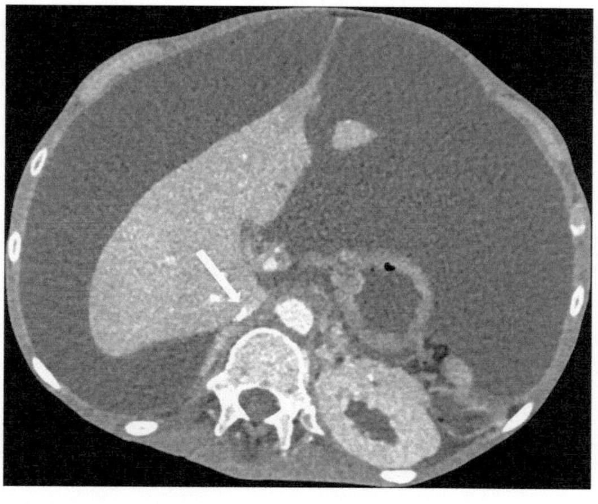

Fig. 18.6 Contrast-enhanced CT exam, axial plane, venous phase. Stretched and collapsed inferior cava vein (white arrow) in a patient with a large amount of ascites and a round shape of the abdomen on the axial plane

18.4.7 Deformation of Solid Abdominal Viscera and Abdominal Wall Hernias

The increase of IAP leads to the compression or displacement of solid abdominal organs, such as the kidneys, manifesting as contour deformities. Additionally, abdominal wall hernias, bilateral inguinal herniation, and pelvic floor descent in a supine position may occur in the case of IAH [39] (Fig. 18.7).

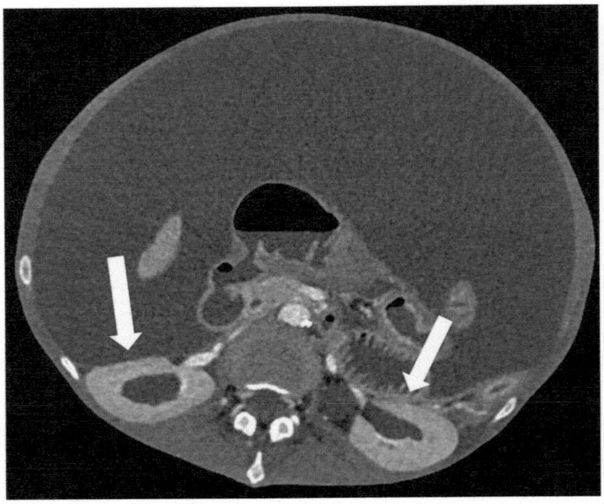

Fig. 18.7 Contrast-enhanced CT exam, axial plane, venous phase. Posterior displacement and contour deformation of the kidneys in a patient with massive ascites

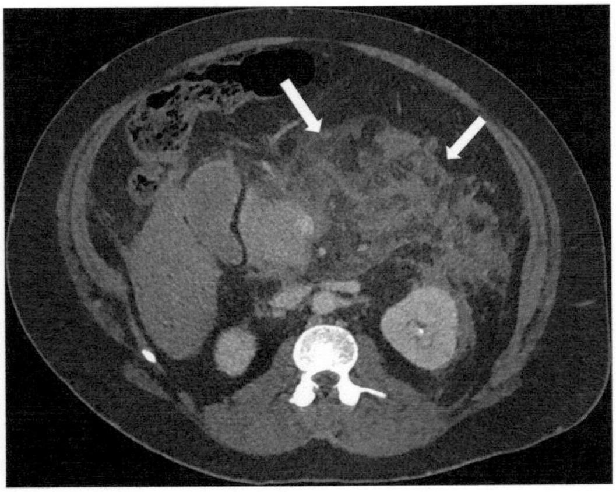

Fig. 18.8 Contrast-enhanced CT exam, axial plane, venous phase. Mesenteric fat stranding (white arrows) in the same patient of Fig. 18.2 with acute necrotizing and hemorrhagic pancreatitis

18.4.8 Mesenteric Fat Stranding

The mesenteric fat stranding is defined as an increased attenuation of mesenteric fat compared to retroperitoneal fat (Fig. 18.8). It can be ill-defined, reticular, or linear [2]. This CT finding is common and not specific to IAH or ACS because it is related to inflammation, edema, fibrosis, or hemorrhage.

Table 18.1 Reports the key points of the ACS, including both pathophysiology and CT findings.

Table 18.1 Key points of abdominal compartment syndrome

Abdominal compartment syndrome (ACS)		
Definition	A persistent intra-abdominal pressure (IAP) greater than 20 mmHg associated with new organ dysfunction and/or organ failure	
Etiology	Acute increased intra-abdominal volume and/or decreased abdominal wall compliance	
		Pathophysiology
Main primary causes	*Traumatic injuries* High-grade parenchymal injuries Massive hemoperitoneum Over-packing	Large amount of blood in abdominal spaces and related inflammatory reaction Excessive increase of intra-abdominal pressure
	Abdominal surgery Liver transplantation	Mismatch donor-recipient Edema of the transplanted liver due to ischemia-reperfusion injury
	Endovascular repair of ruptured abdominal aortic aneurysm	Large amount of blood in abdominal spaces and related inflammatory reaction Edema of the abdominal organs and bowel due to ischemia-reperfusion injury
	Toxic megacolon	Colonic overdistension resulting in excessive increase of intra-abdominal pressure
	Massive ascites in patient with decompensated hepatopathy	Acute excessive increase of intra-abdominal pressure
	Pancreatitis	Excessive increase of intra-abdominal pressure due to large amount of pancreatic ascites and bulky intra-abdominal collection Large amount of blood in abdominal spaces and related inflammatory reaction in case of hemorrhagic pancreatitis
Main secondary causes	*Massive fluid resuscitation* (septic shock, burns) *Massive blood transfusion in case of shock*	Acute excessive increase of intra-abdominal pressure due to large amount of fluid in the peritoneal spaces Bowel wall edema due to intestinal ischemia/reperfusion damage
CT Findings	**Round belly sign**	Ratio of anteroposterior to transverse (AP/T) abdomen diameter at the level where the left renal vein crosses the aorta, excluding the subcutaneous fat (normal value ≦0.80)
	Peritoneal-to-abdominal height ratio	Ratio of anteroposterior peritoneal compartment diameter and anteroposterior abdomen diameter, excluding subcutaneous fat (normal value ≦0.52)
	Bowel wall thickness enhancement	Increased wall thickness of small or large bowel (>3 mm)
	Mosaic liver perfusion sign	Heterogeneous liver parenchyma enhancement with hypodense areas on portal phase
	Narrowing of inferior vena cava	Inferior vena cava width less than 3 mm
	Deformation of solid abdominal viscera	Compression or displacement of solid abdominal viscera
	Elevation of the diaphragm	Dome of the diaphragm at or above the 10th thoracic vertebral body
	Mesenteric fat stranding	Increased CT density of mesenteric fat compared to that of retroperitoneal fat

18.5 Conclusions

Since the diagnosis of ACS is mainly clinical, imaging serves to identify and highlight potential causes and suggestive findings of IAH or ACS. This is particularly crucial for patients managed outside or inside sub-intensive care units. Radiologists therefore need a deep understanding of the disease's pathophysiology and imaging findings. While none of the CT findings are specific to IAH or ACS, their presence in critically ill patients can raise suspicion and serve as non-invasive red flags. This should prompt clinicians to measure IAP invasively to confirm the diagnosis. Imaging also plays a critical role when direct IAP measurement is not feasible or unreliable. However, CT should be viewed as an adjunctive tool in the recognition of patients with IAH/ACS rather than a substitute for direct IAP measurement in high-risk patients.

References

1. Lewis M, Benjamin ER, Demetriades D. Intra-abdominal hypertension and abdominal compartment syndrome. Curr Probl Surg. 2021;58(11):100971. https://doi.org/10.1016/j.cpsurg.2021.100971.
2. Bouveresse S, Piton G, Badet N, Besch G, Pili-Floury S, Delabrousse E. Abdominal compartment syndrome and intra-abdominal hypertension in critically ill patients: diagnostic value of computed tomography. Eur Radiol. 2019;29(7):3839–46. https://doi.org/10.1007/s00330-018-5994-x.
3. Pereira BM. Abdominal compartment syndrome and intra-abdominal hypertension. Curr Opin Crit Care. 2019;25(6):688–96. https://doi.org/10.1097/MCC.0000000000000665.
4. Caruso M, Rinaldo C, Iacobellis F, et al. Abdominal compartment syndrome: what radiologist needs to know. Radiol Med. 2023;128(12):1447–59. https://doi.org/10.1007/s11547-023-01724-4.
5. Brillantino A, Andreano M, Lanza M, et al. Advantages of damage control strategy with abdominal negative pressure and instillation in patients with diffuse peritonitis from perforated diverticular disease. Surg Innov. 2019;26(6):656–61. https://doi.org/10.1177/1553350619857561.
6. Brillantino A, Iacobellis F, Renzi A, et al. Diagnostic value of arterial blood gas lactate concentration in the different forms of mesenteric ischemia. Eur J Trauma Emerg Surg. 2018;44(2):265–72. https://doi.org/10.1007/s00068-017-0805-7.
7. Iacobellis F, Laccetti E, Tamburrini S, et al. Role of multidetector computed tomography in the assessment of pancreatic injuries after blunt trauma: a multicenter experience. Gland Surg. 2019;8(2):184–96. https://doi.org/10.21037/gs.2019.02.02.
8. Brillantino A, Iacobellis F, Festa P, et al. Non-operative management of blunt liver trauma: safety, efficacy and complications of a standardized treatment protocol. Bull Emerg Trauma. 2019;7(1):49–54. https://doi.org/10.29252/beat-070107.
9. Brillantino A, Iacobellis F, Robustelli U, et al. Non operative management of blunt splenic trauma: a prospective evaluation of a standardized treatment protocol. Eur J Trauma Emerg Surg. 2016;42(5):593–8. https://doi.org/10.1007/s00068-015-0575-z.
10. Iacobellis F, Di Serafino M, Brillantino A, et al. Role of MRI in early follow-up of patients with solid organ injuries: how and why we do it? Radiol Med. 2021;126(10):1328–34. https://doi.org/10.1007/s11547-021-01394-0.
11. Iacobellis F, Scaglione M, Brillantino A, et al. The additional value of the arterial phase in the CT assessment of liver vascular injuries after high-energy blunt trauma. Emerg Radiol. 2019;26(6):647–54. https://doi.org/10.1007/s10140-019-01714-y.
12. Ertel W, Oberholzer A, Platz A, Stocker R, Trentz O. Incidence and clinical pattern of the abdominal compartment syndrome after "damage-control" laparotomy in 311 patients with severe abdominal and/or pelvic trauma. Crit Care Med. 2000;28(6):1747–53. https://doi.org/10.1097/00003246-200006000-00008.
13. Biancofiore G, Bindi ML, Romanelli AM, et al. Intra-abdominal pressure monitoring in liver transplant recipients: a prospective study. Intensive Care Med. 2003;29(1):30–6. https://doi.org/10.1007/s00134-002-1552-7.
14. Leppäniemi A, Kemppainen E. Recent advances in the surgical management of necrotizing pancreatitis. Curr Opin Crit Care. 2005;11(4):349–52. https://doi.org/10.1097/01.ccx.0000166398.50517.fb.
15. Golfieri R, Giampalma E, Fusco F, et al. Orthotopic liver transplantation (OLT): contribution of imaging and interventional radiology in preparing the transplantation and managing complications. Part 2: post-OLT complications and their treatment. Radiol Med. 2005;110(5–6):433–83.
16. De Filippo M, Puglisi S, D'Amuri F, et al. CT-guided percutaneous drainage of abdominopelvic collections: a pictorial essay. Radiol Med. 2021;126(12):1561–70. https://doi.org/10.1007/s11547-021-01406-z.
17. Di Serafino M, Viscardi D, Iacobellis F, et al. Computed tomography imaging of septic shock. Beyond the cause: the "CT hypoperfusion complex". A pictorial essay. Insights Imaging. 2021;12(1) Published 2021 Jun 5:70. https://doi.org/10.1186/s13244-021-01006-5.
18. Di Grezia G, Gatta G, Rella R, et al. MDCT in acute ischaemic left colitis: a pictorial essay. Radiol Med. 2019;124(2):103–8. https://doi.org/10.1007/s11547-018-0947-7.

19. Cullen DJ, Coyle JP, Teplick R, Long MC. Cardiovascular, pulmonary, and renal effects of massively increased intra-abdominal pressure in critically ill patients. Crit Care Med. 1989;17(2):118–21. https://doi.org/10.1097/00003246-198902000-00002.
20. Mohmand H, Goldfarb S. Renal dysfunction associated with intra-abdominal hypertension and the abdominal compartment syndrome. J Am Soc Nephrol. 2011;22(4):615–21. https://doi.org/10.1681/ASN.2010121222.
21. Richards WO, Scovill W, Shin B, Reed W. Acute renal failure associated with increased intra-abdominal pressure. Ann Surg. 1983;197(2):183–7. https://doi.org/10.1097/00000658-198302000-00010.
22. Diebel LN, Dulchavsky SA, Wilson RF. Effect of increased intra-abdominal pressure on mesenteric arterial and intestinal mucosal blood flow. J Trauma. 1992;33(1):45–9. https://doi.org/10.1097/00005373-199207000-00010.
23. Joseph DK, Dutton RP, Aarabi B, Scalea TM. Decompressive laparotomy to treat intractable intracranial hypertension after traumatic brain injury. J Trauma. 2004;57(4):687–95. https://doi.org/10.1097/01.ta.0000140645.84897.f2.
24. Cheatham ML, Malbrain ML. Cardiovascular implications of abdominal compartment syndrome. Acta Clin Belg. 2007;62(Suppl 1):98–112. https://doi.org/10.1179/acb.2007.62.s1.013.
25. Sugrue M, Bauman A, Jones F, et al. Clinical examination is an inaccurate predictor of intraabdominal pressure. World J Surg. 2002;26(12):1428–31. https://doi.org/10.1007/s00268-002-6411-8.
26. Kirkpatrick AW, Brenneman FD, McLean RF, Rapanos T, Boulanger BR. Is clinical examination an accurate indicator of raised intra-abdominal pressure in critically injured patients? Can J Surg. 2000;43(3):207–11.
27. Malbrain ML, Deeren D, De Potter TJ. Intra-abdominal hypertension in the critically ill: it is time to pay attention. Curr Opin Crit Care. 2005;11(2):156–71. https://doi.org/10.1097/01.ccx.0000155355.86241.1b.
28. Iacobellis F, Brillantino A, Di Serafino M, et al. Economic and clinical benefits of immediate total-body CT in the diagnostic approach to polytraumatized patients: a descriptive analysis through a literature review. Radiol Med. 2022;127(6):637–44. https://doi.org/10.1007/s11547-022-01495-4.
29. Mulas V, Catalano L, Geatti V, et al. Major trauma with only dynamic criteria: is the routine use of whole-body CT as a first level examination justified? Radiol Med. 2022;127(1):65–71. https://doi.org/10.1007/s11547-021-01430-z.
30. Bottari A, Silipigni S, Carerj ML, et al. Dual-source dual-energy CT in the evaluation of hepatic fractional extracellular space in cirrhosis. Radiol Med. 2020;125(1):7–14. https://doi.org/10.1007/s11547-019-01089-7.
31. Agostini A, Borgheresi A, Mari A, et al. Dual-energy CT: theoretical principles and clinical applications. Radiol Med. 2019;124(12):1281–95. https://doi.org/10.1007/s11547-019-01107-8.
32. Bi Y, Zhu X, Yu Z, Wu G, Han X, Ren J. Interventional radiology protocol for treatment of esophagogastric anastomotic leakage. Radiol Med. 2019;124(12):1253–61. https://doi.org/10.1007/s11547-019-01074-0.
33. Granata V, Fusco R, Cozzi D, et al. Structured reporting of computed tomography in the polytrauma patient assessment: a Delphi consensus proposal. Radiol Med. 2023;128(2):222–33. https://doi.org/10.1007/s11547-023-01596-8.
34. Scaglione M, Masala S, Iacobellis F, et al. Imaging in non-traumatic emergencies. Tomography. 2023;9(3):1133–6. Published 2023 Jun 12. https://doi.org/10.3390/tomography9030093.
35. Berritto D, Iacobellis F, Mazzei MA, et al. MDCT in ischaemic colitis: how to define the aetiology and acute, subacute and chronic phase of damage in the emergency setting. Br J Radiol. 2016;89(1061):20150821. https://doi.org/10.1259/bjr.20150821.
36. Iacobellis F, Ierardi AM, Mazzei MA, et al. Dual-phase CT for the assessment of acute vascular injuries in high-energy blunt trauma: the imaging findings and management implications. Br J Radiol. 2016;89(1061):20150952. https://doi.org/10.1259/bjr.20150952.
37. Iacobellis F, Abu-Omar A, Crivelli P, et al. Current standards for and clinical impact of emergency radiology in major trauma. Int J Environ Res Public Health. 2022;19(1):539. Published 2022 Jan 4. https://doi.org/10.3390/ijerph19010539.
38. Iacobellis F, Narese D, Berritto D, et al. Large bowel ischemia/infarction: how to recognize it and make differential diagnosis? A review. Diagnostics (Basel). 2021;11(6):998. Published 2021 May 30. https://doi.org/10.3390/diagnostics11060998.
39. Pickhardt PJ, Shimony JS, Heiken JP, Buchman TG, Fisher AJ. The abdominal compartment syndrome: CT findings. AJR Am J Roentgenol. 1999;173(3):575–9. https://doi.org/10.2214/ajr.173.3.10470882.
40. Al-Bahrani AZ, Abid GH, Sahgal E, O'shea S, Lee S, Ammori BJ. A prospective evaluation of CT features predictive of intra-abdominal hypertension and abdominal compartment syndrome in critically ill surgical patients. Clin Radiol. 2007;62(7):676–82. https://doi.org/10.1016/j.crad.2006.11.006.
41. Verma S, Rana SS, Kang M, Gorsi U, Gupta R. Computed tomography features predictive of intra-abdominal hypertension in acute necrotizing pancreatitis: a prospective study. Indian J Gastroenterol. 2021;40(3):326–32. https://doi.org/10.1007/s12664-021-01149-9.
42. Epelman M, Soudack M, Engel A, Halberthal M, Beck R. Abdominal compartment syndrome in children: CT findings. Pediatr Radiol. 2002;32(5):319–22. https://doi.org/10.1007/s00247-001-0569-3.

43. Patel A, Lall CG, Jennings SG, Sandrasegaran K. Abdominal compartment syndrome. AJR Am J Roentgenol. 2007;189(5):1037–43. https://doi.org/10.2214/AJR.07.2092.
44. Je BK, Kim HK, Horn PS. Abdominal compartment syndrome in children: clinical and imaging features. AJR Am J Roentgenol. 2019;212(3):655–64. https://doi.org/10.2214/AJR.18.20119.
45. Iacobellis F, Berritto D, Fleischmann D, et al. CT findings in acute, subacute, and chronic ischemic colitis: suggestions for diagnosis. Biomed Res Int. 2014;2014:895248. https://doi.org/10.1155/2014/895248.
46. Reginelli A, Iacobellis F, Berritto D, et al. Mesenteric ischemia: the importance of differential diagnosis for the surgeon. BMC Surg. 2013;13 Suppl 2(Suppl 2):S51. https://doi.org/10.1186/1471-2482-13-S2-S51.

Part IV

Liver and Biliary System

19 Arterial, Portal, Venous Causes of Liver Emergencies

Gianluca Ponticiello, Gaspare Oliva,
Costanza Camillo, Roberto Ronza,
Vittorio Sabatino, and Marco Di Serafino

19.1 Introduction

The liver is a highly vascular organ with unique vascular anatomy: the hepatic artery (HA) and portal vein (PV) provide the main inflow, while the hepatic veins (HV) represent the primary outflow tract. The liver's complex vascular supply and high metabolic activity make it particularly susceptible to circulatory disturbances. The severity and nature of hepatic injury depend on the blood vessels involved and the extent to which the injury is related to passive congestion or reduced perfusion. Vascular disorders of the liver, although affecting less than 5 out of 10.000 patients, encompass a number of rare conditions that represent a significant health problem globally in the field of liver diseases. Furthermore, it is particularly important to note that these patients are usually young and would otherwise have a normal life expectancy, which can be significantly shortened if not properly managed. Awareness of imaging findings in the appropriate clinical context is crucial for prompt and accurate diagnosis, as delays can lead to severe consequences with significant morbidity and mortality. In this chapter, we will discuss the fundamental role of CT angiography in the early detection of various acute non-traumatic vascular emergencies of the liver, including hepatic infarction (HA occlusion or stenosis), HA pseudoaneurysm (PSA), Budd-Chiari syndrome and acute PV thrombosis (non-cirrhotic, non-malignant).

19.2 Hepatic Infarction

Hepatic infarction (HI) is rare due to the liver's dual blood supply from the hepatic artery (HA) and the portal vein (PV). The presence of numerous anastomotic vessels and collateral branches further contributes to the rarity of HI. Despite the PV being the main feeding vessel of the liver, PV occlusion rarely causes HI. HI most commonly occurs in patients with HA occlusion/stenosis or PV thrombosis accompanied by HA occlusion [1]. Given that the clinical manifestations and laboratory abnormalities related to vascular injuries are non-specific, early radiological examination plays a crucial role in making an early diagnosis and establishing the best treatment options [2]. Demonstrating the rarity of liver infarction, the main cause is liver transplantation; hepatic artery occlusion (HAO) is a critical complication of liver allograft dysfunction and failure after liver transplantation (LT), occurring in approximately 4–12% of cases. Usually an early

G. Ponticiello (✉) · G. Oliva · C. Camillo · R. Ronza
V. Sabatino · M. Di Serafino
Department of General and Emergency Radiology, "Antonio Cardarelli" Hospital, Naples, Italy
e-mail: gianluca.ponticiello@aocardarelli.it; gaspare.oliva@aocardarelli.it; costanza.camillo@aocardarelli.it; roberto.ronza@aocardarelli.it; vittorio.sabatino@aocardarelli.it; marco.diserafino@aocardarelli.it

L. Romano et al. (eds.), *CT of Non-Traumatic Body Emergencies*,
https://doi.org/10.1007/978-3-031-84849-0_19

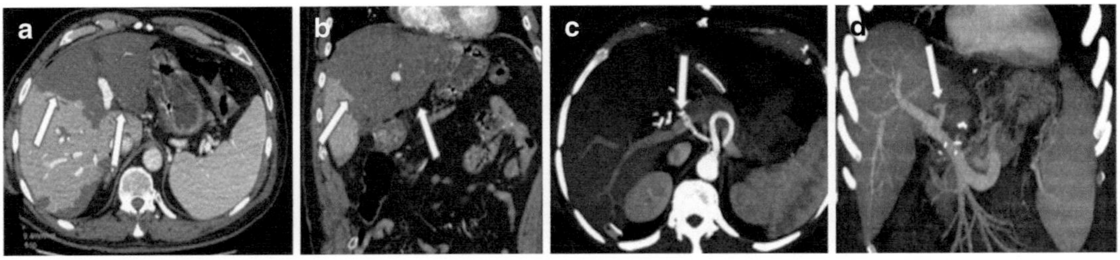

Fig. 19.1 39-year-old male; two days after the orthotopic liver transplantation the patient presented fever, chills, and right upper quadrant pain. (**a** and **b**) Axial and coronal MPR reconstruction showed a large infarcted area in left liver lobe (arrows); (**c**) MIP reconstructions depict the thrombus of the left hepatic artery (arrow) and also the absence of distal flow (**d**) MIP reconstructions venous phase shows thrombosed hepatic veins (arrow)

complication, it can still occur up to 4 months after transplantation [3]. CT angiography (CTA) can complement Doppler ultrasound (US), which has low specificity, and CTA has been considered a second-line tool in diagnosing HAO after LT [4]. When CDUS shows a vascular abnormality, the surgical anatomy is difficult to interpret, or the patient's clinical status is deteriorating, there is a need to complement the study with contrast-enhanced CT. On imaging, hepatic infarction (HI) typically appears on CT as a triangular or wedge-shaped hypoenhancing area with its base adjacent to the liver capsule and its apex pointing toward the liver hilum. Standard postcontrast portal venous phase images are very useful in showing the affected area. Multiplanar reconstructions (MPR) are essential to identify this typical triangular morphology of the infarcted area (Fig. 19.1a and b). In this phase, it is also possible to evaluate the presence of potential sequelae of infarction, such as bile duct necrosis and biloma formation, atrophy of the affected segments, and potentially superimposed infection, which could be suspected if gas is present on imaging. Additional arterial phase images are essential for detecting major arterial occlusion, especially in the patient group thought to benefit from endovascular treatment or revascularization surgery. Several studies have reported the diagnostic performance of CTA in diagnosing hepatic artery occlusion (HAO) with a three-dimensional reformatting technique, such as maximum intensity projection (MIP) or volume rendering [5, 6] (Fig. 19.1c and d).

CT angiography may demonstrate the occlusion of a hepatic artery, characterized by a non-enhancing filling defect; CTA has shown almost perfect sensitivity and specificity for detecting HAO. In modern medical practice, hepatic infarction is primarily attributed to iatrogenic causes; beyond liver transplantation, other iatrogenic causes include surgery, percutaneous embolization (Fig. 19.2), endovascular tumor treatments, and transjugular intrahepatic portosystemic shunt procedures.

HI is particularly a more common complication when treating metastases and hepatocellular carcinoma (HCC). Non-cirrhotic patients appear to have a higher risk of developing locoregional complications post-transarterial chemoembolization (TACE) than patients with liver cirrhosis. This may be due to the hypertrophied peribiliary plexus observed in cirrhotic patients. Predisposing factors for liver infarction include non-selective embolization, large tumor burden, and frequently repeated treatments [7, 8].

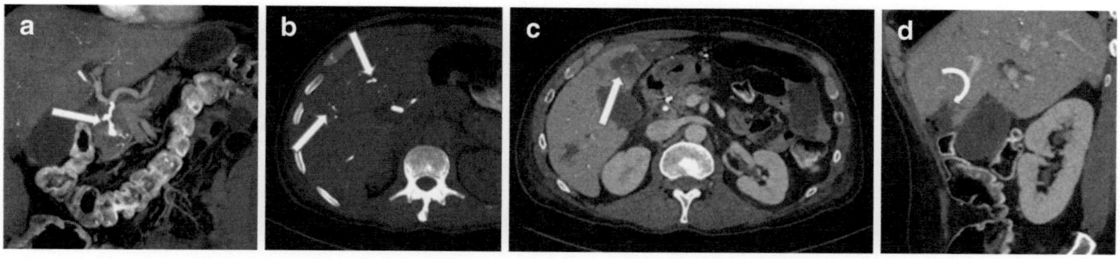

Fig. 19.2 A 65-year-old male patient with gastroduodenal artery pseudoaneurysm was treated with percutaneous embolization 2 days after the embolization, the patient again presented to ER with high fever, hypotension, and severe right upper quadrant pain. (**a**) coronal MPR reconstruction revealed the outcomes of gastroduodenal artery embolizationion (arrow). (**b**) Axial unenhanced CT revealed migration of embolizing material into the intrahepatic arterial branches (arrows) (**c** and **d**) portal venous phase CT revealed some subcapsular infarcted areas (arrow), the major at the level of the IV segment with gas bubbles within this parenchymal (arrowcurved). Axial and sagittal MPR reconstruction The imaging and clinical findings were considered to represent a superinfection of the infarcted parenchyma

19.3 Hepatic Arterial Pseudoaneurysms (PsA)

The initial descriptions of hepatic arterial pseudoaneurysms (PsA) were most often associated with hepatic trauma or infective and inflammatory etiologies; however, the increased use of percutaneous procedures and laparoscopic surgeries has broadened the etiological scope of this condition. Iatrogenic injuries (laparoscopic cholecystectomy, thoracocentesis, percutaneous liver biopsy, pancreaticoduodenectomy, and liver transplantation) currently account for approximately twice as many PsA cases as accidental trauma. Most PsAs are intrahepatic and present with hemobilia; xtrahepatic PsAs may present with abdominal pain, gastrointestinal hemorrhage, and hemobilia. Many PsAs of the hepatic arterial vasculature may be asymptomatic prior to rupture. Depending on the presentation and the time from the inciting factor, diagnosis can be challenging. Management of extrahepatic arterial PsA is not as well defined as for the intrahepatic type [9], with options including embolization, stent-grafting, surgical ligation, and resection. In such cases, contrast-enhanced CT scans may reveal small sacculations. PsAs follow the contrast enhancement pattern of the originating artery: both arterial and portal venous phase images should be acquired, as some pseudoaneurysms with a narrow neck may enhance only in the venous phase and may be easily missed on arterial phase images (Fig. 19.3).

Pseudoaneurysms have very fragile walls prone to rupture. Their contours are typically irregular, and they usually have a saccular shape. Hematomas surrounding the pseudoaneurysms are frequently observed at the time of diagnosis. As imaging findings may be extremely subtle or non-existent in the acute phase, follow-up imaging may be necessary in patients where clinical suspicion for HA pseudoaneurysm is high [10].

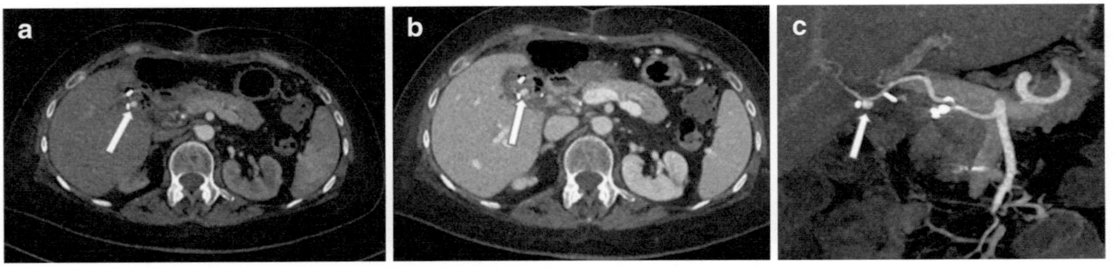

Fig. 19.3 Hepatic artery pseudoaneurysm. 45-year-old woman undergoing cholecystectomy surgery; about 3 days after the procedure, the patient experienced severe right upper quadrant pain, hematemesis, and hypotension. (**a** and **b**) Postcontrast arterial phase and portal phase CT image: presence of 5 mm vascular formation with the same postcontrastographic dynamics at the aorta (arrow): diagnosis of pesudoaneurysm (**c**) MIP reconstructions confirmed the presence of pseudoaneurysm (arrow) originating from the right hepatic artery

19.4 Budd-Chiari Syndrome

BCS is a rare vascular liver disorder characterized by the obstruction of hepatic venous outflow, ranging from small hepatic venules (type III) to the entry of the IVC into the right atrium (type I) [11]. BCS is categorized as either primary, accounting for 75% of cases and caused by thrombosis due to factors like hematologic disorders and thrombotic diathesis, or secondary, often resulting from malignancy (such as HCC, metastases, and cholangiocarcinoma) or compression by space-occupying lesions [12]. The pathophysiological effects include obstruction leading to sinusoidal congestion, ischemia, and ultimately hepatocellular necrosis, which can progress to centrilobular fibrosis, nodular regenerative hyperplasia, and cirrhosis. Early diagnosis is crucial for treatment planning and preventing complications, as peripheral perfusion defects, congestion, and progressive fibrosis seen in BCS may be potentially reversible with prompt endovascular treatments like direct or transjugular intrahepatic portosystemic shunt procedures (TIPS) [13]. Clinically, BCS can manifest in two distinct forms: acute (sudden hepatic outflow obstruction, rarely fulminant) subacute/chronic (long-term effects of hepatic outflow obstruction) and depends on the obstruction site and the affected liver regions [14]. Population studies indicate that ascites is the most common symptom, seen in 62–85% of patients, followed by hepatomegaly (67%), pain (61%), esophageal varices (58%), and gastrointestinal bleeding (5–21%). Approximately 10–15% of patients are asymptomatic, with only abnormal liver function tests and the presence of large hepatic venous collaterals [15]. However, to confirm clinical suspicion, radiological exams are necessary. Contrast-enhanced CT scans should be used to verify the diagnosis of BCS, evaluate the extent of thrombosis and the severity of the disease, plan radiological interventions, characterize hepatic nodules, rule out malignancies, and assess changes in liver morphology [16]. Numerous imaging features are associated with BCS, and their presence depends on the disease stage, making diagnosis challenging. In the acute phase of BCS, the liver is typically enlarged, with affected segments primarily located at the site of congestion and necrosis, appearing hypertrophied. CT scans reveal centrilobular or sinusoidal congestion, characterized by heterogeneous "mosaic" enhancement after contrast administration. This includes reduced peripheral enhancement with stronger central liver enhancement, known as the "flip-flop" or "zonal" enhancement pattern [17] (Fig. 19.4).

Notably, sinusoidal congestion is not hypertrophic but shows better venous enhancement. In BCS, imaging can identify direct and indirect signs, specifically [18]:

1. *Direct signs*: venous anomalies and the visualization of occluded, stagnant, or reversed venous flow in the hepatic veins (HV) or the inferior vena cava (IVC). Postprocessing tools are crucial, and HV visualization is improved

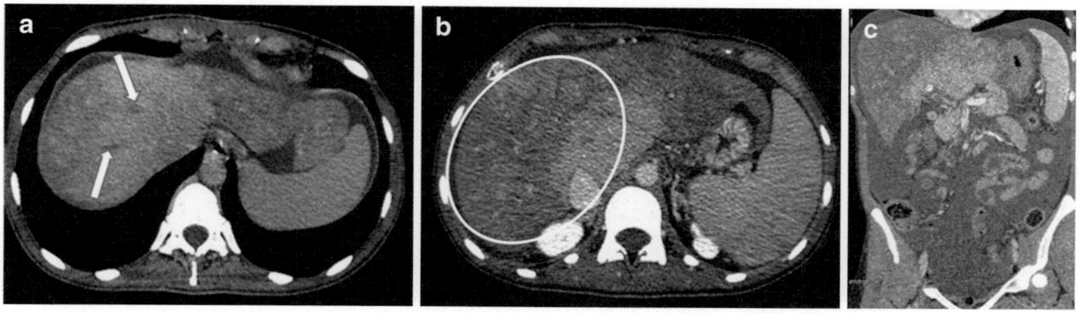

Fig. 19.4 Acute Budd-Chiari syndrome. A 29-year-old female with known polycythemia presented with acute and severe right upper quadrant pain, elevated liver enzymes and abdominal distension. (**a**) On axial portal venous phase CT shows thrombosed hepatic veins (arrows). (**b**) On axial portal venous phase CT images the liver exhibits decreased peripheral enhancement caused by portal and sinusoidal stasis, with stronger central liver enhancement, a pattern called "zonal enhancement" (white circles) (**c**) coronal MPR reconstruction demonstrates hepatomegaly, the typical postcontrastographic impregnation pattern, and diffuse ascites

on thick-section reconstructed images (MIP, maximum intensity projection).

2. *Indirect signs*: These are non-specific and represent the consequences of prolonged hepatic venous impairment, including liver parenchymal changes with fibrosis and atrophy of affected segments, and hypertrophy of unaffected areas (e.g., caudate lobe hypertrophy).

In the subacute phase, increasing fibrosis leads to portal hypertension, manifesting classically with esophageal varices, dilated superficial veins on the trunk, varicosities in the lower limbs, intra- or extrahepatic collaterals, and splenomegaly. Portal vein thrombosis can develop in subacute/chronic BCS due to underlying thrombophilia or stagnation of portal flow caused by outflow blockage. Signs of portal hypertension include the presence of various intra and extrahepatic collateral vessels (Fig. 19.5).

In the chronic phase, fibrosis will be the dominating aspect, with consequent alteration of liver morphology, atrophy of the affected segments, and hypertrophy of the spared ones [19].

Focal liver lesions have a reported prevalence of 60–80% in chronic BCS [20]. Characterization of liver nodules associated with BCS influences the patient's prognosis. The presence of multiple (>10) nodules, with a typical diameter of 0.5–4 cm, is usually indicative of regenerative nodules (RN).

The chronic parenchymal congestion with the formation of focal parenchymal nodules may eventually cause a classical morphological situation also called as the "nut meg liver".

RN originate from vascular disturbances and tend to increase in number and size, and change their imaging features over time. RN are usually hyperattenuating on pre-contrast CT, markedly and homogeneously hypervascular in arterial phase, and remain slightly hyperattenuating on portal venous and delayed phases [21] (Fig. 19.6).

Although benign lesions usually do not exhibit washout, many studies have reported washout in regenerative nodules in BCS, complicating the differential diagnosis with hepatocellular carcinoma (HCC). Traditional guidelines for non-invasive HCC diagnosis are not applicable in this context, and no pathognomonic pattern has been universally identified on CT. However, imaging features that favor HCC in BCS include solitary lesions, generally larger than regenerative nodules (over 30 mm), and hypoattenuating on pre-contrast CT [22]. Biopsy is recommended for patients with three or fewer nodules, nodules with a diameter of 3 cm or more, heterogeneity or washout in the venous phase, changes observed in two consecutive imaging studies, or increased alpha-fetoprotein levels [23] .

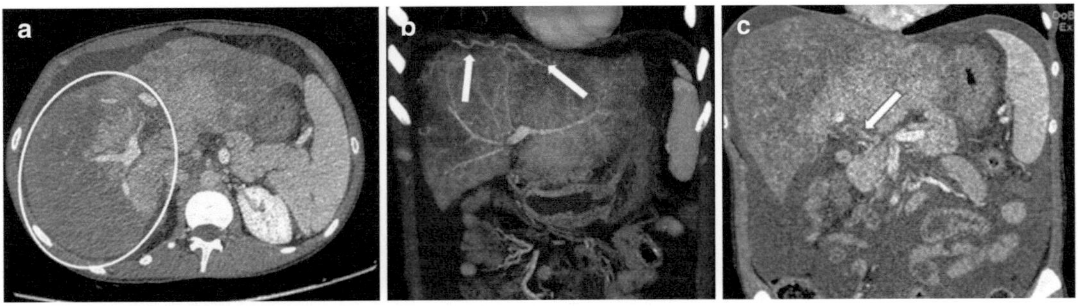

Fig. 19.5 (**a**) In subacute BCS morphological changes and fibrosis occur in the liver and regions of hypoperfused parenchyma can still be seen with the so-called "mosaic" enhancement pattern characterized by reticular enhancement (white circles); (**b**) the growing amount of fibrosis leads to portal hypertension with all its classical manifestations: esophageal varices, dilated superficial veins in trunk and varicosities in the lower limbs, intra- or extrahepatic collaterals (arrows), and splenomegaly. (**c**) Portal vein thrombosis can develop in subacute BCS as the result of underlying thrombophilia or stagnation of portal flow caused by an outflow block (arrow)

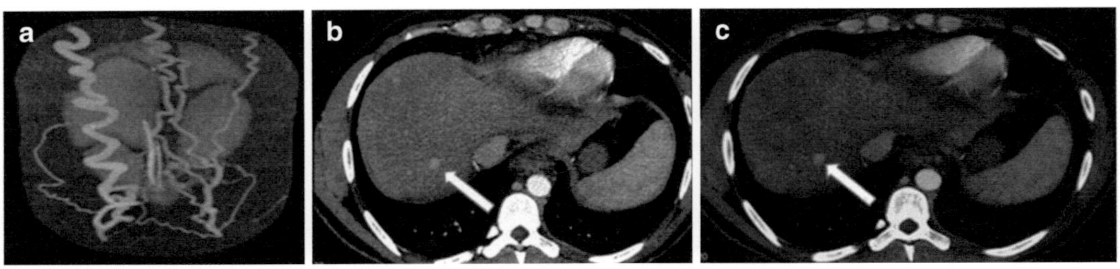

Fig. 19.6 (**a**) MIP coronal CT image: abdominal wall venous collaterals in a patient with chronic BCS. Regenerative nodules in the chronic phase of BCS exhibit typical dynamic behavior after intravenous contrast administration (**b** and **c**) homogeneously hypervascular on arterial and portal venous phases (arrow) and remain slightly hyperattenuating on delayed phases

19.5 Acute Portal Vein Thrombosis (Non-cirrhotic, Non-malignant)

The portal vein (PV) is the primary blood supplier to the liver parenchyma, formed by the convergence of the splenic vein (SV) and the superior mesenteric vein (SMV). It acts as a filter for blood coming from the digestive system, spleen, pancreas, and gallbladder. Portal vein thrombosis (PVT) is the most common cause of prehepatic portal hypertension and is defined as the partial or complete obstruction of the portal vein lumen. Anatomically, PVT can occur in the intrahepatic or extrahepatic portal venous tract and may involve the superior mesenteric vein, splenic vein, or both [24]. Factors contributing to PVT include the components of the Virchow triad (hypercoagulability, endothelial dysfunction, and stasis), with liver cirrhosis and neoplastic conditions, particularly hepatocellular carcinoma (HCC), being significant predisposing factors [25]. Clinically, PVT is categorized into acute and chronic forms, which represent different stages of the same disease, sharing similar causes but differing in management [26]. Determining whether the thrombosis is acute or chronic is crucial for prognosis and therapeutic decision-making, as portal hypertension and liver failure can develop without proper treatment. This chapter focuses on the primary emergency concerning the portal vein: acute PVT occurring in the absence of malignancy and cirrhosis. Acute portal vein thrombosis (PVT) is defined as the recent formation (less than 30 days) of a thrombus within the main portal vein or its branches.

Although it is an uncommon diagnosis, acute PVT can lead to significant morbidity, including bowel infarction, and even mortality. The clinical presentation can vary widely, from asymptomatic cases in partial PVT to sepsis and hypotension in patients with acute complete PVT. Generally, liver function remains normal even in extensive cases of PVT [27]. The severity of the presentation depends on the cause and extent of the thrombosis, with acute extension of the thrombus into the superior mesenteric vein being more likely to cause bowel ischemia and infarction [28]. Prompt diagnosis is crucial to prevent severe short-term complications such as bowel infarction, sepsis, and potential death. Several factors increase the risk of developing acute PVT: local factors (21–30% of cases) include cancer in any abdominal organ, extrinsic compression of the portal vein and/or its branches, postoperative status, and abdominal infections or inflammations such as pancreatitis or inflammatory bowel disease; systemic factors, including prothrombotic disorders, are present in up to 70% of patients with acute PVT [29]. Classification of PVT can be evaluated based on its:

- *Extension*: intrahepatic, extrahepatic, or both; monodistrictual or polidistrictual.
- *Degree*: partial or complete.
- *Onset*: acute or chronic.

The percentage of lumen occlusion is crucial in PVT classification as it impacts the treatment approach. PVT severity ranges from partial occlusion to cavernous transformation [30]. Differentiating between partial and complete PVT involves the following criteria: partial PVT is defined by the presence of a residual lumen in the vein with a peripheral circulating channel, whereas complete PVT is defined by a completely obstructed vein. The degree of occlusion correlates with the increasing severity of clinical manifestations. From a radiological perspective, PVT can be classified into four categories based on the involvement of:

1. Intrahepatic portal vein.
2. Extrahepatic portal vein.
3. Both intrahepatic and extrahepatic portal veins.
4. Superior mesenteric vein (SMV) and/or splenic vein (SV).

Due to non-specific symptoms, diagnosis is typically made through imaging, with contrast-enhanced computed tomography (CT) being the primary method. CT is used to establish the diagnosis, determine the etiology, and identify complications of acute PVT, with sensitivity and specificity rates ranging from 80% to 100% [31]. In addition to determining the extent of thrombosis, CT is also used to map portosystemic collaterals for possible intervention. Many findings are easily identified on portal venous phase images, though multiphase imaging, including non-contrast, arterial, portal venous, and potentially delayed phases, can optimize the information obtained from the examination. On CT, acute PVT features include increased attenuation in the PV on unenhanced scans and a lack of enhancement after IV contrast administration; the absence of contrast enhancement within the thrombus is a key finding for distinguishing bland PVT from malignant PVT (Fig. 19.7).

Transient hepatic attenuation differences related to altered hepatic perfusion can also be demonstrated, with geographic areas of increased attenuation at the periphery of the liver during arterial phase imaging. These differences are due to decreased portal venous perfusion and compensatory increased arterial perfusion from the liver periphery [26]. Enlargement of pre-existing veins in the porta hepatis and around biliary structures can be seen within a few days of acute PVT onset. This is especially noticeable in the gallbladder wall, which appears thickened and enhanced after contrast injection and should be carefully distinguished from acute cholecystitis [32]. Venous collaterals may form within just a few weeks after the initial PVT. CT is superior to CDUS in assessing the extension of thrombus within the portal venous system due to its higher sensitivity and accuracy in detecting thrombosis of the superior mesenteric vein (SMV) and splenic vein. Venous mesenteric infarction is challenging to recognize because clinical and

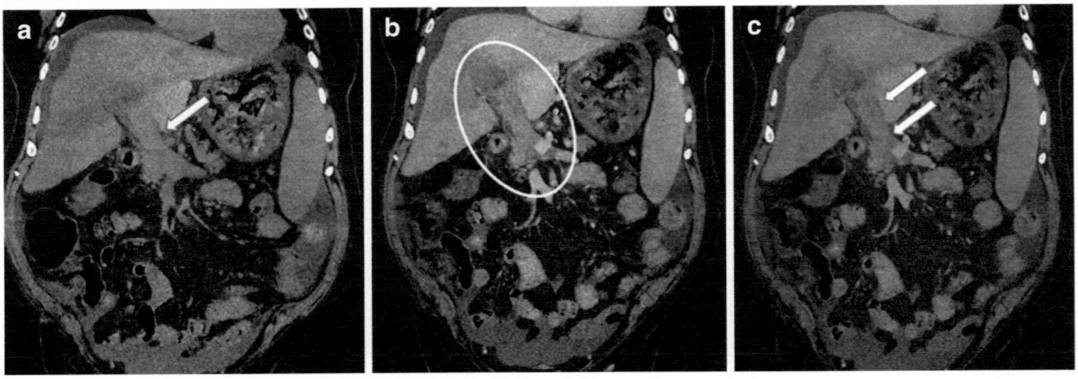

Fig. 19.7 CT images of a 62-year-old male affected by myelofibrosis, presented with intense abdominal pain. (**a**) Precontrast coronal CT image shows increased portal vein caliber and attenuation (arrow) (**b** and **c**) portal phase: CT coronal image better shows the extension of the portal vein thrombosis (white circles); enhancing walls of the main portal vein and a low attenuating thrombus within the lumen, consistent with acute portal vein thrombosis (arrows)

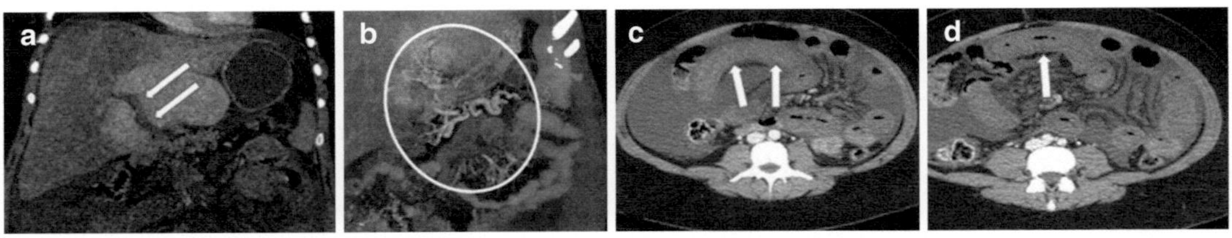

Fig. 19.8 CT of a 39-year-old female with polycythemia who presented with intense acute abdominal pain. (**a**) Portal phase coronal CT image shows acute massive thrombosis of the main portal vein and the extension of the thrombus to the superior mesenteric vein (arrows). (**b**) MIP CT image shows portal cavernomatosis and multiple mesenteric collateral circles (whitw circles) (**c** and **d**) Portal phase axial CT images show severe mesenteric edema.and thickening of small bowel (arrows) suggestive of venous bowel ischemia. Emergent surgery confirmed imaging findings and the patient underwent extensive bowel resection

biological manifestations are non-specific. However, persistent severe abdominal pain despite adequate anticoagulation, organ failure (such as shock, renal failure, metabolic acidosis, elevated arterial lactates), massive ascites, and rectal bleeding are suggestive of infarction. CT scan provides crucial additional information regarding the extent of thrombus into the mesenteric veins and arches, the presence of local factors, and signs of bowel congestion and ischemia (Fig. 19.8).

Distal thrombosis (occlusion of second-order branches of the superior mesenteric vein), bowel anomalies (homogeneous or heterogeneous hypoattenuating or hyperattenuating wall thickening, dilatation, abnormal or absent wall enhancement), mesenteric stranding, large ascites, pneumatosis, and portal venous gas are frequently observed in patients requiring intestinal resection [33]. If acute and complete portal vein thrombosis (PVT) is not resolved, it can progress to chronic PVT, resulting in cavernous transformation of the portal vein. This often leads to the development of massive esophageal, gastric, gastroesophageal, or ectopic varices, which can potentially bleed. Additionally, patients may experience refractory ascites and/or hydrothorax. In the absence of cirrhosis or other concurrent causes of portal hypertension, signs such as ascites, splenomegaly, and portosystemic collaterals suggest chronicity of PVT [34]. CT imaging plays a crucial role in confirming the presence of chronic PVT. The thrombosed vessel may appear obliterated or attenuated, with the incorporation of a clot into the vessel wall. Chronic venous thrombus can also exhibit linear areas of calcification within the thrombus. Furthermore, CT enables visualization of features associated with portal hypertension, including ascites, splenomegaly, and portosystemic shunts.

References

1. Virmani V, Ramanathan S, Virmani VS, Kielar A, Sheikh A, Ryan J. Non-neoplastic hepatic vascular diseases: spectrum of CT and MRI appearances. Clin Radiol. 2014;69(5):538–48.
2. Giovine S, Pinto A, Crispano S, Lassandro F, Romano L. Retrospective study of 23 cases of hepatic infarction: CT findings and pathological correlations. Radiol Med. 2006;111(1):11.
3. Pérez-Saborido B, Pacheco-Sánchez D, Barrera-Rebollo A, et al. Incidence, management, and results of vascular complications after liver transplantation. Transplant Proc. 2011;43:749.
4. Kim JS, Kim KW, Lee J, Kwon HJ, Kwon JH, Song GW, et al. Diagnostic performance for hepatic artery occlusion after liver transplantation: computed tomography angiography versus contrast-enhanced ultrasound. Liver Transpl. 2019;25:1651–60.
5. Karaosmanoglu A, Onder O, Kizilgoz V, Kantarci HP, M, Ozmen M, Karcaaltincaba M., Akata D. Infarcts and ischemia in the abdomen: an imaging perspective with an emphasis on cross-sectional imaging findings. Abdom Radiol. 2023;48:2167–95.
6. Delgado-Moraleda J, Ballester-Vallés C, Marti-Bonmat L. Role of imaging in the evaluation of vascular complications after liver transplantation. Insights Imaging. 2019;10
7. Marcacuzco Quinto A, et al. Complications of transarterial chemoembolization (TACE) in the treatment of liver tumors. Cirugía Español. 2018;96(9):560–7.
8. Sun Z, et al. Hepatic and biliary damage after transarterial chemoembolization for malignant hepatic tumors: incidence, diagnosis, treatment, outcome and mechanism. Crit Rev Oncol Hematol. 2011;79(2):164–74.
9. Jeng KS, Huang CC, Lin CK, et al. Early detection of a hepatic artery pseudoaneurysm after liver transplantation is the determinant of survival. Transplant Proc. 2016;48(4):1149–55.
10. Madhusudhan KS, Venkatesh HA, Gamanagatti S, Garg P, Srivastava DN. Interventional Radiology in the management of visceral artery pseudoaneurysms: a review of techniques and embolic materials. Korean J Radiol. 2016;17(3):351–63.
11. Li Y, De Stefano V, Li H, Zheng K, Bai Z, Guo X, Qi X. Epidemiology of Budd-Chiari syndrome: a systematic review and meta-analysis. Clin Res Hepatol Gastroenterol. 2019;43:468–74.
12. Sabol TP, Molina M, Wu GY. Thrombotic venous diseases of the liver. J Clin Transl Hepatol. 2015;3(3):189–94.
13. Sharma A, Keshava SN, Eapen A, Elias E, Eapen CE. An update on the management of Budd-Chiari syndrome. Dig Dis Sci. 2021;66:1780–90.
14. Thuluvath PJ, Alukal JJ, Zhang T. Acute liver failure in Budd-Chiari syndrome and a model to predict mortality. Hepatol Int. 2021;15:146–54.
15. Darwish Murad S, Plessier A, Hernandez-Guerra M, Fabris F, Eapen CE, Bahr MJ, Trebicka J, Morard I, Lasser L, Heller J, et al. EN-Vie (European Network for Vascular Disorders of the Liver). Etiology, management, and outcome of the Budd-Chiari syndrome. Ann Intern Med. 2009;151:167–75.
16. Gupta P, Bansal V, Kumar-M P, Sinha SK, Samanta J, Mandavdhare H, Sharma V, Dutta U, Kochhar R. Diagnostic accuracy of Doppler ultrasound, CT and MRI in Budd Chiari syndrome: systematic review and meta-analysis. Br J Radiol. 2020;93:20190847.
17. Brancatelli G, Vilgrain V, Federle MP, Hakime A, Lagalla R, Iannaccone R, Valla D. Budd-Chiari syndrome: spectrum of imaging findings. AJR Am J Roentgenol. 2007;188:W168–76.
18. Bansal V, Gupta P, Sinha S, et al. Budd-Chiari syndrome: imaging review. Br J Radiol. 2018;91(1092):20180441.
19. Van Wettere M, Bruno O, Rautou PE, Vilgrain V, Ronot M. Diagnosis of Budd-Chiari syndrome. Abdom Radiol. 2018;43:1896–907.
20. Flor N, Zuin M, Brovelli F, Maggioni M, Tentori A, Sardanelli F, Cornalba GP. Regenerative nodules in patients with chronic Budd-Chiari syndrome: a longitudinal study using multiphase contrast-enhanced multidetector CT. Eur J Radiol. 2010;73:588–93.
21. Brancatelli G, Federle MP, Grazioli L, Golfieri R, Lencioni R. Benign regenerative nodules in Budd-Chiari syndrome and other vascular disorders of the liver: radiologic-pathologic and clinical correlation. Radiographics. 2002;22:847–62.
22. Kim JA, Ahn HS, Park H, Seo YR, Seo JH, Kim CW, Kim HY. Hepatocellular carcinoma hidden by multiple infarcted regenerative nodules. Korean J Intern Med. 2016;31:1178–80.
23. Ren W, Qi X, Yang Z, Han G, Fan D. Prevalence and risk factors of hepatocellular carcinoma in Budd-Chiari syndrome: a systematic review. Eur J Gastroenterol Hepatol. 2013;25:830–41.
24. Young K, Wong R. Evaluation and management of acute and chronic portal vein thrombosis in patients with cirrhosis. Clin Liver Dis (Hoboken). 2018;10:152–6.
25. Primignani M, Martinelli I, Bucciarelli P, et al. Risk factors for thrombophilia in extrahepatic portal vein obstruction. Hepatology. 2005;41(03):603–6.
26. Margini C, Berzigotti A. Portal vein thrombosis: the role of imaging in the clinical setting. Dig Liver Dis. 2017;49:113–20.

27. Sheen CL, Lamparelli H, Milne A, Green I, Ramage JK. Clinical features, diagnosis and outcome of acute portal vein thrombosis. QJM. 2000;93(08):531–4.
28. Amitrano L, Guardascione MA, Scaglione M, et al. Prognostic factors in noncirrhotic patients with splanchnic vein thromboses. Am J Gastroenterol. 2007;102:2464–70.
29. Plessier A, Darwish-Murad S, Hernandez-Guerra M, et al; European Network for Vascular Disorders of the Liver (EN-Vie). Acute portal vein thrombosis unrelated to cirrhosis: a prospective multicenter follow-up study. Hepatology. 2010;51(01):210–8.
30. Teng F, Sun KY, Fu ZR. Tailored classification of portal vein thrombosis for liver transplantation: focus on strategies for portal vein inflow reconstruction. World J Gastroenterol. 2020;26:2691–701.
31. Canellas R, Mehrkhani F, Patino M, et al. Characterization of portal vein thrombosis (neoplastic versus bland) on CT images using software-based texture analysis and thrombus density (Hounsfield units). AJR Am J Roentgenol. 2016;207:W81–7.
32. Moomjian LN, Winks SG. Portal cavernoma cholangiopathy: diagnosis, imaging, and intervention. Abdom Radiol. 2017;42:57–68.
33. Fernandes T, Oliveira MI, Castro R, Araújo B, Viamonte B, Cunha R. Bowel wall thickening at CT: simplifying the diagnosis. Insights Imaging. 2014;5(2):195–208.
34. Berzigotti A, Garcia-Criado A, Darnell A, et al. Imaging in clinical decision-making for portal vein thrombosis. Nat Rev Gastroenterol Hepatol. 2014;11:308–16.

Acute Cholecystitis and Cholangitis

20

Riccardo Ferrari, Margherita Trinci, Valeria Lonardo, Antonio Galluzzo, and Michele Galluzzo

20.1 CT in Acute Cholecystitis and Cholangitis

Acute biliary tract inflammatory disease may involve intra-hepatic and extra-hepatic biliary duct called cholangitis or the gallbladder configuring the pathology known as cholecystitis.

20.1.1 Acute Cholecystitis

Acute gallbladder inflammatory disease is called acute cholecystitis (AC), and is distinguished into lithiasic (ALC) and alithiasic (AAC).

20.1.1.1 Litiasic Acute Cholecystitis

ALC is responsible for approximately 95% of all acute cholecystitis cases, representing the most common cause of acute upper quadrant abdominal pain. Annually, it affects about 200,000 individuals in the United States and poses a significant life-threatening risk; although mortality rates have decreased from around 5% in the 1980s, to less than 1% today, it remains the primary reason for emergency cholecystectomies [1, 2]. In the United States, gallstones affect over 25 million people [3]. While 80% of these individuals exhibit no symptoms, 15% experience non-specific symptoms such as bloating and nausea. Conversely, the remaining 5% develop symptoms indicative of ALC, including a clinical triad of colicky or continuous right hypochondriac pain, lasting approximately 30 min, hyper-pyrexia, and mild leukocytosis, with patients often testing positive for Murphy's sign and exhibiting nausea and occasionally palpable swelling or subsequent jaundice [4].

The major risk factors for ALC are summarized by the four 'Fs': Forties, Female, Fat, and Fair. Age and female gender are linked to higher stone production, while obesity directly and indirectly increases the risk of cholecystitis. The incidence of stones and cholecystitis significantly arises with a Body Mass Index (BMI) greater than 34 in women and 38 in men [5]. During pregnancy, the risk of gallstone formation increases due to hormonal changes inducing biliary stasis, making AC the second most common non-gynecological condition for surgical intervention (prevalence about 3%) [5–7]. The risk of

R. Ferrari · M. Galluzzo (✉)
Department of Emergency Radiology, San Camillo- Forlanini Hospital, Rome, Italy
e-mail: mgalluzzo@sirm.org

M. Trinci
Department of Radiology, S. Giovanni di Dio Hospital, Orbetello, Italy

V. Lonardo
Advanced Biomedical Sciences Department, University of Naples Federico II, Naples, Italy

A. Galluzzo
Department of Radiology, Careggi University Hospital, Florence, Italy
e-mail: antonio.galluzzo@unifi.it

L. Romano et al. (eds.), *CT of Non-Traumatic Body Emergencies*,
https://doi.org/10.1007/978-3-031-84849-0_20

forming calculi increases with the number of pregnancies and decreases with longer breast-feeding time.

Various medications, including hormonal therapies such as contraceptives, Ceftriaxone, Octreotide, and immunotherapies, have been associated with increased stone production [8].

Cystic bile duct obstruction by stones is the main etiopathogenesis, though not all obstructions lead to acute cholecystitis. If the obstruction is transient and brief, patients may experience biliary colic that resolves within a few hours; however, prolonged obstruction can lead to the rise of intracolecystits pressure with mucosal damage and activation of inflammatory mediators, culminating in bacterial superinfection similar to cholangitis [4].

Histological studies have shown arterial occlusion from thrombotic formations in branches of the cystic artery, causing ischemic necrosis in parts of the gallbladder. Clinically, the size of the gallstone correlates with inflammation severity, smaller stones typically cause mild or no inflammation, whereas large stones causing cystic duct obstruction increase internal pressure, leading to clot formation and subsequent cholecystitis [9].

Cholecystitis progresses through four distinct but linked phases:

1. Initial congestion and edema (days 1–4): Characterized by congestion and wall edema due to the gallstone wedged in the cystic duct.
2. Necrotizing phase (days 3–5): Peak circulatory disorders result in tissue necrosis and potential gallbladder perforation with biliary peritonitis.
3. Purulent phase (days 5–14): Leucocytes infiltration into necrotic tissue leads to production of purulent fluid inside the gallbladder.
4. Chronic phase (post 2–3 weeks): Following repeated mild attacks, the gallbladder presents a contracted aspect and hypertrophic walls; the chronic inflammation is characterized by gallbladder wall fibrosis and intramural abscesses; bile concentration and calcific crystals production is possible [9].

20.1.1.2 Alitiasic Acute Cholecystitis

Alitiasic acute cholecystitis (ACC) is present in the remaining 5–10% of patients, 80% of these patients are male and developed the disease after surgery.

Main causes of ACC in adult patient populations are summarized as

1. Severe complications inducing hypoxic-based wall ischemia such as trauma, cardiovascular interventions, septic shock, hypovolemic shock, and burns.
2. Chronic conditions such as prolonged fasting, parenteral nutrition, or congenital malformations.

Infectious diseases including bacteria (gram-negative or anaerobic), viruses (EBV, hepatotrophic virus), disseminated candidiasis, leptospirosis, chronic biliary tract carriers of typhoid and non-typhoid Salmonella, cholera, and tuberculosis, less often malaria, brucellosis, and dengue fever. AIDS infection is correlated to bile duct and gallbladder inflammation.

3. AAC has been reported to 0.7–0.9% of patients undergoing open abdominal aortic reconstruction, 0.5% of patients undergoing cardiac surgery, and 4% of patients undergoing bone marrow transplantation [10, 11].

In the pediatric population, ACC accounts for 50–70% of the flogistic gall bladder pathology with multifactorial pathogenesis.

The pathological chain that leads to ACC is started by bile stasis with biliary sludge formation and bile inspissation that directly creates toxic damage to the gallbladder epithelium. Microvascular occlusion of the gallbladder vasculature occurs secondary to endothelial injury, leading to gallbladder ischemia, which may occur in critically ill patients. AAC can also progress to gangrene, gallbladder empyema, and perforation in up to 50% of patients. Cholecystic flogosis may also be directly attributable to transcatheter chemotherapy [11–13].

20.1.2 Acute Cholangitis

Acute cholangitis (ACG) is a systemic disease characterized by increased bile duct pressure and bacterial overinfection [5]. Bile is normally sterile, the presence of bacteria in the biliary system, termed bacterobilia, is a necessary but not sufficient event to determine ACG due to the protection mechanisms of bile duct system. The release of IgA and mucus by the epithelium has anti-adhesion activity, and prevents bacteriostasis, which is physiologically induced by bile salts. Kupffer cells and the tight junction between the cholangiocytes prevent the translocation of bacteria from the hepatobiliary system into the portal venous system. Bacteria can also be carried into the duodenum by the regular flow of bile, while the sphincter of Oddi prevents the retrograde flow of bile. Any cause of obstruction in the biliary tract can therefore lead to bile stasis, which inevitably causes an increase in intraductal pressure that underlies the inflammatory event. In this case, the tight junctions widen, and there is dysfunction of the Kupffer cells and a reduction in the production of IgA [14–17]. The normal intraductal bile pressure should be between 7 and 14 cm of water and it is maintained by the sphincter of Oddi. When bile pressure exceeds 25 cm of water, cholangiovenous and cholangiolymphatic reflux can occur, leading to bacteremia and endotoxemia. That condition causes the release of systemic inflammatory mediators, such as tumor necrosis factor (TNF) and interleukin receptors; the cascade leads to a hemodynamic compromise [18].

The main causes of bile duct obstruction are:

1. Benign:

Post-surgical obstruction; biliary stent obstruction; acute or chronic pancreatitis; autoimmune cholangitis; primary sclerosing cholangitis; complicated calculosis; Mirizzi's Syndrome (a stone impacted in the cystic duct or gallbladder neck causing compression on the common bile duct or common hepatic duct); congenital anomalies; Lemmel Syndrome (peri-ampullary diverticulum causing distal biliary obstruction); haemophilia

2. Malignant:

Pancreatic cancer; gallbladder cancer; cholangiocarcinoma; neoplasms of the small intestine or liver metastases

3. Infectious:

Parasitic infections or AIDS (typically found in individuals with an average age of 37 years) [5, 18].

The main pathogens isolated after bacterial over infection are *Escherichia Coli* (25–50%), Klebsiella species (15–20%), Enterococcus species (10–20%), and Enterobacter species (5–10%) [19].

The most frequent cause of ACG is choledocho-lithiasis, US gallstones are present in 10–15% of the white population and of patients hospitalized for complications 6–9% are diagnosed with acute cholangitis. Less than 200,000 cases of ACG occur in the US per year [20]. Clinical evaluation of these patients varies according to the severity of ACG. Historically, the term "hepatic fever" was coined by Charcot in 1887, who described a clinical triad: high fever lasting more than 24 h, mild abdominal pain, and jaundice.

The term "acute obstructive cholangitis" has been introduced to describe a more severe cholangitis disease that includes hypotension and deterioration of the general condition (Reynold's Pentad, 1959). Charcot's Triad is not diagnostic due to its low sensitivity (26.4%) despite its high specificity (95.9%). A recent Tokyo guideline was established that includes laboratory and imaging parameters for the final diagnosis [21].

The ACG has a clinical-laboratory-instrumental classification into three different degrees of severity [5, 12, 20] (Table 20.1).

ACG is a life-threatening pathology: whereas before the 1980s the mortality rate was around 50%, it is now between 2.7% and 10%, also due to improved diagnostic criteria [5]. Although

Table 20.1 Grades and treatmens of cholangitis

Grade I (Mild acute cholangitis)	No organ dysfunction No criteria of moderate acute cholangitis	Antibiotic treatment
Grade II (Moderate acute cholangitis)	No organ dysfunction No response to the initial antibiotic treatment. *Any two of the five conditions should be present:* Leukocytosis (WBC >12,000/cmm) or leukopenia (WBC <4000/cmm); High temperature (≥39 °C); Elderly (age >75 years); Hyperbilirubinemia (total bilirubin ≥5 mg/dL); Hypoalbuminemia (< 0.7 × lower limit of normal).	Biliary drainage should be considered if the patient does not respond to initial treatment. Early endoscopic or percutaneous biliary drainage is indicated.
Grade III (Severe acute cholangitis)	Patients do not respond to initial medical treatment Organ dysfunction in at least one of the following organs/systems: (1) Cardiovascular system: hypotension requiring dopamine infusion ≥5 μg/kg per minute, or any dose of norepinephrine; (2) Nervous system: disturbance of consciousness; (3) Respiratory system: PaO2/FiO2 ratio <300; (4) Renal system: oliguria, serum creatinine >2 mg/dL; (5) Hepatic system: Platelet international normalized ratio (INR) >1.5; and (6) Hematological system: Platelet count <100000/cm	Appropriate respiratory/circulatory management Biliary drainage as soon as possible after the patient's general condition has improved

acute cholangitis is a rarer condition than cholecystitis, it has a higher proportion of severe cases, about 12.3% compared to 6% of severe cases of cholecystitis. According to the latest guidelines, mild ACG requires initial treatment with antibiotics, which is usually sufficient. Biliary drainage should be considered if the patient does not respond to initial treatment [22]. In moderate acute cholangitis, early endoscopic or percutaneous biliary drainage is indicated. Any treatment of the aetiological cause requires an improvement in the patient's general condition. In severe ACG, appropriate respiratory/circulatory management is required and biliary drainage should be performed as soon as possible after the patient's general condition has improved [22].

20.2 Diagnostic Workflow

The diagnostic workflow in biliary tract pathology requires a multimodality approach.

Ultrasound is the first-line imaging modality for suspected acute cholecystitis due to its accessibility, lack of ionizing radiation, and ability to detect gallstones, one of the primary causes of the condition. It can identify gallbladder wall thickening, pericholecystic fluid, and a positive sonographic Murphy's sign an exquisite tenderness over the gallbladder upon probe pressure, highly suggestive of acute cholecystitis [23].

Computed Tomography Scan, which is readily available in Emergency Departments, is a pan-exploration method that allows images of great anatomical detail to be obtained in a very short time. The speed of the currently available volumetric CT equipment, by reducing the acquisition time and the patient's apnea time, allows to production of images that are rarely affected by respiratory movement artefacts with the further possibility to obtain multiplanar (MPR) maximum intensity projection (MIP) and three-dimensional reconstructions (3D VR) of high quality. Volumetric acquisition with increased acquisition speed allows to optimize and reduce the contrast agent dose to the patient.

A study by Werts et al. concluded that CT was more sensitive than ultrasound for the diagnosis of acute colecistytis, but stated that they are complementary and should be used if US is negative and clinical suspicion remains high [24].

It is also indicated in patients with suspected cholangitis, in extra-biliary gallstone pathologies, in the search for possible complications such as abscesses or pancreatitis, in doubtful or negative ultrasound cases, in patients with right quadrant pain, fever, and leukocytosis, and in the assessment of non-specific abdominal pain.

It is recommended to perform the examination under basal conditions and after the administration of the contrast medium, with the aim of promoting a correct evaluation.

Magnetic Resonance Imaging (MRI) and Magnetic Resonance Cholangiopancreatography (MRCP) provide excellent contrast resolution and are particularly useful for characterizing biliary and pancreatic pathology without the use of ionizing radiation. MRCP, a specialized MRI technique, produces detailed images of the bile ducts and pancreatic ducts and can be instrumental in diagnosing cholangitis and identifying the cause of biliary obstruction. Its high contrast resolution allows optimal evaluation of coledocal litiasis, and it is therefore the gold standard for this type of pathology.

Although endoscopic retrograde cholangiopancreatography (ERCP) is primarily a therapeutic tool, it can also have a diagnostic role, particularly in acute cholangitis. It allows for direct visualization, diagnosis, and simultaneous treatment of biliary tract diseases, including stone removal and stent placement to relieve obstructions.

Despite the high sensitivity and specificity of these imaging techniques, certain challenges remain. For instance, the presence of very small stones or biliary sludge may be missed by ultrasound, and non-calcified stones can be difficult to detect by CT. Moreover, conditions like AAC might show minimal or atypical imaging findings, requiring a high index of suspicion and correlation with clinical and laboratory data.

The choice of imaging technique is influenced by the clinical presentation and suspected diagnosis based on initial evaluation. Imaging findings must be integrated with clinical and laboratory data to tailor management plans, whether conservative, interventional, or surgical. Early and accurate diagnosis through imaging is crucial to improving outcomes in patients with acute cholecystitis and cholangitis, reducing the risk of complications such as gallbladder rupture or severe infection.

20.3 Computed Tomography (CT) in Acute Cholecystitis: Technique and Diagnostic Signs

20.3.1 CT Imaging Technique

Computed tomography (CT) is a crucial diagnostic tool in the evaluation of acute cholecystitis, particularly when ultrasound findings are inconclusive or the patient's body habitus limits ultrasound visibility. The standard protocol for a CT aimed at diagnosing acute cholecystitis includes:

- *Precontrast phase*: This initial scan can identify calcified gallstones and gas within the gallbladder wall or lumen, which are signs of emphysematous cholecystitis, a more severe form of the disease.
- Contrast-enhanced phases: scans should be performed, in both the arterial and portal venous phases. The use of intravenous contrast helps delineate the gallbladder wall from the surrounding liver tissue and enhances the visualization of the gallbladder's vascularity, inflammation, and any adjacent complications.
- Scanning parameters: High-resolution images with thin slices (e.g., 2.5 mm or less) are preferred to accurately assess the gallbladder wall and nearby structures.

MPR reconstructions are indicated.

20.4 CT Main Findings and Signs

Main CT Signs of Cholecystitis Are

1. *Presence of Gallstones:* CT scan gallstones detection is correlated to their composition. Stones with Calcium content are hyperdense and thus easily identified (70%) inside the bile fluid; a percentage of stones consist of cholesterol with low or similar density relative to bile and are therefore undetectable. Recent literature proposes the use of multi-energy CT technique to increase the likelihood of stones identifying with different compositions [25]. The limit of CT is the identification of stones inside the choledochal duct; Some authors have shown that post-contrast enhancement of the walls of the cystic duct gives a better picture of the presence of choledocal lithiasis [26] (Figs. 20.1a, b and 20.2a, b).
2. *Gallbladder Distention—hydrops.* The gallbladder is considered distended if it measures more than 4 cm along the short axis and more than 9 cm along the long axis.
3. *Wall Thickening:* Focal or diffuse. The wall is considered thickened if the diameter is more than 3 mm. The use of intravenous contrast increases the contrast between the normally thin (<3 mm), rim-enhancing gallbladder wall and adjacent tissues (Fig. 20.3a and b).
4. *Wall Enhancement:* Mural or mucosal enhancement after contrast media administration. Wall hypodensity due to subserosal oedema and enhancement of the inner mucosa after ev mdc is called the "halo sign" typically with circumferential distribution (Fig. 20.4) [27].
5. *Fluid Collections in the Gallbladder Bed and/or Perihepatic Space, in the Absence of Ascitis.*
6. *Change in the Density of the Intraluminal Bile*, in the presence of sludge or hyperdense material.
7. *Alteration in Pericholecystic Fat Cell Density,* characterized by fluid in the pericholestic space or changing of the density of fat tissue.
8. *Increased Vascularization of the Pericholecystic Hepatic Parenchyma:* Enhancement of adjacent liver parenchyma due to reactive hyperemia is a useful sign for early diagnosis. Pericholecystic liver parenchyma enhancement after CM injection caused by reactive hyperemia, is particularly visible during arterial phase imaging. This sign has been attributed to increased blood flow in the cystic vein [28, 29].

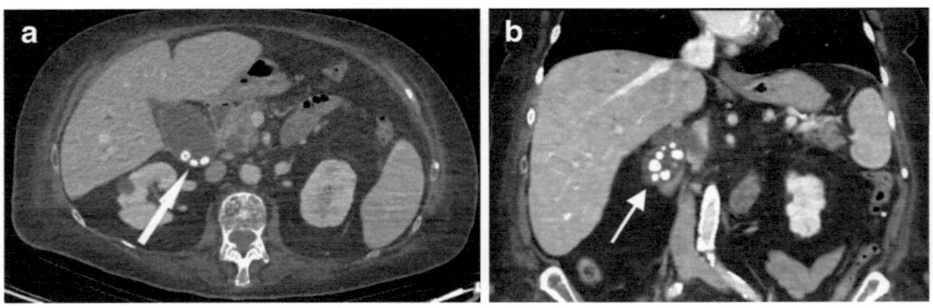

Fig. 20.1 (**a** and **b**) CT scan evidences gallbladder gallstones with calcium content. Because they are hyperdense are easily identified inside the bile fluid

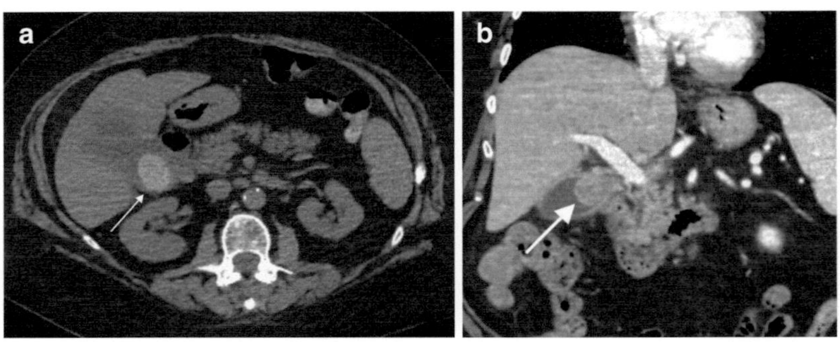

Fig. 20.2 (**a** and **b**) Gallbladder infundibular gallstone

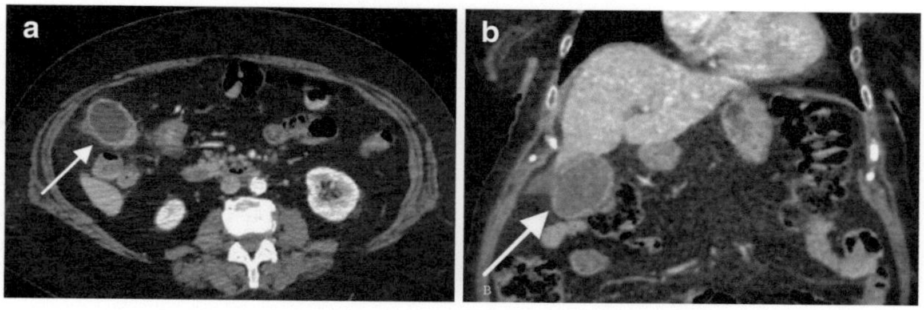

Fig. 20.3 (**a** and **b**) Gallbladder wall thickened (>3 mm) (arrow). After intravenous contrast administration there is a rim-enhancing of gallbladder wall (arrow)

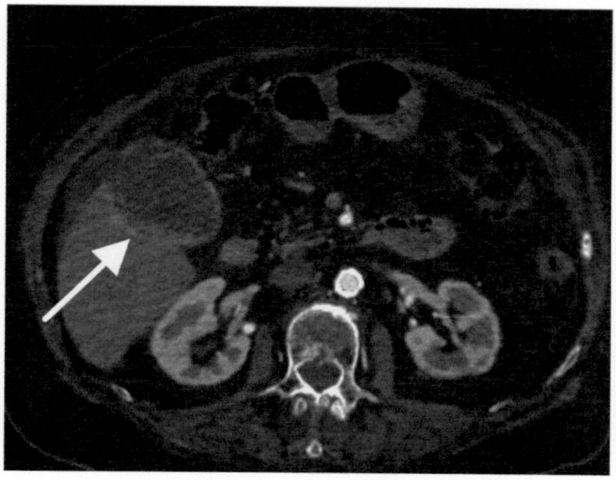

Fig. 20.4 Halo sign with the enhancement of perycolecistic hepatic parenchyma (arrow)

9. *Tensile Gallbladder Fundus Sign:* In the absence of other features, is considered an "early"sign (sensivity: 75%; specificity: 95%). The fundus of the gallbladder can be seen to bulge into the anterior wall of the abdomen [28, 30].

Mirvis et al. suggested cholecystitis CT diagnostic criteria that are summarized in Table 20.2.

Table 20.2 Main CT findings Mirvis criteria

CT findings
1. Gallstones
2. Gallbladder distention
3. Thickened gallbladder wall
4. Wall enhancement
5. Halo sign—subserosal edema
6. Pericholecystic fluid collections
7. Density of the intraluminal bile
8. Fat stranding
9. Enhancement of adjacent liver parenchyma
10. Tensile gallbladder fundus sign

Table 20.3 Main CT findings Mirvis criteria, major and minor criteria

Major criteria	Minor criteria
Gallstones	Gallbladder distention
Thickened gallbladder wall	Sludge
Pericholecystic fluid collections	
Subserosal edema	

Diagnosis of acute cholecystitis can be supported if one major and two minor criteria are present [31, 32] (Table 20.3).

20.5 CT Sign of Complicated Cholecistis

Patterns of gallbladder mucosal enhancement on CT can be used for distinguishing acute uncomplicated from gangrenous cholecystitis (Table 20.4).

Gangrenous cholecystitis (GC) is defined as necrosis and perforation of the gallbladder wall, the result of ischemia following progressive vascular insufficiency. The incidence of gangrenous cholecystitis ranges from 2% to 38%, generally in elderly patients, and is an emergency condition that can cause organ damage if its diagnosis is delayed, requiring prompt surgical treatment and a high rate of conversion from laparoscopic to open treatment.

Bennet et al., suggest some CT criteria for gangrenous cholecystitis diagnosis, some of which are similar to acute cholecystitis diagnosis with the addition of air bubbles inside or within the wall of gallbladder [33, 34].

Emphysematous cholecystitis is caused by a secondary infection of the gallbladder wall, with gas-forming organisms, and is commonly seen in diabetic patients. CT is considered the most sensitive and specific imaging technique for the diagnosis and is recommended for the diagnosis, whose course is extremely rapid, with potentially fatal complications such as intra-abdominal abscess, generalized peritonitis, gas gangrenous of the abdominal wall, and sepsis with distributive septic shock. CT shows low-attenuation foci consistent with gas within the gallbladder wall or lumen. Axial unenhanced CT is useful, where gas appears clearly hypodense within the gallbladder wall, and to differentiate between intraluminal and intramural gas also after biliary surgery or sphincterotomy [29, 35].

A suppurative condition is when high attenuation material consistent with pus is identified within the distended gallbladder lumen and is indistinguishable from sludge.

Hemorrhagic cholecystitis, will manifest as high-attenuation material within the gallbladder lumen. Vicarious excretion of recently administered iodinated contrast material in the bile is a potential mimic and an appropriate history should be obtained to avoid this pitfall [30, 32].

Acute cholecystitis is often complicated with pericholecystic abscess formation (3–19% of cases), and can be present as intramural and pericholecystic rim-enhancing fluid collections (Fig. 20.5a–c).

Other complications of cholelithiasis include biliary fistula, gallstone ileus, and Mirizzi's syndrome.

In a fistula, gallstones can erode into adjacent hollow visceral organs and migrate into the duodenum at the terminal ileum, causing stenosis and leading to the so-called biliary-ileus (Fig. 20.6a–c).

Table 20.4 CT signs of gangrenous cholecystitis

Gangrenous cholecystitis
Gas in the wall: (100%)
Membranous structures within the lumen (intraluminal flap or Intraluminal membrane), (99.5%)
Irregular thickening of the gallbladder wall (97.6%)
Irregular, discontinuous, and poor contrast enhancement of gallbladder wall (Interrupted rim sign) (73%)
Abscess (96.6%)
Increased density of fat around the gallbladder
Adjacent hepatic parenchyma hyperenhancement

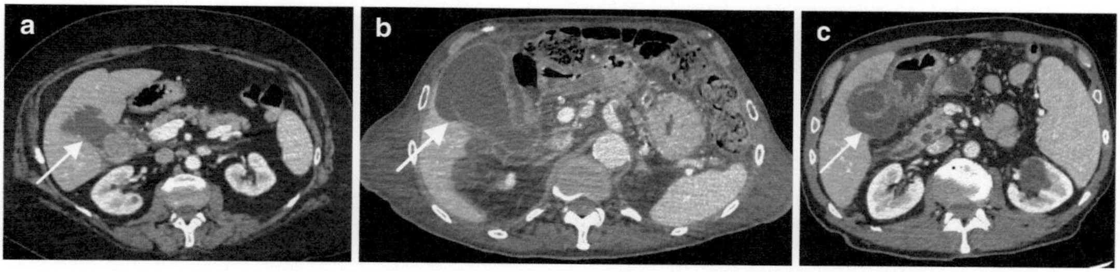

Fig. 20.5 Pericolecystic abscess in liver parenchyma (arrows)

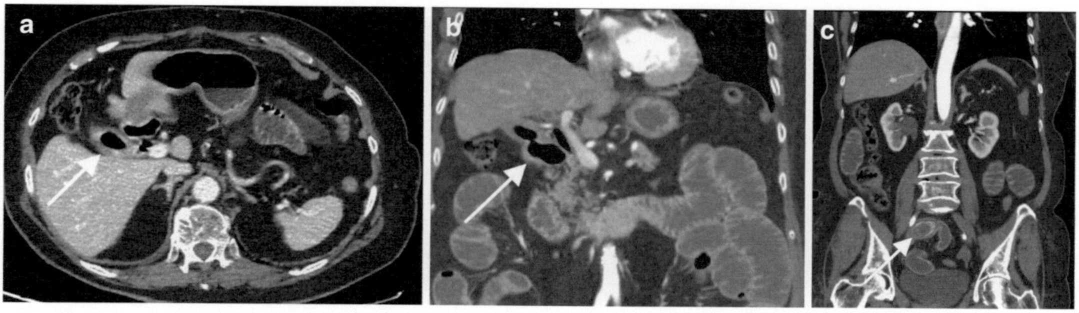

Fig. 20.6 (**a** and **b**) Cholecystic-duodenal fistula in biliary ileus: axial (**a**) and coronal (**b**) plane demonstrates the presence of air in the lumen of gallbladder (arrows). (**c**) The abdominal coronal reconstruction CT scan evidences biliary ileus with cholecystic calculus (arrow) migrated to small bowel lumen through cholecystic-duodenal fistula

20.6 CT Sign of Cholangytis

In the case of cholangitis, imaging allows accurate anatomical assessment of the location and severity of the disease, in particular, obstruction and inflammation of the bile duct need to be precisely evaluated. The role of CT in cholangitis is lower compared to MRI. Even though transient hepatic attenuation differences (THADs) could be a specific sign of inflammation of the peribiliary space. It appears as focal or diffuse hyperdense areas in the peribiliary spaces visible in the hepatic arterial phase. Thad's incidence varies from 71% to 98% and correlates with clinical parameters of inflammation. Pneumobilia is a finding in the history of endoscopic or surgical intervention and may progress to cholangitis caused by gas-forming organisms. Signs of atrophy and changes in parenchymal attenuation are often seen as chronic, flogosis consequences. Inhomogeneous enhancement is a useful complementary sign, often seen in the early phase of dynamic imaging and disappearing after treatment [31, 34].

Abscesses may be seen (20% of pyogenic cholangitis), often multiple, septate with peripheral rim enhancement. This sign allows differential diagnosis with a biloma, which appears hypodense and sometimes contains stones. This type of collection may not communicate with the biliary tree [33, 35].

CT is therefore useful for the diagnosis of bile duct stenosis, in particular in the differential diagnosis between neoplasia and fibrosis. In case of the suspect of bile duct neoplasia late venous phase should be performed as fibrous component of cholangiocarcinoma enhanced in the late venous phase.

Bibliography

1. Friedman GD. Natural history of asymptomatic and symptomatic gallstones. Am J Surg. 1993;165(4):399–404. https://doi.org/10.1016/s0002-9610(05)80930-4.
2. Shaffer EA. Epidemiology and risk factors for gallstone disease: has the paradigm changed in the 21st century? Curr Gastroenterol Rep. 2005;7(2):132–40. https://doi.org/10.1007/s11894-005-0051-8.
3. Everhart JE, Khare M, Hill M, Maurer KR. Prevalence and ethnic differences in gallbladder disease in the United States. Gastroenterology. 1999;117(3):632–9. https://doi.org/10.1016/s0016-5085(99)70456-7.
4. Roncacci A, Rende C, Buquicchio GL, Sessa B, Miele V. Colecistite acuta. Radiol Med. 2010;115(Suppl):S90–9. https://doi.org/10.1007/s11547-000-0000-0.
5. Sharp HT. The acute abdomen during pregnancy. Clin Obstet Gynecol. 2002;45:405–13.
6. Liu B, Beral V, Balkwill A, Million Women Study Collaborators. Childbearing, breastfeeding, other reproductive factors and the subsequent risk of hospitalization for gallbladder disease. Int J Epidemiol. 2009;38(1):312–8. https://doi.org/10.1093/ije/dyn174. Epub 2008 Sep 4
7. Salari N, Hasheminezhad R, Heidarisharaf P, Khaleghi AA, Azizi AH, Shohaimi S, Mohammadi M. The global prevalence of gallstones in pregnancy: a systematic review and meta-analysis. Eur J Obstet Gynecol Reprod Biol X. 2023;19:100237. https://doi.org/10.1016/j.eurox.2023.100237.
8. Jpn. Societ. Gastroenterol. Practice guidelines of the gallstone disease. Tokyo: Dai Nippon Printing Co., Ltd; 2009. p. 30–1. (in Japanese, clinical practice guidelines CPGs)
9. Adachi T, Eguchi S, Muto Y. Pathophysiology and pathology of acute cholecystitis: A secondary publication of the Japanese version from 1992. J Hepatobiliary Pancreat Sci. 2022;29(2):212–6. https://doi.org/10.1002/jhbp.912. Epub 2021 Mar 27
10. Botea F, Kraft A, Popescu I. Pathophysiology and diagnosis of acute acalculous cholecystitis. In: Di Carlo I, editor. Difficult acute cholecystitis. Cham: Springer; 2021. https://doi.org/10.1007/978-3-030-62102-5_3.
11. Markaki I, Konsoula A, Markaki L, Spernovasilis N, Papadakis M. Acute acalculous cholecystitis due to infectious causes. World J Clin Cases. 2021;9(23):6674–85. https://doi.org/10.12998/wjcc.v9.i23.6674.
12. Kimura Y, Takada T, Kawarada Y, Nimura Y, Hirata K, Sekimoto M, Yoshida M, Mayumi T, Wada K, Miura F, Yasuda H, Yamashita Y, Nagino M, Hirota M, Tanaka A, Tsuyuguchi T, Strasberg SM, Gadacz TR. Definitions, pathophysiology, and epidemiology of acute cholangitis and cholecystitis: Tokyo Guidelines. J Hepatobiliary Pancreat Surg. 2007;14(1):15–26. https://doi.org/10.1007/s00534-006-1152-y.
13. Gallaher JR, Charles A. Acute cholecystitis: a review. JAMA. 2022;327(10):965–75. https://doi.org/10.1001/jama.2022.2350.
14. Parks RW, Clements WD, Smye MG, Pope C, Rowlands BJ, Diamond T. Intestinal barrier dysfunction in clinical and experimental obstructive jaundice and its reversal by internal biliary drainage. Br J Surg. 1996;83(10):1345–9. https://doi.org/10.1002/bjs.1800831007.
15. Flemma RJ, Flint LM, Osterhout S, Shingleton WW. Bacteriologic studies of biliary tract infection. Ann Surg. 1967;166(4):563–72. https://doi.org/10.1097/00000658-196710000-00005.
16. Sung JY, Costerton JW, Shaffer EA. Defense system in the biliary tract against bacterial infection. Dig Dis Sci. 1992;37(5):689–96. https://doi.org/10.1007/BF01296423.
17. Lan Cheong Wah D, Christophi C, Muralidharan V. Acute cholangitis: current concepts. ANZ J Surg. 2017;87(7–8):554–9. https://doi.org/10.1111/ans.13981. Epub 2017 Mar 24
18. Buyukasik K, Toros AB, Bektas H, Ari A, Deniz MM. Diagnostic and therapeutic value of ERCP in acute cholangitis. ISRN Gastroenterol. 2013;2013:191729. https://doi.org/10.1155/2013/191729.
19. Weber A, Schneider J, Wagenpfeil S, Winkle P, Riedel J, Wantia N, Feihl S, Römmler F, Baur DM, Schmid RM, Algül H, Huber W. Spectrum of pathogens in acute cholangitis in patients with and without biliary endoprosthesis. J Infect. 2013;67(2):111–21. https://doi.org/10.1016/j.jinf.2013.04.008. Epub 2013 Apr 17
20. Ahmed M. Acute cholangitis – an update. World J Gastrointest Pathophysiol. 2018;9(1):1–7. https://doi.org/10.4291/wjgp.v9.i1.1.
21. Takada T, Strasberg SM, Solomkin JS, et al. TG13: Updated Tokyo Guidelines for the management of acute cholangitis and cholecystitis. Hepatobiliary Pancreat Sci. 2013;20:1–7. https://doi.org/10.1007/s00534-012-0566-y.
22. Takada T, Kawarada Y, Nimura Y, Yoshida M, Mayumi T, Sekimoto M, Miura F, Wada K, Hirota M, Yamashita Y, Nagino M, Tsuyuguchi T, Tanaka A, Kimura Y, Yasuda H, Hirata K, Pitt HA, Strasberg SM, Gadacz TR, Bornman PC, Gouma DJ, Belli G, Liau KH. Background: Tokyo Guidelines for the management of acute cholangitis and cholecystitis. J Hepatobiliary Pancreat Surg. 2007;14(1):1–10. https://doi.org/10.1007/s00534-006-1150-0. Epub 2007 Jan 30
23. Ralls PW, et al. Sonographic evaluation of gallbladder volume and contraction. Radiology. 1985;155(3):767–71. https://doi.org/10.1148/radiology.155.3.3890007.
24. Wertz JR, et al. Comparing the diagnostic accuracy of ultrasound and CT in evaluating acute cholecystitis. AJR Am J Roentgenol. 2018;211(2):W92–7. https://doi.org/10.2214/AJR.17.18884. Epub 2018 Apr 27

25. Paulson EK. Acute cholecystitis: CT findings. Semin Ultrasound CT MR. 2000;21(1):56–63. https://doi.org/10.1016/s0887-2171(00)90013-1.
26. Kim SV, et al. Cystic Duct Enhancement: A Useful CT Finding in the Diagnosis of Acute Cholecystitis Without Visible Impacted Gallstones. AJR Am J Roentgenol. 2015;205(5):991–8. https://doi.org/10.2214/AJR.15.14403.
27. Runner GJ, et al. Gallbladder wall thickening. AJR Am J Roentgenol. 2014;202(1):W1–W12. https://doi.org/10.2214/AJR.12.10386.
28. Park AC, et al. Usefulness of the tensile gallbladder fundus sign in the diagnosis of early acute cholecystitis. AJR Am J Roentgenol. 2013;201(2):340–6. https://doi.org/10.2214/AJR.12.9919.
29. Bortoff AG et al. Gallbladder Stones: imaging and intervention radiographics 2000;20(3):751–766. https://doi.org/10.1148/radiographics.20.3.g00ma16751.
30. Murphy MC, Gibney B, Gillespie C, Hynes J, Bolster F. Gallstones top to toe: what the radiologist needs to know. Insights Imaging. 2020;11:13. https://doi.org/10.1186/s13244-019-0825-4.
31. Pötter-Lang S, Ba-Ssalamah A, Bastati N, Messner A, Kristic A, Ambros R, Herold A, Hodge JC, Trauner M. Modern imaging of cholangitis. Br J Radiol. 2021;94(1125):20210417. https://doi.org/10.1259/bjr.20210417. Epub 2021 Jul 20
32. Fidler J, Paulson EK, Layfield L. CT evaluation of acute cholecystitis: findings and usefulness in diagnosis. American Journal of Roentgenology 1999;166(5):1085–88. https://doi.org/10.2214/ajr.166.5.8615248.
33. Heffernan EJ, Geoghegan T, Munk PL, Ho SG, Harris AC. Recurrent pyogenic cholangitis: from imaging to intervention. AJR Am J Roentgenol. 2009;192(1):W28–35. https://doi.org/10.2214/AJR.08.1104.
34. Bennett GL, Rusinek H, Lisi V, Israel GM, Krinsky GA, Slywotzky CM, Megibow A. CT findings in acute gangrenous cholecystitis. AJR Am J Roentgenol. 2002;178(2):275–81. https://doi.org/10.2214/ajr.178.2.1780275 PMID: 11804880.
35. Lallemand B, De Keuleneer R, Maassarani F. Emphysematous cholecystitis Acta Chir Belg. 2003;103(2):230–2. https://doi.org/10.1080/00015458.2003.11679413. PMID: 12768870..

Part V

Pelvis

21 Pelvic Inflammatory Diseases

Pietro Valerio Foti, Massimo Tonolini, Renato Farina, Luca Mammino, and Antonio Basile

21.1 Introduction

Pelvic inflammatory disease (PID) represents an infection-related inflammatory spectrum spanning from the uterine cervix to the peritoneal cavity (cervicitis, endometritis, salpingitis, pelvic peritonitis), determined by ascending microbes from the lower genital tract. Categories of patients at risk of PID are sexually active women ≤25 years old and high-risk women >25 years old (multiple sexual partners and/or previous sexually transmitted infections) [1]; symptomatic partner, new sexual partners, unprotected sexual intercourse, early sexual intercourse (<15 years of age), low socioeconomic status, intrauterine devices (especially in the first 20 days after insertion) and douching are other risk factors for PID [2–4]. The commonest pathogenic agents responsible for sexually transmitted infections, recognized as etiologic agents of PID are, in order of frequency: *Chlamydia trachomatis*, gram-negative bacteria, mycoplasmas and *Neisseria gonorrhoeae*; in over 50% of cases PID results from polymicrobial infection [5]. According to World Health Organization data, in 2020 the incidence of *Chlamydia trachomatis* and *Neisseria gonorrhoeae* infections worldwide was 129 million and 82 million respectively [6, 7], nevertheless, it is conceivable that the real incidence of PID is undervalued due to the difficulties in diagnosing this disease in patients with atypical symptoms, and due to limited availability of recommended diagnostic tests in low-income countries [1, 8, 9]. Postabortion and postpartum intrauterine manoeuvres and, more in general, gynecologic surgery are other risk factors for PID to take into account [10, 11]. PID seldom may be caused by atypical pathogens such as *Mycobacterium tuberculosis* and *Actinomyces. Mycobacterium tuberculosis* usually spreads to the genital tract haematogenously or lymphatically; actinomycosis is instead related to the use of intrauterine devices [11].

Patients with mild-to-moderate PID (about 90% of cases) are generally managed as outpatients; on the other hand, severe PID requires hospitalization in order to rule out and/or promptly treat pelvic abscesses and peritonitis, representing its major acute complications [1, 12]. Among benign gynecological diseases, PID

P. V. Foti · R. Farina · A. Basile (✉)
Department of Medical Surgical Sciences and Advanced Technologies "G.F. Ingrassia" – Radiology I Unit, University Hospital Policlinico "G. Rodolico-San Marco", Catania, Italy
e-mail: pietrovalerio.foti@unict.it; antonio.basile@unict.it

M. Tonolini
Department of Radiology, "Luigi Sacco" University Hospital, Milan, Italy
e-mail: massimo.tonolini@asst-fbf-sacco.it

L. Mammino
Department of Diagnostic Radiology, Neuroradiology and Interventional Radiology, "Garibaldi Centro" Hospital, Catania, Italy
e-mail: lmammino@arnasgaribaldi.it

L. Romano et al. (eds.), *CT of Non-Traumatic Body Emergencies*,
https://doi.org/10.1007/978-3-031-84849-0_21

is the main cause of hospitalization in women of reproductive age and, together with its clinical sequelae (infertility, ectopic pregnancy and chronic pelvic pain), entails a considerable social and economic burden [13]. Rising antibiotic resistance is another emerging global concern regarding PID treatment [4].

21.2 Pathophysiology

Numerous factors contribute to the pathophysiological complexity of PID. Although the vagina and cervix are continuously exposed to various commensal and pathogenic microorganisms, the action of the mucosal immune system of the female genital tract ensures that infections are relatively uncommon [1]. The mucosal immune system consists of resident epithelial cells, supportive stromal cells and also immune cells migrating into the female reproductive tract [14]. Bacterial vaginosis, found in about 30% of women of reproductive age and in more than 60% of cases of PID [15], is a subversion of the vaginal microbiota that occurs when the physiologic dominant vaginal flora, composed of lactic acid-producing bacteria, is superseded by an anaerobic prevailing flora (including *Gardnerella vaginalis*, *Megasphaera* spp. and *Atopobium vaginae*). The alteration of this dynamic balance determines the establishment of an inflammatory process that, together with infection-related epithelium damage, can promote an ascending infection by vaginal and cervical microbes, causing cervicitis and endometritis [1, 4, 16]. If inflammation is limited to the lower genital tract and uterus (vaginitis, cervicitis and endometritis), long-term morbidity is extremely limited. If infection-induced inflammation extends to the fallopian tube, then dysfunction of mucosal ciliated cells, submucosal inflammatory oedema, occlusion of the fallopian tubes and stagnation of luminal secretions occur, thus resulting in salpingitis. This latter can lead to long-term complications such as tubal factor infertility and ectopic pregnancy.

The involvement of the peritoneal cavity with the deposition of fibrinoid exudate on the serosal surface of the various pelvic compartments characterizes the pelvic peritonitis of genital origin. This peritoneal exudate determines the coalescence of the uterus, adnexa, small bowel loops, sigmoid colon and rectum; fibrotic adhesions that may result are often a cause of chronic pelvic pain [1, 17].

21.3 Diagnosis

The diagnosis of PID relies on four pillars, including medical history, physical examination, laboratory tests and imaging studies, and is considerably hampered by the wide variety and different severity degree of symptoms as well as by the variable clinical course (acute, chronic or subclinical) [1, 4]. Although the typical, full-blown PID causes acute pelvic pain and fever, both of these symptoms are often absent, since approximately only 40% of women diagnosed with PID are symptomatic [8] and less than one-third experience fever [1]. Therefore, given the common subtle presentation of the disease, clinicians have to investigate the possible presence of other nonspecific and more blurred symptoms: nausea/vomiting, anomalous vaginal discharge, metrorrhagia, intermenstrual and/or postcoital bleeding, dyspareunia, dysuria, pollakiuria, rectal symptoms, lumbago and right hypochondrial pain (Table 21.1) [1, 4, 10, 18].

At physical bimanual pelvic examination, motion-induced pelvic organ tenderness, in particular cervical tenderness, uterine tenderness (indicative of endometritis) or adnexal tenderness (indicative of salpingitis) is the clinical signs suggesting a diagnosis of PID [1, 10]. Concomitant rectal signs or evidence of a pelvic mass may be an expression of complicated PID with an abscess in the rectouterine pouch [10]. Abdominal tenderness may also be lacking, especially if salpingitis and peritonitis are not present [1].

Visual inspection of the cervix should be performed in the search for mucopus (yellow or green), cervical friability, erythema and oedema. Endocervical samples (or vaginal samples, should the former not be possible) are recommended to achieve a microbiological diagnosis. Microbiological samples aim to search for etio-

Table 21.1 Main symptoms in patients with PID [1, 4, 10]

Disease severity	Clinical symptoms
Mild-to-moderate PID	No symptoms (only histologic evidence)
	Malaise
	Nausea/vomiting
	Anomalous vaginal discharge
	Metrorrhagia
	Intermenstrual bleeding
	Postcoital bleeding
	Dyspareunia
	Dysuria and pollakiuria
	Rectal symptoms
	Lumbago
	Mild bilateral lower abdominal pain
Moderate-to-severe PID	Acute pelvic pain
	Fever
	Rectal symptoms
	Right hypochondrial pain worsened by movement and breathing

logic agents most commonly responsible for PID. The assessment for bacterial vaginosis implies microscopy and laboratory tests of the vaginal secretions (vaginal pH, wet mount, clue cells, whiff test and leukorrhea: more than 1 leukocyte per epithelial cell) [1, 4, 10].

As for laboratory blood tests, a complete blood count, C-reactive protein and erythrocyte sedimentation rate are recommended; hyperleukocytosis coupled with high levels of C-reactive protein may indicate a complicated PID or also a differential diagnosis (acute appendicitis) [1, 10]. In addition, high C-reactive protein levels are associated with poor clinical outcomes among patients hospitalized for PID [19]. Nevertheless, peripheral white blood cell count may often be in the standard; therefore, it is important to remember that lack of hyperleukocytosis, a normal C-reactive protein concentration and even negative microbiological results do not allow to rule out a diagnosis of PID. Moreover, screening for human immunodeficiency virus (HIV) should be performed in patients with clinically suspected PID [1, 10].

Diagnostic imaging is definitely helpful to noninvasively confirm the gynecological origin of the disease and to rule out competing differential diagnoses, nevertheless awaiting the carrying out of specific imaging examinations should not delay the beginning of antibiotic treatment [4, 10]. Overall indications for imaging are as follows: patients with nonspecific symptoms, the ineffectiveness of pharmacological therapy, assessment of suspected complications (i.e. abscesses), treatment planning (percutaneous drainage) of a known abscess [2].

Ultrasound (US) should generally represent the ideal noninvasive first-line imaging approach to investigate abdominal and pelvic pain, particularly in young women. In clinically severe PID and when a pelvic mass is suspected at bimanual pelvic examination, US is recommended to search for signs of complicated upper genital tract inflammation (thickened fluid-filled tubes or polymorphous fluid collections); however, US demonstrates poor sensitivity (30%) and specificity (67%) in patients with mild-to-moderate uncomplicated PID [20].

Computed tomography (CT) examination of the abdomen and pelvis with intravenous injection of contrast agent is useful to rule out urinary and gastrointestinal causes of acute abdomen, such as obstructive uropathy, appendicitis and diverticulitis [1, 2, 10], although the overall sensitivity of CT findings for the diagnosis of acute PID is poor [21].

When allowed by stable clinical conditions and scanner availability, magnetic resonance imaging (MRI) should be used to clarify inconclusive US/CT findings and suspected gynaecologic abnormalities. Its advantages include intrinsic multiplanar capabilities, lack of ionising radiation, multi-parametric imaging with excellent soft tissue contrast, including detection of fat and blood products [11]. MRI has a sensitivity of 95% and specificity of 89% in the diagnosis of acute PID [22]; the sensitivity, in particular, rises to 98.4% when diffusion-weighted imaging (DWI) is added to conventional MR sequences [23].

In patients with suspicion of PID, laparoscopy can confirm the diagnosis through the visual evidence of signs of acute tubal inflammation (redness, oedema, thickening, dilatation and purulent exudate) in about 65% of the cases, nevertheless laparoscopic procedure is not recommended for purely diagnostic purposes, because of its invasiveness and the inability to achieve a correct diagnosis in patients with cervicitis and/or endometritis without salpingitis; therefore it is rarely used in mild-to-moderate PID and in the early stage of the disease [1, 2, 10, 18, 21].

21.4 CT Imaging

Nowadays, in emergency care settings multidetector CT represents the mainstay "workhorse" examination to investigate patients with symptoms and signs of acute abdominal and pelvic disease; its advantages include widespread availability on a 24/7 basis, short examination time, and comprehensive assessment of the abdominopelvic cavity [24]. Although clinical examination remains the gold standard for the diagnosis of PID, in an emergency department a specialistic gynecological examination is not continuously available. In this setting, where the emergency physician is often called upon to clinically assess and diagnose this condition, multidetector CT plays a crucial role, since early diagnosis of PID is key for effective management of acute disease and reduces the risk of sequelae [17, 21, 22].

21.4.1 CT Imaging Protocol and Technical Considerations

Unless contraindicated by allergy or impaired renal function, iodinated contrast medium should be administered to provide comprehensive assessment and differential diagnosis of acute pelvic conditions such as suspected PID. According to recent studies, contrast dose should be adjusted based on lean body weight [25]. Since PID generally affects premenopausal women, radiologists should advise against liberal use of CT in reproductive age. When CT is deemed necessary to provide a prompt diagnosis in emergency care setting, in young women with unspecific abdominal complaints we suggest to order a single CT acquisition in the portal venous phase, 70–80 s after intravenous contrast administration at a 2.5–3 mL/s flow rate, in order to limit the erogated ionising radiation dose. If available, state-of-the art techniques to further reduce radiation dose should be used, such as iterative reconstruction algorithms. Additionally, preliminary unenhanced acquisition should be included when suspected cystic, neoplastic or haemorrhagic genital condition is suspected, as it may provide a confident measurement of attenuation (Hounsfield units, HU) of fluid versus blood in the peritoneal effusion and genital structures, and confident detection of contrast enhancement in normal structures and lesions. Respectively, arterial-dominant and excretory phases should be acquired only when concern for bleeding or involvement of urinary tract is suspected [24].

21.4.2 CT Anatomy of the Female Pelvis

On current multidetector CT scanners, almost isotropic submillimeter voxels are acquired, resulting in the reconstruction of multiplanar high-resolution images. In females, routine reformations of 3–5 mm thick images along three planes are advised: sagittal viewing is particularly beneficial to assess size, morphology and contrast enhancement of the uterus, which largely varies according to age, menstrual phase and timing of acquisition [26]. Albeit the characteristic uterine zonal anatomy as depicted by MRI is not perceptible at CT, the uterus should be evaluated for size, position, dilatation and content of its cavity. Additionally, coronal or oblique-coronal reformations facilitate the assessment of adnexal structures (fallopian tubes and ovaries) [24, 27].

In normal conditions, the ovaries measure approximately 3 × 3 × 2 cm, and show a more or less recognizable follicular structure on contrast-enhanced CT images. They are identified by their position close to external iliac vessels and located posterior to the round ligaments; differently from lymphadenopathies, they lie anteromedially to the pelvic ureters [24]. The nondilated (calibre <4 mm) fallopian tubes are generally not recognizable at CT, unless delineated by pelvic effusion [5, 17]; when dilated by intraluminal fluid, blood or pus, they may be identified as tubular, C- or S-shaped juxta-uterine structures with variably fluid or sovrafluid density content [24].

Importantly, unsuspected gynaecologic abnormalities, including PID changes, may be encountered in unenhanced abdominal CT performed under alternative presumptive diagnosis, particularly renal colic/urolithiasis. Therefore, we recommend careful scrutiny of female genital structures, because it may happen to detect peritoneal cul-de-sac fluid (limited amount is normal in reproductive age) or blood, fallopian tube dilatation or adnexal enlargement; in these situations, gynaecologic consultation followed by MRI or contrast-enhanced CT should be advised.

21.4.3 Spectrum of CT Imaging Findings

In a recently published meta-analysis, contrast-enhanced CT demonstrated a sensitivity of 79% and a specificity of 99% in the diagnosis of acute PID in an emergency care setting. This relatively low sensitivity is due to the heterogeneity in the severity degree of acute PID, so contrast-enhanced CT may fail to detect the disease at its early stage of onset and/or cases of mild-to-moderate PID [22], that is when CT findings may be subtle or non-specific. Among the CT findings for the diagnosis of acute PID, fallopian tube bilateral thickening represents the most specific (95.1%), whereas mid-pelvic fat stranding is the most sensitive (60.4%) [21]. The different disease manifestations are illustrated below; their CT findings are summarized in Table 21.2.

21.4.3.1 Cervicitis

Cervicitis refers to the inflammation of the uterine cervix and represents an early, and sometimes subclinical, stage of PID. When present, symptoms may include pelvic pressure and/or pain, vaginal discharge and postcoital bleeding. If appreciable, CT findings include an enlarged oedematous uterine cervix, an overly enhancing endocervical canal, occasionally with complex fluid inside, parametrial and mesorectal fat stranding. Peritoneal effusion in the posterior cul-de-sac may occasionally be seen. Multiple round cystic alterations, centrally located within the cervix, characterize cystic cervicitis, a distinct form of infectious cervicitis.

As regards differential diagnosis, the integrity of the cervical stroma allows us to distinguish cervicitis from cervical cancer [28, 29].

21.4.3.2 Endometritis

Endometritis represents the inflammation of the endometrial mucosa and may likewise have a subclinical course. Endometritis is more often diagnosed during pregnancy or puerperium, whereas in nonpregnant patients, its main causes are PID and invasive diagnostic and therapeutic gynecologic procedures.

CT findings of endometritis encompass an enlarged uterus, fluid-filled endometrial cavity, abnormal endometrial enhancement (exceeding that of the surrounding inner myometrium) and indistinct uterine borders (Fig. 21.1). In milder cases, the endometrium may show a normal appearance as well [21, 28–30].

Uterine empyema (pyometra) refers to the distension of the uterine cavity by purulent content. It usually represents a chronic form of endometritis and can have various causes such as endometrial polyps, factors resulting in cervical stenosis and postsurgical infections. Pyometra mainly affects the postmenopausal population, in which incontinence is a risk factor to consider. At CT imaging uterine empyema presents with distention of the uterine cavity by complex fluid, with or without gas bubbles, fluid-fluid and air-fluid levels [29].

21.4.3.3 Salpingitis

Salpingitis is the early acute form of PID and is characterized by an inflammation of one or both fallopian tubes. At this stage, inflammation leads to oedema and congestion of the fallopian tube, whereas tubal distention is typically lacking.

At CT imaging the tube is thickened (axial diameter ≥5 mm) and shows mucosal enhancement; haziness of the pelvic fat and free fluid in the pouch of Douglas may also be observed (Fig. 21.2a and b). However, it must be remem-

Table 21.2 CT findings of PID [2, 4, 11, 17, 21, 28, 29]

Disease manifestation	CT findings
Cervicitis	Enlarged uterine cervix with overly enhancing endocervical canal
	parametrial fat stranding
Endometritis	Enlarged uterus
	Fluid-filled endometrial cavity
	Abnormal endometrial enhancement (more than the surrounding inner myometrium)
	Indistinct uterine borders
Salpingitis	Fallopian tube thickening (diameter ≥5 mm) with mucosal enhancement
	Haziness of the pelvic fat
Pyosalpinx (tubal empyema)	Fallopian tube dilatation (incomplete septa) with complex internal fluid
	Tubal wall thickening and enhancement
Oophoritis	Enlarged ovary (short axis diameter >3 cm) with polycystic appearance
	Iperenhancement of the ovary
	Periovarian oedema
Tubo-ovarian abscess	Uni/bilateral hypodense, multilocular, thick-walled complex adnexal mass
	Enhancing walls and internal septa
	Gas bubbles within the cystic loculations
	Thickening of pelvic ligaments
	Broad ligament anterior displacement
	Perivisceral fat stranding
	Hydroureteronephrosis
	Lymphadenopathies
Pelvic peritonitis	Peritoneal thickening and enhancement
	Intraperitoneal fluid collections (abscesses)
	Haziness/stranding of mesentery, greater omentum and mesosigma
	Fascial planes and pelvic ligaments thickening and enhancement
	Paralytic ileus
Fitz-Hugh–Curtis syndrome	Liver capsule thickening and enhancement
	Arterial phase subglissonian enhancement disappearing in subsequent phases
	Free/loculated perihepatic fluid
	Perihepatic peritoneal septa
	Periportal oedema
	Fluid along the right paracolic gutter
	Gallbladder wall thickening
Ovarian vein thrombophlebitis	Dilated ovarian vein (mainly right) with hypodense central filling defects
	Perivascular fat stranding
Hydrosalpinx	Fallopian tube dilatation with fluid-attenuation content
	No tubal wall thickening/enhancement
Haematosalpinx	Fallopian tube dilatation with high attenuation content (>30 HU)
	No tubal wall thickening/enhancement

bered that, at a very early stage, the fallopian tube may also show a normal appearance at diagnostic imaging methods. If left untreated, tubal inflammation may lead to intra- and peri-tubal adhesions. Adhesions, in turn, may cause, acutely, the evolution to the stage of tubal empyema, or result in chronic sequelae such as infertility and ectopic pregnancy [13, 29].

21.4.3.4 Pyosalpinx (or Tubal Empyema)

Pyosalpinx represents the next stage of PID after salpingitis; it occurs when the infection gets further complicated by the obstruction of the tubal lumen and is characterized by the distension of the lumen by purulent content.

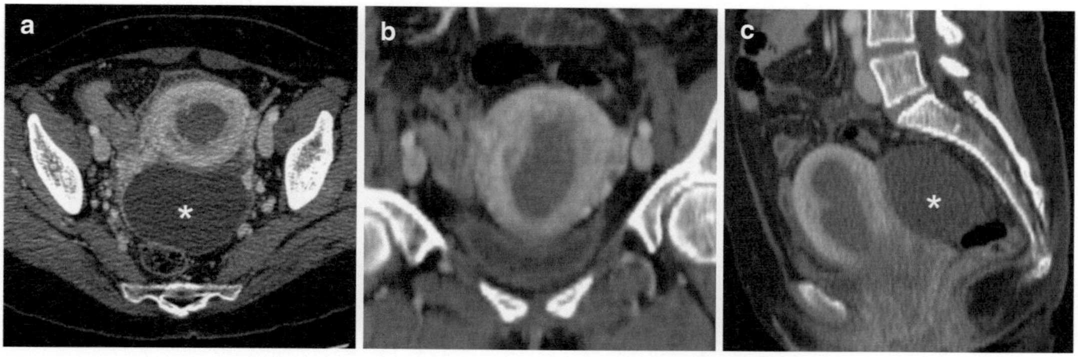

Fig. 21.1 Endometritis. Axial (**a**), coronal (**b**) and sagittal (**c**) contrast-enhanced CT images of the pelvis showing inhomogeneous contrast enhancement of the myometrium and markedly dilated uterine cavity filled by heterogeneous fluid. Associated effusion with thin serosal hyperenhancement in the pelvic cul-de-sac consistent with loculated peritonitis (*). (Adapted from: Foti et al. [30], licensed under CC-BY 4)

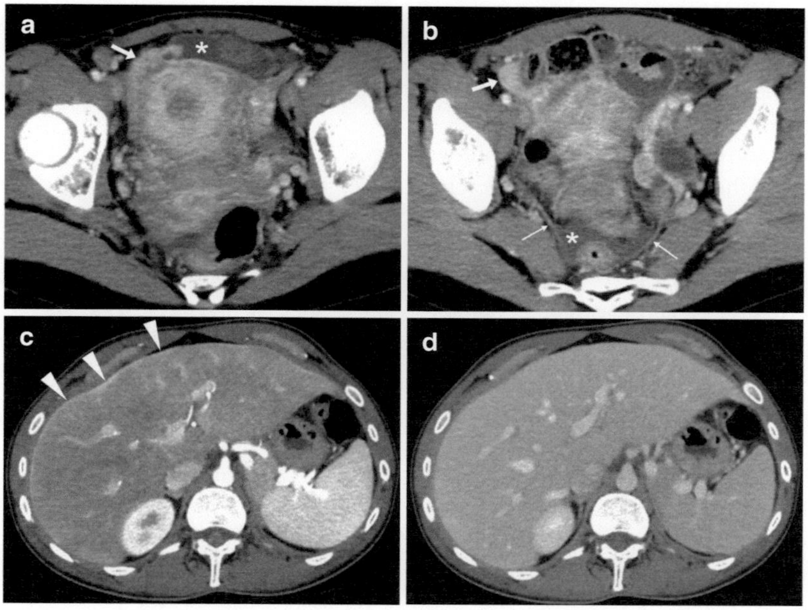

Fig. 21.2 Salpingitis-related Fitz-Hugh-Curtis syndrome in a 37-year-old woman with acute pelvic pain, right hypochondrial pain, severe constipation and leucocytosis. Axial contrast-enhanced CT images of the pelvis (**a** and **b**) show thickening and enhancement of the right fallopian tube (arrows), a finding consistent with acute salpingitis. A fluid collection (* in **a**) adjacent to the right tube and free fluid in the pouch of Douglas (* in **b**) are easily detectable. Note the mild thickening and enhancement of the parietal peritoneum of the pelvic sidewall (thin arrows in **b**). Arterial phase CT image of the upper abdomen (**c**) demonstrates thickening and enhancement of the liver capsule and of the underlying subglissonian parenchyma (arrowheads), that disappear in the subsequent portal-venous phase (**d**). (Courtesy of Dr. Giovanni Scavone and Dr. Andrea Conti, Department of Diagnostic Radiology, "Garibaldi Centro" Hospital, Catania, Italy)

At CT imaging the typical finding is represented by a tortuous dilated tubular juxtauterine mass, distended by complex internal fluid, with thickening and noticeable enhancement of the tubal walls (Fig. 21.3). Other nonspecific signs of PID, such as pelvic effusion, thickening of the uterosacral ligaments and oedema of the perivisceral fat may be seen as well [11, 29].

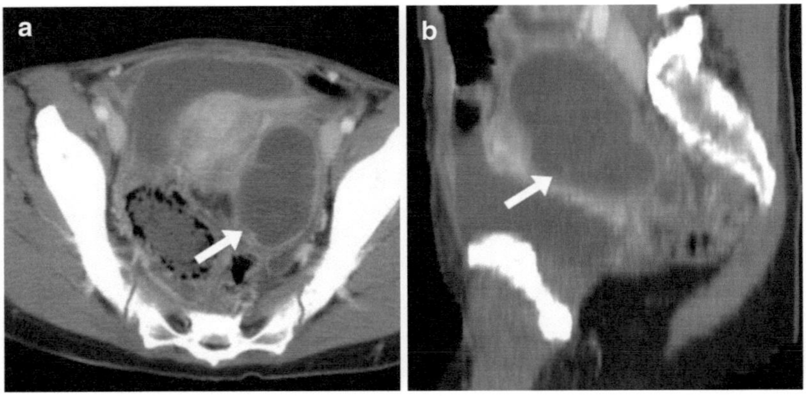

Fig. 21.3 Surgically proven pyosalpinx. Axial (**a**) and sagittal (**b**) contrast-enhanced CT images of the pelvis showing markedly dilated left-sided fallopian tube (arrows) filled by heterogeneous fluid, with enhancing, moderately thickened walls

21.4.3.5 Oophoritis

Oophoritis, described as inflammation of one or both ovaries, is almost always associated with salpingitis and pyosalpinx since it occurs when inflammation and infection spread by contiguity from the fallopian tubes to the ovaries.

CT findings of oophoritis are as follows: enlarged ovary (short axis diameter >3 cm), oedema and hyperemia of the ovarian stroma, the polycystic-like appearance of the ovary (multiple follicles with a diameter of 2–10 mm), iperenhancement of the ovary and periovarian oedema (Fig. 21.4).

The main differential diagnosis of oophoritis is with ovarian torsion because of a certain amount of overlap in the imaging findings, in particular the oedema of the ovarian stroma [28, 29].

Adnexal torsion is a gynecologic emergency that occurs when the ovary, the fallopian tube or both twist, partially or completely, on their vascular pedicle. Although possible at any age, adnexal torsion usually occurs in women of reproductive age, in which a benign ovarian mass (>5 cm), such as a large cyst or a mature cystic teratoma, serves as a lead point for torsion. Abrupt-onset lower quadrant pain is the most common clinical presentation, although intermittent pain may also be observed, likely due to torsion and detorsion; nonspecific symptoms such as nausea and vomiting often coexist. The right side is more involved due to the contralateral protection provided by the sigmoid colon. CT findings of ovarian torsion include: unilaterally enlarged edematous ovary (diameter >5 cm), ipsilateral uterine deviation, wall thickening of an adnexal mass, dilated enhancing ovarian blood vessels, periovarian fat stranding and free fluid in the cul-de-sac (Fig. 21.5). The pathognomonic twisted pedicle, containing the thickened fallopian tube, may demonstrate either a spiral configuration or a solid-like appearance (Fig. 21.5b and c). If torsion persists over time, then haemorrhagic alterations occur in the form of hyperattenuating areas; at this late stage, adnexal contrast enhancement may be minimal or absent [24, 31].

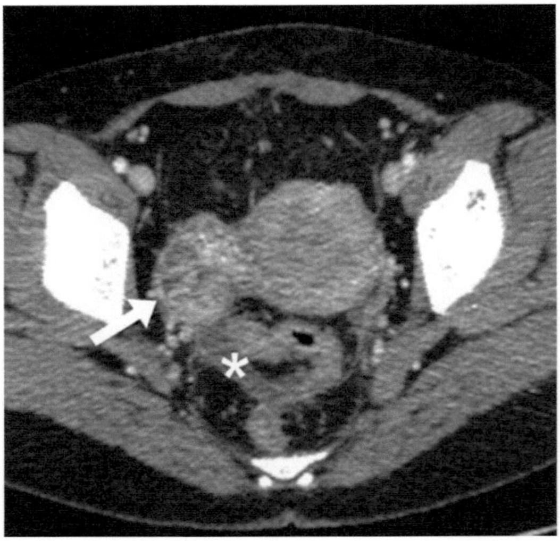

Fig. 21.4 Oophoritis. Axial contrast-enhanced CT image showing a heterogeneously enhancing, unilaterally enlarged right ovary (arrow). Note minimal fluid (*) in the pelvic cul-de-sac. Findings were consistent with clinical outcome of uncomplicated PID. (Adapted from: Foti et al. [30], licensed under CC-BY 4.0)

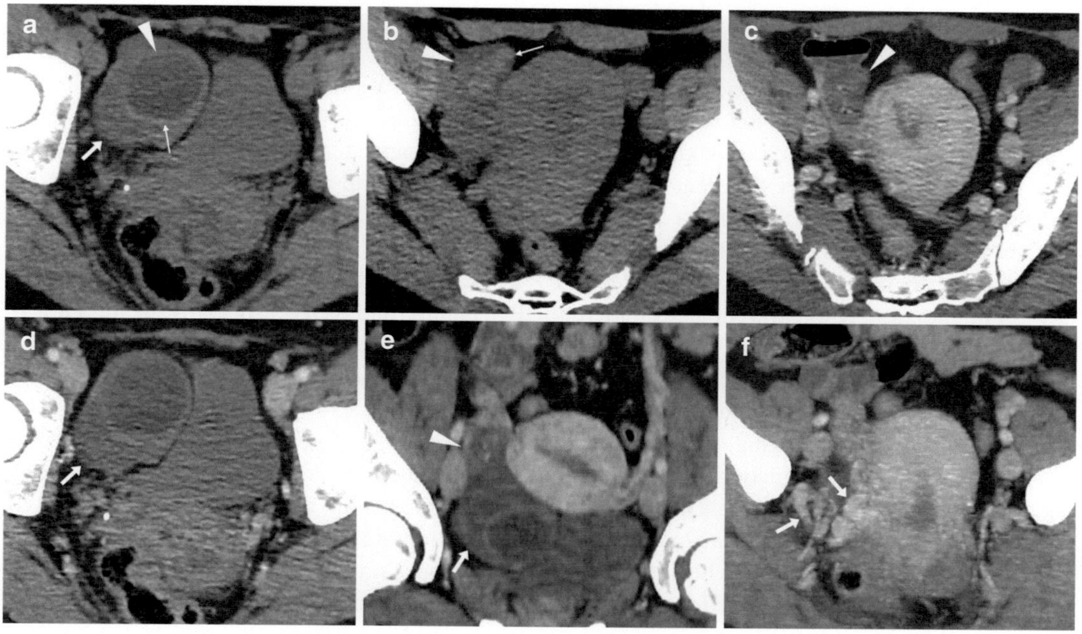

Fig. 21.5 Adnexal torsion in a 43-year-old woman with acute pelvic pain and vomiting. Axial plain CT image of the pelvis (**a**) demonstrates an enlarged (diameter 7 cm) edematous right ovary (arrow) with a unilocular cyst (diameter 5 cm) (arrowhead). Note the thin peripheral hyperdense rim (thin arrow). Axial plain CT image (**b**) (obtained cranial to a) shows a solid component in the cranial part of the adnexa (arrowhead) adjacent to the uterus, likely representing the twisted pedicle. Note, here too, the slightly hyperdense area (thin arrow). Axial contrast-enhanced CT scans (**c**, **d**) and coronal reformatted CT image (**e**) display minimal contrast enhancement of both the right ovary (arrows in **d** and **e**) and the twisted pedicle (arrowheads in **c** and **e**). Oblique coronal MIP image (**f**) showing dilated enhancing blood vessels along the right margin of the uterus (arrows)

21.4.3.6 Tubo-ovarian Abscess (TOA)

Tubo-ovarian abscess represents a late complication of PID and complicates about 10–34% of hospitalized cases of PID [13, 29, 31]. At this stage, the fallopian tube and ovary cannot be clearly and separately identified at imaging, due to the loss of fat planes between the adnexa and adjacent pelvic structures, and the subversion of normal ovarian parenchyma as a result of necrotic alterations; the mass may be uni- or bilateral.

CT findings of TOA include a low-attenuation multilocular cystic complex adnexal mass with thickened and strikingly enhancing walls and internal septa (Fig. 21.6), thickening of pelvic ligaments, extensive adjacent fat stranding and fluid in the cul-de-sac. The occasional finding of gas bubbles within the mass can suggest the anaerobic source of the infection, but may also indicate a fistulization to the gastrointestinal tract. Anterior displacement of the ipsilateral broad ligament (Fig. 21.6), due to the posterior

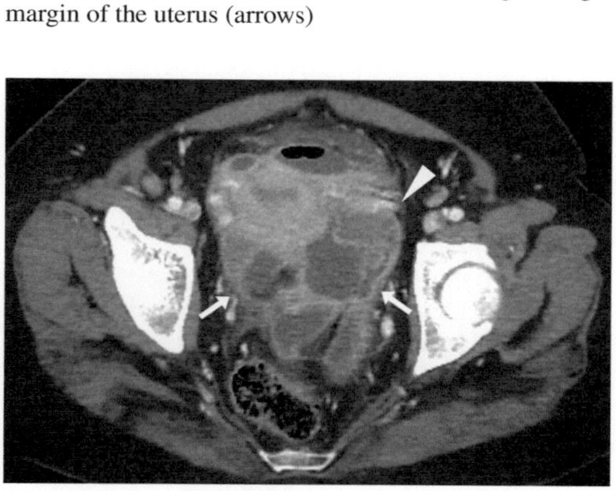

Fig. 21.6 Tubo-ovarian abscesses in a 48-year-old woman with intellectual disability and history of sexual abuse. Contrast-enhanced CT scan demonstrates bilateral low-attenuation multilocular cystic complex adnexal masses bordered by thickened and enhancing walls, with internal septa (arrows). Note the anterior displacement of the left uterine vessels contained in the ipsilateral broad ligament (arrowhead), representing an important diagnostic finding of TOA

location of the mesovarium, may often be seen and represents a useful diagnostic sign to discriminate a TOA from a pelvic abscess from other sources (appendix, colon and less often bladder) in which this finding is lacking; in addition, pelvic abscesses of a different origin are located farther away from the adnexa and generally show thicker walls. Hydroureteronephrosis, abdominal abscesses (secondary to rupture) and bowel inflammation with paralytic ileus may further complicate TOAs.

In the presence of ascites and lymphadenopathies, distinguishing a TOA from an ovarian epithelial tumor may be challenging, nevertheless in ovarian malignancies tubal dilation is usually missing; in addition, an appropriate clinical history may address towards a correct diagnosis [2, 11, 27–32].

TOA is among the criteria for hospitalization in women with PID (Table 21.3). Drainage of TOA can be performed through laparotomy, laparoscopy or image-guided percutaneous access. Indications for surgical drainage include: ineffectiveness of antibiotic therapy within 48–72 h, persistent fever, persistent/increasing leucocytosis and an increase in the size of the abscess [1, 30].

Table 21.3 Criteria for hospitalization in women with PID [1]

Criteria for hospitalization in women with PID
Impossibility to rule out surgical emergencies (i.e. appendicitis)
Pregnancy
Ineffectiveness of oral antibiotic therapy
Inability to follow or tolerate an outpatient oral antibiotic treatment
Severe illness, nausea/vomiting, high fever
Tubo-ovarian abscess

21.4.3.7 Peritonitis

Pyosalpinx and TOA, especially in the case of rupture with leakage of pus into the peritoneal cavity, may lead to peritonitis, a life-threatening emergency.

CT findings of peritonitis include thickening and enhancement of parietal and visceral peritoneum, thickening and enhancement of pelvic and abdominal fascial planes, intraperitoneal collections, fat stranding of the mesentery, greater omentum and mesosigma, inflammatory changes of the bowel wall and paralytic ileus (Fig. 21.7). Pleural effusion and systemic symptoms, such as respiratory distress may also be observed [28, 29].

21.4.3.8 Fitz–Hugh–Curtis Syndrome (Perihepatitis)

Fitz–Hugh–Curtis syndrome, also called perihepatitis, is a complication of PID, caused by the spread of pelvic infection through the clockwise peritoneal circulation along the right paracolic gutter toward the ipsilateral upper abdominal

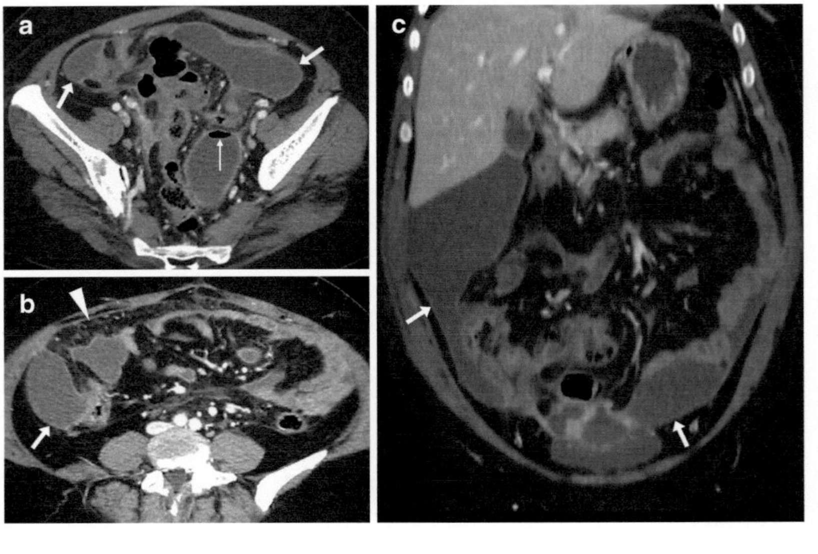

Fig. 21.7 TOA-related peritonitis in a 48-year-old woman. The same patient as in Fig. 21.6. Axial contrast-enhanced CT scans (**a** and **b**) and coronal reformatted CT image (**c**) show multiple abdominal intraperitoneal collections (abscesses) (arrows). Note the gas bubble within the pelvic abscess (thin arrow in **a**). Also of note is the thickening and fat stranding of the greater omentum (arrowhead in **b**)

quadrant. It is characterized by an inflammation of the liver peritoneal capsule and perihepatic adhesions. Perihepatitis clinically manifests with sudden onset of right hypochondrial pain and tenderness (positive Murphy's sign), exacerbated with deep inhalation and movement, sometimes associated with right shoulder pain; on the basis of clinical presentation, the differential diagnosis includes pneumonia, pleuritis and mainly cholecystitis. Pelvic symptoms are often minimal or even absent, making the diagnosis more difficult.

CT findings of Fitz–Hugh–Curtis syndrome encompass thickening and enhancement of the liver capsule, subglissonian and periportal areas of enhancement in the arterial phase disappearing in subsequent phases, free and/or loculated perihepatic fluid, periportal oedema, fat stranding and fluid along the right paracolic gutter, gallbladder wall thickening and peritoneal septa in the form of typical "violin string" adhesions connecting the liver capsule with the anterior abdominal wall (Figs. 21.2c–d and 21.8). The arterial phase subglissonian enhancement (a perfusion related pseudolesion or transient hepatic attenuation differences THAD), albeit characteristic, is not pathognomonic of Fitz-Hugh-Curtis syndrome, being also observable in other clinical conditions such as acute cholecystitis, cholelithiasis, cholangitis, liver abscess, congenital hepatic fibrosis, acute pancreatitis, appendicitis, peritonitis, peritoneal carcinomatosis, superior vena cava

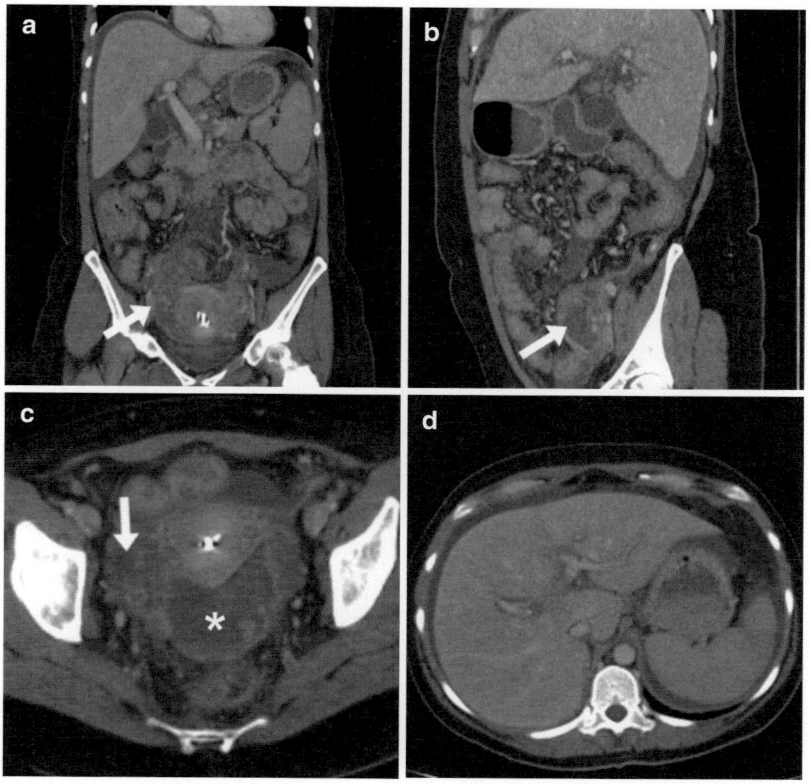

Fig. 21.8 PID-associated Fitz-Hugh-Curtis syndrome. Panoramic coronal (**a**) and sagittal (**b**) contrast-enhanced CT images showing moderate multi-compartmental ascitic fluid, median medium-sized uterus with intracavitary metal IUD. In the pelvis, sagittal (**b**) and axial (**c**) images show a sizeable, predominantly fluid-attenuating right parauterine structure with enhancing walls (arrows), and pelvic cul-de-sac effusion with enhancing walls (* in **c**). Additionally, in axial portal venous phase image (**d**) inhomogeneous liver perfusion with periportal oedema was noted. Urgent surgery confirmed peritonitis from PID including right-sided pyosalpinx, treated with salpingo-oophorectomy. (Adapted from Tonolini M. EuroRAD Case 10,088. Severe pelvic inflammatory disease with peritonitis as a complication of IUD positioning in an HIV-infected woman)

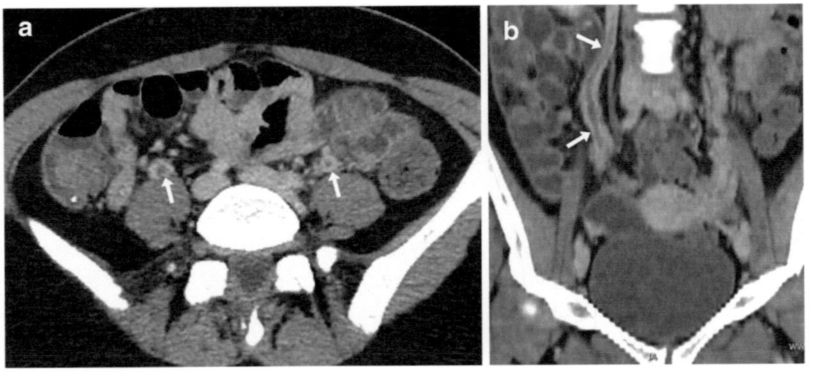

Fig. 21.9 Ovarian vein thrombophlebitis with bilateral involvement in a 47-year-old woman with vomiting, fever and epigastric pain. Axial portal venous phase CT scan (**a**) shows dilated right and left ovarian veins with hypodense central filling defects within the vessel lumen (arrows). Coronal reformatted CT image (**b**) demonstrates the thrombus inside the right ovarian vein in its full longitudinal extension (arrows)

obstruction. Therefore, a thorough patient history and careful physical examination are key to diagnosing this clinically challenging condition, that should be suspected in sexually active women with right hypochondrial pain. However, it should not be forgotten that Fitz–Hugh–Curtis syndrome, albeit rarely, may occur also in male patients [2, 17, 28, 29, 33–35].

21.4.3.9 Ovarian Vein Thrombophlebitis

Ovarian vein (syn. gonadal vein) thrombophlebitis may represent a complication of PID. This condition is fostered by inflammation, insufficient blood flow, heightened blood coagulation and vein compression. Risk factors other than PID include pregnancy, puerperium, estrogen therapy, malignancy, thrombophilia, recent surgery and hospitalization. The right ovarian vein is most involved (80–90% of cases), whereas the left ovarian vein and bilateral ovarian vein involvement are reported in 6% and 14% of cases, respectively. The predilection for the right ovarian vein may be due to the anterograde direction of the blood flow on the right side, which fosters bacterial infection, conversely from the retrograde bloodstream in the left ovarian vein. Clinically, ovarian vein thrombophlebitis may manifest with pain in lower abdominal quadrants, generally on the affected side, sometimes radiating to the flank or groin; hematuria has been reported as well.

CT findings encompass a dilated ovarian vein with wall enhancement, hypodense central filling defects within the vessel lumen and tortuous collateral veins; perivascular fat stranding and free fluid may also be seen (Fig. 21.9). If misdiagnosed and untreated, ovarian vein thrombophlebitis is life-threatening because of the risk of septic pulmonary embolism (3–33% of the cases) [28, 29, 36, 37].

21.4.3.10 Chronic PID (Hydrosalpinx)

Hydrosalpinx is defined as a serous fluid-filled dilatation of the fallopian tube due to fimbrial obstruction. Adhesions resulting from prior episodes of PID are the main cause of hydrosalpinx, this latter indeed may represent the evolution of a pyosalpinx after proteolysis of pus induced by antibiotic treatment.

CT findings of hydrosalpinx include a dilated, tortuous fluid-attenuation tubular juxtauterine structure, anatomically distinct from the ovary, bounded by a subtle nonenhancing, nonhyperemic wall. When the long axis of the fallopian tube is perpendicular to the scan plane and the longitudinal folds of the tube are thickened, the pathognomonic "cogwheel" appearance of hydrosalpinx can be observed.

The term haematosalpinx indicates a dilatation of the fallopian tubes by blood products. Haematosalpinx is associated with endometriosis, ectopic pregnancy, malignancy, PID, adnexal torsion and trauma. At CT imaging the tubal content demonstrates high attenuation (>30 HU) reflecting the presence of haemorrhagic fluid. In noninfectious haematosalpinx and hydrosalpinx the fallopian tube wall is thin with slight or no enhancement, conversely from the thickened and briskly enhancing tubal wall of pyosalpinx [2, 11, 24, 28–30].

21.5 Sequelae

Clinical sequelae of PID encompass greater risk of recurrent infection, ectopic pregnancy, tubal factor infertility and chronic pelvic pain (defined as menstrual/nonmenstrual pain lasting for at least 6 months) [1]. PID represents the most common cause of distal tubal obstruction; it is estimated that a previous PID is responsible for about 30–40% of cases of infertility and 50% of cases of ectopic pregnancy [5, 11]. In particular, the likelihood of tubal factor infertility increases with the number of episodes of PID: 8%, 20% and 40% of patients after one, two and three episodes respectively [3].

In addition, it should be noted that an association has been found between clinical history of PID and increased risk of some histotypes of epithelial ovarian cancer (serous epithelial ovarian cancer, high-grade serous carcinoma and clear cell carcinoma), thus confirming the role of chronic inflammation in the oncogenic process [38].

References

1. Soper DE. Pelvic inflammatory disease. Obstet Gynecol. 2010;116(2 Pt 1):419–28. https://doi.org/10.1097/AOG.0b013e3181e92c54.
2. Rezvani M, Shaaban AM. Fallopian tube disease in the nonpregnant patient. Radiographics. 2011;31(2):527–48. https://doi.org/10.1148/rg.312105090.
3. Sam JW, Jacobs JE, Birnbaum BA. Spectrum of CT findings in acute pyogenic pelvic inflammatory disease. Radiographics. 2002;22(6):1327–34. https://doi.org/10.1148/rg.226025062.
4. Curry A, Williams T, Penny ML. Pelvic Inflammatory Disease: Diagnosis, Management, and Prevention. Am Fam Physician. 2019;100(6):357–64.
5. Thomassin-Naggara I, Perrot N, Salem C, Marsault C, Bazot M. Pathologie tubaire. EMC Encyclopédie Médico-Chirurgicale (Elsevier SAS, Paris); 2006. Radiodiagnostic – Urologie-Gynécologie, 34–610-A-10
6. Rodrigues R, Vieira-Baptista P, Catalão C, Borrego MJ, Sousa C, Vale N. Chlamydial and gonococcal genital infections: a narrative review. J Pers Med. 2023;13(7):1170. https://doi.org/10.3390/jpm13071170.
7. WHO. Sexually Transmitted Infections (STIs). Available online: https://www.who.int/news-room/fact-sheets/detail/sexually-transmitted-infections-(stis). Accessed on 18 March 2024.
8. Kreisel K, Flagg EW, Torrone E. Trends in pelvic inflammatory disease emergency department visits, United States, 2006–2013. Am J Obstet Gynecol. 2018;218(1):117.e1–117.e10. https://doi.org/10.1016/j.ajog.2017.10.010.
9. Lillis R, Kuritzky L, Huynh Z, Arcenas R, Hansra A, Shah R, Yang B, Taylor SN. Outpatient sexually transmitted infection testing and treatment patterns in the United States: a real-world database study. BMC Infect Dis. 2023;23(1):469. https://doi.org/10.1186/s12879-023-08434-2.
10. Brun JL, Castan B, de Barbeyrac B, Cazanave C, Charvériat A, Faure K, Mignot S, Verdon R, Fritel X, Graesslin O, CNGOF; SPILF. Pelvic inflammatory diseases: updated French guidelines. J Gynecol Obstet Hum Reprod. 2020;49(5):101714. https://doi.org/10.1016/j.jogoh.2020.101714.
11. Revzin MV, Moshiri M, Katz DS, Pellerito JS, Mankowski Gettle L, Menias CO. Imaging evaluation of fallopian tubes and related disease: a primer for radiologists. Radiographics. 2020;40(5):1473–501. https://doi.org/10.1148/rg.2020200051.
12. Kim HY, Yang JI, Moon C. Comparison of severe pelvic inflammatory disease, pyosalpinx and tubo-ovarian abscess. J Obstet Gynaecol Res. 2015;41(5):742–6. https://doi.org/10.1111/jog.12617.
13. Paik CK, Waetjen LE, Xing G, Dai J, Sweet RL. Hospitalizations for pelvic inflammatory disease and tuboovarian abscess. Obstet Gynecol. 2006;107(3):611–6. https://doi.org/10.1097/01.AOG.0000200595.92385.07.
14. Wira CR, Fahey JV, Rodriguez-Garcia M, Shen Z, Patel MV. Regulation of mucosal immunity in the female reproductive tract: the role of sex hormones in immune protection against sexually transmitted pathogens. Am J Reprod Immunol. 2014;72(2):236–58. https://doi.org/10.1111/aji.12252.
15. Allsworth JE, Peipert JF. Prevalence of bacterial vaginosis: 2001–2004 National Health and Nutrition Examination Survey data. Obstet Gynecol. 2007;109(1):114–20. https://doi.org/10.1097/01.AOG.0000247627.84791.91.
16. Ravel J, Moreno I, Simón C. Bacterial vaginosis and its association with infertility, endometritis, and pelvic inflammatory disease. Am J Obstet Gynecol.

2021;224(3):251–7. https://doi.org/10.1016/j.ajog.2020.10.019.

17. Franco PN, García-Baizán A, Aymerich M, Maino C, Frade-Santos S, Ippolito D, Otero-García M. Gynaecological causes of acute pelvic pain: common and not-so-common imaging findings. Life (Basel). 2023;13(10):2025. https://doi.org/10.3390/life13102025.
18. Workowski KA, Bachmann LH, Chan PA, et al. Sexually transmitted infections treatment guidelines, 2021. MMWR Recomm Rep. 2021;70(RR-4):1–187. https://doi.org/10.15585/mmwr.rr7004a1.
19. Terao M, Koga K, Fujimoto A, Wada-Hiraike O, Osuga Y, Yano T, Kozuma S. Factors that predict poor clinical course among patients hospitalized with pelvic inflammatory disease. J Obstet Gynaecol Res. 2014;40(2):495–500. https://doi.org/10.1111/jog.12189.
20. Gaitán H, Angel E, Diaz R, Parada A, Sanchez L, Vargas C. Accuracy of five different diagnostic techniques in mild-to-moderate pelvic inflammatory disease. Infect Dis Obstet Gynecol. 2002;10(4):171–80. https://doi.org/10.1155/S1064744902000194.
21. Jung SI, Kim YJ, Park HS, Jeon HJ, Jeong KA. Acute pelvic inflammatory disease: diagnostic performance of CT. J Obstet Gynaecol Res. 2011;37(3):228–35. https://doi.org/10.1111/j.1447-0756.2010.01380.x.
22. Okazaki Y, Tsujimoto Y, Yamada K, Ariie T, Taito S, Banno M, Kataoka Y, Tsukizawa Y. Diagnostic accuracy of pelvic imaging for acute pelvic inflammatory disease in an emergency care setting: a systematic review and meta-analysis. Acute Med Surg. 2022;9(1):e806. https://doi.org/10.1002/ams2.806.
23. Li W, Zhang Y, Cui Y, Zhang P, Wu X. Pelvic inflammatory disease: evaluation of diagnostic accuracy with conventional MR with added diffusion-weighted imaging. Abdom Imaging. 2013;38(1):193–200. https://doi.org/10.1007/s00261-012-9896-0.
24. Tonolini M, Foti PV, Costanzo V, Mammino L, Palmucci S, Cianci A, Ettorre GC, Basile A. Cross-sectional imaging of acute gynaecologic disorders: CT and MRI findings with differential diagnosis-part I: corpus luteum and haemorrhagic ovarian cysts, genital causes of haemoperitoneum and adnexal torsion. Insights Imaging. 2019;10(1):119. https://doi.org/10.1186/s13244-019-0808-5.
25. Zanardo M, Doniselli FM, Esseridou A, Agrò M, Panarisi NAR, Monti CB, Di Leo G, Sardanelli F. Lean body weight versus total body weight to calculate the iodinated contrast media volume in abdominal CT: a randomised controlled trial. Insights Imaging. 2020;11(1):132. https://doi.org/10.1186/s13244-020-00920-4.
26. Yitta S, Hecht EM, Mausner EV, Bennett GL. Normal or abnormal? Demystifying uterine and cervical contrast enhancement at multidetector CT. Radiographics. 2011;31(3):647–61. https://doi.org/10.1148/rg.313105057.
27. Bennett GL, Slywotzky CM, Giovanniello G. Gynecologic causes of acute pelvic pain: spectrum of CT findings. Radiographics. 2002;22(4):785–801. https://doi.org/10.1148/radiographics.22.4.g02jl18785.
28. Revzin MV, Mathur M, Dave HB, Macer ML, Spektor M. Pelvic inflammatory disease: multimodality imaging approach with clinical-pathologic correlation. Radiographics. 2016;36(5):1579–96. https://doi.org/10.1148/rg.2016150202.
29. Shibuki S, Saida T, Hoshiai S, Ishiguro T, Sakai M, Amano T, Abe T, Yoshida M, Mori K, Nakajima T. Imaging findings in inflammatory disease of the genital organs. Jpn J Radiol. 2024;42(4):331–46. https://doi.org/10.1007/s11604-023-01518-8.
30. Foti PV, Tonolini M, Costanzo V, Mammino L, Palmucci S, Cianci A, Ettorre GC, Basile A. Cross-sectional imaging of acute gynaecologic disorders: CT and MRI findings with differential diagnosis-part II: uterine emergencies and pelvic inflammatory disease. Insights Imaging. 2019;10(1):118. https://doi.org/10.1186/s13244-019-0807-6.
31. Iraha Y, Okada M, Iraha R, Azama K, Yamashiro T, Tsubakimoto M, Aoki Y, Murayama S. CT and MR imaging of gynecologic emergencies. Radiographics. 2017;37(5):1569–86. https://doi.org/10.1148/rg.2017160170.
32. Potter AW, Chandrasekhar CA. US and CT evaluation of acute pelvic pain of gynecologic origin in nonpregnant premenopausal patients. Radiographics. 2008;28(6):1645–59. https://doi.org/10.1148/rg.286085504.
33. Shibata J, Ofuchi Y, Yonezawa N. Fitz-Hugh-Curtis syndrome: the diagnostic role of the arterial phase CT scan. BMJ Case Rep. 2023;16(9):e257417. https://doi.org/10.1136/bcr-2023-257417.
34. Joo SH, Kim MJ, Lim JS, Kim JH, Kim KW. CT diagnosis of Fitz-Hugh and Curtis syndrome: value of the arterial phase scan. Korean J Radiol. 2007;8(1):40–7. https://doi.org/10.3348/kjr.2007.8.1.40.
35. Ramanathan S, Raghu V, Virmani V, Sheikh A, Al Heidous M, Tirumani S. Unveiling the unreal: comprehensive imaging review of hepatic pseudolesions. Clin Imaging. 2021;80:439–53. https://doi.org/10.1016/j.clinimag.2021.09.008.
36. Arora E, Mujumdar V, Martin A, Tuli S. Ovarian vein thrombosis in a non-puerperal patient. Eur J Case Rep Intern Med. 2022;9(5):003351. https://doi.org/10.12890/2022_003351.
37. Setia A, Adili F, Ludwig K, Herold J. Acute abdominal pain as a result of an isolated left ovarian vein thrombosis. Case Rep Med. 2023;2023:9528088. https://doi.org/10.1155/2023/9528088.
38. Jonsson S, Jonsson H, Lundin E, Häggström C, Idahl A. Pelvic inflammatory disease and risk of epithelial ovarian cancer: a national population-based case-control study in Sweden. Am J Obstet Gynecol. 2024;230(1):75.e1–75.e15. https://doi.org/10.1016/j.ajog.2023.09.094.

22 Pelvic Hemorrhagic Diseases

Francesco Giurazza, Pietro Roccatagliata, Claudio Carrubba, Fabio Corvino, and Raffaella Niola

22.1 Introduction

Spontaneous pelvic hemorrhage is defined as the presence of intra-abdominal bleeding without a traumatic cause. This condition is rare but can be catastrophic if not promptly diagnosed and treated. It may present with severe pelvic pain and distension, a decreased hematocrit level, or, more rarely, hypovolemic shock [1]. However, these signs might not always be present or may be ambiguous, and the hematocrit level in an initial serum sample may not accurately reflect the severity of the bleeding [2]. Common sources of spontaneous abdomino-pelvic hemorrhage include visceral (gastrointestinal), gynecologic, and vascular diseases [3, 4]. As with traumatic hemoperitoneum, it is crucial to identify any active bleeding in cases of nontraumatic hemoperitoneum. Radiological imaging plays a pivotal role in this scenario; while ultrasound is the first line examination and allows mainly for fluid detection suggesting bleeding, contrast-enhanced Computed Tomography allows detailed detection of the site of bleeding and identification of the feeding vessels. If active bleeding is detected, conservative management should be abandoned in favor of surgical or endovascular intervention. Once active bleeding has been excluded, a thorough search for the source of the hemoperitoneum should be conducted [3].

F. Giurazza (✉) · C. Carrubba · F. Corvino · R. Niola
Vascular and Interventional Radiology Department, AORN "A. Cardarelli", Naples, Italy
e-mail: francesco.giurazza@aocardarelli.it; claudio.carrubba@aocardarelli.it; fabio.corvino@aocardarelli.it; raffaella.niola@aocardarelli.it

P. Roccatagliata
Department of Precision Medicine, University of Campania "L. Vanvitelli", Naples, Italy

22.2 Role of Radiology in Pelvic Hemorrhage

Identifying and localizing the source of acute pelvic hemorrhage is one of the primary challenges during the early diagnostic phase of acute intraperitoneal bleeding. This is crucial for providing timely hemostasis via transarterial embolization or surgery. Radiologists play an increasingly significant role in diagnosing and treating pelvic hemorrhage. Several imaging techniques are now available to identify the source of bleeding, including ultrasound (US), computed tomography (CT) with intravenous contrast (IVC), and dual-energy CT [5, 6].

22.2.1 Ultrasound

This is the initial imaging technique, particularly useful for unstable patients or when

L. Romano et al. (eds.), *CT of Non-Traumatic Body Emergencies*,
https://doi.org/10.1007/978-3-031-84849-0_22

abdominal bleeding of gynecological origin is suspected [5, 6]. Haemoperitoneum may appear non-specific on US and can be hypoechoic, isoechoic, or hyperechoic. It might also present as heterogeneous collections or with a fluid-fluid level. If haemoperitoneum is hypoechoic, it can be indistinguishable from ascites. The presence of clots (grouped echogenic content) near an organ can help pinpoint the bleeding source. However, US has limitations as it cannot detect active bleeding or provide adequate acoustic windows to assess deep peritoneal and retroperitoneal spaces.

22.2.2 CT

CT is the technique of choice, offering high sensitivity and specificity in locating the hemorrhage, differentiating between arterial and venous origins, and enabling non-invasive vascular assessment. The standard protocol includes a basal acquisition and three contrast-enhanced phases extending from the diaphragm to the pubic symphysis. An additional late phase can be included if needed at the radiologist's discretion [5, 7]. Recently, dual-energy CT has been introduced as an essential tool in emergency radiology and it is particularly effective for detecting abdominal bleeding. It offers advantages such as eliminating the need for a baseline acquisition without contrast through virtual non-contrast reconstruction mapping, reducing scanning and radiation time. It also accurately assesses contrast extravasation and iodine quantification, thereby reducing the required dose of IVC.

22.3 CT and Blood Attenuation

The utility of CT for the detection of pelvic bleeding lies in its ability to depict the difference between low-attenuation fluid and blood, which has a higher attenuation. Attenuation measurements at CT can help differentiate among simple ascites, hematoma, urine, chyle, and active bleeding. Blood usually has higher measured attenuation than other body fluids; however, its attenuation may vary, and its CT appearance often depends on the age, extent, and location of the hemorrhage. The measured attenuation of clotted blood is 45–70 HU. The body attempts hemostasis by forming a blood clot at the site of injury. Thus, on CT images, the highest-attenuation hematoma, or sentinel clot, is closest to the site of bleeding, whereas lower-attenuation unclotted blood is located further from the source. The sentinel clot sign is useful for identifying the dominant source of hemoperitoneum in patients with multiple injuries from trauma and it also may be valuable in cases of nontraumatic hemoperitoneum. Active arterial extravasation of contrast material is depicted at CT with a measured attenuation value higher than that of free or clotted blood, a feature indicative of the presence of intravenous contrast material in the blood, progressively increasing during the acquisition phases.

22.4 Causes of Non-traumatic Pelvic Bleedings

Main etiologies of non-traumatic pelvic bleeding are intestinal, vascular and gynecologic diseases (Table 22.1).

Table 22.1 Main causes of non-traumatic pelvic bleedings and related CT findings

Main causes of non-traumatic pelvic bleedings	CT Findings
Intestinal (diverticulitis, hemorrhoid diseases)	Outpouching from a colonic parietal defect with hyperdense intraluminal contents that after contrast injection enlarge suggesting active bleeding; congestion of the rectal wall with diffuse parietal enhancement increasing in contrastographic phases
Vascular lesion (aneurysm or pseudoaneurysm of visceral artery)	Accumulation of contrast material within an apparent aneurysmal sac surrounded by high-attenuation free fluid
Gynecologic condition (ruptured ovarian cyst, ectopic or scar pregnancy, AVM uterine, HELLP syndrome)	Fluid with internal echogenicity or high attenuation around the uterus and adnexa; associated mixed- attenuation adnexal mass with a high-attenuation component or fluid-fluid level

22.4.1 Intestinal

Acute intestinal hemorrhage is a critical condition with a high mortality rate, which can reach up to 40% in cases of massive bleeding and even higher rates in elderly patients with comorbidities. These hemorrhages can be classified as either upper or lower based on their location, depending on whether they originate proximally or distally to the Treitz ligament. In 75% of cases, it is an upper gastrointestinal hemorrhage, presenting clinically with hematemesis or melena. The most common cause is peptic ulcer disease and in patients with portal hypertension, esophageal varices. Lower gastrointestinal bleeding, originating between the Treitz ligament and the rectum, accounts for approximately 25% of cases, presenting clinically with rectal bleeding and hematochezia. The main causes are diverticular and hemorrhoidal disease. Other causes include vascular lesions (such as colonic angiodysplasia), cancer, inflammatory colitis, infections, and benign ano-rectal lesions.

22.4.1.1 Diverticulitis

Acute colonic diverticulitis (ACD) is the most common complication of diverticular disease and represents an abdominal emergency. It includes a variety of conditions, extending from localized diverticular inflammation to intraperitoneal bleeding. Representing the diverticulum as an outpouching from a parietal defect from where the blood vessels penetrate, diverticular bleeding can be an occurrence (Figs. 22.1 and 22.2), more appreciable in chronic diverticulitis [8, 9]. On unenhanced CT, hyperdense intraluminal contents can suggest bleeding; after contrast medium, the presence of active contrast extravasation with enlarging contrast volume on the portal venous phase represents the finding of active bleeding.

22.4.1.2 Hemorrhoid Disease

HD is the most prevalent benign anorectal condition. The functional unit of hemorrhoids is the corpus cavernosum recti (CCR) (Figs. 22.3 and 22.4). The rectum receives blood supply from three primary arteries: the superior rectal artery (SRA), the middle rectal artery (MRA), and the

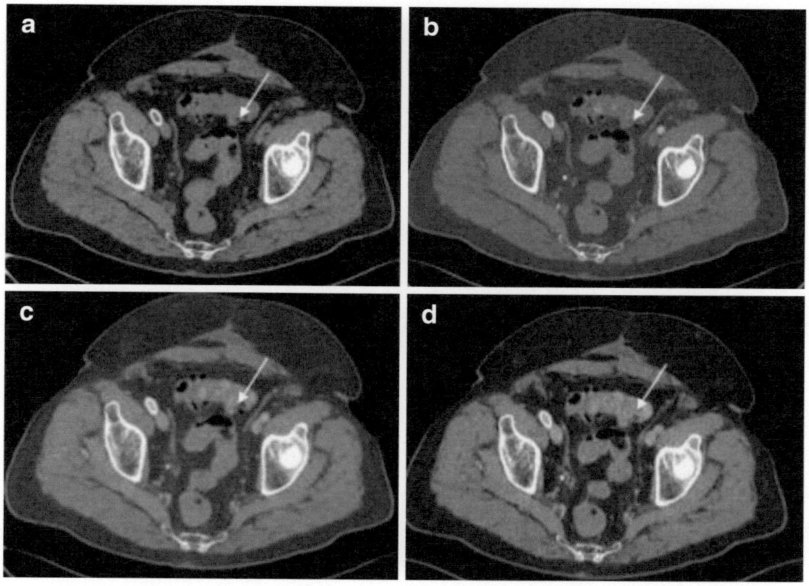

Fig. 22.1 84-year-old male, uptaking antiplatelet therapy because of right external iliac stenting, affected by bleeding diverticulitis. Axial CT scan: (**a**) basal acquisition showing sigmoidal diverticula (white arrow) with inner lumen full of isodense material, slightly hyperdense into the diverticula, suggesting blood material; arterial (**b**), venous (**c**) and delayed (**d**) phases showing intraluminal contrast extravasation (white arrows) with progressive intraluminal extravasation increase

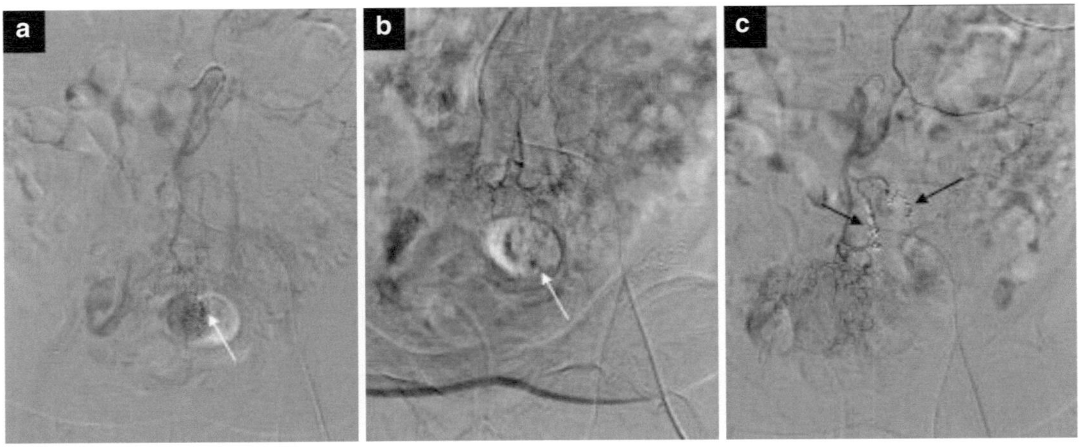

Fig. 22.2 Same patient as Fig. 22.1. An endovascular embolization approach was applied in this patient. (**a**) Diagnostic digital subtraction arteriography (DSA) from inferior mesenteric artery detecting contrast extravasation (white arrow) in the middle portion of sigma, corresponding to CT findings. (**b**) Superselective distal sigmoidal DSA confirming diverticular bleeding (white arrow). (**c**) DSA acquired after coils embolization (black arrows) showing bleeding disappearance

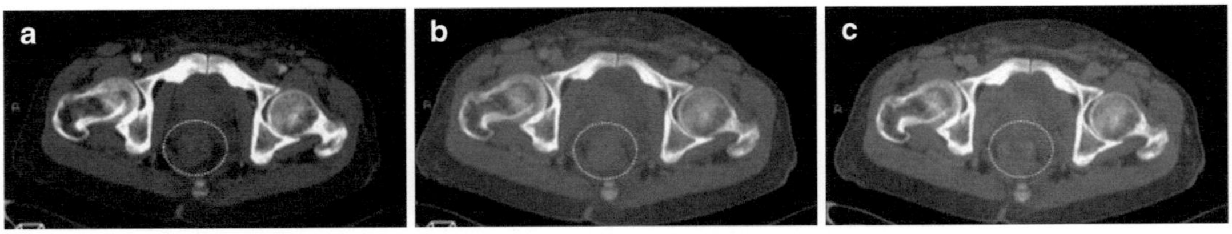

Fig. 22.3 64-year-old male, cirrhotic because of hepatitis virus beta infection, previously undergoing transjugular portosystemic shunt, affected by rectal variceal hemorrhoidal bleeding. Axial contrast-enhanced CT scan: arterial (**b**), venous (**c**), and delayed (**c**) phases showing intraluminal contrast extravasation (white dotted circle) with progressive intraluminal extravasation increase

inferior rectal artery (IRA). The SRA, branching from the inferior mesenteric artery (IMA), is the main supplier of blood to the CCR. The IRA, originating from the internal pudendal artery, supplies the anal canal and anus. The MRA exhibits variability in its origin, deriving from the internal pudendal artery in 40% of cases and the inferior gluteal artery in 26% of cases [8]. Most patients find relief through medical or office-based treatments, such as injection sclerotherapy, rubber band ligation, infrared photocoagulation, and bipolar diathermy. Surgical or endovascular embolization is required in approximately 10% of cases. Recently, vascular embolization using coils has gained importance. Typically, metallic microcoils or microparticles are applied to occlude all branches of the SRA above the pubic symphysis [10]; this technique, named "Emborrhoid" proof to be effective in both patients with chronic hemorrhoidal bleeding and portal hypertension related hemorroids.

22.4.2 Vascular

CT is usually performed in patients with known abdominal aortic aneurysm (AAA) presenting with abdominal pain to exclude rupture or to identify other causes for the patient's symptoms. An early contained rupture may manifest with the "draped aorta" sign, which is considered present when the posterior wall of the aorta is not identifiable as distinct from adjacent structures. Rupture is usually associated with a large retroperitoneal

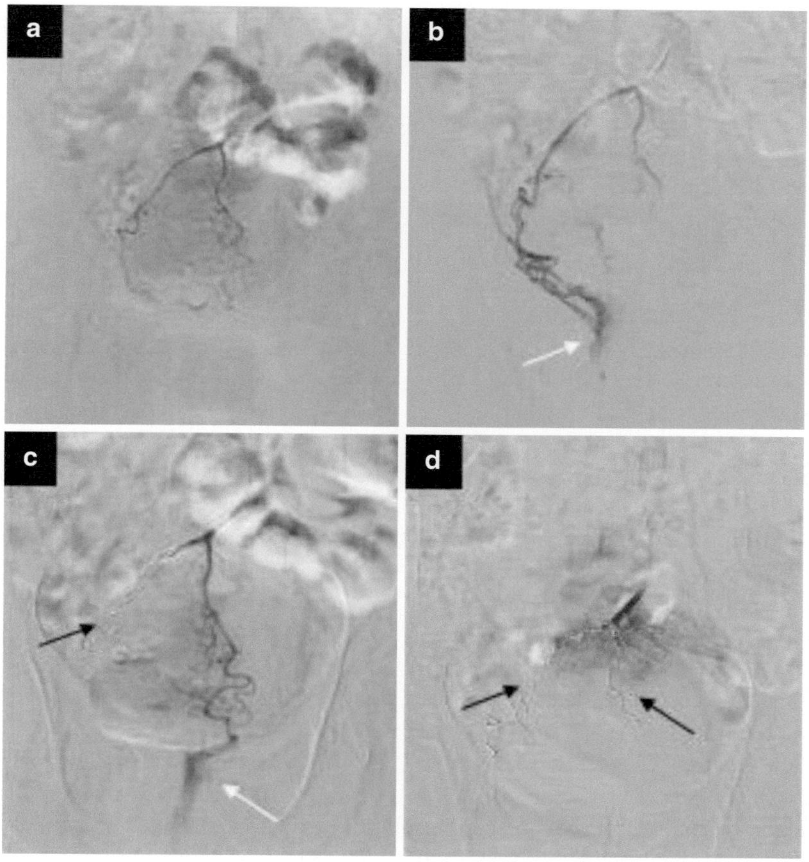

Fig. 22.4 Same patient of Fig. 22.3. An endovascular embolization approach was applied in this patient. (**a**) Diagnostic digital subtraction arteriography (DSA) of superior hemorrhoidal artery detecting vessels tortuosity, typical of hemorrhoidal bleeding; (**b**) Superselective distal DSA of right anterior hemorrhoidal branch showing corpus cavernosum recti (white arrow); (**c**) after coiling of right hemorrhoidal branches (black arrow), left branches were investigated confirming corpus cavernosum recti opacification (white arrow); (**d**) Post coils embolization (black arrows) DSA of showing devascularization of the superior hemorrhoidal plexus, healthy rectal tissues vascularized by inferior hemorrhoidal branches

hematoma adjacent to the aneurysm. Bleeding can extend to the intraperitoneal compartment if the rupture occurs on the anterior wall of the aortic aneurysm. If contrast extravasation is detected, it is an unequivocal sign of aneurysm rupture.

22.4.3 Gynaecologic

The most common gynecologic sources of bleeding are ectopic pregnancy and ruptured ovarian cyst in women in childbearing age [11], while pelvic malignancies are in non-childbearing age women. Hemoperitoneum also has been seen in the setting of endometriosis and uterine rupture, but such occurrences are uncommon.

22.4.3.1 Hemorrhagic Ovarian Cyst

A hemorrhagic ovarian cyst is a frequent cause of acute pelvic pain in women of childbearing age [11]. The most common underlying etiology is a corpus luteal or follicular cyst. Hemorrhage into an ovarian cyst is a relatively common occurrence, but few hemorrhagic ovarian cysts rupture and cause hemoperitoneum [12]. Fluid with internal echogenicity or high attenuation can be seen surrounding the uterus in the presence of recent bleeding, and an associated mixed-attenuation adnexal mass with a high-attenuation component and at times a fluid-fluid level may be present [11]. Ovarian carcinoma may also cause ascites, sometimes of hemorrhagic characteristics, but the clinical setting and identification of peritoneal tumor implants should assist in the correct diagnosis [13].

22.4.3.2 Ectopic Pregnancy (EP)

EP can cause life-threatening bleeding and therefore must be considered in every woman of childbearing age who presents with abdominal or pelvic pain. Ectopic pregnancy accounts for up to 1% of pregnancies, with 97% of occurrences located in either the ampullary (most common) or the isthmic portion of the fallopian tube [14]. Risk factors include previous ectopic pregnancy, pelvic inflammatory disease, in vitro fertilization, use of an intrauterine device, and tubal surgery [14, 15]. In the context of a positive human chorionic gonadotropin level of more than 2000 IU/L and no intrauterine pregnancy, the finding of an extraovarian mass is highly suggestive of an ectopic pregnancy. On the other hand, scar pregnancy (SP) is secondary to implantation of a gestational sac on a previous cesarean section scar. SP- and CP-related hemorrhage can be lethal and often needs a hysterectomy.

Early diagnosis is performed by using transvaginal sonography and pelvic magnetic resonance imaging (MRI); this may allow conservative uterine-sparing medical and surgical treatment [16, 17]. Local methotrexate (MTX) injection and systemic infusion, US-guided uterine drainage, hysteroscopic resection, and uterine arteries embolization (UAE), among other options, have been reported as a conservative treatment for SP and CP [18]. UAE is mainly performed on C-SP patients who fulfill the following criteria: high arterial flow related to the gestational sac, a myometrial thickness between the sac and urinary bladder below 2 mm, serum b-hCG level of more than 10,000 mIU/ mL [19]. UAE can be associated with the administration of methotrexate, given systemic or locally through transarterial injection in the uterine artery with the aim to reduce collateral effects.

UAE leads to acute ischemic degradation of the gestational sac due to extensive blockage of the uterine vascularity. MTX is a folic acid antagonist that blocks the division of trophoblast cells and inhibits trophoblast proliferation, so it stops embryonic development.

After treatment, monitoring is done by serial serum quantitative b-hCG level and repeated sonography and color Doppler imaging.

Technical success is determined by the absence of uterine arterial flow on bilateral iliac arteriography and cessation of active vaginal bleeding, while clinical success is defined as reduced sac size without active vaginal rebleeding and with steadily declining b-hCG level. Non-surgical therapy has become the favored option for patients with a cesarean scar or cervical ectopic pregnancy, especially for women who wish to maintain fertility.UAE and intra-arterial MTX infusion result in the resolution of cesarean and cervical ectopic pregnancies with hemorrhage control and uterine preservation.

22.4.3.3 Uterine Arteriovenous Malformations (AVM)

AVM are divided into congenital and acquired [20] (Figs. 22.5 an 22.6); an acquired uterine AVM is characterized by a single arteriovenous communication between the branches of the uterine artery and the myometrial venous plexus; it is typically confined to the uterus; congenital AVMs extend over the uterus with filler involving other pelvic districts and present with a much more complex angioarchitecture. The most common presenting symptoms are menorrhagia and metrorrhagia. Bleeding is often intermittent and torrential. These patients may also present with anemia and hypotension, secondary to acute blood loss. Imaging plays a pivotal role. Transvaginal color Doppler US is typically the initial imaging study of choice for abnormal uterine bleeding. MRI is recommended for the evaluation beyond US for uterine AVM when indicated. Angiography should be offered in consideration for a possible therapeutic option following diagnostic confirmation. The typical findings of a uterine AVM by angiography include high arterial flow with early venous filling. A single direct

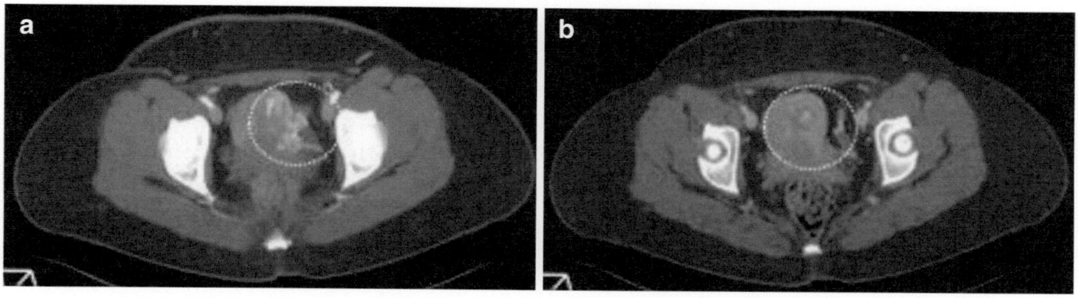

Fig. 22.5 24 years old lady, two previous pregnancies and one previous abortion, complaining vaginal bleeding for 2 months after the abortion. Axial CT scan in arterial (**b**) and venous (**b**) phases showing aberrant vascularization of the left portion of the uterus with multiple tortuosous vessels, suggesting AVM

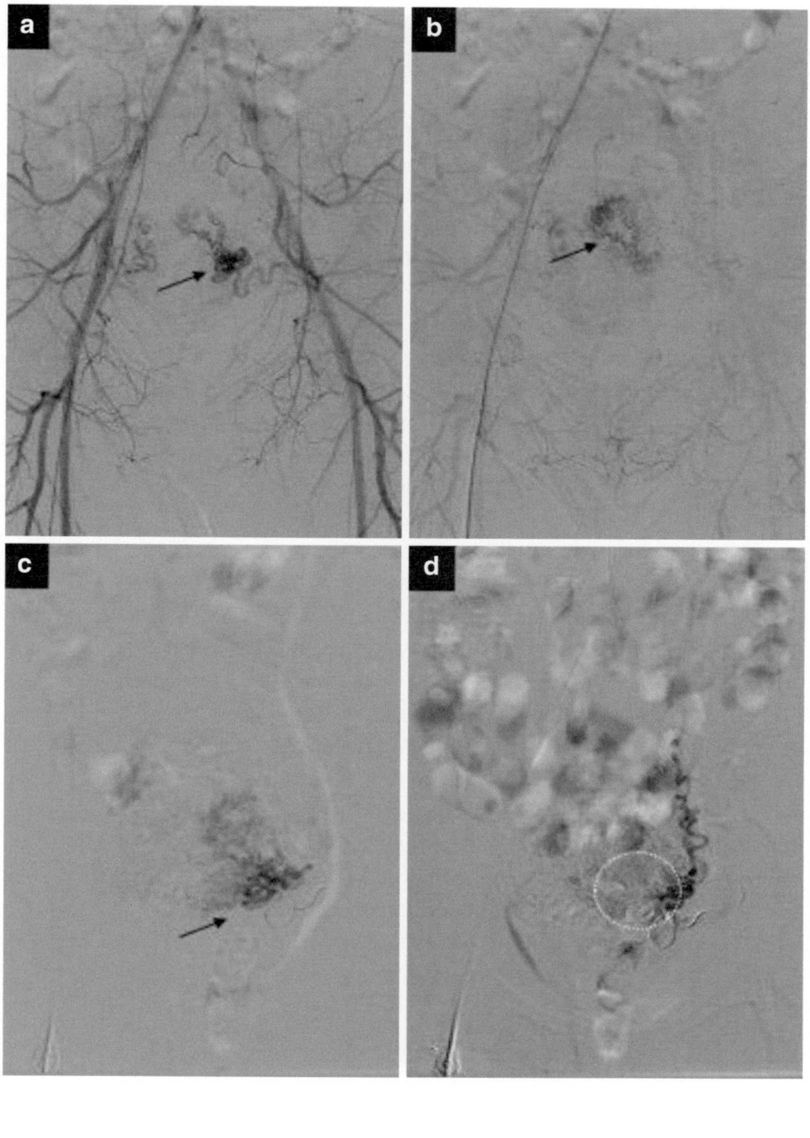

Fig. 22.6 Same patient in Fig. 22.5. (**a**) Pelvic early DSA showing anomalous vascularization of the left uterine artery refurnishing multiple tortuosous vessels (black arrow), corresponding to acquired uterine AVM; no anomalies detected on the right side; (**b**) Pelvic delayed DSA confirming left uterine AVM with precocious venous opacification (black arrow); (**c**) Superselective distal DSA of the left uterine artery showing AVM nidus (black arrow); (**d**) After microparticles embolization, distal DSA showed AVM disappearance (white dotted circle), with concomitant left ovarian artery hypertrophy refurnishing healthy uterine tissues

fistulous communication to the venous structures may be identified. The embolization technique, as for all AVM, is based on nidus embolization. Transcatheter embolization with superselective angiography allows to properly identify and occlude the nidus. A variety of embolic agents and combination of embolic agents have been used for treatment in the reviewed cases, and the choices of the embolic agents are largely based on the preference of the interventional radiologists. Liquids are the most effective [21] in both the dimethyl sulfoxide (DMSO) family and glues. Coils and particles should be avoided, as for all AVM. The follow-up is both clinical and imaging.

22.4.3.4 Postpartum Hemorrhage (PPH)

PPH is commonly defined as greater than 500 mL blood loss during and following vaginal delivery, and greater than 1000 mL blood loss for cesarean section [22, 23]. Primary PPH occurs within the first 24 h after delivery; secondary PPH occurs after 24 h.

Multiple conservative treatments and minimally invasive techniques including UAE and uterine balloon tamponade aim to prevent these complications and have successfully and progressively reduced the rate of peripartum hysterectomy from 1/1000 to 1/2000 in the last 20 years.

Pregnancy increases circulating blood volume by 50% to perfuse the low-resistance uteroplacental unit and to compensate for blood loss at delivery. Upon delivery, contraction of the myometrium compresses the spiral arteries, leading to hemostasis.

The most common cause of PPH is the failure of mechanical compression of the spiral arteries caused by uterine atony. Uterine atony accounts for 70% of cases of primary PPH and often results in hemorrhagic shock, which can progress to disseminated intravascular coagulation (DIC). Additional causes of PPH include retained products of conception, abnormally invasive placenta, uterine rupture, lower genital tract laceration, and coagulopathy [24].

22.5 Conclusions

Non-traumatic pelvic hemorrhages can represent a life-threatening scenario; radiology plays a pivotal role in their clinical management. Its goal is twofold, both diagnostic and operative: contrast-enhanced CT represents the best diagnostic radiological examination able to detect both the source of bleeding and the feeding vessels; interventional radiology with embolization procedures allows the treatment of the source of bleeding.

References

1. McCort JJ. Intraperitoneal and retroperitoneal hemorrhage. Radiol Clin North Am. 1976;14:391–405.
2. Scott WW, Fishman EK, Siegelmann SS. Anticoagulants and abdominal pain: the role of computed tomography. JAMA. 1984;252:2053–6.
3. Lucey BC, Varghese JC, Soto JA. Spontaneous hemoperitoneum: causes and significance. Curr Probl Diagn Radiol. 2005;34:182–95.
4. Mortele KJ, Cantisani V, Brown DL, Ros PR. Spontaneous intraperitoneal hemorrhage: imaging features. Radiol Clin North Am. 2003;41:1183–201.
5. Furlan A, Fakhran S, Federle MP. Spontaneous abdominal hemorrhage, causes, CT findings, and clinical implications. AJR Am J Roentgenol. 2009;193:1077–87.
6. Vidal V, Louis G, Bartoli J, Sielezneff I. Embolization of the hemorrhoidal arteries (the emborrhoid technique): a new concept and challenge for interventional radiology. Diagn Interv Imaging. 2014;95:307–15.
7. Sugi MD, Sun DC, Menias CO, Prabhu V, Choi HH. Acute diverticulitis: key features for guiding clinical management. Eur J Radiol. 2020;128:109026.
8. Vu KN, Kaitoukov Y, Morin-Roy F, Kauffmann C, Giroux MF, Thérasse E, et al. Rupture signs on computed tomography, treatment, and outcome of abdominal aortic aneurysms. Insights Imaging. 2014;5:281–93. https://doi.org/10.1007/s13244-014-0327-3.
9. Schreyer A, Layer G. S2k guidlines for diverticular disease and diverticulitis: diagnosis, classification, and therapy for the radiologist. Fortschr Röntgenstr. 2015;187:676–84.
10. Lestar B, Penninckx F, Kerremans R. The composition of anal basal pressure: an in vivo and in vitro study in man. Int J Color Dis. 1989;4:118–22.
11. Hertzberg BS, Kliewer MA, Paulson EK. Ovarian cyst rupture causing hemoperitoneum: imaging fea-

tures and potential for misdiagnosis. Abdom Imaging. 1999;24:304–8.
12. Hallatt JG, Steele CH, Snyder M. Ruptured corpus luteum with hemoperitoneum: a study of 173 surgical cases. Am J Obstet Gynecol. 1984;149:5–9.
13. Hertzberg BS, Kliewer MA, Paulson EK. Ovarian cyst rupture causing hemoperitoneum: imaging features and potential role for misdiagnosis. Abdom Imaging. 1999;24:304–8.
14. Della-Giustina D, Denny M. Ectopic pregnancy. Emerg Med Clin North Am. 2003;21:565–84.
15. Hallatt JG, Steele CH, Snyder M. Ruptured corpus luteum with hemoperitoneum: a study of 173 surgical cases. Am J Obstet Gynecol. 1984;149:5–8.
16. Martinelli P, Maruotti GM, Oppedisano R, Agangi A, Mazzarelli LL, Votino C, et al. Is uterine artery embolization for cervical ectopic pregnancy always safe? J Minim Invasive Gynecol. 2007;14:758–63.
17. Zhang B, Jiang ZB, Huang MS, Guan SH, Zhu KS, Qian JS, et al. Uterine artery embolization combined with methotrexate in the treatment of cesarean scar pregnancy: results of a case series and review of the literature. J Vasc Interv Radiol. 2012;23:1582–8.
18. Zhang S, Yan H, Ji WT. Uterine artery embolization combined with intra-arterial MTX infusion: its application in treatment of cervical pregnancy. Arch Gynecol Obstet. 2016;293:1043–7.
19. Kanat-Pektas M, Bodur S, Dundar O, Bakır VL. Systematic review: what is the best first-line approach for cesarean section ectopic pregnancy? Taiwan J Obstet Gynecol. 2016;55:263–9.
20. Yoon DJ, Jones M, Taani JA, Buhimschi C, Dowell JD. A systematic review of acquired uterine arteriovenous malformations: pathophysiology, diagnosis, and Transcatheter treatment. AJP Rep. 2016;6:e6–14.
21. Giurazza F, Corvino F, Paladini A, Borzelli A, Scognamiglio D, Frauenfelder G, et al. Uterine arteriovenous fistula with concomitant pelvic varicocele: endovascular embolization with Onyx-18®. Case Rep Vasc Med. 2017;2017:3548271.
22. World Health Organization. WHO recommendations for the prevention and treatment of postpartum haemorrhage. Geneva: World Health Organization; 2012.
23. Kumar N. Postpartum hemorrhage; a major killer of woman: review of current scenario. Obstet Gynecol Int J. 2016;4:00116.
24. Lindquist JD, Vogelzang RL. Pelvic artery embolization for treatment of postpartum hemorrhage. Semin Intervent Radiol. 2018;35:41–7.

Part VI

Retroperitoneum

Aortic Emergencies

23

Chiara Rinaldo, Andrea Maria Rinaldo,
Dario Grimaldi, Martina Caruso, Antonio Raucci,
and Francesca Iacobellis

23.1 Introduction

Non-traumatic aortic emergencies (NTAE) include a range of rare but potentially fatal conditions. Compared to myocardial infarction and stroke, aortic emergencies are less frequent but have a similarly high mortality rate if not promptly diagnosed and treated. The main non-traumatic aortic emergencies include acute aortic syndromes (aortic dissection, intramural hematoma, and penetrating atherosclerotic ulcer) and rupture/instability of an aortic aneurysm. Clinical presentation of aortic emergencies is highly variable, with the most common symptom being acute stabbing thoraco-abdominal pain, sometimes migratory. Due to the non-specific clinical presentation, imaging is essential for a rapid and accurate diagnosis. MDCT is the first-choice imaging modality, with a sensitivity of 100% and specificity of 98–99%. MDCT is also readily available in most emergency departments and can be performed quickly. Accurate diagnosis and classification of aortic emergencies facilitate the selection of the most appropriate treatment, guiding the patient towards open surgery, endovascular treatment, or solely pharmacological management.

C. Rinaldo (✉) · D. Grimaldi · M. Caruso
A. Raucci · F. Iacobellis
Department of General and Emergency Radiology, "Antonio Cardarelli" Hospital, Naples, Italy

A. M. Rinaldo
University of Naples Federico II, Department of Advanced Biomedical Sciences, Naples, Italy

23.2 Acute Aortic Syndromes

Initially coined by Vilacosta and Roman, the term "acute aortic syndromes" (AAS) encompasses three interrelated entities:

- Aortic dissection (AD)
- Intramural hematoma (IMH)
- Penetrating atherosclerotic ulcer (PAU)

A common denominator among these conditions is the compromise of the aortic wall integrity (Fig. 23.1).

The incidence of AAS is 5 cases per 100,000 per year, with a mean age of onset of 63 years and a marked predominance in males (65%). The most significant risk factor is arterial hypertension, particularly in patients with poorly controlled blood pressure. Additional risk factors include connective tissue disorders (Marfan syndrome, Ehlers-Danlos syndrome), bicuspid aortic valve, Takayasu arteritis, substance abuse (e.g., cocaine), and iatrogenic causes (e.g., aortic surgery, interventional procedures) [1, 2–4].

Patients typically present with severe, tearing chest pain that may be migratory. The pain's location correlates with the site of the pathologi-

L. Romano et al. (eds.), *CT of Non-Traumatic Body Emergencies*,
https://doi.org/10.1007/978-3-031-84849-0_23

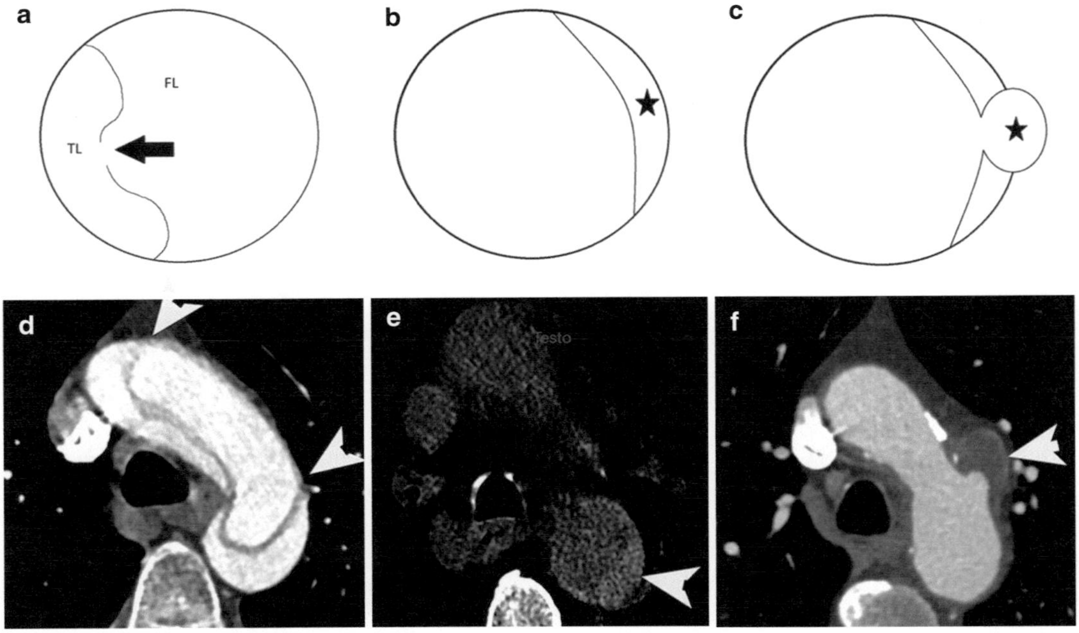

Fig. 23.1 SAA. (**a** and **d**) Drawing and contrast-enhanced CT scan study of the chest demonstrate AD. The intimal tear (arrow) allows blood flow to penetrate the wall thickness, separating the intima and part of the media, resulting in the formation of two lumens (TL = true lumen; FL = false lumen). (**b** and **e**) Drawing and contrast-enhanced CT scan study of the chest demonstrates IMH. Hematoma of the aortic media without the intimal tear characteristic of AD (star). (**c and f**) Drawing and contrast-enhanced CT scan study of the chest demonstrates PAU. An atherosclerotic ulcer penetrates the elastic lamina (star) and is frequently linked to hematoma formation in the aortic media

cal process. Anterior chest or neck and jaw pain typically indicates involvement of the ascending aorta, whereas back and abdominal pain suggest pathology in the descending aorta [5]. Involvement of the aortic root or ascending aorta may present with shock, hypotension, and congestive heart failure [6].

Symptoms may overlap with those of an acute coronary syndrome, pulmonary embolism, or even acute abdomen. MDCT is the first-choice modality for diagnosing AAS due to its availability and rapid execution. MDCT demonstrates very high sensitivity and specificity, enabling simultaneous evaluation of the neck, thorax, and abdomen, all potentially affected regions [7].

23.3 Aortic Dissection

Aortic dissection (AD) is the most common AAS. It was first described in 1760 by Dr. Frank Nicholls, who identified it as the cause of King George II's death through autopsy [8].

Histologically, AD originates from an intimal tear or primary intimal lesion that allows blood to penetrate the aortic wall, destroying the media layer. This results in the formation of a false lumen (FL) within the aortic wall, separate from the true lumen (TL) (Fig. 23.2). The FL generally has higher pressure than the TL, promoting pathological progression both axially and longitudinally [5].

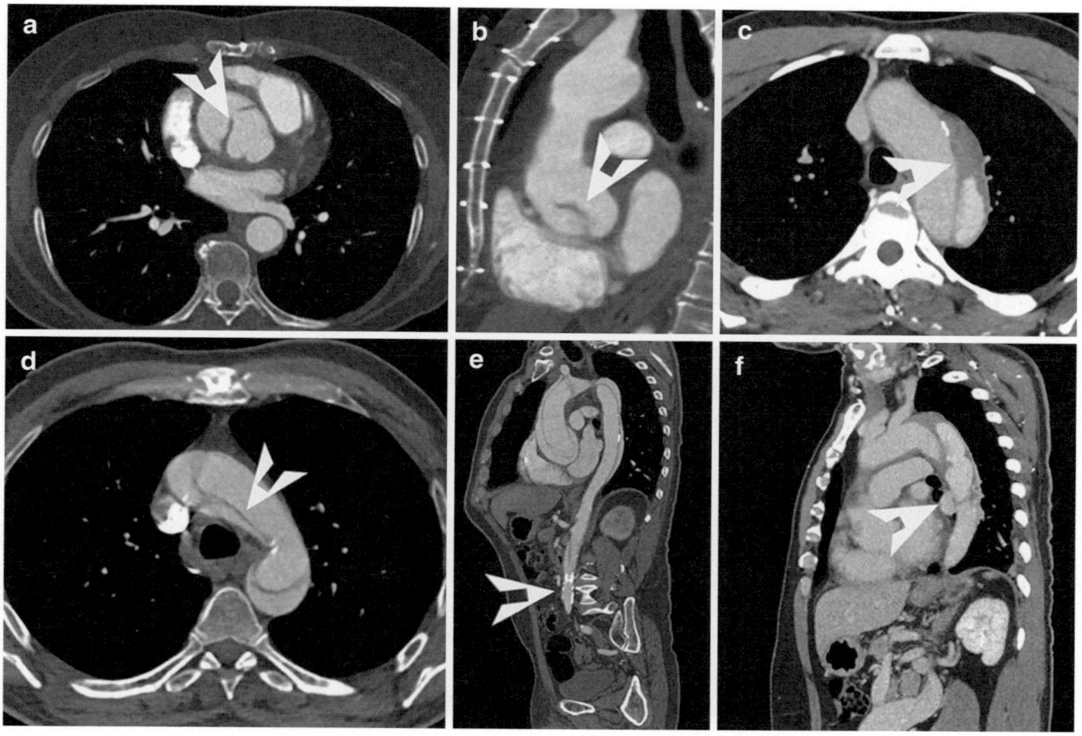

Fig. 23.2 Stanford classification of AD. (**a** and **b**) Contrast-enhanced CT scan study of the chest shows AD originating from the valvular plane, consistent with type A AD. (**d** and **e**) Contrast-enhanced CT scan study of the chest and abdomen demonstrates AD originating from the proximal third of the aortic arch extending to the infrarenal aortic segment; this is also classified as type A AD. (**c** and **f**) Contrast-enhanced CT scan study of the chest and abdomen demonstrates AD originating downstream of the left subclavian artery, consistent with type B AD

The typical lesion is transverse and does not involve the entire aortic circumference [9]. Since the dissection flap comprises the intima and inner two-thirds of the media, the term "medio-intimal flap" is more accurate [9, 10]. The intima is displaced into the lumen, sometimes with associated calcifications. The extent of the medio-intimal flap can vary both longitudinally and circumferentially. The entry tear may progress anterogradely or, less commonly, retrogradely along the aortic lumen. As the percentage of the media layer involved in the intimal-medial flap increases, the outer wall of the false lumen becomes thinner, raising the risk of aortic rupture.

23.3.1 Risk Factors, Clinical Presentation, and Classification

The most common comorbidity in AD is severe arterial hypertension. Chronic high-pressure exposure leads to aortic wall degeneration. Other less common risk factors include connective tissue disorders, inflammatory processes affecting the vessel wall (vasculitis), structural aortic abnormalities, Turner syndrome, or iatrogenic causes [11]. Risk factors are summarized in Table 23.1.

AD symptoms have a sudden onset, typically presenting as severe chest or back pain, described as tearing or knife-like, in elderly (sixth or seventh decade) with history of uncontrolled arterial hypertension. There is a broad spectrum of pathological conditions associated with AD due to the variable extent of dissection along the blood vessel (Table 23.2).

Table 23.1 Predisposing factors for non-traumatic aortic dissection

Predisposing factors	Description
Hypertension	Chronic high blood pressure increases stress on the aortic wall
Genetic conditions	Marfan syndrome, Ehlers-Danlos syndrome, and other connective tissue disorders
Bicuspid aortic valve	A congenital heart defect that affects the aortic valve
Atherosclerosis	Build-up of plaque in the arteries can weaken the aortic wall
Inflammatory diseases	Conditions like giant cell arteritis or Takayasu arteritis that affect blood vessels
Pre-existing aortic aneurysm	A weakened and enlarged section of the aorta that is more prone to dissection
Cocaine or amphetamine use	These substances can increase blood pressure and stress on the aorta
Previous cardiac surgery	Surgery involving the aorta or aortic valve can increase dissection risk

Based on symptom onset, aortic dissection is classified into three phases [12, 13]:

- Acute: within 14 days of symptom onset.
- Subacute: 14 days to 3 months.
- Chronic: more than 3 months after initial symptoms.

The clinical diagnosis of aortic dissection is challenging because the symptoms are nonspecific and there are no biomarkers; therefore, imaging is essential. Imaging not only confirms or excludes the diagnosis but also defines the morphology and extent of dissection, essential for classification and management.

The most commonly used classification for aortic dissection is the Stanford classification system proposed by Dailey et al., identifying two types of dissection [14] (Fig. 23.3):

- Type A: involves the ascending aorta regardless of the origin and extent of dissection. This type requires urgent surgical treatment due to possible complications, including hemopericardium with cardiac tamponade risk, coronary artery dissection, and aortic insufficiency with valve involvement [1, 9, 15].
- Type B: the medio-intimal flap originates distal to the left subclavian artery. Type B dissections are usually managed medically [1, 9, 15].

Table 23.2 Pathological conditions associated with aortic dissection

Pathological condition	Description	Location
Aortic regurgitation	Backflow of blood into the left ventricle due to valve dysfunction	Often associated with Type A dissection
Malperfusion syndromes	Ischemia of organs due to compromised blood flow	Can occur if dissection involves renal and mesenteric arteries
Pericardial effusion/tamponade	Accumulation of blood in the pericardial sac	Often associated with Type A dissection
Stroke	Disruption of blood flow to the brain	Can occur if dissection involves carotid arteries
Renal failure	Impaired kidney function due to reduced blood flow	Often associated with Type B dissection
Angina and myocardial infarction	Chest pain and heart attack due to compromised coronary artery blood flow	Often associated with involvement of coronary arteries

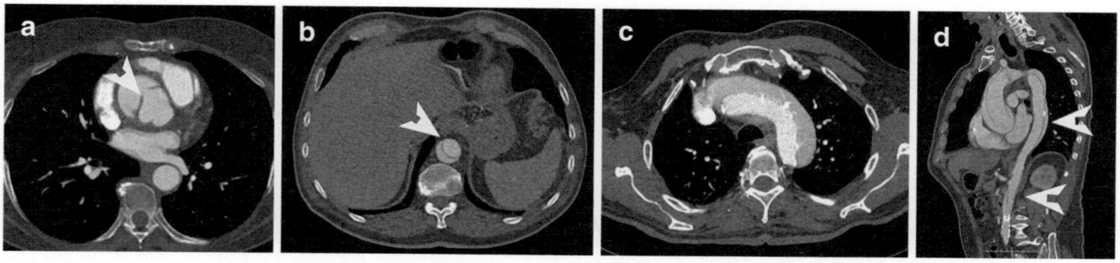

Fig. 23.3 CT Signs of aortic dissection (AD). (**a** and **b**) Contrast-enhanced CT scan study of the chest demonstrates an entry tear of the medio-intimal flap originating from the aortic root and extending to the descending thoracic aorta, with evidence of both true and false lumens. (**c**) Contrast-enhanced CT scan study of the chest demonstrates greater enhancement of the true lumen compared to the false lumen and intraluminal displacement of intimal calcifications. (**d**) Contrast-enhanced CT scan study of the chest and abdomen in sagittal reconstruction demonstrates the characteristic spiral course of the AD

Table 23.3 Key features of true and false lumen in aortic dissection: CT findings

Characteristic	True lumen	False lumen
Size	Often compressed by the false lumen, thus generally smaller.	Generally larger due to higher luminal pressures.
External wall calcifications	Visible and useful in acute dissections.	Not visible.
Enhancement	Early and homogeneous.	Delayed opacification.
Communication	Direct communication between the true lumen and the non-dissected aorta	Not present.
Beak sign	Not present.	Acute angle formed by the false lumen edge on axial CT images.
Cobweb sign	Not present.	
Typical location	Posterolateral left side of the ascending aorta, anterolateral right side of the descending aorta	Anterolateral right side of the ascending aorta, posterolateral left side of the descending aorta.
Origin of main branches	Often surrounded by the false lumen	Frequently surrounds the true lumen

Complicated Type B AD refers to persistent or recurrent pain and uncontrolled hypertension despite therapy, increasing aortic diameters, organ hypoperfusion, and signs of rupture (hemothorax, mediastinal hematoma), often managed with endovascular repair using a stent graft (TEVAR) [16, 17].

Accurate imaging and reporting are crucial in determining the therapeutic strategy, and guiding patients toward surgical or non-surgical treatment.

23.3.2 Imaging

CT is the preferred method for studying aortic dissection. Contrast-enhanced CT not only diagnoses and classifies dissection but also evaluates potential organ complications (Table 23.3).

Non-contrast CT findings of AD may be subtle but can include intramural hematoma, discussed in the following section. Displacement of atherosclerotic intimal calcifications into the lumen is a frequent finding in dissections.

Contrast-enhanced CT provides excellent detail. Findings include [11, 18, 19] (Fig. 23.2 and Table 23.6):

- Intimal flap
- Double lumen (true and false lumens).
- "Mercedes-Benz sign": in triple-barreled dissections, three lumens are seen in axial images, two false lumens, and one true lumen.
- "Windsock sign": complete intimal dissection at the aortic arch with the false lumen entirely surrounding the true lumen.
- Organ complication findings (e.g., organ ischemia).

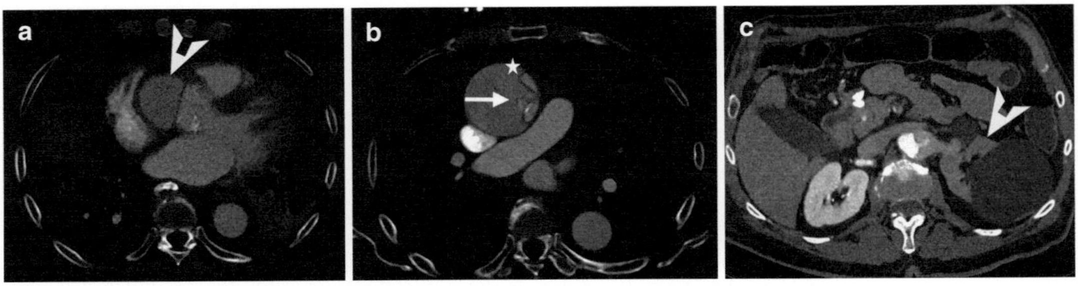

Fig. 23.4 CT Signs of true lumen and false lumen. (**a** and **b**) Contrast-enhanced CT scan study of the chest demonstrates the typical anterolateral right side location of the false lumen in the ascending aorta; additionally, the false lumen can be identified by delayed opacification, "beak sign" (star), and "cobweb sign" (arrow). (**c**) The left renal artery usually originates from the false lumen. In this contrast-enhanced CT scan study of the abdomen, consequent hypoperfusion of the left kidney is clearly evident

A crucial part of AD evaluation is identifying the true lumen, especially for endovascular treatment. Distinguishing between the true and false lumens can be challenging without direct communication between the true lumen and the non-dissected aorta. However, several signs can guide radiologists in correct identification [6, 19] (Fig. 23.4 and Table 23.3):

23.3.2.1 True Lumen

- Often compressed by the false lumen, which has higher pressures, thus generally smaller.
- Shows external wall calcifications (especially in acute dissections).
- Early and homogeneous enhancement.
- Often contiguous with the aortic root.
- Celiac trunk, superior mesenteric artery, and right renal artery usually originate from the true lumen.

23.3.2.2 False Lumen

- Generally larger due to higher luminal pressures.
- Delayed opacification.
- Typical location: anterolateral right side of the ascending aorta, posterolateral left side of the descending aorta.
- "Beak sign": an acute angle formed by the false lumen edge on axial CT images.
- "Cobweb sign": fine linear low-attenuation structures within the false lumen indicating media remnants.
- The left renal artery usually originates from the false lumen.
- The false lumen frequently surrounds the true lumen in Stanford type A dissections.

23.3.3 Perfect Report

The radiologic CTA report should include:

- Stanford classification (A vs B)
- Presence of rupture signs (periaortic stranding or hematoma)
- Entry tear location
- Longitudinal extent of the medio-intimal flap
- Aortic root involvement
- True and false lumen identification
- Presence of thrombosis in the false lumen
- Origin of branch vessels
- Signs of organ ischemia or vascular occlusion
- Aortic diameters and anatomical characteristics, including diameters and status of access arteries (common femoral artery and external iliac artery)

23.4 Intramural Hematoma

Intramural hematoma (IMH) is defined as a hematoma within the tunica media of the aortic wall due to a rupture of the vasa vasorum. The rupture of the vasa vasorum can be spontaneous

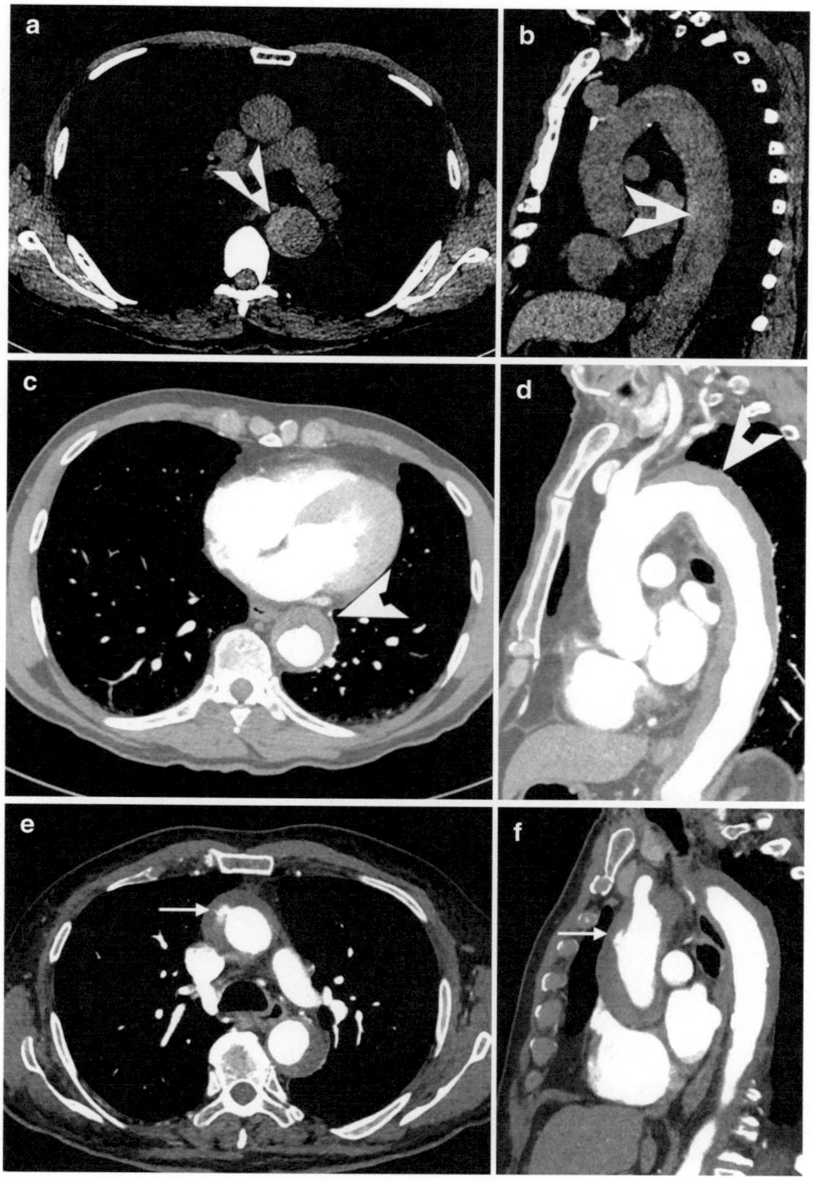

Fig. 23.5 IMH. (**a, b**) Noncontrast CT scan study of the chest demonstrates a typically hyperdense, crescent-shaped wall. (**c, d**) Contrast-enhanced CT scan study of the chest demonstrates the lack of opacification of the IMH. (**e, f**) Contrast-enhanced CT scan study of the chest demonstrates the presence of a "primary intimal tear" within the context of the IMH (arrow)

or the consequence of a penetrating ulcer. Thanks to the increased resolution of imaging techniques, it has been recognized that IMH can also develop following a small intimal tear with a thrombosed false lumen, and, for this reason, it can be considered a variant of AD. Indeed, the current opinion on IMH is that it may be a variant or a precursor of AD with a small intimal defect and thrombosed false lumen without a re-entry tear. This type is also referred to as "thrombosed-type acute AD", where the separation of the aortic wall layers is occupied by thrombus rather than by freely flowing blood, which would typically fill the false lumen in a classic dissection [2]. A circular or crescent-shaped thickening >5 mm of the aortic wall in the absence of detectable blood flow suggests an IMH [2] (Fig. 23.5).

23.4.1 Risk factor, Clinical Presentation, and Classification

As with aortic dissection, the primary risk factor for intramural hematoma is hypertension [11, 18].

The main clinical features of IMH are those of acute aortic syndromes, namely chest pain radiating to the back. Due to the similarities with AD, IMHs are also classified and treated according to the Stanford classification [20].

23.4.2 Imaging

CT is the gold standard modality for the study of intramural hematoma. In pre-contrast CT studies, a typically hyperdense, crescent-shaped, or circular wall alteration (60 +/− 15 HU) with a thickness between 5 and 15 mm is observed [21]. Post-contrast administration usually does not show contrast enhancement of the wall lesion nor the presence of an intimal flap (Fig. 23.5 and Table 23.6).

A fundamental role of imaging is to identify, if present, a micro entry tear, which would change patient management towards endovascular treatment (TEVAR) or open surgery [22].

To distinguish between IMH and a thrombotic variant of AD, in addition to searching for an intimal lesion, the longitudinal distribution of the lesion can be evaluated, being more linear in IMH and typically spiral-shaped in the thrombotic variant of AD. The required imaging details include the location and extent of aortic wall thickening, the coexistence of atherosclerotic disease (displacement of calcifications), and the presence of small intimal lesions. Patients need close monitoring during the first 30 days. If there is lumen dilation, penetrating ulcer, IMH enlargement, or dissection, surgical or endovascular treatment should be considered [22].

The findings of an IMH with a dissection variant include a small intimal rupture termed "primary intimal tear" (PIT) or "ulcer-like projections/lesions" which is a small blood-filled sac protruding from the true lumen (with which it communicates) into the thrombosed false lumen of the aorta (Fig. 23.5). This finding is an indicator of potential communication formation between the two lumens, possibly resulting in an AD [23]. These lesions should not be confused with "intramural blood pools" (IBP), which do not impact patient prognosis and thus management. An IBP appears as a small focus of enhancement within the hematoma without visible communication with the true lumen, often with a peripheral connection to an intercostal or lumbar artery [24]. IBPs are usually benign and self-limiting, not associated with an unfavorable prognosis; most IBPs spontaneously regress in size over time and/or completely disappear in follow-up MDCT [24].

23.4.3 Perfect Report

In the report, the radiologist should indicate:

- Location
- Wall thickness
- Maximum diameter of the affected aortic lumen
- Presence of "primary intimal tear" (PIT) or "ulcer-like projections/lesions"
- Longitudinal extension
- Involvement of supra-aortic and abdominal branches
- Any complications

23.5 Penetrating Atherosclerotic Ulcer

A penetrating atherosclerotic ulcer (PAU) is defined as an ulceration of an atherosclerotic plaque that erodes through the intima and internal elastic lamina into the media of the aortic wall [1, 15, 26] (Fig. 23.6). This condition typically occurs in elderly individuals with multiple cardiovascular risk factors. PAUs account for approximately 7.5% (range 2.3–11%) of all acute aortic syndromes [25].

PAU predominantly affects the aortic arch and the descending thoracic aorta in 90% of cases.

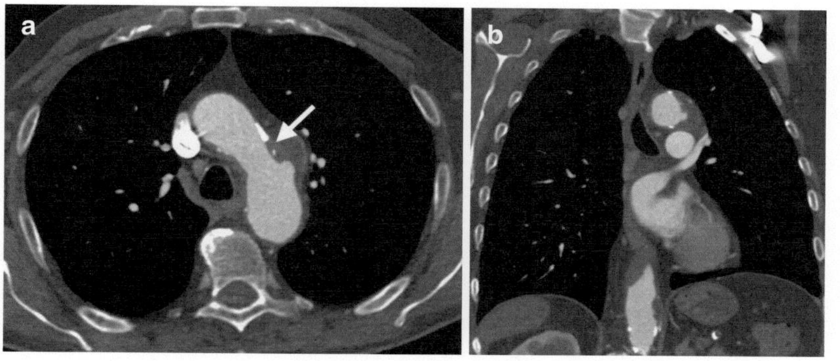

Fig. 23.6 PAU. (**a** and **b**) Contrast-enhanced CT scan study of the chest shows a small PAU in the middle third of the aortic arch with associated IMH. The image also reveals intimal calcification (arrow), confirming the diagnostic suspicion of PAU

While a PAU can remain stable, it has the potential to progress to aortic dissection, pseudoaneurysm, and spontaneous aortic rupture [26].

There is no consensus on the specific depth or diameter of an ulcer that would necessitate treatment. Currently, no "cut-off" values exist to determine the depth and diameter of the PAU neck that justify intervention. However, recent studies indicate that a depth >20 mm or a neck diameter >10 mm are associated with higher complication rates [27, 28]. Intervention, often endovascular due to the patient's comorbidities and the lesion's location, is indicated for recurrent symptoms, rapid size increase, or signs of contained rupture such as periaortic hematoma and associated pleural effusion. In asymptomatic or chronic cases, observation with periodic imaging assessment is recommended [29].

23.5.1 Risk Factors, Clinical Presentation, and Classification

PAUs typically occur in elderly male patients with a history of hypertension (up to 92%), smoking (up to 77%), coronary artery disease (up to 46%), and chronic obstructive pulmonary disease [25]. Symptomatic patients usually present with acute, intense chest pain, often described as tearing, ripping, migrating, or pulsating [25]. PAUs are also frequently diagnosed incidentally in asymptomatic patients. Similar to aortic dissection, PAUs are classified using the Stanford system.

23.5.2 Imaging

On contrast-enhanced CT, a PAU is characterized by an ulcerative lesion penetrating the intima and reaching the media within an atherosclerotic plaque. This is often accompanied by a slightly jagged outward bulging of the aortic wall profile (Fig. 23.6 and Table 23.6). Non-contrast CT may show a hematoma surrounding the ulceration [30]. Imaging modalities cannot reliably determine if an ulcer has penetrated the internal elastic lamina, making it challenging to differentiate between an ulcerated plaque and a PAU in some cases. However, certain imaging characteristics can aid in differentiation [7, 31]:

- Ulcerated plaques present a wavy interface and are overlaid by thrombus, whereas PAUs have a smooth interface and may be associated with intramural hematoma.
- In a PAU, contrast extends beyond the intimal calcification (Fig. 23.6).

23.5.3 Perfect Report

The radiologist's report should include:

- Location
- Length extension
- Maximum depth of the PAU
- Size of the entry tear
- Presence and thickness of any associated intramural hematoma
- Presence of other complications such as pseudoaneurysm and aortic rupture

23.6 Rupture and Unstable Aortic Aneurysm

Aortic aneurysms are focal dilations of the aorta that are 50% larger than the vessel's normal diameter (Table 23.4) [32, 33]. Most aortic aneurysms (AA) are true aneurysms. A true aortic aneurysm involves all three layers (intima, media, and adventitia) of the vessel wall. A pseudoaneurysm (false aneurysm) is a blood collection in direct communication with the arterial lumen but not contained by the normal vessel wall, being held by the adventitia or surrounding soft tissues [32, 33].

The most common etiologies of AA are degenerative and inflammatory (Table 23.5). Aneurysms can develop in any segment of the aorta, but the majority involve the infrarenal segment [31, 34].

The most significant complication of AA is aortic rupture. The mortality rate for ruptured AA is 50%; therefore, accurate diagnosis is critical for timely surgical intervention. CT imaging can reveal both aortic aneurysm rupture and signs of impending wall instability indicating imminent rupture. Recognizing these findings suggests the need for urgent treatment (open surgery or TEVAR) [33].

Table 23.4 Normal aortic diameters at different anatomical levels

Level of aorta	Normal diameter (cm)
Ascending aorta	3
Aortic arch	2.5
Descending thoracic aorta	2.5
Abdominal aorta (above renal arteries)	2.4
Abdominal aorta (below renal arteries)	2
Common iliac arteries	1

Table 23.5 Causes of aortic aneurysm

Causes of aortic aneurysm	Description
Degenerative causes (most common)	Atherosclerosis and chronic hypertension lead to plaque build-up and weakening of the aortic wall.
Infection	Infections such as syphilis and salmonella can infect the aortic wall (mycotic aneurysm).
Inflammatory diseases	Diseases like giant cell arteritis and Takayasu arteritis that cause inflammation of blood vessels.
Genetic disorders	Conditions such as Marfan syndrome, Ehlers-Danlos syndrome, and bicuspid aortic valve.

23.6.1 Risk Factors and Clinical Presentation

The prevalence of aneurysms increases with age. Approximately 10% of patients over 65 have an aortic aneurysm, with males being more affected than females (male-to-female ratio 4:1) [31]. Concomitant coronary artery disease and peripheral vascular disease, as well as a family history of aortic aneurysm, are strong risk factors for this condition [31].

An AA is considered unstable when there are signs of imminent rupture. Symptomatic unstable AA is clinically indistinguishable from AD, IMH, or PAU [35]. Most stable AAs are asymptomatic. Large aneurysms may present as a pulsatile abdominal mass in some patients. In cases of rupture, the classic triad of pain, hypotension, and a pulsatile abdominal mass is observed in 25–50% of patients.

23.6.2 Imaging

As with acute aortic syndromes, the gold standard for studying aortic aneurysmal disease is CT. Various CT signs can indicate the unstable nature of an aneurysm (Table 23.6). However, CT findings of contained rupture or impending aneurysm rupture can be subtle and easily overlooked, so a thorough knowledge of these findings is crucial for prompt treatment.

CT signs of imminent rupture include [36] (Fig. 23.7):

- Rapid size increase (>10 mm/year)
- Focal discontinuities of intimal calcifications (missing calcium sign)
- Eccentric aortic lumen shape
- Crescent-shaped hyperattenuation area (crescent sign), seen on non-contrast MDCT as a

localized, usually curvilinear area of higher attenuation in the thrombus, caused by fresh blood first infiltrating the mural thrombus and then penetrating the aortic wall

Table 23.6 CT findings in non-traumatic aortic emergencies

Pathological condition	CT findings
Aortic dissection	Intimal Flap: A thin, linear structure within the aorta, separating true and false lumens. Double Lumen Sign: Presence of two lumens (true and false) within the aorta. Displacement of intimal calcification Delayed enhancement of false lumen Ischemia of distal organs
Intramural hematoma	Crescentic or circumferential high-attenuation area within the aortic wall Aortic wall thickening Absence of intimal flap.
Penetrating atherosclerotic ulcer	Focal outpouching of contrast from the aortic lumen into the aortic wall Adjacent aortic wall thickening Often associated with intramural hematoma
Aortic rupture	Periaortic stranding and hematoma Extravasation of contrast
Unstable aortic aneurysm	Rapid size increase (>10 mm/year); Missing calcium sign Eccentric aortic lumen shape; Crescent sign Draped sign Periaortic stranding

- Thrombotic fissuration
- Poorly defined posterior aortic wall closely adhering to the spine (draping sign)
- Periaortic stranding

In the event of aortic rupture, the primary CT signs are periaortic hematoma, visible even in the precontrast phase, and contrast extravasation (Fig. 23.8). Thoracic aorta rupture may present with mediastinal hematoma, hemopericardium, and hemothorax. Abdominal aorta rupture typically shows an extensive retroperitoneal hematoma involving the psoas and peri- and pararenal spaces (Table 23.6). Intraperitoneal hemorrhage can be an immediate or delayed finding.

23.6.3 Perfect Report

A comprehensive radiological report on AA should include the following features, especially if it is a new or undocumented finding:

- Size and shape
  - Fusiform or saccular
  - Maximum transverse diameter of the aneurysmal sac, measured perpendicular to the aorta's longitudinal axis
  - Longitudinal extent of the aneurysmal sac
  - Luminal diameter if a mural thrombus is present
  - Aortic caliber proximally and distally to the aneurysm

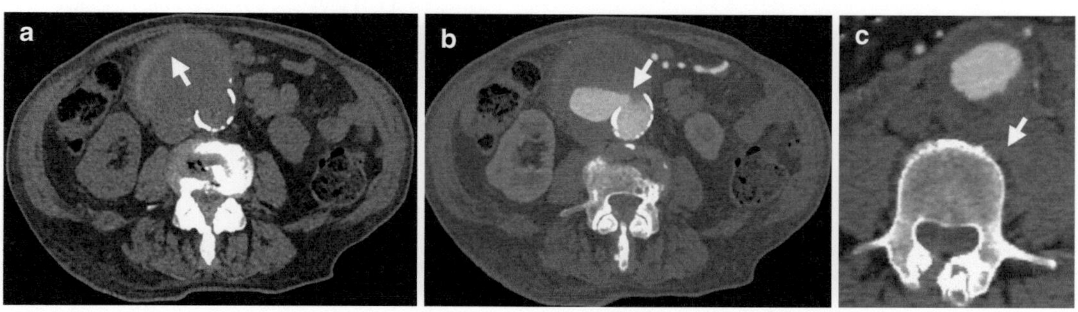

Fig. 23.7 CT signs of imminent rupture. (**a**) Non-contrast CT scan study of the abdomen demonstrates a large subrenal abdominal aortic aneurysm with a crescent-shaped hyperattenuation area (crescent sign) (arrow). (**b**) Contrast-enhanced CT scan study of the abdomen shows focal discontinuities of intimal calcifications (missing calcium sign) (arrow). (**c**) Contrast-enhanced CT scan study of the abdomen shows a poorly defined posterior aortic wall closely adhering to the spine (draping sign) (arrow) and periaortic stranding

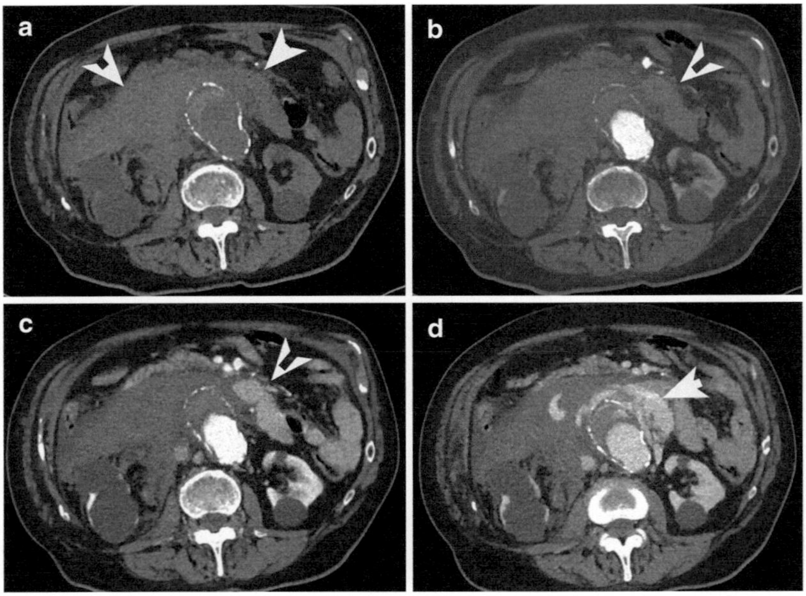

Fig. 23.8 Rupture aortic aneurysm. (**a**) Non-contrast CT scan study of the abdomen demonstrates a large abdominal aortic aneurysm with a periaortic hematoma. (**b–d**) After contrast administration, progressive contrast extravasation is observed

- Wall characteristics
  - Mural calcification
  - Presence of parietal thrombotic apposition
- Location and relationship to involved branches/structures:
  - Renal arteries:

    Involvement of renal artery origins or distance from the most caudal renal artery origin

    Presence of accessory and/or aberrant renal arteries
  - Splanchnic arteries
  - Supra-aortic vessels
- Possible etiology characterization:
  - Degenerative
  - Mycotic
- Signs of aortic rupture or impending rupture
- Presence of organ damage (e.g., renal or splenic infarction)
- Status and diameters of access arteries (common femoral artery and external iliac artery) and diameters and any anatomical characteristics of the aorta

References

1. Hiratzka LF, Bakris GL, Beckman JA, Bersin RM, Carr VF, Casey DE Jr, Eagle KA, Hermann LK, Isselbacher EM, Kazerooni EA, Kouchoukos NT, Lytle BW, Milewicz DM, Reich DL, Sen S, Shinn JA, Svensson LG, Williams DM, American College of Cardiology Foundation/American Heart Association Task Force on Practice Guidelines; American Association for Thoracic Surgery; American College of Radiology; American Stroke Association; Society of Cardiovascular Anesthesiologists; Society for Cardiovascular Angiography and Interventions; Society of Interventional Radiology; Society of Thoracic Surgeons; Society for Vascular Medicine. 2010 ACCF/AHA/AATS/ACR/ASA/SCA/SCAI/SIR/STS/SVM guidelines for the diagnosis and management of patients with Thoracic Aortic Disease: a report of the American College of Cardiology Foundation/American Heart Association Task Force on Practice Guidelines, American Association for Thoracic Surgery, American College of Radiology, American Stroke Association, Society of Cardiovascular Anesthesiologists, Society for Cardiovascular Angiography and Interventions, Society of Interventional Radiology, Society of Thoracic Surgeons, and Society for Vascular Medicine. Circulation. 2010;121(13):e266–369.

https://doi.org/10.1161/CIR.0b013e3181d4739e. Epub 2010 Mar 16. Erratum in: Circulation. 2010 Jul 27;122(4):e410
2. Valente T, Rossi G, Lassandro F, Rea G, Marino M, Muto M, Molino A, Scaglione M. MDCT evaluation of acute aortic syndrome (AAS). Br J Radiol. 2016;89(1061):20150825. https://doi.org/10.1259/bjr.20150825. Epub 2016 Apr 1
3. Howard DP, Banerjee A, Fairhead JF, Perkins J, Silver LE, Rothwell PM, Oxford Vascular Study. Population-based study of incidence and outcome of acute aortic dissection and premorbid risk factor control: 10-year results from the Oxford Vascular Study. Circulation. 2013;127(20):2031–7. https://doi.org/10.1161/CIRCULATIONAHA.112.000483. Epub 2013 Apr 18
4. Yuan X, Mitsis A, Tang Y, Nienaber CA. The IRAD and beyond: what have we unravelled so far? Gen Thorac Cardiovasc Surg. 2019;67(1):146–53. https://doi.org/10.1007/s11748-017-0817-6. Epub 2017 Sep 6
5. Vilacosta I, San Román JA. Acute aortic syndrome. Heart. 2001;85(4):365–8. https://doi.org/10.1136/heart.85.4.365.
6. Ko JP, Goldstein JM, Latson LA Jr, Azour L, Gozansky EK, Moore W, Patel S, Hutchinson B. Chest CT angiography for acute aortic pathologic conditions: pearls and pitfalls. Radiographics. 2021;41(2):399–424. https://doi.org/10.1148/rg.2021200055.
7. Chiu KW, Lakshminarayan R, Ettles DF. Acute aortic syndrome: CT findings. Clin Radiol. 2013;68(7):741–8. https://doi.org/10.1016/j.crad.2013.03.001. Epub 2013 Apr 11
8. Nicholls F. Observations concerning the body of His Late Majesty. Philos Trans Lond. 1761;52:265–74. https://doi.org/10.1098/rstl.1761.0052.
9. Nienaber CA, Powell JT. Management of acute aortic syndromes. Eur Heart J. 2012;33(1):26–35b. https://doi.org/10.1093/eurheartj/ehr186. Epub 2011 Aug 2
10. Braverman AC, Thompson RW, Sanchez LA. Diseases of the aorta. In: Bonow RO, Mann DL, Zipes DP, Libby P, editors. Braunwald's heart disease. 9th ed. Philadelphia: Elsevier Saunders; 2012. p. 1309–37. https://doi.org/10.1007/978-1-84996-362-6_22.
11. Macura KJ, Corl FM, Fishman EK, Bluemke DA. Pathogenesis in acute aortic syndromes: aortic dissection, intramural hematoma, and penetrating atherosclerotic aortic ulcer. AJR Am J Roentgenol. 2003;181(2):309–16. https://doi.org/10.2214/ajr.181.2.1810309.
12. Dake MD, Thompson M, van Sambeek M, Vermassen F, Morales JP, DEFINE Investigators. DISSECT: a new mnemonic-based approach to the categorization of aortic dissection. Eur J Vasc Endovasc Surg. 2013;46(2):175–90. https://doi.org/10.1016/j.ejvs.2013.04.029. Epub 2013 May 28
13. Saremi F, Hassani C, Lin LM, Lee C, Wilcox AG, Fleischman F, Cunningham MJ. Image predictors of treatment outcome after thoracic aortic dissection repair. Radiographics. 2018;38(7):1949–72. https://doi.org/10.1148/rg.2018180025. Epub 2018 Oct 12
14. Daily PO, Trueblood HW, Stinson EB, Wuerflein RD, Shumway NE. Management of acute aortic dissections. Ann Thorac Surg. 1970;10(3):237–47. https://doi.org/10.1016/s0003-4975(10)65594-4.
15. Erbel R, Aboyans V, Boileau C, Bossone E, Bartolomeo RD, Eggebrecht H, Evangelista A, Falk V, Frank H, Gaemperli O, Grabenwöger M, Haverich A, Iung B, Manolis AJ, Meijboom F, Nienaber CA, Roffi M, Rousseau H, Sechtem U, Sirnes PA, Allmen RS, Vrints CJ, ESC Committee for Practice Guidelines. 2014 ESC Guidelines on the diagnosis and treatment of aortic diseases: document covering acute and chronic aortic diseases of the thoracic and abdominal aorta of the adult. The Task Force for the Diagnosis and Treatment of Aortic Diseases of the European Society of Cardiology (ESC). Eur Heart J. 2014;35(41):2873–926. https://doi.org/10.1093/eurheartj/ehu281. Epub 2014 Aug 29. Erratum in: Eur Heart J. 2015 Nov 1;36(41):2779. https://doi.org/10.1093/eurheartj/ehv178
16. Fattori R, Cao P, De Rango P, Czerny M, Evangelista A, Nienaber C, Rousseau H, Schepens M. Interdisciplinary expert consensus document on management of type B aortic dissection. J Am Coll Cardiol. 2013;61(16):1661–78. https://doi.org/10.1016/j.jacc.2012.11.072.
17. Grabenwöger M, Alfonso F, Bachet J, Bonser R, Czerny M, Eggebrecht H, Evangelista A, Fattori R, Jakob H, Lönn L, Nienaber CA, Rocchi G, Rousseau H, Thompson M, Weigang E, Erbel R, European Association for Cardio-Thoracic Surgery (EACTS); European Society of Cardiology (ESC); European Association of Percutaneous Cardiovascular Interventions (EAPCI). Thoracic Endovascular Aortic Repair (TEVAR) for the treatment of aortic diseases: a position statement from the European Association for Cardio-Thoracic Surgery (EACTS) and the European Society of Cardiology (ESC), in collaboration with the European Association of Percutaneous Cardiovascular Interventions (EAPCI). Eur J Cardiothorac Surg. 2012;42(1):17–24. https://doi.org/10.1093/ejcts/ezs107. Epub 2012 May 4
18. Sebastià C, Pallisa E, Quiroga S, Alvarez-Castells A, Dominguez R, Evangelista A. Aortic dissection: diagnosis and follow-up with helical CT. Radiographics. 1999;19(1):45–60; quiz 149–50. https://doi.org/10.1148/radiographics.19.1.g99ja0945.
19. LePage MA, Quint LE, Sonnad SS, Deeb GM, Williams DM. Aortic dissection: CT features that distinguish true lumen from false lumen. AJR Am J Roentgenol. 2001;177(1):207–11. https://doi.org/10.2214/ajr.177.1.1770207.
20. Schlatter T, Auriol J, Marcheix B, Lebbadi M, Marachet MA, Dang-Tran KD, Tran M, Honton B, Gardette V, Rousseau H. Type B intramural hematoma of the aorta: evolution and prognostic value of intimal erosion. J Vasc Interv Radiol. 2011;22(4):533–41. https://doi.org/10.1016/j.jvir.2010.10.028.

21. Holden A. The value of narrow CT window settings in the recognition of subtle acute aortic intramural haematoma. Australas Radiol. 2000;44(1):128–9. https://doi.org/10.1046/j.1440-1673.2000.00769.x.
22. von Kodolitsch Y, Csösz SK, Koschyk DH, Schalwat I, Loose R, Karck M, Dieckmann C, Fattori R, Haverich A, Berger J, Meinertz T, Nienaber CA. Intramural hematoma of the aorta: predictors of progression to dissection and rupture. Circulation. 2003;107(8):1158–63. https://doi.org/10.1161/01.cir.0000052628.77047.ea.
23. Kitai T, Kaji S, Yamamuro A, Tani T, Kinoshita M, Ehara N, Kobori A, Kim K, Kita T, Furukawa Y. Detection of intimal defect by 64-row multidetector computed tomography in patients with acute aortic intramural hematoma. Circulation. 2011;124(11 Suppl):S174–8. https://doi.org/10.1161/CIRCULATIONAHA.111.037416.
24. Wu MT, Wang YC, Huang YL, Chang RS, Li SC, Yang P, Wu TH, Chiou KR, Huang JS, Liang HL, Pan HB. Intramural blood pools accompanying aortic intramural hematoma: CT appearance and natural course. Radiology. 2011;258(3):705–13. https://doi.org/10.1148/radiol.10101270. Epub 2011 Jan 6
25. Lansman SL, Saunders PC, Malekan R, Spielvogel D. Acute aortic syndrome. J Thorac Cardiovasc Surg. 2010;140(6 Suppl):S92–7; discussion S142-S146. https://doi.org/10.1016/j.jtcvs.2010.07.062.
26. Nathan DP, Boonn W, Lai E, Wang GJ, Desai N, Woo EY, Fairman RM, Jackson BM. Presentation, complications, and natural history of penetrating atherosclerotic ulcer disease. J Vasc Surg. 2012;55(1):10–5. https://doi.org/10.1016/j.jvs.2011.08.005. Epub 2011 Nov 1
27. Evangelista A, Carro A, Moral S, Teixido-Tura G, Rodríguez-Palomares JF, Cuéllar H, García-Dorado D. Imaging modalities for the early diagnosis of acute aortic syndrome. Nat Rev Cardiol. 2013;10(8):477–86. https://doi.org/10.1038/nrcardio.2013.92. Epub 2013 Jun 25
28. Patatas K, Shrivastava V, Ettles DF. Penetrating atherosclerotic ulcer of the aorta: a continuing debate. Clin Radiol. 2013;68(8):753–9. https://doi.org/10.1016/j.crad.2012.11.014. Epub 2013 Mar 27
29. Botta L, Buttazzi K, Russo V, Parlapiano M, Gostoli V, Di Bartolomeo R, Fattori R. Endovascular repair for penetrating atherosclerotic ulcers of the descending thoracic aorta: early and mid-term results. Ann Thorac Surg. 2008;85(3):987–92. https://doi.org/10.1016/j.athoracsur.2007.10.079.
30. Baikoussis NG, Apostolakis EE. Penetrating atherosclerotic ulcer of the thoracic aorta: diagnosis and treatment. Hell J Cardiol. 2010;51(2):153–7.
31. Maddu KK, Shuaib W, Telleria J, Johnson JO, Khosa F. Nontraumatic acute aortic emergencies: Part 1, Acute aortic syndrome. AJR Am J Roentgenol. 2014;202(3):656–65. https://doi.org/10.2214/AJR.13.11437.
32. Booher AM, Eagle KA. Diagnosis and management issues in thoracic aortic aneurysm. Am Heart J. 2011;162(1):38–46.e1. https://doi.org/10.1016/j.ahj.2011.04.010. Epub 2011 Jun 15
33. Guo DC, Papke CL, He R, Milewicz DM. Pathogenesis of thoracic and abdominal aortic aneurysms. Ann N Y Acad Sci. 2006;1085:339–52. https://doi.org/10.1196/annals.1383.013.
34. Isselbacher EM. Thoracic and abdominal aortic aneurysms. Circulation. 2005;111(6):816–28. https://doi.org/10.1161/01.CIR.0000154569.08857.7A.
35. Ueda T, Chin A, Petrovitch I, Fleischmann D. A pictorial review of acute aortic syndrome: discriminating and overlapping features as revealed by ECG-gated multidetector-row CT angiography. Insights Imaging. 2012;3(6):561–71. https://doi.org/10.1007/s13244-012-0195-7. Epub 2012 Nov 6
36. Rakita D, Newatia A, Hines JJ, Siegel DN, Friedman B. Spectrum of CT findings in rupture and impending rupture of abdominal aortic aneurysms. Radiographics. 2007;27(2):497–507. https://doi.org/10.1148/rg.272065026.

24 Other Vascular Emergencies

Fabio Corvino, Francesco Giurazza, Antonio Corvino, Massimo Galia, and Raffaella Niola

24.1 Spontaneous Retroperitoneal Haemorrhage

24.1.1 Introduction

Spontaneous retroperitoneal hematoma (SRH) is a potentially fatal and difficult-to-diagnose clinical entity defined as bleeding into the retroperitoneal space without any triggers such as trauma, invasive procedures and abdominal aortic aneurysm. SRH usually occurs in the elderly population that generally takes anticoagulants or antiplatelet therapy; moreover, in only one-third of patients had a pathological value of aPTT or INR associated with SRH. They may also be a result of haemodialysis, haemophilia or abnormal retroperitoneal formations (as vascular retroperitoneal lesions such as cysts, aneurysms, tumors, or lipomas). Bleeding can occur in any retroperitoneal vessels and organs; a specific section for the more representative ones, as iliopsoas haemorrhage, will be discussed in a specific section (see Sect. 24.2) [1]. To date, the SRH pathogenesis is still unclear, it may be caused by microvessel arteriosclerosis, vascular direct lesions such as segmental arterial mediolysis or unrecognized micro-trauma. However, the bleeding cause is often unclear [2] (Table 24.1).

24.1.2 Clinical Presentation

SRH has a very pleiomorphic presentation and it may be considered in all cases with lumbar pain associated with hypovolemia, where another plausible ethology is not found.

The most common symptoms are pain (especially in the abdomen, back or legs) and weakness, leg numbness or pulselessness. Rarely, flank ecchymoses or masses may be present. Moreover, in case of massive bleeding symptoms due to hypovolemia may be present as weakness or syncope up to haemorrhagic shock [2, 3].

F. Corvino (✉)
Interventional Radiology Department, AORN "A. Cardarelli", Naples, Italy

Section of Radiology, Department of Biomedicine, Neuroscience and Advanced Diagnostics (BiND), University Hospital "Paolo Giaccone", Palermo, Italy
e-mail: fabio.corvino@aocardarelli.it

F. Giurazza · R. Niola
Interventional Radiology Department, AORN "A. Cardarelli", Naples, Italy
e-mail: francesco.giurazza@aocardarelli.it; raffaella.niola@aocardarelli.it

A. Corvino
Motor Science and Wellness Department, University of Naples "Parthenope", Naples, Italy
e-mail: antonio.corvino@uniparthenope.it

M. Galia
Section of Radiology, Department of Biomedicine, Neuroscience and Advanced Diagnostics (BiND), University Hospital "Paolo Giaccone", Palermo, Italy
e-mail: massimo.galia@unipa.it

L. Romano et al. (eds.), *CT of Non-Traumatic Body Emergencies*,
https://doi.org/10.1007/978-3-031-84849-0_24

Table 24.1 Clinical presentation and typical CT findings in those vascular emergencies

Vascular emergencies	Signs/symptoms	Ct findings
Spontaneous retroperitoneal haemorrhage	Pain (especially in the abdomen, back or legs) and Weakness, leg numbness or pulselessness. Anemia Tachycardia Hypotension Haemorrhagic shock	Hazy margin with fluid tracking through the retroperitoneum Acute and subacute hematoma: high attenuation in basal phase Chronic hematoma: low attenuation in basal phase Cause of the bleeding: hemorrhagic cyst, bleeding tumor, pancreatico-duodenal aneurysm rupture, pseudoaneurysm
Ilio-psoas hematoma	Groin or thight pain omolateral to hematoma Muscle dysfunction Paresthesia Nerve palsy Ecchymosis Anemia Tachycardia Hypotension	Muscle hyperdense hematoma in non-contrast CT scan Fluid-fluid level Active bleeding in post-contrast phase
IVC thrombosis	Bilateral lower extremity swelling Dilation of superficial abdominal vessels Phlegmasia cerulea dolens Venous gangrene Fever	Absence of enhancement in IVC without vessel expansion in case of bland thrombosis Presence of enhancement in IVC with vessel expansion in case of neoplastic thrombosis Acute or chronic deep vein thrombosis associated Pericaval or periaortic collateral veins in case of chronic thrombosis

24.1.3 Imaging

CT scan is the gold standard to studying the retroperitoneum in the case of SRH, especially in an emergency setting. In the CT study, the retroperitoneal structures may present a hazy margin with fluid tracking through the retroperitoneum. A possible differentiation between acute or subacute and chronic hematomas could be related to the CT attenuation in the non-contrast phase: in acute or subacute cases the haematoma present itself generally with high attenuation differentiating from the chronic cases where the hematoma presents with low attenuation. In a post-contrast phase CT study, the hematoma should be present with a well-defined margin generally with hyperaemic walls; in addition to it there should be the presence or the absence of active bleeding or vascular lesions (as pseudoaneurysm, cyst, tumour, etc.) that will guide the subsequent treatment [4, 5].

24.1.4 Differential Diagnosis

SRH must be differentiated from other acute haemorrhagic lesions, firstly a ruptured acute abdominal aorta must be ruled out; moreover, it's mandatory to recognize the cause of haemorrhage in retroperitoneal region such as a bleeding tumour (e.g. renal angiomyolipoma or adrenal gland haemorrhage). In the case of acute hematoma, an abscess or a mass, malignant or benign, could be excluded by the administration of contrast media it is essential for a correct diagnosis. In the case of a chronic haematoma, the CT images' appearance could be confused with an abscess or a necrotic mass and only a direct percutaneous aspiration allows to differentiate them [1–6].

24.1.5 Interventional Radiology Therapeutic Option

Thought to principally occur as a rare phenomenon in elderly anticoagulated patients, SRH has a low published incidence of under 0.6% but a relatively high overall mortality of up to 22% based on case series published to date [7].

SRHs management is still debated; however, in hemodynamically stable patients with negative CT studies for bleeding, a conservative treatment is the preferred approach with volume support with blood products, reverse anticoagulation, and pain relief. In case of clinical condition worsening or in case of active bleeding at CT study the endovascular embolization treatment should be preferred to open surgical one [8].

One of the main risk factors for death is the volume of hematoma; there is still debate in literature if an embolization treatment in an earlier phase should be preferred to a conservative one [9].

24.2 Iliopsoas Haemorrhage

24.2.1 Introduction

Hemorrhage of the iliopsoas muscle leading to hematoma formation is an uncommon occurrence. The incidence of this condition is reported to be between 0.003% and 0.6% inpatient series with predisposing factors for hemorrhage or hematoma formation [1]. This incidence varies depending on patient-specific factors such as a history of hemophilia, age, and anticoagulation status. The iliopsoas compartment is a retroperitoneal space that is located posterior to the abdomen and pelvic region extending into the thigh. It contains the greater psoas, smaller psoas and iliac muscles; all of them extend from the diaphragm region to the lesser trochanter of the femur. The greater psoas fibres are the most significant muscles that overlie the vertebral column. The greater psoas muscles originate from on either side of the vertebral column with a deeper segment from the first four lumbar vertebrae and a superficial segment from the lateral surface of the thoracic vertebrae and from adjacent intervertebral discs. They reach the lesser pelvic region, where combining with iliac muscle fibres, form the iliopsoas muscle that inserts distally on the lesser trochanter of the femur with the common tendon (Fig. 24.1). The smaller psoas muscle is more medial and anterior to the greater one, originating from the vertical fascicles inserted on the last thoracic and first lumbar

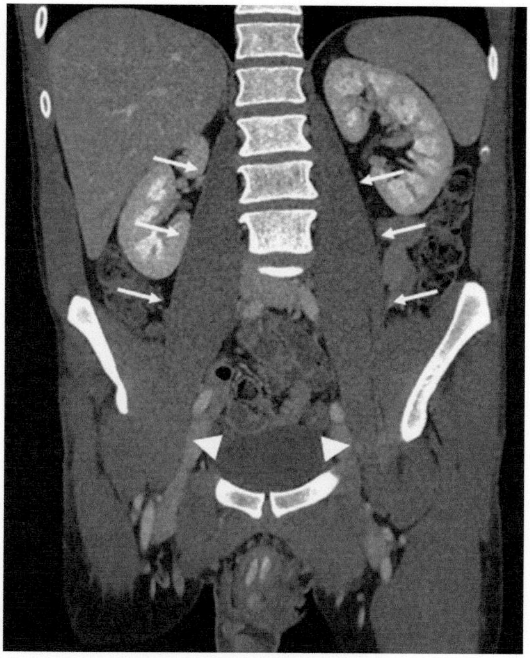

Fig. 24.1 Ileopsoas muscle: The greater psoas originates bilaterally from the vertebral column (arrows) and its insertion attaches distally to the lesser trochanter of the femur combining itself with the iliac muscle fibers (arrowheads)

vertebrae inserting itself to the innominate line and the iliopectineal eminence. Finally, the iliac muscle originates from the surface of the iliac fossa and anterior inferior iliac spine, and combining with greater psoas fibres, insert itself into the lesser trochanter of the femur with the common tendon [10].

The inflammatory and haemorrhagic ones are the most common pathologic processes that involve this compartment, with a very low rate of neoplasm processes generally secondary to adjacent spread and rarely primary (liposarcoma, fibrosarcoma and leiomyosarcoma). Iliopsoas haemorrhage could be spontaneous or secondary to trauma, anticoagulant therapy, inflammatory disease, tumour or iatrogenic due to surgery or biopsy. One of the major contributors to haemorrhage, especially in elderly population for their muscular fatty involution, is microangiopathy and vascular fragility that enhance the risk for the intramuscular tears and bleeding [11]. The iliopsoas muscles are supported by different arteries: collateral rami of the lumbar arteries, by the iliolumbar arteries, circumflex iliac artery, obturator artery, and femoral artery. Knowledge of them is crucial for a subsequent embolization treatment session [12].

24.2.2 Clinical Presentation

Iliopsoas hematomas typically present with groin or thigh pain, muscle dysfunction, numbness or paresthesia of the unilateral lower extremity, and occasionally nerve palsy, most commonly affecting the femoral nerve. Motor weakness can occur in cases of chronic or large hematomas. Ecchymosis may also appear in the periumbilical area (Cullen's sign) or on the flanks (Grey-Turner's sign). It may also give systemic findings such as decreased haematocrit, tachycardia, and hypotension secondary to bleeding [3]. Nerve palsy due to iliopsoas hematoma is a rare condition but it may often present with subtle symptoms such as a tender lower abdominal mass, anemia, inguinal ecchymosis, constipation, a flexed and externally rotated hip, pain with hip range of motion, and varying degrees of lower extremity pain [13].

24.2.3 Imaging

Hematomas could be unilateral or occasionally bilateral (in this case the bleeding occurs as a consequence of coagulopathy due to anticoagulant medication or haemophilia); it tends to involve the iliopsoas muscle along its extension, causing enlargement or a mass-effect of high attenuation on non-enhanced CT scans (Fig. 24.2) [14]. When there is blood in different time of degradation there could be a fluid-fluid level (also known as hematocrit effect), better highlighted in post-contrast scans (Fig. 24.3). The use of contrast media allows to identify the presence of an active bleeding inside the hematoma, with the demonstration of a focal blush during arterial phase, with the typical pooling during the venous and late phases (Fig. 24.4) [6].

24.2.4 Differential Diagnosis

See the Sect. 24.1.4.

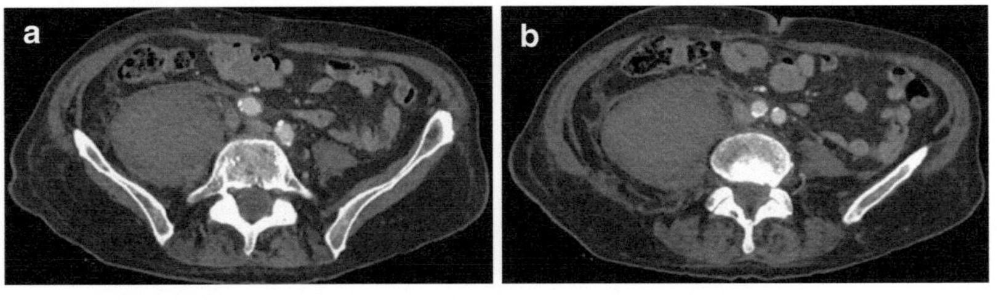

Fig. 24.2 Spontaneous hematoma in a 68-year-old male patient receiving Dabigatran. CT scan shows right ilio-psoas hematoma spontaneously hyperdense without bleeding after contrast media administration

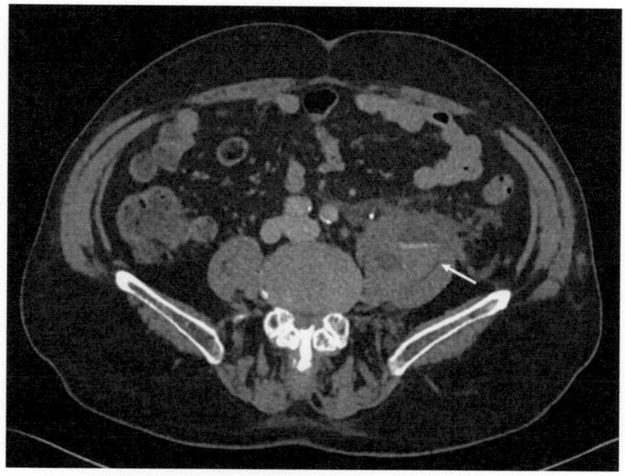

Fig. 24.3 Fluid-fluid level with direct extravasation (arrow) in the post-contrast portal phase

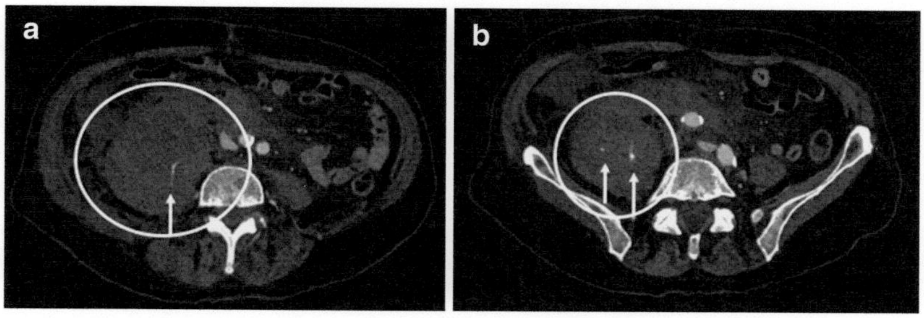

Fig. 24.4 Spontaneous retroperitoneal bleeding in a 75-year-old male patient patient receiving Rivaroxaban. CT scan shows enlargement of the right psoas with higher attenuation (circle) and multiple bleeding sites (arrow)

24.2.5 Interventional Radiology Therapeutic Option

A conservative management is the first approach in patients with spontaneous retroperitoneal haemorrhage, including the discontinuation of anticoagulant therapy, correction of coagulopathy and supportive/resuscitative measures. Embolization is becoming more common as an alternative to open surgery in treating retroperitoneal bleeding following iatrogenic injuries, after procedures such as percutaneous lumbar sympathectomy, renal biopsy, and percutaneous nephrostomy, or following iatrogenic iliofemoral vessel injuries. Open surgery is indicated if the patient remains unstable despite adequate fluid and blood product resuscitation, or if interventional radiology is either unsuccessful or unavailable [15]. In cases where the MDCT study demonstrated the presence of a bleeding, Interventional Radiology with intra/arterial embolization is the gold-standard, when the blood clotting laboratory's values allow a percutaneous approach. To date, there is no specific embolic material that promotes clot formation and the stop of the bleeding in retroperitoneal region. Anatomically, there is a rich network of collateral arteries between the different lumbar arteries and new arterial pathways may develop after obliteration of the lumbar arteries; to prevent technical failure or re-bleeding it's crucial to embolize both proximal and distal vascular bed. The use of coil or other embolic material that embolize proximally might not be sufficient; for this reason, these embolic materials are associated with the use of a liquid embolic agent that allows the embolization of the entire arterial segment as small-sized polyvinyl alcohol particles or Gelfoam that is an inexpensive and usually temporary embolic agent, with recanalization after usually occurring within 5–20 days [16, 17] (Fig. 24.5).

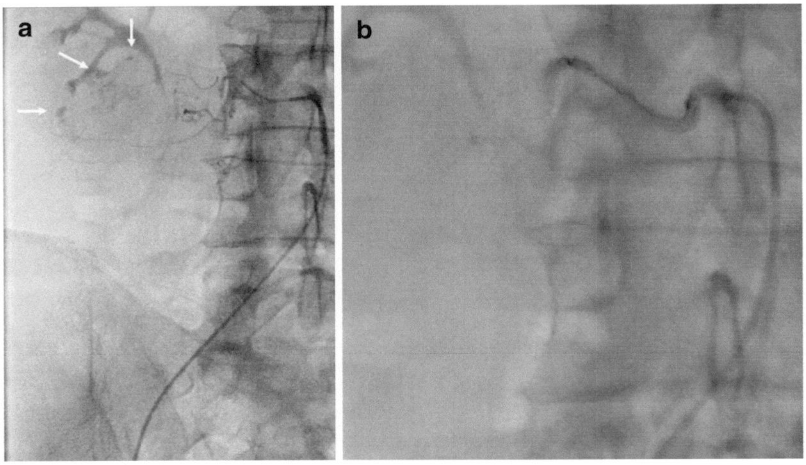

Fig. 24.5 Same patient of Fig. 24.4. (**a**). Angiographic study of the third right lumbar artery showed the presence of multiple haemorrhagic spot (arrow). (**b**). Final angiogram after embolization with 500–700 um PVA particles and coils demonstrated occlusion of the artery with the absence of further haemorrhagic spots

24.3 Inferior Vena Cava (IVC) Thrombosis

24.3.1 Introduction

Lifetime incidence of deep vein thrombosis (DVT) is 0.1% with a 4–15% incidence of IVC thrombosis in patients with a confirmed DVT. IVC thrombosis can be divided into congenital versus acquired; isolated or associated with deep venous thrombosis of the lower extremities from where the thrombus can spread. According to the Virchow triad, the clot formation may be secondary to a hypercoagulable state as malignancies or to a venous stasis due to local compression by adenopathy, fibrosis or large retroperitoneal masses or to a foreign body such as central venous catheters or IVC filters, that function as a trigger for thrombus formation. Bland thrombus is the leading cause of IVC obstruction, which places the patient at high risk for pulmonary embolism (PE) [18, 19].

24.3.2 Clinical Presentation

The clinical presentation of IVC thrombosis varies based on the thrombosis level (from the iliac confluence to the right atrium) and the degree of cava occlusion. Typically, patients exhibit bilateral lower extremity swelling and dilation of superficial abdominal vessels, although this classic presentation occurs in only about half of symptomatic cases [20]. If the thrombus is limited to the IVC, excluding the iliac or femoral systems, collateral pathways develop along the posterior abdominal wall. However, if the distal systems are involved, dilated veins can appear on the abdominal wall between the groin and axillae within days. Extension of the thrombosis to the pelvic and femoral veins increases the risk of phlegmasia cerulea dolens and venous gangrene. Additionally, fever can be present, as noted by Tsuji et al., who observed that 40% of their series of 10 patients were febrile at presentation [21].

24.3.3 Imaging

The portal-venous phase of a contrast-enhanced CT (60–80 s after contrast administration of a 100–120 ml of non-ionic contrast material injected at a rate of 3–5 ml/s) is the better phase to evaluate the IVC. A dynamic multiphasic imaging is performed if indicated; however, to confirm the presence of thrombus a late phase is useful to confirm total absence of enhancement [22]. During the portal-venous phase, the amount of contrast material in the suprarenal IVC is much more than the lower portion due to the venous return from the kidneys. The presence of a persistent filling defect within the column of contrast material leads to the diagnosis of bland thrombus. The bland thrombus lacks of luminal

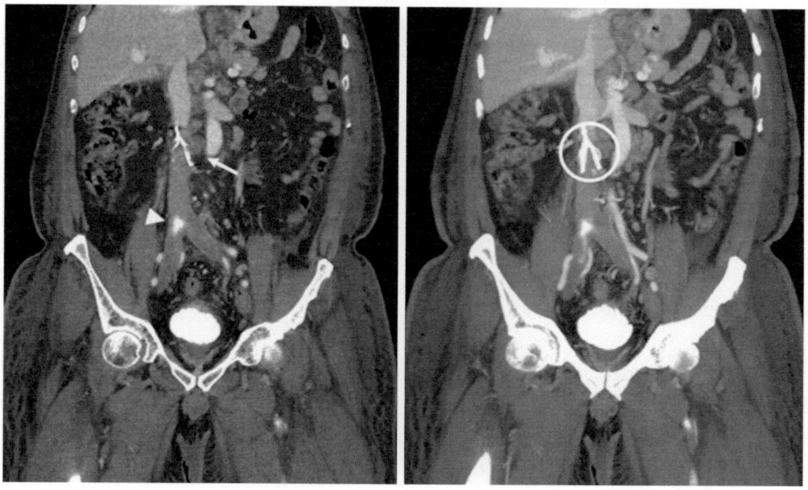

Fig. 24.6 A 55-year-old male patient with a bleeding gastric malignant neoplasm with lymph node spread (arrow) presented to our emergency department with a right lower extremity DVT. Due to the impossibility of carrying out anticoagulant therapy, the patient underwent an IVC filter placement (circle). However, the association of lymph node adjacent compression and foreign body hypercoagulability brings a complete IVC and bilateral lower extremities thrombosis. The arrowhead shows residual contrast into the IVC after an unsuccessful attempt at endovascular recanalization with mechanical thrombectomy devices

expansion and enhancement (Fig. 24.6); while imaging features consistent with tumor thrombus on CT include the presence of enhancement (the most specific sign) with the appearance of vessel expansion (generally evident also in bland thrombosis) and the extension into the vessel from an adjacent neoplasm. The differentiation of bland and neoplastic thrombosis is crucial in the setting of neoplasia, impacting the subsequent staging and treatment approach. In case of acute deep thrombus formation, it's difficult to see a collateral pathway that forms a natural bypass obstruction; those cases are emergent conditions, similar to arterial ones that could bring the patient to an irreversible ischemic condition of lower extremities. On the other hand, when the IVC thrombus becomes chronic a collateral pathway, that bypass the obstruction, could be formed by the pericaval and periaortic collateral veins [23].

24.3.4 Differential Diagnosis

One of the main challenges of IVC imaging is the risk of confusing artifacts with IVC thrombus. One such artifact, the pseudolipoma, is a volume-averaging artifact caused by prominent pericaval fat above the caudate lobe, often observed in patients with cirrhosis. Another artifact, the admixture artifact, could be seen in the renal veins when contrast-enhanced blood from the kidneys mixes with non-enhanced blood from the lower extremities. This artifact may also occur due to retrograde contrast flow into the IVC as a result of right heart failure or an injection rate exceeding 3 mL/sec [24].

24.3.5 Interventional Radiology Therapeutic Option

Pharmacologic anticoagulation, when clinically feasible, remains the mainstay of treatment for DVT with or without IVC thrombosis. However, anticoagulation may have little effect on regression or resolution of IVC thrombus or a decrease in the occurrence of PE in those patients [25].

In addition to anticoagulation, to prevent pulmonary embolism arising from a DVT, a possible additional treatment is vena cava filter placement. Anatomically, the correct position of the vena cava filter is below the ostium of the renal veins;

for this reason, in case of an IVC thrombosis that involves the suprarenal tract the filter placement is contraindicated, except in some clinical conditions presented after. The absolute indication is the presence of DVT or PE with any of these conditions:–Contraindication to any anticoagulation treatment, both prophylactic and therapeutical dose;–Recurrent PE in spite of anticoagulation treatment;–Complications related to anticoagulation treatment. Extended indications include specific risks for complications from PE or anticoagulation and are summarized in the following:–subrenal iliocaval DVT or large free-floating proximal DVT;–Massive PE treatment with DVT in patients at risk of further episode of PE;–Limited cardiac reserve in patient with PE and DVT;–Prophylaxis in patients with severe trauma, spinal cord injury, or paraplegia;–Poor compliance with anticoagulation treatment. However, even if the placement of vena cava filter above the renal veins is very rare, due to the risk of misplacement toward the right hearth, there are some indications about this use:–Renal vein thrombosis monolateral or bilateral;–EP due to gonadic vein thrombosis;–Extended thrombosis above a previous filter positioned in IVC subrenal region [26, 27].

In addition to the placement of caval filter, other therapeutical options could be useful in ilio-femoral DVT treatment with extension into IVC; specifically, multiple endovascular methods like catheter-directed therapy (CDT) with or without mechanical thrombectomy (MT), balloon angioplasty and stent placement, are reported to be safe and effective in the short term, in terms of PE presentation, and in the long term, in terms of evolution rate in chronic post-thrombotic syndrome [28].

References

1. Dohan A, Sapoval M, Chousterman BG, di Primio M, Guerot E, Pellerin O. Spontaneous soft-tissue hemorrhage in anticoagulated patients: safety and efficacy of embolization. AJR Am J Roentgenol. 2015;204(6):1303–10. https://doi.org/10.2214/AJR.14.12578.
2. Sunga KL, Bellolio MF, Gilmore RM, Cabrera D. Spontaneous retroperitoneal hematoma: etiology, characteristics, management, and outcome. J Emerg Med. 2012;43(2):e157–61. https://doi.org/10.1016/j.jemermed.2011.06.006.
3. Rodriguez-Merchan EC, De la Corte-Rodriguez H. Iliopsoas hematomas in people with hemophilia: diagnosis and treatment. Expert Rev Hematol. 2020;13(8):803–9. https://doi.org/10.1080/17474086.2020.1787146.
4. Caleo O, et al. Spontaneous non-aortic retroperitoneal hemorrhage: etiology, imaging characterization and impact of MDCT on management. A multicentric study. Radiol Med. 2015;120(1):133–48. https://doi.org/10.1007/s11547-014-0482-0.
5. Sahu KK, Mishra AK, Lal A, George SV, Siddiqui AD. Clinical spectrum, risk factors, management and outcome of patients with retroperitoneal hematoma: a retrospective analysis of 3-year experience. Expert Rev Hematol. 2020;13(5):545–55. https://doi.org/10.1080/17474086.2020.1733963. Epub 2020 Mar 3. Erratum in: Expert Rev Hematol. 2020 Jun;13(6):i. doi: 10.1080/17474086.2020.1771654.
6. Landecy M, Paquette B, Revel L, Behr J, Badet N, Delabrousse E. Does IV contrast extravasation on CT in anticoagulant-related rectus sheath and iliopsoas hematoma predict hematoma expansion and patient outcomes? Abdom Radiol (NY). 2016;41(11):2241–7. https://doi.org/10.1007/s00261-016-0818-4.
7. Tiralongo F, Toscano S, Mosconi C, et al. Spontaneous retroperitoneal hematoma treated with transarterial embolization: a systematic review and metanalysis. CVIR Endovasc. 2024;7:50. https://doi.org/10.1186/s42155-024-00462-6.
8. Klausenitz C, Kuehn JP, Noeckler K, Radosa CG, Hoffmann RT, Teichgraeber U, Mensel B. Efficacy of transarterial embolisation in patients with life-threatening spontaneous retroperitoneal haematoma. Clin Radiol. 2021;76(2):157.e11–8. https://doi.org/10.1016/j.crad.2020.10.003.
9. Barral M, Pellerin O, Tran VT, Gallix B, Boucher LM, Valenti D, Sapoval M, Soyer P, Dohan A. Predictors of mortality from spontaneous soft-tissue hematomas in a large multicenter cohort who underwent percutaneous transarterial embolization. Radiology. 2019;291(1):250–8. https://doi.org/10.1148/radiol.2018181187.
10. Torres GM, Cernigliaro JG, Abbitt PL, Mergo PJ, Hellein VF, Fernandez S, Ros PR. Iliopsoas compartment: normal anatomy and pathologic processes. Radiographics. 1995;15(6):1285–97. https://doi.org/10.1148/radiographics.15.6.8577956.
11. Tonolini M, Campari A, Bianco R. Common and unusual diseases involving the iliopsoas muscle compartment: spectrum of cross-sectional imaging findings. Abdom Imaging. 2012;37(1):118–39. https://doi.org/10.1007/s00261-011-9764-3.

12. Cronin CG, Lohan DG, Meehan CP, Delappe E, McLoughlin R, O'Sullivan GJ, McCarthy P. Anatomy, pathology, imaging and intervention of the iliopsoas muscle revisited. Emerg Radiol. 2008;15(5):295–310. https://doi.org/10.1007/s10140-008-0703-8.
13. Guild TT, Crawford AM, Striano BM, Mortensen S, Wixted JJ. The epidemiology and management of iliopsoas hematoma with femoral nerve palsy: a descriptive systematic review of 174 cases. Injury. 2023;54(2):280–7. https://doi.org/10.1016/j.injury.2022.11.057.
14. Lenchik L, Dovgan DJ, Kier R. CT of the iliopsoas compartment: value in differentiating tumor, abscess, and hematoma. AJR Am J Roentgenol. 1994;162(1):83–6. https://doi.org/10.2214/ajr.162.1.8273696.
15. Touma L, Cohen S, Cassinotto C, Reinhold C, Barkun A, Tran VT, Banon O, Valenti D, Gallix B, Dohan A. Transcatheter arterial embolization of spontaneous soft tissue hematomas: a systematic review. Cardiovasc Intervent Radiol. 2019;42(3):335–43. https://doi.org/10.1007/s00270-018-2086-x.
16. Lucatelli P, De Rubeis G, Citone M, Lucarelli NM, Pasqualini V, Sturiale M, Giuliani S, Rosati M, Ceccherini C, Corona M, Mosconi C, Utili A, Argirò R. Heparin-related major bleeding in Covid-19-positive patient: perspective from the outbreak. Cardiovasc Intervent Radiol. 2020;43(8):1216–7. https://doi.org/10.1007/s00270-020-02532-3.
17. Palumbo D, Guazzarotti G, De Cobelli F. Spontaneous major Haemorrhage in COVID-19 patients: a proposal for a pathophysiology-based angiographic treatment. Cardiovasc Intervent Radiol. 2021;44(8):1289–90. https://doi.org/10.1007/s00270-021-02842-0.
18. Yamashita Y, Morimoto T, Kimura T. Venous thromboembolism: recent advancement and future perspective. J Cardiol. 2022;79(1):79–89. https://doi.org/10.1016/j.jjcc.2021.08.026.
19. Benedetti R, Marino S, Tangianu F, Imberti D. Inferior vena cava filters: a clinical review and future perspectives. J Clin Med. 2024;13(6):1761. https://doi.org/10.3390/jcm13061761.
20. Huynh K, Sanchala A, Ekiz A. Recurrent deep vein thrombosis (DVT) and inferior vena cava (IVC) filter: should a computed tomography (CT) Venogram and inferior vena Cavogram be the standard of care? Cureus. 2024;16(4):e58529. https://doi.org/10.7759/cureus.58529.
21. Tsuji Y, Inoue T, Murakami H, Hino Y, Matsuda H, Okita Y. Deep vein thrombosis caused by congenial interruption of the inferior vena cava–a case report. Angiology. 2001;52(10):721–5. https://doi.org/10.1177/000331970105201010.
22. Teter K, Schrem E, Ranganath N, Adelman M, Berger J, Sussman R, Ramkhelawon B, Rockman C, Maldonado TS. Presentation and management of inferior vena cava thrombosis. Ann Vasc Surg. 2019;56:17–23. https://doi.org/10.1016/j.avsg.2018.08.082.
23. Partovi S, Kalva SP, Walker TG, Taj SM, Ganguli S. Long term follow-up of endo-vascular recanalization of chronic inferior vena cava occlusion secondary to inferior vena cava filters. Vasa. 2017;46(2):121–6. https://doi.org/10.1024/0301-1526/a000593.
24. Wang Y, Gu J, Lu L, Yang Y, Zhang W, Huang C. Endovascular strategy for inferior vena cava thrombosis secondary to deep venous thrombosis of the lower extremities: early experience from two Centres. Vasc Endovasc Surg. 2023;57(7):689–96. https://doi.org/10.1177/15385744231167668.
25. Jiang J, Jiao Y, Zhang X. The short-term efficacy of vena cava filters for the prevention of pulmonary embolism in patients with venous thromboembolism receiving anticoagulation: meta-analysis of randomized controlled trials. Phlebology. 2017;32(9):620–7. https://doi.org/10.1177/0268355516669004.
26. Visconti L, Celi A, Carrozzi L, Tinelli C, Crocetti L, Daviddi F, De Caterina R, Madonna R, Pancani R. Inferior vena cava filters: concept review and summary of current guidelines. Vasc Pharmacol. 2024;155:107375. https://doi.org/10.1016/j.vph.2024.107375.
27. Haddad P, Peng J, Drake M, Rahimi M. Inferior vena cava filters: an overview. Methodist Debakey Cardiovasc J. 2024;20(3):49–56. https://doi.org/10.14797/mdcvj.1346.
28. Kim KA, Choi SY, Kim R. Endovascular treatment for lower extremity deep vein thrombosis: an overview. Korean J Radiol. 2021;22(6):931–43. https://doi.org/10.3348/kjr.2020.0675.

25 Pancreatitis

Giuliana Giacobbe, Martina Caruso, Piero Trovato, Chiara Rinaldo, Dario Grimaldi, and Marco Di Serafino

25.1 Introduction

Acute pancreatitis (AP) is a sudden inflammation of the pancreas. It is a potentially life-threatening condition, characterized by various stages of severity as well as the possible onset of local and/or systemic complications [1]. Generally, the symptomatology manifests itself with an onset of sudden and violent acute abdominal pain, mainly localized in the epi-mesogastric region and with irradiation to the dorsal region in about 50% of cases, associated with loss of appetite, nausea, and/or vomiting. In mild pancreatitis, these symptoms tend to be limited and resolve within a few days or a week. In more severe forms, however, pancreatitis may progress to acute failure of one or more organs (e.g. cardiovascular failure, respiratory failure, and/or acute kidney damage) until shock with possible death (>5% of cases) [2]. The main causes of AP are cholelithiasis and alcohol abuse. Less frequent etiological conditions include metabolic disorders, iatrogenic causes, autoimmune diseases, and neoplasms; in about 20% of cases, no specific cause is identified (Table 25.1) [3, 4].

G. Giacobbe (✉) · M. Caruso · C. Rinaldo
D. Grimaldi · M. Di Serafino
Department of General and Emergency Radiology, "Antonio Cardarelli" Hospital, Naples, Italy
e-mail: giuliana.giacobbe@aocardarelli.it; martina.caruso@aocardarelli.it; chiara.rinaldo@aocardarelli.it; dario.grimaldi@aocardarelli.it; marco.diserafino@aocardarelli.it

P. Trovato
Division of Radiology, "Istituto Nazionale Tumori IRCCS Fondazione Pascale—IRCCS", Naples, Italy
e-mail: piero.trovato@istitutotumori.na.it

L. Romano et al. (eds.), *CT of Non-Traumatic Body Emergencies*,
https://doi.org/10.1007/978-3-031-84849-0_25

Table 25.1 Causes of acute pancreatitis

Calculosis of the biliary tract (about 15%)
Idiopathic (about 20%)
Alcohol abuse
Metabolic disorders (e.g. hypertriglyceridaemia, hypercalcaemia)
Autoimmune
Penetrating peptic ulcer
Trauma
Iatrogenic (e.g. Endoscopic retrograde cholangiopancreatography, ERCP)
Slow-growing neoplasm
Malnutrition
Hereditary pancreatitis (e.g. SPINK 1 gene mutation)
Infections
Toxic (e.g. poisons)
Drugs (e.g. steroids, tetracyclines)
Others (e.g. cystic fibrosis, SLE)

25.2 Diagnosis

Prior to the widespread use in clinical practice of imaging methods in the evaluation of AP, clinical scoring systems, including Ranson, Glasgow, and the APACHE II (Acute Physiology and Chronic Health Evaluation) score, were mainly used. These scoring systems proved useful for predicting disease severity but not for predicting the development of local complications, organ failure, or mortality.

The Atlanta classification, initially developed in 1992, provided for the first time standardized terms for AP and its associated complications [5].

However, the 1992 nomenclature often proved confusing, leading to incorrect use of these terms in clinical practice and research. Furthermore, advances in imaging and understanding of pathophysiology necessitated a substantial revision of the classification system, leading to the development of the 2012 Atlanta Revised Classification (RAC) [6].

Currently, according to the RAC guidelines (2012), the diagnosis of AP requires the presence of at least two of the following three features:

- acute, intense, and persistent epigastric pain often radiating to the back;
- serum lipase or amylase activity at least three times higher than the upper limit of normal;
- findings characteristic of AP on Contrast-enhanced Computed Tomography (CECT) and, less commonly, on magnetic Resonance Imaging (MRI) or Ultrasound (US).

Although imaging may not be required in the presence of the clinical and laboratory criteria, it may be of paramount importance in defining etiopathogenesis and identifying possible complications.

The RAC also classifies AP on the basis of time criterion, severity, and morphological. In particular, it identifies two temporal phases of AP: early and late phases.

The early phase is represented by the first week from the onset of symptoms; in this phase, it is only the clinical parameters, determined by the systemic inflammatory response syndrome (SIRS), that are crucial for correct treatment planning.

The late phase, on the other hand, generally begins in the 2nd week, lasting up to several months, and only occurs in patients with moderate or severe pancreatitis, who may develop persistent organ failure and/or local complications. In these cases, the clinical parameters associated with the imaging findings determine the patient's management [6].

With the 2012 RAC, the concept of severity was also redefined. In fact, the 1992 classification of AP distinguished two degrees of disease, mild or severe, based on the presence or absence of organ failure [7].

According to the 2012 classification, three categories are distinguished:

- mild—no organ failure and no local or systemic complications;
- moderate—presence of transient organ failure of less than 48 h and/or presence of local complications;
- severe (15–20% of cases) - persistent organ failure >48 h.

Patients with mild pancreatitis generally do not develop organ failure and/or local complications and are usually discharged within the first week; in these cases, the main role of imaging is in defining the etiopathogenesis of the disease [8].

Moderate and/or severe AP manifests with organ failure lasting less than or more than 48 h and/or with local or systemic complications. In these cases, imaging plays a crucial role in the proper management of the patient [6].

The modified Marshall scoring system (Table 25.2) was approved in the RAC as the primary method for determining organ failure [9].

This system, taking into account the functionality of the three main systems involved (respiratory, cardiovascular and renal), assigns a score based on the results obtained: a value ≥2 for any system indicates a condition of organ failure.

In RAC, two sub-categories of AP were also identified on the basis of imaging findings: acute interstitial edematous pancreatitis and acute necrotizing pancreatitis.

Interstitial edematous pancreatitis represents the most frequent form (approximately 90–95% of cases) and is often referred to as the uncomplicated form. Acute necrotizing pancreatitis, on the other hand, occurs more rarely (in about 5–10% of cases).

25.3 The Role of the CT

The diagnosis of AP is essentially based on clinical and laboratory criteria; early CECT may be indicated in cases where there is clinical-laboratory discordance or where early complications such as ischemia or intestinal perforation are suspected [10, 11].

CECT can also be used to clarify the etiopathogenesis and to assess the morphology of AP findings although its main role is to define the extent and severity of inflammation and to identify possible complications.

Early stratification of patients with AP on the basis of the severity of the disease is of paramount importance. In mild forms, as previously mentioned, the main role of imaging is s to help identify the cause of pancreatitis. In these cases, US and MRI can also play a pivotal role; in particular, US makes it possible to identify the presence of gallstones and biliary tract stones with the limitation, however, of visualizing the terminal choledochal, which is better visualized by cholangial MRI [12]. In the more severe forms, the role of imaging, specifically CECT examination, is of fundamental importance in the classification, staging, and follow-up of the disease: the identification and quantification of pancreatic necrosis, the identification and assessment of the extent of intra-pancreatic and/or peri-pancreatic collections and their possible over-infection,

Table 25.2 Modified Marshall scoring system for organ dysfunction

Organ system	Score 0	Score 1	Score 2	Score 3	4
Respiratory (PaO_2/FiO_2 ratio)	>400	301–400	201–300	101–200	≤101
Renal (serum creatinine)	<1.4 mg/dL	1.4–1.8 mg/dL	1.9–3.6 mg/dL	3.6–4.9 mg/dL	>4.9 mg/dL
Cardiovascular (systolic blood pressure, pH)	>90 mm Hg	<90 mm Hg, fluid responsive	<90 mm Hg, not fluid responsive	<90 mm Hg, pH < 7.3	<90 mm Hg, pH < 7.2

A score of ≥2 in any system defines the presence of organ failure. Transient organ failure: organ failure resolving after ≤48 h; Persistent organ failure: organ failure persisting >48 h and finally the identification of hemorrhagic complications [13].

In the latter two situations (collections and hemorrhage), Interventional Radiology can also be of fundamental importance in the management of the patient, through the use of percutaneous drainage procedures of the collections (especially if infected) and embolization in situations of arterial hemorrhage. It is therefore essential for a correct evaluation of the radiological findings to know the timing of the onset of pancreatitis symptoms so that the radiological image can be correlated with the evolution of the disease itself [5].

A crucial fact to take into account, in fact, is that in the very early stages of inflammatory disease, radiological findings correlate very poorly with the severity of the disease and there is little sensitivity in identifying the presence of necrosis. CT examination is therefore essential at least 72 h after the onset of symptoms, at which time complications and possible pancreatic necrosis are better distractible and assessable [6].

In this regard, in the acute setting and thus within 72 h of symptom onset, CECT has been shown to be non-superior to clinical scoring systems by underestimating the presence of pancreatic/peripancreatic necrosis and its severity. Therefore, early CECT rarely changes patient management and does not improve clinical outcomes. However, there are exceptions that mainly include equivocal results of laboratory tests: for instance, alcohol-induced pancreatitis and hypertriglyceridemia may present with a lower elevation of serum amylase and lipase.

In 1990, a severity index was developed on the basis of CECT findings, called CT severity index (CTSI), which combines Balthazar grades (0–4 points) with the extent of pancreatic necrosis (0–6 points) on a severity scale ranging from 0 to 10 (Table 25.3); these scoring systems are designed to guide the management of patients with AP. A higher severity index score is associated with increased morbidity and mortality [13–15].

In particular, the CTSI of AP, assessed a combination of primary CECT findings including peripancreatic inflammation and inflammatory collections and the extent of pancreatic necrosis: less than 30%, 30–50%, and more than 50% of the pancreas. A significant direct correlation has been found between the CTSI and both the morbidity and mortality of AP.

Table 25.3 CT severity index

Pancreatic inflammation	**Points**
Normal pancreas	0
Pancreas enlargement	1
Peripancreatic inflammation	2
1 peripancreatic fluid collection	3
>1 peripancreatic fluid collection	4
Pancreatic necrosis	**Points**
None	0
<30%	2
30–50%	4
>50%	6

In 2004, Mortele et al. suggested a modified version of CTSI (mCTSI) by simplifying the assessment of pancreatic inflammation and quantification of the amount of necrosis (<30% or >30% only) and adding assessment of extra-pancreatic complications including pleural effusion, ascites, vascular, parenchymal, or gastrointestinal tract complications to the conventional CTSI (Table 25.4) [16].

Recently, comparative studies between the RAC, CTSI, and mCTSI have been reported. In general, there is good agreement between RAC, CTSI, and mCTSI; however, the mCTSI was found more sensitive but less specific than the CTSI in differentiating mild from more severe cases of AP [17].

In another series, however, the mCTSI was reported to be more accurate, easier to calculate, and with lower inter-observer variation than the CTSI in the management of patients with AP [18]. Another study considered two distinct clinical uses for the mCTSI and the CTSI, suggesting mCTSI for predicting short-term mortality and CTSI for predicting the need for intervention [19].

The role of dual-energy CECT has also been reported in the context of AP, although research is currently still limited. Early studies suggest that dual-energy techniques may allow better definition of residual parenchyma, necrotic debris, and

Table 25.4 Modified CT severity index of acute pancreatitis developed by Mortele et al.

Inflammation (points)	Necrosis (points)	Extra-pancreatic complications (one or more, 2 points)
Normal pancreas (0)	None (0)	Pleural effusion, ascites, vascular complications, parenchimal complications, gastrointestinal tract involvement
Intrinsic pancreatic abnormalities with or without inflammatory changes in peripancreatic fat (2)	<30% (2)	Pleural effusion, ascites, vascular complications, parenchimal complications, gastrointestinal tract involvement
Pancreatic or peripancreatic fluid collection or peripancreatic fat necrosis (4)	>30% (4)	Pleural effusion, ascites, vascular complications, parenchimal complications, gastrointestinal tract involvement

Modified severity index is defined by points of inflammation plus point of necrosis and points of extra-pancreatic complications (score 0–2: mild acute pancreatitis; 4–6: moderate acute pancreatitis; 8–10: severe acute pancreatitis)

possible hematoma; it may also be useful in the detection of non-calcific gallstones as a cause of AP using virtual single-energy imaging [20, 21]. Finally, in today's age of artificial intelligence (AI), machine learning algorithms have been developed to accurately predict severity, complications, recurrence, mortality, and even optimal timing of surgery for AP patients [22–25].

In particular, a study developed an AI tool with automatic pancreas segmentation and measurement of morphological information of the pancreas on CT images to facilitate better and faster diagnosis in AP [26].

Other studies, on the other hand, have devised machine-learning models by integrating clinical data with radiomic features extracted from CT images that can make an early diagnosis of the severity of acute gallstone pancreatitis or predict organ failure in acute hyperlipidemic pancreatitis (HLAP) [27, 28]. However, further validation and standardization are needed before widespread clinical application.

25.4 CT Semeiotics

25.4.1 Acute Interstitial Edematous Pancreatitis

Interstitial edematous pancreatitis is the most frequent form (approximately 90–95% of cases). Most patients with acute interstitial edematous pancreatitis present on CT scans with diffuse (or local) enlargement of the pancreatic gland. At CECT, homogeneous enhancement is generally

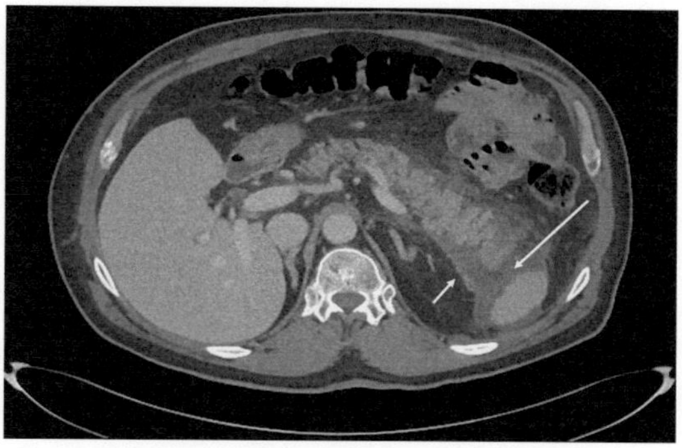

Fig. 25.1 Acute interstitial edematous pancreatitis. The contrast-enhanced CT axial scan in the portal phase shows moderate free fluid in the peripancreatic region (long arrow) with associated reactive thickening of the peritoneal fasciae (short arrow). Pancreas appears edematous and enlarged, especially at the level of the body-tail region. No evidence of parenchymal necrosis or any vascular complications. No visible gallstones

present, although this enhancement may often be less intense than that of the normal pancreas due to interstitial edema [29, 30].

In addition, the peripancreatic fat usually shows some inflammatory changes and therefore takes on a thickened and fuzzy appearance [29]. Free peripancreatic fluid and/or well-defined collections of homogeneous, non-necrotic fluid content may also be present (Figs. 25.1 and 25.2).

25.4.2 Acute Necrotizing Pancreatitis

The necrotizing form occurs in 5–10% of cases. We refer to a necrotizing form when both the glandular parenchyma and the peripancreatic tissues are affected. Depending on the areas involved, acute necrotizing pancreatitis can be classified into three subcategories:

- pancreatic only
- peripancreatic only
- combined pancreatic and peripancreatic

Combined acute necrotizing pancreatitis with involvement of the pancreatic gland and peripancreatic adipose cell is the most frequent subcategory (approximately 75% of cases).

On CECT, the combined subtype is manifested by a lack of enhancement at the level of the glandular parenchyma as well as by the visibility of peripancreatic collections of heterogeneous content, typically localized at the level of the retrocavity of the epiploons and/or along the anterior pararenal fascia. In peripancreatic necrosis alone (approximately 20% of cases), the glandular parenchyma shows preserved enhancement while the necrosis involves only the peripancreatic tissue with evidence of collections containing variable amounts of fluid with an inhomogeneous, corpuscular appearance [29, 30].

Pancreatic necrosis alone is the least common subtype, occurring in 5% of cases; it has no peripancreatic collections (Fig. 25.3).

Since the development of impaired pancreatic perfusion and peripancreatic necrosis takes several days, early CECT may underestimate the extent of pancreatic and peripancreatic necrosis. In the early days of the disease, the perfusion pattern of the pancreatic parenchyma may be normal and/or slightly attenuated. After the first week of the disease, an area of pancreatic parenchyma that does not strengthen should be considered necrotic [29, 30].

It is therefore necessary to perform a CT examination with contrast medium no earlier than 72 h after the onset of symptoms for an accurate diagnosis of necrotizing pancreatitis.

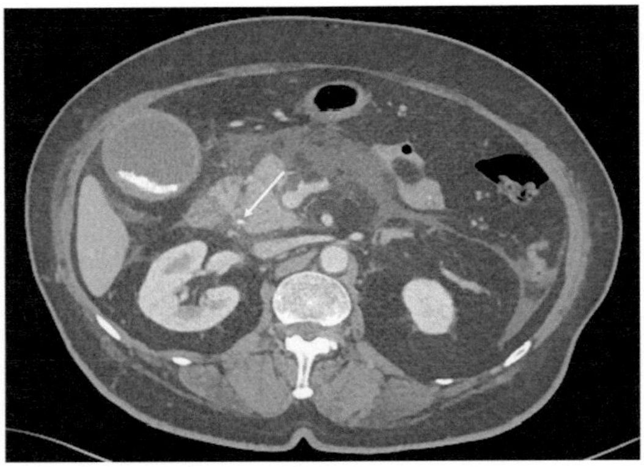

Fig. 25.2 Gallstone pancreatitis. The contrast-enhanced CT axial scan in the portal phase shows acute interstitial pancreatitis evidenced by unorganized, acute peripancreatic fluid/stranding. No areas of hypoenhancement to suggest a necrotizing component. Calcified gallstone at the distal common bile duct near the major duodenal papilla (arrow). The bile ducts and the main pancreatic duct are not dilated. Over-stretched, diffusely thickened walled gallbladder with lithiased content

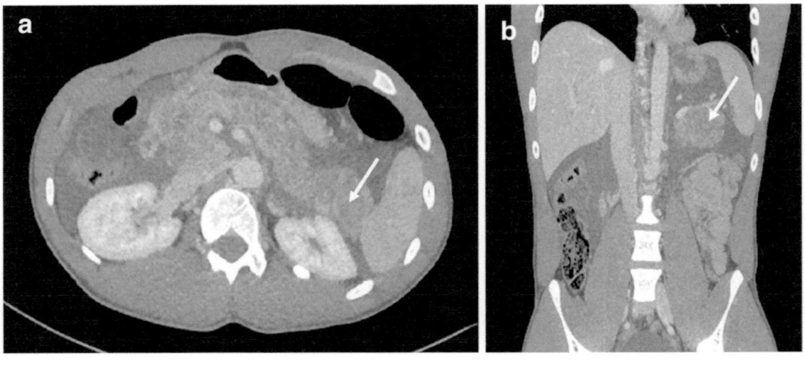

Fig. 25.3 Necrotizing pancreatitis. Axial (**a**) and coronal (**b**) CT images with contrast show a swollen pancreas with unenhanced areas in the body and tail of the pancreas (arrow, **a** and **b**); concomitant peripancreatic fluid, and mesenteric fat filaments. Free abdominal fluid is also observed

25.5 Local Complication

25.5.1 Pancreatic and Peripancreatic Collections

The RAC in 2012 distinguishes 4 types of peripancreatic collections in AP according to content, degree of encapsulation, and time [5–7].

In particular, the new Atlanta classification first abandons terms that are misleading in clinical practice such as 'acute pseudocyst' and/or 'abscess' to describe any peripancreatic collection in a setting of acute pancreatic inflammation, and makes an important distinction between collections with homogeneous fluid content (typical of acute interstitial edematous pancreatitis) and collections with an inhomogeneous appearance that contain necrotic debris (typical of necrotizing pancreatitis).

Therefore, the revised classification includes new definitions that more accurately describe the various types of collections found; in particular, it introduces terms such as APFC (Acute Peripancreatic Fluid Collection), ANC (Acute Necrotic Collection), Pseudocysts e WON (walled-off necrosis) based on the time course (<4 weeks or >4 weeks from the onset of pain), the degree of encapsulation and the presence or absence of necrosis on imaging (Table 25.5) [5].

APFCs represent collections that contain fluid only and are not or only partially encapsulated; they tend to conform to retroperitoneal spaces. They are seen within 4 weeks in interstitial edematous pancreatitis. Frequently they regress spontaneously and usually their drainage is not recommended because of the high risk of over-infection. APFC are always peripancreatic. If a collection of similar appearance is found within the pancreatic parenchyma, it is by definition an ANC and the diagnosis is no longer interstitial edematous pancreatitis but acute necrotizing pancreatitis [29, 30].

If an APFC does not resolve within four weeks, it takes on a more organized appearance and is called a pseudocyst. The pseudocyst has a well-defined capsule showing contrast enhancement on CT scan and typically has a peripancreatic location, although in some cases it may show an intrapancreatic location (e.g. in the case of a disconnected duct in a previous necrosectomy). The contents are always homogeneous fluid (Fig. 25.4) [29, 30]. Pseudocysts may have a connection with the pancreatic ductal system, which may be evident on CT examination although it is better seen on cholangial-MRI due to its better contrast resolution [29, 30].

ANC, on the other hand, are collections that occur within the first four weeks after the onset of symptoms in acute necrotizing pancreatitis. They are poorly organized, inhomogeneous in content, necrotic in appearance with varying amounts of non-liquefied debris such as solid-looking components and fat globules. Typically they may be either extra-pancreatic in location in the pararenal spaces with possible extension to the pelvis, or intrapancreatic where they merge with areas of intraglandular necrosis; they are often multiple [29, 30].

Table 25.5 Classification of collections in acute pancreatitis

Collections	Time elapsed since the onset of symptoms (weeks)	Subcategory of acute pancreatitis	Localization	Imaging features
APFC	<4	Interstitial edematous	Extrapancreatic	Homogeneous, content fluid, no walls, occupying the retroperitoneal structures
ANC	<4	Necrotizing	Intra- and/or extrapancreatic	Homogeneous/inhomogeneous, content not solely liquid (solid or fatty), free of walls
PSEUDOCYSTS	>4	Interstitial edematous	Extrapancreatic	Homogeneous, fluid, circumscribed and delimited by walls
WON	>4	Necrotizing	Intra- and/or extrapancreatic	Inhomogeneous, dense and non-liquid, bounded by walls

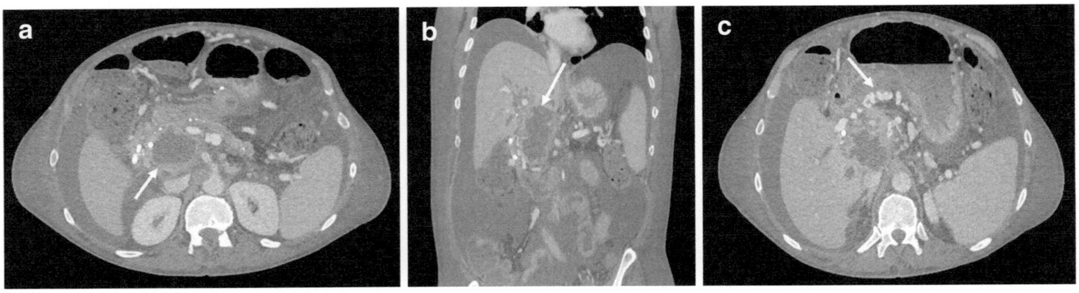

Fig. 25.4 CT scan in the portal phase shows a circumscribed pseudocyst occupying the head of the pancreas, with homogeneous fluid content (arrow, axial image **a**); there is no enhancement of its wall. The remaining pancreatic gland appears hypoatrophic with evidence of some sporadic parenchymal microcalcifications, as from chronic inflammatory outcomes. The cystic-looking formation also appears to fistulize in the liver parenchyma (arrow, coronal image **b**). Chronic thrombosis of the portal olive and superior mesenteric vein is associated with the development of portal cavernomatosis (arrow, axial image **c**)

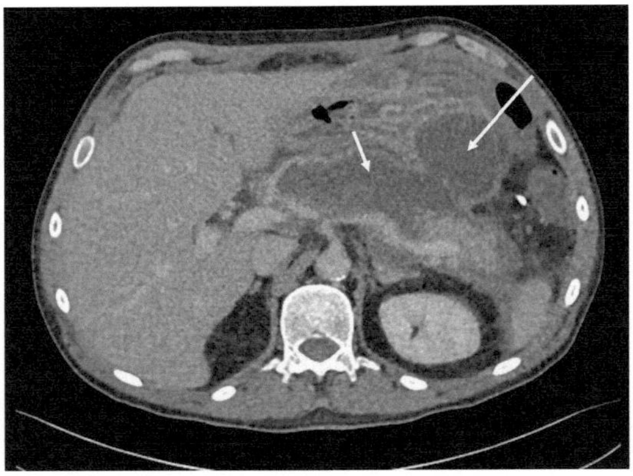

Fig. 25.5 53-year-old male with combined pancreatic and peripancreatic necrotizing pancreatitis with evidence of WON. CT portal phase shows a voluminous encapsulated formation located at the level of the body of the pancreas, compatible with an area of necrosis (short arrow). This area appears in continuity with a further necrotic collection located at the anterior peripancreatic site (long arrow). A small area of spared pancreatic parenchyma is evident at the level of the tail. No gas foci within the collection. The findings are indicative of walled pancreatic necrosis

In the early phase of pancreatitis, the differentiation between APFC and ANC can often be difficult to assess.

Imaging at 2 weeks is usually helpful in distinguishing an APFC from an ANC. Any peripancreatic collection associated with pancreatic parenchymal necrosis should be defined as an ANC, even if it is homogeneous and does not contain non-liquefied debris.

After 4 weeks, an ANC tends to organize and typically develops a thick wall with contrast enhancement, at which point the collection is termed a WON (Fig. 25.5). It, like APFC, can have both intra- and extra-pancreatic localization and take on a markedly inhomogeneous appearance [29, 30].

25.6 Infection

Any of the collection subtypes described above can be sterile and/or suffer from bacterial over-infection, especially in the case of necrotic collections. Over-infection is quite rare in the first week and is identifiable on CT scan as the presence of multiple air bubbles in the context of the collections, often secondary to colonization by Gram-negative enteric bacilli [31].

Infected collections may also be the consequence of a pancreatic-enteric fistula resulting from necrotic collections that may, although in rare cases, erode the intestinal wall, most commonly of the colon and duodenum [32].

However, the presence of gas within the pancreatic duct may also mimic an infected pancreatic collection, although in general, gas within the pancreatic duct tends to assume a more linear distribution as well as typically occurring in the clinical setting of a recent endoscopic pancreatography and/or after stent insertion.

To date, there is also debate regarding image-guided fluid collection or fine-needle aspiration of necrotic tissue to confirm the presence of infection prior to necrosectomy; however, due to the countless disadvantages (high number of false positives due to possible contamination as well as high number of false negatives due to too early sampling), these procedures have fallen into disuse in recent years and there has been a move towards more conservative management involving the insertion of a percutaneous drain with culture analysis that could delay and/or avoid invasive surgery [5].

25.7 Pancreatitis and Mass Effect on Adjacent Organs

AP and in particular the necrotizing form, with its associated inflammatory changes and collections, can lead to a compressive effect on adjacent organs with possible mechanical occlusion in the stomach or intestines; hydronephrosis can also be a consequence of this mass effect, as can biliary obstruction [29, 30]. The latter may also be secondary to a fibrotic evolution of the biliary tract due to pancreatic inflammation.

Inflammatory changes may also secondarily affect the intestine and in particular the adjacent duodenum, which may appear diffusely thickened and stratified on CT scan with evidence of mucosal hyperemia and submucosal edema.

Furthermore, patients with voluminous collections are at risk of abdominal compartment syndrome, in which increased intra-abdominal pressure may be responsible for organ ischemia with further possible necrotic evolution [29, 30].

25.8 Pancreatic Duct Complications

In about 40% of patients with pancreatic necrosis, an additional complication called a disconnected pancreatic duct may occur. This can be the result of the necrosis itself or be due to iatrogenic causes. On CT scan or even MRI, the presence of a disconnected duct is suggested by a large and persistent collection that tends to increase and often involves the neck or body of the pancreas [29, 30]. Often the remaining upstream glandular parenchyma appears viable with the duct that may or may not appear dilated at that level; moreover, it can sometimes be seen communicating directly and in a perpendicular orientation with the collection itself and this represents a pathognomonic sign.

Sometimes the presence of a disconnected pancreatic duct may evolve into pancreatic ascites or a pancreatic-pleural fistula [33].

If a pancreatic duct lesion is suspected, it can be confirmed with ERCP and/or MRCP.

Another possible late complication of necrotizing pancreatitis is stenosis of the pancreatic duct, which may develop as a consequence of the inflammation itself or healing following drainage of necrotic collections [34].

25.9 Vascular Complications

Vascular complications in AP occur in about 25% of cases and are responsible for high morbidity and mortality. The survival of patients with pancreatitis and vascular complications is closely dependent on early diagnosis of these as well as timely therapeutic management.

Hemorrhage represents one of the most fatal vascular complications in pancreatitis. It recognizes a multifactorial etiopathogenesis.

One factor is undoubtedly the severe inflammation of the glandular parenchyma, which leads to a massive release of proteolytic and lipolytic enzymes and is responsible for damage to the vascular walls, which are thus rendered susceptible to rupture or subsequent formation of pseudoaneurysmal lesions [35].

The splenic artery, portal vein, splenic vein, and other small peripancreatic vessels are the most common sources of hemorrhage, while the artery most frequently involved in the formation of pseudoaneurysms in cases of necrotizing pancreatitis is the splenic artery (up to 10% of patients), followed by the gastroduodenal artery, the pancreaticoduodenal artery, the hepatic artery and the left gastric artery [36].

Spontaneous hemorrhage as well as pseudoaneurysms can be seen in the context of the pancreatic parenchyma, collections, or in the lumen of the gastrointestinal tract. Bleeding may also show intra- and/or retro-peritoneal spread.

At CECT, active bleeding presents as a blush with different morphology, of high attenuation (hyperdensity) after administration of endovenous contrast, which tends to increase in the later phases of the dynamic study. The pseudoaneurysm, on the other hand, is identified on CT as a circumscribed area, with globular morphology, characterized by enhancement synchronous to the vessels.

A further, albeit later pathogenetic mechanism responsible for active bleeding and/or especially pseudoaneurysm formation is mediated by long-lasting pseudocysts. The vessels in this case may be eroded due to persistent compression or by the elastolytic action of the enzymatic content of the pseudocysts themselves [37].

Rupture of a pseudoaneurysm and/or a vessel within a pseudocyst transforms it into a voluminous pseudoaneurysmal pseudocyst ('pulsatile pseudocyst'), which in turn may eventually open into the retroperitoneum or peritoneal cavity or may communicate with adjacent hollow structures such as the stomach, jejunum, colon and Wirsung's duct (the latter occurrence is referred to as pancreatic hemosuccus, Figs. 25.6 and 25.7) [38].

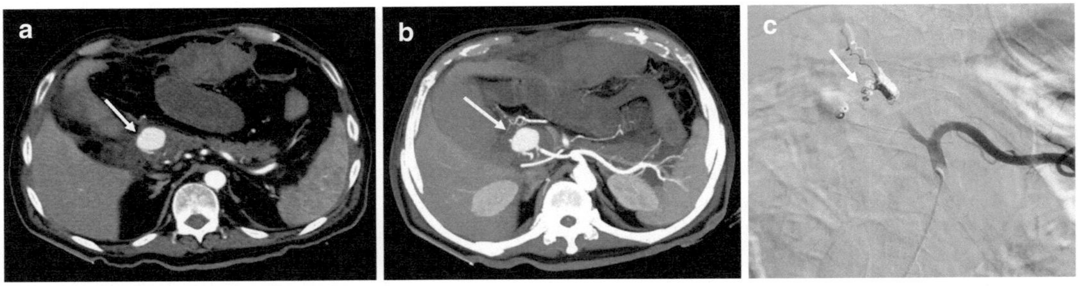

Fig. 25.6 62-year-old male with hemosuccus pancreaticus. The contrast-enhanced CT axial scan in the arterial phase (**a**) and its maximum intensity projection axial reconstruction (**b**) shows a large pancreaticoduodenal artery pseudoaneurysm (arrow; **a**, **b**). The bleeding vessel was subsequently embolized using coil (arrow; **c**)

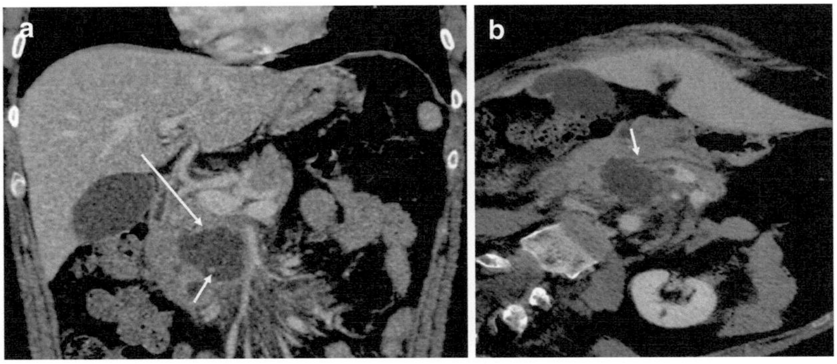

Fig. 25.7 54-year-old female with necrotic pancreatitis and hemosuccus pancreaticus. The contrast-enhanced CT scan coronal reconstruction in the portal phase (**a**) shows a large pancreatic necrotic head collection (long arrow; **a**) with a low-flow hemorrhagic focus inside (short arrow; **a**). Axial-oblique minimum intensity projection contrast-enhanced CT scan reconstruction in the portal phase (**b**) shows a disconnected pancreatic duct (arrow; **b**)

Local inflammation with prothrombotic effect, reduced venous flow as well as the mass effect on neighboring venous structures by pancreatic and peripancreatic collections are also responsible for venous thrombosis. Acute venous thrombosis presents itself as a focal complete and/or partial opacification defect of the vessel lumen, which appears ectasic at this level.

In chronic cases, however, the affected vein takes on a filiform appearance with the development of multiple collateral vessels. The splenic vein is the site most commonly affected by the presence of a thrombus (>23% of cases), while the superior mesenteric vein and portal vein are less commonly affected [39, 40].

References

1. Lee DW, Cho CM. Predicting severity of acute pancreatitis. Medicina (Kaunas). 2022;58(6)
2. Mergener K, Baillie J. Acute pancreatitis. BMJ. 1998;316(7124):44–8.
3. Mitchell RMS, Byrne MF, Baillie J. Pancreatitis. Lancet (London, England). 2003;361(9367):1447–55.
4. Wang G-J, Gao C-F, Wei D, Wang C, Ding S-Q. Acute pancreatitis: etiology and common pathogenesis. World J Gastroenterol. 2009;15(12):1427–30.
5. Foster BR, Jensen KK, Bakis G, Shaaban AM, Coakley FV. Revised Atlanta classification for acute pancreatitis: a pictorial essay. Radiogr A Rev Publ Radiol Soc North Am Inc. 2016;36(3):675–87.
6. Banks PA, Bollen TL, Dervenis C, Gooszen HG, Johnson CD, Sarr MG, et al. Classification of acute pancreatitis--2012: revision of the Atlanta classification and definitions by international consensus. Gut. 2013;62(1):102–11.
7. Bradley EL 3rd. A clinically based classification system for acute pancreatitis. Summary of the international symposium on acute pancreatitis, Atlanta, Ga, September 11 through 13, 1992. Arch Surg. 1993;128(5):586–90.
8. Singh VK, Bollen TL, Wu BU, Repas K, Maurer R, Yu S, et al. An assessment of the severity of interstitial pancreatitis. Clin Gastroenterol Hepatol Off Clin Pract J Am Gastroenterol Assoc. 2011;9(12):1098–103.
9. Marshall JC, Cook DJ, Christou NV, Bernard GR, Sprung CL, Sibbald WJ. Multiple organ dysfunction score: a reliable descriptor of a complex clinical outcome. Crit Care Med. 1995;23(10):1638–52.
10. Tüney D, Altun E, Barlas A, Yegen C. Pancreatico-colonic fistula after acute necrotizing pancreatitis. Diagnosis with spiral CT using rectal water soluble contrast media. JOP. 2008;9(1):26–9.
11. Kochhar R, Jain K, Gupta V, Singhal M, Kochhar S, Poornachandra KS, et al. Fistulization in the GI tract in acute pancreatitis. Gastrointest Endosc. 2012;75(2):436–40.
12. Whitcomb DC. Clinical practice. Acute Pancreatitis N Engl J Med. 2006;354(20):2142–50.
13. Balthazar EJ. Acute pancreatitis: assessment of severity with clinical and CT evaluation. Radiology. 2002;223(3):603–13.
14. Balthazar EJ, Robinson DL, Megibow AJ, Ranson JH. Acute pancreatitis: value of CT in establishing prognosis. Radiology. 1990;174(2):331–6.
15. Banday IA, Gattoo I, Khan AM, Javeed J, Gupta G, Latief M. Modified computed tomography severity index for evaluation of acute pancreatitis and its correlation with clinical outcome: a tertiary care hospital based observational study. J Clin Diagn Res. 2015;9(8):TC01–5.
16. Mortele KJ, Wiesner W, Intriere L, Shankar S, Zou KH, Kalantari BN, et al. A modified CT severity index for evaluating acute pancreatitis: improved correlation with patient outcome. AJR Am J Roentgenol. 2004;183(5):1261–5.
17. Sahu B, Abbey P, Anand R, Kumar A, Tomer S, Malik E. Severity assessment of acute pancreatitis using CT severity index and modified CT severity index: correlation with clinical outcomes and severity grading as per the revised Atlanta classification. Indian J Radiol Imaging. 2017;27(2):152–60.
18. Raghuwanshi S, Gupta R, Vyas MM, Sharma R. CT evaluation of acute pancreatitis and its prognostic correlation with CT severity index. J Clin Diagn Res. 2016;10(6):TC06–11.
19. Sidhu HS, Benigno S, Ganeshan B, Dikaios N, Johnston EW, Allen C, et al. Textural analysis of multiparametric MRI detects transition zone prostate cancer. Eur Radiol. 2017;27(6):2348–58.
20. Murray N, Darras KE, Walstra FE, Mohammed MF, McLaughlin PD, Nicolaou S. Dual-energy CT in evaluation of the acute abdomen. Radiogr A Rev Publ Radiol Soc North Am Inc. 2019;39(1):264–86.
21. George E, Wortman JR, Fulwadhva UP, Uyeda JW, Sodickson AD. Dual energy CT applications in pancreatic pathologies. Br J Radiol. 2017;90(1080):20170411.
22. Hu J-X, Zhao C-F, Wang S-L, Tu X-Y, Huang W-B, Chen J-N, et al. Acute pancreatitis: a review of diagnosis, severity prediction and prognosis assessment from imaging technology, scoring system and artificial intelligence. World J Gastroenterol. 2023;29(37):5268–91.
23. Liang H, Wang M, Wen Y, Du F, Jiang L, Geng X, et al. Predicting acute pancreatitis severity with enhanced computed tomography scans using convolutional neural networks. Sci Rep. 2023;13(1):17514.
24. Chen Z, Wang Y, Zhang H, Yin H, Hu C, Huang Z, et al. Deep learning models for severity prediction of acute pancreatitis in the early phase from abdominal nonenhanced computed tomography images. Pancreas. 2023;52(1):e45–53.

25. Rocca A, Brunese MC, Santone A, Varriano G, Viganò L, et al. Radiomics and 256-slice-dual-energy CT in the automated diagnosis of mild acute pancreatitis: the innovation of formal methods and high-resolution CT. Radiol Med. 2024;129(10):1444–53. https://doi.org/10.1007/s11547-024-01878-9. Epub 2024 Aug 30. PMID: 39214954; PMCID: PMC11480164.
26. Pan X, Jiao K, Li X, Feng L, Tian Y, Wu L, et al. Artificial intelligence-based tools with automated segmentation and measurement on CT images to assist accurate and fast diagnosis in acute pancreatitis. Br J Radiol. 2024;97(1159):1268–77.
27. Ma Y, Yue P, Zhang J, Yuan J, Liu Z, Chen Z, et al. Early prediction of acute gallstone pancreatitis severity: a novel machine learning model based on CT features and open access online prediction platform. Ann Med. 2024;56(1):2357354.
28. Lin W, Huang Y, Zhu J, Sun H, Su N, Pan J, et al. Machine learning improves early prediction of organ failure in hyperlipidemia acute pancreatitis using clinical and abdominal CT features. Pancreatol Off J Int Assoc Pancreatol. 2024;24(3):350–6.
29. Brizi MG, Perillo F, Cannone F, Tuzza L, Manfredi R. The role of imaging in acute pancreatitis. Radiol Med. 2021;126(8):1017–29. https://doi.org/10.1007/s11547-021-01359-3. Epub 2021 May 12. PMID: 33982269; PMCID: PMC8292294.
30. Di Serafino M, Ronza R, D'Auria D, Fiorentino R, Arundine D, et al. Stocky/packed pancreas: a case of focal drug-induced acute pancreatitis mimicking cancer. Tomography. 2022;8(4):2073–82. https://doi.org/10.3390/tomography8040174. PMID: 36006072; PMCID: PMC9414187.
31. Beger HG, Rau B, Mayer J, Pralle U. Natural course of acute pancreatitis. World J Surg. 1997;21(2):130–5.
32. Freeny PC, Lewis GP, Traverso LW, Ryan JA. Infected pancreatic fluid collections: percutaneous catheter drainage. Radiology. 1988;167(2):435–41.
33. Fung C, Svystun O, Fouladi DF, Kawamoto S. CT imaging, classification, and complications of acute pancreatitis. Abdom Radiol (New York). 2020;45(5):1243–52.
34. Oza VM, Kahaleh M. Endoscopic management of chronic pancreatitis. World J Gastrointest Endosc. 2013;5(1):19–28.
35. Stroud WH, Cullom JW, Anderson MC. Hemorrhagic complications of severe pancreatitis. Surgery. 1981;90(4):657–65.
36. Kalas MA, Leon M, Chavez LO, Canalizo E, Surani S. Vascular complications of pancreatitis. World J Clin Cases. 2022;10(22):7665–73.
37. Flati G, Salvatori F, Porowska B, Talarico C, Flati D, Proposito D, et al. Severe hemorrhagic complications in pancreatitis. Ann Ital Chir. 1995;66(2):233–7.
38. Vujic I. Vascular complications of pancreatitis. Radiol Clin North Am. 1989;27(1):81–91.
39. Bernades P, Baetz A, Lévy P, Belghiti J, Menu Y, Fékété F. Splenic and portal venous obstruction in chronic pancreatitis. A prospective longitudinal study of a medical-surgical series of 266 patients. Dig Dis Sci. 1992;37(3):340–6.
40. Rattner DW, Warshaw AL. Venous, biliary, and duodenal obstruction in chronic pancreatitis. Hepato-Gastroenterology. 1990;37(3):301–6.

Urologic Emergencies

26

Dario Grimaldi, Pierantonio Grimaldi,
Chiara Rinaldo, Giuliana Giacobbe,
Vittorio Sabatino, and Marco Di Serafino

26.1 Introduction

Urological emergencies represent a significant challenge in clinical practice, requiring rapid and accurate diagnosis to ensure timely and effective treatment. Computed tomography (CT) is a fundamental diagnostic tool in this context, due to its ability to provide detailed images of the urinary tract and surrounding structures. This chapter explores the use of CT in urological emergencies, highlighting the main indications and radiological characteristics of the most common conditions, such as complicated urinary infections, acute urinary obstructions, and vascular emergencies. Through clinical cases and illustrations, best practices for interpreting CT images will be illustrated to improve clinical management and patient outcomes.

26.2 Obstructive Uropathy

Obstructive uropathy consists of a structural or functional blockage of normal urinary flow, which can impair urinary function [1]. Numerous pathological conditions can cause obstructive uropathy (Table 26.1). The most common causes vary with age. In children and young adults, anatomical abnormalities are predominant. In young adults, the most frequent cause is urolithiasis. In the elderly, the main causes include benign prostatic hyperplasia or prostate cancer, retroperitoneal or pelvic tumors, and urolithiasis (Fig. 26.1) [2]. The obstruction can occur at any level, from the renal tubules to the external urethral meatus. In patients with good renal function, unilateral obstruction can be compensated by the contralateral kidney. However, in patients with reduced renal function, even unilateral obstruction can lead to significant renal function impairment. Symptoms and signs vary based on the location, degree, and onset speed of the obstruction. Pain is common when the obstruction acutely distends the bladder, collecting system, or renal capsule. Complete acute ureteral obstruction causes

The original version of the chapter has been revised. A correction to this chapter can be found at https://doi.org/10.1007/978-3-031-84849-0_32

D. Grimaldi (✉) · C. Rinaldo · G. Giacobbe
V. Sabatino · M. Di Serafino
Department of General and Emergency Radiology, "Antonio Cardarelli" Hospital, Naples, Italy
e-mail: dariogrimaldi@me.com; chiara.rinaldo@aocardarelli.it; giuliana.giacobbe@aocardarelli.it; vittorio.sabatino@aocardarelli.it; marco.diserafino@aocardarelli.it

P. Grimaldi
Department of Mental and Physical Health and Preventive Medicine, University of Campania "Luigi Vanvitelli", Naples, Italy
e-mail: pierantonio.grimaldi@studenti.unicampania.it

L. Romano et al. (eds.), *CT of Non-Traumatic Body Emergencies*,
https://doi.org/10.1007/978-3-031-84849-0_26

severe pain accompanied by nausea and vomiting. Infections complicating the obstruction can cause dysuria, pyuria, urgency and frequency of urination, renal and ureteral pain, and fever. Imaging plays a crucial role in guiding the diagnosis and management [3].

Table 26.1 Most common causes of urinary obstruction

Category	Causes
Urolithiasis	Renal and ureteral stones
Intrinsic causes	Urethral strictures, tumors
Extrinsic causes	Tumor compression, masses, aneurysms
Prostatic diseases	BPH, prostate cancer
Infections	Periureteral abscesses, TB
Trauma and injuries	Ureteral/urethral injuries, fractures
Congenital anomalies	Urethral valves, ureterocele
Iatrogenic	Catheter damage, post-radiotherapy
Neurological conditions	Neurogenic bladder, MS
Other	Blood clots, scar tissue

26.2.1 Urolithiasis

Urolithiasis is by far the most common cause of obstructive uropathy. It is estimated that up to 12% of men and 10% of women develop urinary stones by the age of 70. The composition of the stones varies, but in Western countries, about 85% of stones are composed of calcium, 10% of uric acid, and the remainder are composed of struvite and cystine (Table 26.2) [4]. The formation of stones in the urinary tract is a complex process believed to start with the supersaturation of salts in the urine, leading to the formation of crystalline nuclei. Urine contains substances that promote and inhibit crystal formation, and alterations in these substances favor the aggregation of crystals (Table 26.3). Subsequent mineral deposits on the crystals lead to stone formation [5]. Symptoms, as mentioned in the previous paragraph, are related to the location of the obstruction and the onset of potential complications. Generally, the condition presents with severe

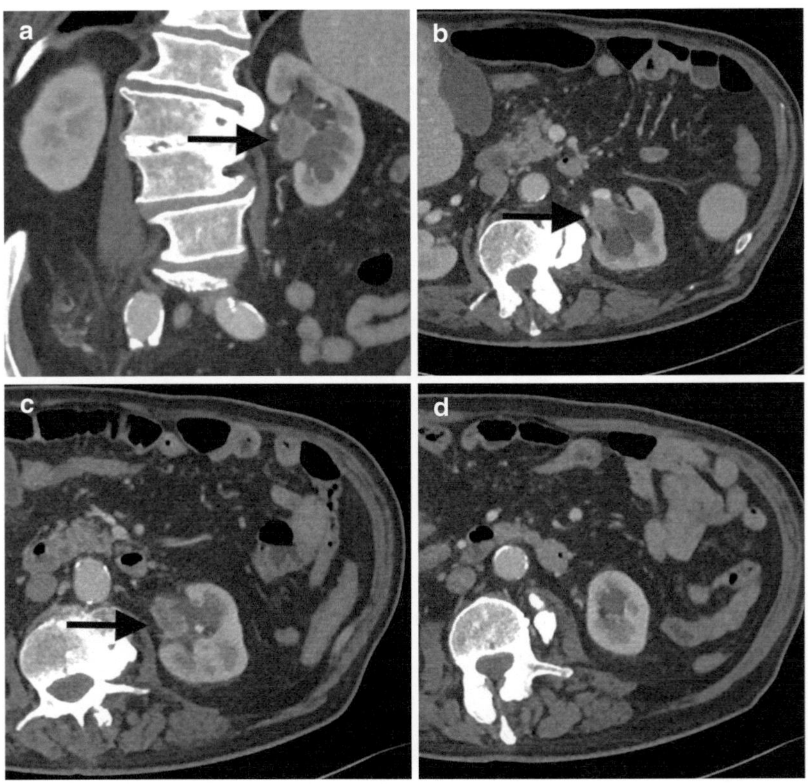

Fig. 26.1 A 60-year-old man presented to our emergency department with a sensation of heaviness in his left flank. The CT scan with contrast (**a**, **b**, **c**, **d**) demonstrates the presence of solid vascularized tissue developing in the renal pelvis (arrows), causing dilation of all calyceal groups. The CT findings are confirmed by histological examination, which documents the presence of a urothelial tumor

Table 26.2 Types of stones, frequency, and radiological appearance

Type of stone	Percentage of frequency	Behavior
Calcium (oxalate and phosphate)	85%	Radiopaque
Uric acid	10%	Radiolucent
Struvite (infection)	2–3%	Radiopaque
Cystine	1–2%	Radiolucent
Xanthine	<1%	Radiolucent

Table 26.3 Promoters and inhibitors of stone formation

Promoters	Inhibitors
Calcium	Citrate
Oxalate	Magnesium
Uric acid	Phytate
Sodium	Pyrophosphate
Phosphate	Glycosaminoglycans

pain accompanied by nausea and vomiting, hematuria, dysuria, and increased urinary frequency [6].

26.2.1.1 Imaging

CT is the gold standard imaging modality for patients suspected of having obstructive uropathy. Indeed, CT scans can identify the cause of obstruction in almost all cases. Noncontrast CT (NCCT) has a sensitivity of 95–98% and a specificity of 96–100% in detecting stones [7]. NCCT requires no patient preparation and is an extremely rapid examination. The most frequent findings include dilation of the collecting system or ureter, the "bulky" appearance of the kidney, and perirenal and periureteral stranding [8]. In CT evaluation for suspected ureteral stones, attention should be focused on the most common sites of obstruction, which include the physiological narrowing of the ureter at the ureterovesical junction, the crossing of the ureter and iliac vessels, and the ureteropelvic junction. However, it should be noted, as reported in Table 26.2, that some types of stones may be radiolucent. If the NCCT evaluation is negative or equivocal, the examination is completed with a contrast-enhanced study (CTU) [9]. CT urography allows for a detailed assessment of the caliceal anatomy, particularly in cases of anatomical anomalies or variants that may predispose to obstructive pathology. After contrast administration, renal parenchymal edema, typical of the acute obstructive phase, can be easily identified. This may be associated with a delay in contrast excretion in the collecting system or ureter beyond the obstruction level, thus indicating the "transition point." Contrast-enhanced evaluation also enables the identification of pathological wall thickening of the excretory pathways or any extrinsic compressions. In Box 26.1, NCCT and CTU are compared in the diagnosis of urolithiasis. The introduction of dual-energy CT has enabled the use of a technique that allows the determination of stone composition by studying the attenuation of stones at two different kVp levels (Table 26.4). Each CT system has its own dedicated algorithm for determining the composition. Dual-energy CT has been shown to successfully predict the effectiveness of extracorporeal shock wave lithotripsy [10].

Box 26.1: Within the Summary Box, We Can Compare NCCT to CTU in the Diagnosis of Urolithiasis

Characteristic	NCCT (Non-contrast CT)	CTU (computed tomography urography)
Visibility and detection of stones	Excellent for high-density stones (radiopaque) and provides clear visualization of stones, especially those with higher density compared to surrounding tissues	Improved visibility of stones and better highlighting, particularly if they are in the process of passing or if complications are present
Detection of complications	Limited to indirect signs of obstruction and inflammation	Greater detail for assessing complications such as hydronephrosis and peri-renal inflammation
Tissue differentiation	Limited in distinguishing between soft tissues and stones	Better differentiation between soft tissues and complex structures due to the use of contrast
Ureter evaluation	Might be difficult to visualize specific changes or lesions in the ureter	Enhanced visualization of the ureter and any related lesions or obstructions
Anatomical detail	Provides good visualization of structures and stones	Offers more detailed views of anatomical structures and the relationships between stones and surrounding tissues
Execution time	Generally quicker and less complex	Requires extra time for contrast administration and distribution
Patient preparation	Minimal, with no special preparation needed	Requires preparation, such as contrast administration and possibly pre-CT medications

Table 26.4 Composition of urinary stones and attenuation coefficients

Stone type	Dual-energy CT characteristics	Attenuation coefficient (HU)
Calcium oxalate	High attenuation on both low and high kVp images.	400–600 HU
Calcium phosphate	Similar to calcium oxalate.	400–600 HU
Uric acid	Lower attenuation on low kVp images.	100–200 HU
Struvite	Intermediate attenuation.	Variable
Cystine	Moderate attenuation.	100–200 HU

26.2.1.2 Complication

Urinary tract obstruction leads to urine stasis and damage to the renal parenchyma. In the early stages, however, if the obstruction is promptly resolved, renal damage is minimal. When dealing with urolithiasis, the morphology and size of the stone should be considered. Stones smaller than 5 mm can often be managed conservatively, as they generally pass spontaneously. It is important to note that struvite stones, in addition to being generally larger, tend to cause frequent and significant infections. Hypertension resulting from the obstruction can lead to the rupture of the excretory system, potentially forming a urinoma and, in some cases, complicated infections and abscesses. Over time, the obstructive process results in reduced renal function (Fig. 26.2) [11].

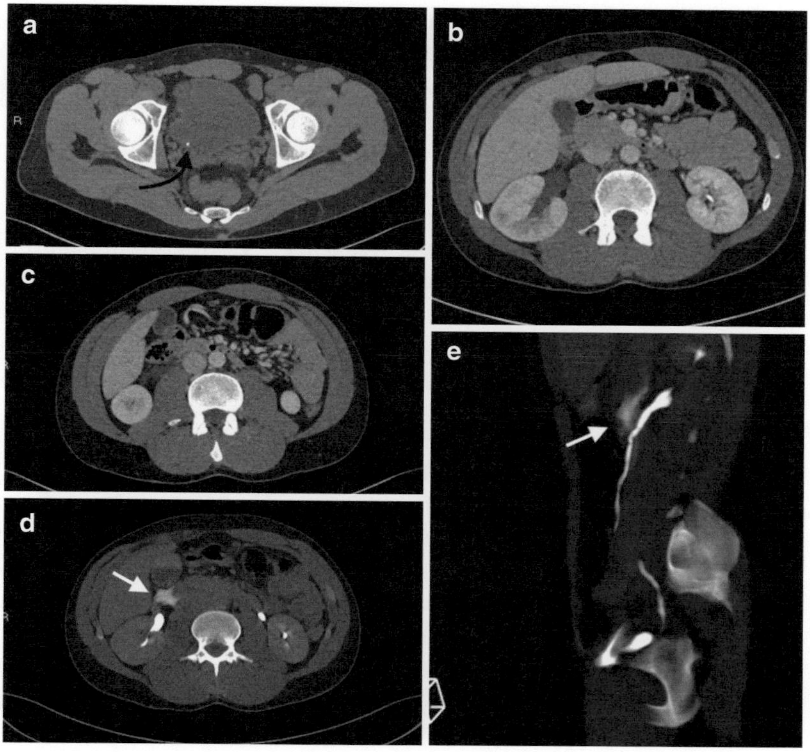

Fig. 26.2 A young patient presents with severe right flank pain. (**a**) A very small urinary stone is located at the ureterovesical junction (black arrow), causing right hydronephrosis (**b**). (**c**) On venous phase imaging, a small fluid collection is observed near the proximal ureter. (**d**, **e**) In the delayed phase, there is contrast-enhanced leakage of urine around the ureter (white arrows)

26.3 Infections

Symptomatic urinary tract infections (UTIs) are extremely common occurrences. It is estimated that in the United States, at least one million patients visit the emergency department due to a UTI. The infection can be localized in the lower urinary tract, involving the bladder and/or urethra, or extend to the upper urinary tract, involving the ureter, pelvis, and renal parenchyma. The microorganisms responsible for the infection typically enter through one of two pathways. The most frequent pathway is through the lower urinary tract, from where the infection ascends and sometimes reaches the kidneys. However, hematogenous spread, usually involving the kidneys, is also possible. UTIs are caused in 85% of cases by bacteria from the intestines or vagina, with the vast majority being E. coli. Lower urinary tract bacterial infections are extremely common among young sexually active women. For this reason, this group is also the most frequently affected by upper urinary tract infections. Finally, it is important to consider the existence of several factors that contribute to an increased risk of UTIs. These include the presence of obstructive urinary tract pathology (such as urolithiasis or other causes), anatomical abnormalities of the upper and lower urinary tracts, the presence of diverticula, and the presence of urinary drainage devices (such as catheters).

26.3.1 Acute Pyelonephritis

Pyelonephritis is a bacterial infection that affects one or both kidneys. As mentioned in the previous paragraph, this condition is significantly more common in women and is caused by *Escherichia* coli in approximately 90% of cases. The infection almost always results from bacteria ascending from the genital area through the urethra, reaching the bladder, ureters, and finally the kidneys. Typically, the flow of urine helps to flush out microorganisms that manage to ascend. However, certain conditions, such as urinary obstruction or anatomical variations, can impede the normal clearance of the urinary tract, facilitating infection. Additionally, some individuals, including diabetic and immunocompromised patients, are more susceptible to developing pyelonephritis and experiencing more severe cases. Common symptoms of pyelonephritis include fever with chills, flank pain, frequency and dysuria, general malaise, nausea, and vomiting [12] [13].

26.3.1.1 Imaging

Usually, clinical presentation and laboratory tests are sufficient to guide the clinician toward a diagnosis. Imaging is not necessary if the patient responds well to antibiotic treatment. However, imaging is required for patients with a kidney transplant, diabetics or immunocompromised individuals, the elderly, those with known anatomical abnormalities or variants, recurrent pyelonephritis, and those with a history of urolithiasis [12]. In noncontrast CT (NCCT) scans performed to rule out stones and related hydronephrosis, the kidney may appear "bulky," with thickening of the perirenal fat and the fascial complex [12]. However, these signs are quite nonspecific and do not allow for a definitive diagnosis. The detection of gas within the renal parenchyma or the collecting system may be indicative of emphysematous pyelonephritis. Contrast-enhanced CT remains the best imaging modality for diagnosing pyelonephritis. Postcontrast images will show one or more (unifocal, multifocal, diffuse) wedge-shaped areas of swollen parenchyma, extending from the papilla to the renal cortex, with reduced enhancement compared to the adjacent healthy tissue. Focal vasospasm, tubular obstruction, and edema are factors underlying these CT-findings [14]. The "rim sign" is useful for differentiating between acute pyelonephritis and renal infarction; the cortical region of infarcted parenchyma appears hyperemic (unlike the nephritic focus) because it is vascularized by capsular branches. In the excretory phase, the presence of a "striated nephrogram" can be observed. This sign indicates the persistence of contrast within edematous tubules alternating with hypoperfused regions (with reduced enhancement) due to debris and inflammatory material occupying the tubule lumen. These signs, as noted in the NCCT evaluation, may be associated with thickening of the perirenal fat and the renal fascial complex, as well as hydronephrosis linked to possible obstructions. Another possible finding that can be evaluated after contrast administration is the thickening and hyperemia of the excretory tract (Fig. 26.3) [15]. In Box 26.2, NCCT and CTU are compared in the diagnosis of pyelonephritis.

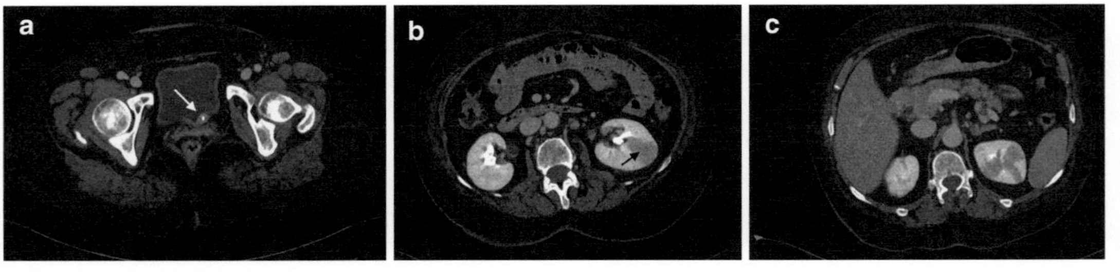

Fig. 26.3 45-year-old patient presents with left flank pain and fever. CT imaging reveals a small urinary stone (white arrow) at the left ureterovesical junction (**a**). Additionally, extensive hypovascular foci are observed, indicative of nephritic involvement (black arrows), affecting large portions of the renal parenchyma (**b**, **c**)

Box 26.2: Within the Summary Box, We Can Compare NCCT and CTU in the Diagnosis of Pyelonephritis

Characteristic	NCCT (non-contrast CT)	CTU (computed tomography urography)
Visibility of inflammation	Good for identifying signs of inflammation and renal edema	Greater detail in evaluating inflammation and involvement of the urinary tract
Renal anatomy detail	Provides clear visualization of renal structure and inflammation-related changes	Offers detailed views of renal structures and urinary tract due to contrast use
Complication visualization	Limited, primarily showing indirect signs of complications like abscesses or hydronephrosis	Better at detecting complications such as renal abscesses, hydronephrosis, and other changes in the urinary tract
Detection of renal stones	Excellent for detecting renal stones, if present, which may contribute to the infection	Useful for assessing stones and their relationship to inflammation or complications
Urinary tract evaluation	Limited in detailed visualization of the urinary tract	Excellent for visualizing the urinary tract, including detecting obstructions or abnormalities associated with pyelonephritis
Contrast detail	No contrast used, therefore less detailed for vascular structures and urinary tract	Uses contrast for clearer visualization of vascular structures and urinary tract
Execution time	Generally quicker and less complex	Requires more time for contrast injection and distribution

26.3.1.2 Complication

The initiation of appropriate antibiotic therapy effectively resolves the infection in most patients. However, the increasing problem of antibiotic resistance, which now affects nearly all microorganisms responsible for pyelonephritis, must be taken into account. Additionally, certain patient populations are at higher risk for resistant infections and frequent complications. Diabetic patients, immunocompromised individuals, and those with known struvite stones exhibit elevated rates of complications and recurrent infections. Common complications include renal and perirenal abscesses and emphysematous pyelonephritis. A rarer complication is renal vein thrombosis [14].

26.3.2 Renal Abscess

Renal abscesses are the most common complication of pyelonephritis, where severe vasospasm and inflammation can lead to liquefactive necrosis and abscess formation. The microorganisms most frequently involved are *E. coli* and Proteus mirabilis. Predisposing factors include diabetes mellitus, urinary tract stones (particularly struvite stones), and ureteral obstructions. Typically, abscesses complicate ascending pyelonephritis. However, in rare cases, abscesses can result from a systemic infection that spreads to the kidneys via the bloodstream. In such cases, multiple abscesses affecting both kidneys are more common. The clinical presentation is similar to that of pyelonephritis. The presence of an abscess complication should be suspected if there is no response to antibiotics after 72 h [16].

26.3.2.1 Imaging

Contrast-enhanced CT is considered the gold standard method for diagnosing and monitoring renal abscesses. On CT evaluation, the abscess will appear as a well-defined, often rounded, low-attenuation mass with thick, typically irregular walls and peripheral enhancement (Fig. 26.4). The presence of gas within the collection strongly suggests an abscess. Hypovascular areas may be observed in the adjacent parenchyma, and uncomplicated nephritic foci may also be present within the same kidney. Often, there is associated

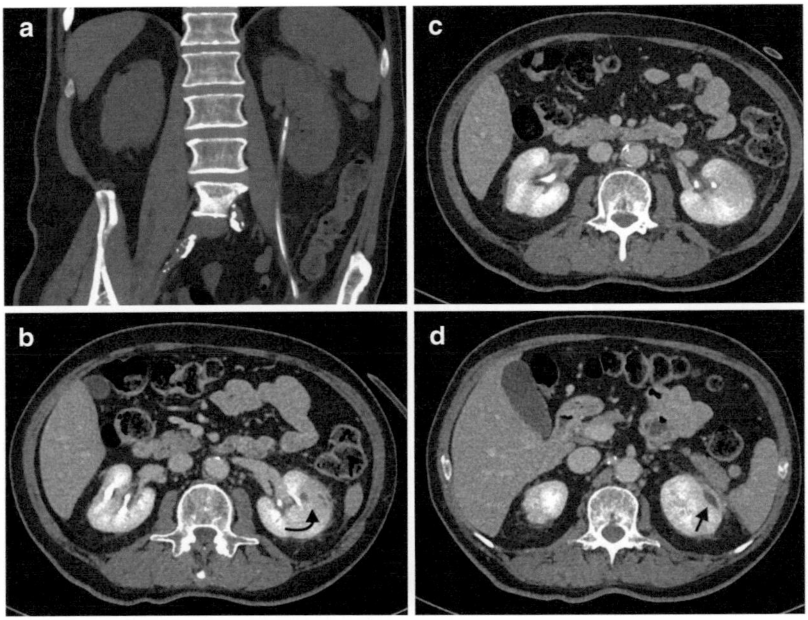

Fig. 26.4 A 50-year-old man with a left ureteral stent presents with fever unresponsive to standard antibiotics. (**a**) On non-contrast CT evaluation, the kidney demonstrates a globular appearance with perirenal fat stranding. In the delayed post-contrast images (**b**, **c**, and **d**), extensive hypovascular areas are observed, indicative of renal inflammation, with the presence of abscess cavities within these areas (black arrows)

fascial thickening and marked perirenal fat stranding. The most common complication is abscess rupture. The abscess collection can extend into the calyceal system and renal pelvis, leading to pyonephrosis, into the perirenal space, resulting in a perinephric abscess, into the anterior or posterior pararenal space (beyond the perirenal fascia), resulting in a paranephric abscess, or into the peritoneal cavity, leading to a subdiaphragmatic or pelvic abscess [12].

26.3.3 Emphysematous Pyelonephritis

Emphysematous pyelonephritis is a severe, necrotizing infection of the kidneys, characterized by the presence of gas produced by bacteria within the renal parenchyma and collecting system. It is associated with high mortality rates and, like other inflammatory conditions of the urinary tract, is significantly more common in women. This condition is typically caused by gas-producing bacteria, most commonly *E.coli* and *Klebsiella pneumoniae*, with other enterobacteria being less frequently involved. These bacteria ferment glucose in the infected tissues, leading to gas production. Consequently, this pathology is frequently associated with uncontrolled diabetes mellitus (approximately 90% of cases), where there is significant urinary excretion of glucose. Other conditions that favor the development of emphysematous infection include urinary obstructions, immunosuppression, and recurrent urinary infections. It is important to differentiate emphysematous pyelonephritis from emphysematous pyelitis, a condition where gas is present only in the excretory pathways (renal calices and pelvis). Although both conditions share similar risk factors and etiology, emphysematous pyelitis is considered to have a more favorable prognosis. The clinical presentation of emphysematous pyelonephritis is similar to that of acute pyelonephritis. The most common symptoms include high fever and chills, flank pain, general malaise, nausea, vomiting, dysuria, and urinary symptoms.

26.3.3.1 Imaging

CT is the preferred diagnostic tool for detecting emphysematous pyelonephritis. Common CT findings include renal enlargement and a "bulky" appearance, the presence of gas within the renal parenchyma in the form of "streaks" or "bubbles," and gas-containing abscesses. Additionally, typical findings of pyelonephritis and renal abscesses may be present. The infection can extend beyond the renal parenchyma to the perirenal space. The presence of free gas in the retroperitoneum indicates a rupture of Gerota's fascia [12, 17].

CT evaluation allows for a definitive diagnosis of emphysematous pyelonephritis and distinguishes between two main types of findings:

Type I: Involvement and destruction of more than one-third of the renal parenchyma, with intraparenchymal gas present but without associated renal or perirenal fluid collections.

Type II: Involvement and destruction of less than one-third of the renal parenchyma, with gas present in the renal parenchyma associated with abscesses or renal collections, and possibly accompanied by perirenal collections.

The presence of liquefied tissue, indicative of abscesses or collections, suggests an effective immune response and is associated with a lower mortality rate (approximately 20% for Type II) compared to the high mortality rate of Type I (70%) [12, 18].

26.3.4 Emphysematous Cystitis

Emphysematous cystitis is an infectious condition characterized by the formation of gas within the bladder wall by gas-producing bacteria, most commonly Escherichia coli, Enterobacter aerogenes, Proteus mirabilis, Clostridium perfringens, and Klebsiella pneumoniae. This condition is rare and typically confined to specific subgroups of patients such as the elderly, debilitated, and bedridden individuals. It is more common in women and generally associated with poorly controlled diabetes mellitus, where urinary excretion of glucose provides a favorable environment for gas-producing bacteria. Other predisposing factors include renal transplantation, urinary tract obstructions, immunosuppression, and prolonged catheterization [19]. Symptoms and signs are similar to those of typical cystitis, including suprapubic pain, general malaise, and fever. Sometimes, more specific urinary symptoms are present, such as dysuria and hematuria. Pneumaturia, or the passage of gas in the urine, is not a common symptom.

26.3.4.1 Imaging

CT imaging is highly sensitive, capable of detecting even minimal amounts of intraluminal or intramural gas. Intraluminal gas bubbles are often associated with recent catheterization, bladder washouts, or, less commonly, fistulas involving the genital or intestinal tract. In such cases, CT enables accurate differential diagnosis. The presence of intramural gas is pathognomonic for emphysematous cystitis [17].

26.4 Vascular Emergencies

Renal vascular emergencies include bleeding, more often related to the presence of neoplasms or complicated infections, renal infarctions, and renal vein thrombosis. These conditions usually require rapid intervention, and therefore, a prompt diagnosis is essential. In all these cases, contrast-enhanced CT is the gold standard.

26.4.1 Renal Infarction

Renal infarction is secondary to reduced or absent blood supply to a part or the entire kidney. Generally, infarction is caused by atherosclerosis or thromboembolism and, therefore, is more common in the elderly population. The most frequent causes of infarction are thromboembolism, dissection, fibromuscular dysplasia, and trauma. Table 26.5 lists the main causes and associated mechanisms determining renal infarction. The clinical presentation of renal infarction is nonspecific. Generally, small renal infarctions do not cause significant symptoms. More extensive renal infarction can present with severe flank pain, nausea, vomiting, hematuria, and proteinuria [20].

Table 26.5 Most common causes of renal infarction

Cause of renal infarction	Description
Thromboembolism (most common)	From cardiac valve, ventricular or atrial thrombus, aorta
Aortic dissection	Disruption of the aortic wall
Renal artery dissection	Disruption of the renal artery wall
Fibromuscular dysplasia (FMD)	Abnormal development of the blood vessel wall
Iatrogenic	Caused by medical procedures (e.g., angiography)
Vasculitis	Inflammation of blood vessels
Malignant hypertension	Extremely high blood pressure causing organ damage
Renal vein occlusion (rare)	Observed in childhood due to severe dehydration
Torsion of the transplanted kidney	Twisting of the blood vessels of the transplanted kidney

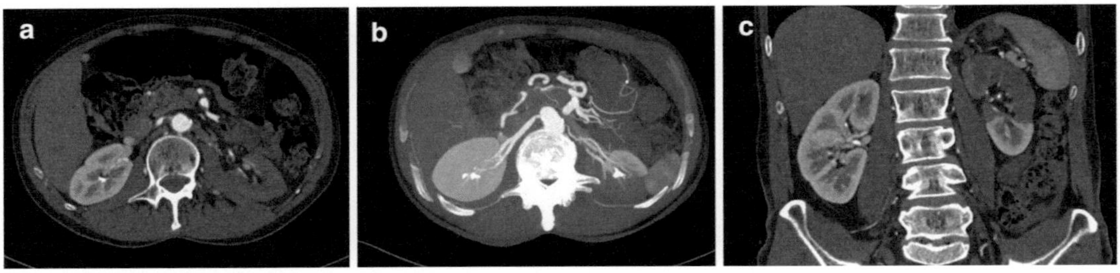

Fig. 26.5 A 60-year-old patient with atrial fibrillation presented to our emergency department with intense left flank pain. Contrast-enhanced CT evaluation (**a**) demonstrated complete vascular occlusion of the left renal artery, resulting in renal ischemia. Images **b** and **c** reveal that the presence of an accessory inferior polar artery maintains blood flow to the lower pole of the kidney, which therefore appears normally perfused

26.4.1.1 Imaging

Contrast-enhanced CT is the gold-standard examination for the evaluation of renal infarction. Evaluation during the arterial phase can, in some cases, highlight the opacification defect of an artery and the consequent hypo-enhancement of the affected territory. If the renal artery is involved, the entire kidney will be hypoperfused. Infarctions are easily identifiable during the cortical phase, where one or more wedge-shaped hypoperfused areas extending from the medullary region to the cortical surface can be observed (Fig. 26.5). In about half of the cases, a thin peripheral enhancement border due to capsular perfusion by extrarenal vessels can be detected. The so-called "rim sign," however, is not immediately present in the event of an infarction, as cortical reperfusion generally occurs after a few hours or even days. The differential diagnosis of renal infarctions, as previously described, includes infectious foci. Careful clinical evaluation and the presence of the rim sign assist in the differential diagnosis. Renal infarction results in a cortical scar [21].

26.4.2 Renal Vein Thrombosis

Renal vein thrombosis may result from either a neoplastic thrombus or a bland thrombus. There are various underlying conditions that can lead to the formation of a thrombus within the renal vein, with the most common being membranous glomerulonephritis, nephrotic syndrome, and other hypercoagulable states. Table 26.6 lists the main causes of renal venous thrombosis, categorized according to the age of onset. Renal vein thrombosis predominantly affects the left renal vein. This predilection is due to the anatomical positioning of the vena cava, which, being located to the right of the aorta, requires the left renal vein to traverse a longer and more tortuous path before joining the vena cava. Clinically, renal vein thrombosis often presents with nonspecific symptoms, correlating with the degree of renal parenchymal compromise. Symptoms may include flank pain, hematuria, and diminished or lost renal function. Frequent complications include renal papillary necrosis, renal atrophy, embolization of thrombus fragments leading to pulmonary embolism [22].

26.4.2.1 Imaging

On contrast-enhanced computed tomography (CT), a bland thrombus is typically visualized as a filling defect within the renal vein during the venous phase of imaging. The affected vein may exhibit a "thickened" appearance. In contrast, a neoplastic thrombus generally demonstrates heterogeneous enhancement post-contrast administration [21]. In cases of renal vein thrombosis, the kidney may appear enlarged ("glistening"), with persistent or absent cortical enhancement, reduced or absent contrast excretion, perinephric fat stranding, and thickening of the renal fascia (Fig. 26.6) [20]. Rarely, perinephric hemorrhage may be observed. In the chronic phase of renal vein thrombosis, the affected vein often appears attenuated due to thrombus retraction [22]. Box 26.3 summarizes the main findings observable on CT with contrast in cases of renal venous thrombosis.

Table 26.6 Most common causes of vein thrombosis

Adults	Children
Nephrotic syndrome	Dehydration
Systemic lupus erythematosus	Sepsis
Amyloidosis	Sickle cell disease
Glomerulonephritis	Polycythemia
Collagen vascular disease	Maternal diabetes
Diabetes mellitus	Indwelling umbilical venous catheters
Renal sepsis (thrombophlebitis)	
Tumor thrombus	
Renal cell carcinoma	
Lymphoma	
Urinary obstruction (rare)	

Box 26.3: Imaging Findings for Renal Vein Thrombosis on Contrast-Enhanced CT

Enlarged kidney
Persistent cortical enhancement and lack of parenchymal enhancement
Delayed, diminished, or absent calyceal opacification
Attenuation changes, focal or diffuse
Perinephric fat stranding due to edema and thickening of renal fascia
Perinephric hemorrhage
Chronic phase: attenuated renal vein due to clot retraction
Collateral vessels around the kidney in chronic cases

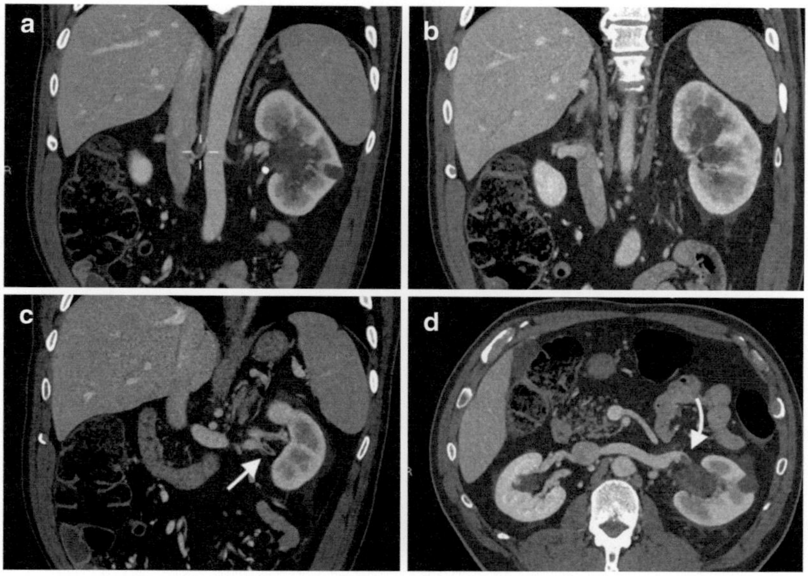

Fig. 26.6 A 40-year-old patient with intense left flank pain. CT evaluation reveals the presence of a small lithiasic nucleus (**a**) causing mild hydronephrosis (**a**, **b**). Images (**c**) and (**d**) show the presence of renal vein thrombosis associated with lithiasic obstruction (white arrows)

26.5 Other Urological Emergencies

26.5.1 Non-traumatic Bladder Rupture

Non-traumatic rupture of the urinary bladder is an infrequent event that nearly always occurs in the presence of pre-existing pathologies. It is considered an emergency due to the potential for severe complications. There are three types of bladder lesions: intraperitoneal lesions, which account for approximately 10–20% of cases; extraperitoneal lesions, which constitute about 80–90% of cases; and combined lesions, which are less common, at around 10%. Spontaneous urinary bladder perforation is extremely rare, making up less than 1% of all bladder injuries, with an overall mortality rate of around 50%. The risk factors are numerous, with the most common being infections, bladder calculi, urinary retention, bladder diverticula, and malignancies. Table 26.7 summarizes the main predisposing factors for bladder rupture, clarifying their pathophysiological mechanisms. Excluding traumatic causes, bladder ruptures can be classified as iatrogenic or spontaneous. Spontaneous rupture of the urinary bladder is usually intraperitoneal. Signs and symptoms of spontaneous bladder rupture are often vague. Most patients present with pelvic pain, dysuria, hematuria, renal failure, and sepsis. Clinical suspicion should be raised in cases of acute abdomen with free peritoneal fluid and an unexplained rise in serum urea and creatinine levels [23].

Table 26.7 Predisposing factors and mechanisms of bladder rupture

Risk factor	Description
Inflammatory cystitis	Inflammation of the bladder lining, which can weaken the bladder wall.
Infection	Bladder infections, including tuberculosis and schistosomiasis, can compromise the integrity of the bladder wall.
Bladder calculi	Bladder stones can cause irritation and weaken the bladder wall, leading to an increased risk of rupture.
Urinary retention	Chronic retention of urine can distend the bladder and make it more susceptible to rupture.
Bladder diverticulum	Outpouchings of the bladder wall that can rupture under pressure.
Malignancy	Bladder cancer can invade and weaken the bladder wall, increasing the risk of rupture.
Intra-arterial chemotherapy	Chemotherapy delivered directly into the arteries can damage the bladder wall.
Atherosclerotic emboli	Blockages in the arteries supplying the bladder can lead to ischemia and weakening of the bladder wall.
Radiation	Previous radiation therapy to the pelvic area can cause fibrosis and weakening of the bladder wall.
Diabetes mellitus	Diabetes can lead to neuropathy and poor bladder function, contributing to an increased risk of bladder rupture.
Hemophilia	Bleeding disorders can lead to hematuria and bladder wall damage, increasing the risk of rupture.
Connective tissue disorders	Conditions such as Ehlers-Danlos syndrome can cause structural weakness in the bladder wall.
Neurogenic bladder	Conditions that impair bladder sensation and contractility, leading to overdistension and increased risk of rupture.
Alcoholism	Chronic alcohol abuse can lead to bladder dysfunction and increased risk of rupture.

26.5.2 Imaging

CT with contrast, completed with delayed phases, and CT cystography are the gold-standard exams for diagnosing bladder rupture. In the case of intraperitoneal rupture, CT shows free fluid in the peritoneum, a possible defect in the bladder wall, or an abnormal position of a Foley catheter. Typically, peritoneal urine collection tends to be multiloculated. The presence of contrast medium in the peritoneum and between the intestinal loops confirms the diagnosis (Fig. 26.7). In extraperitoneal rupture, contrast medium is found around the bladder, in the perivesical space, and

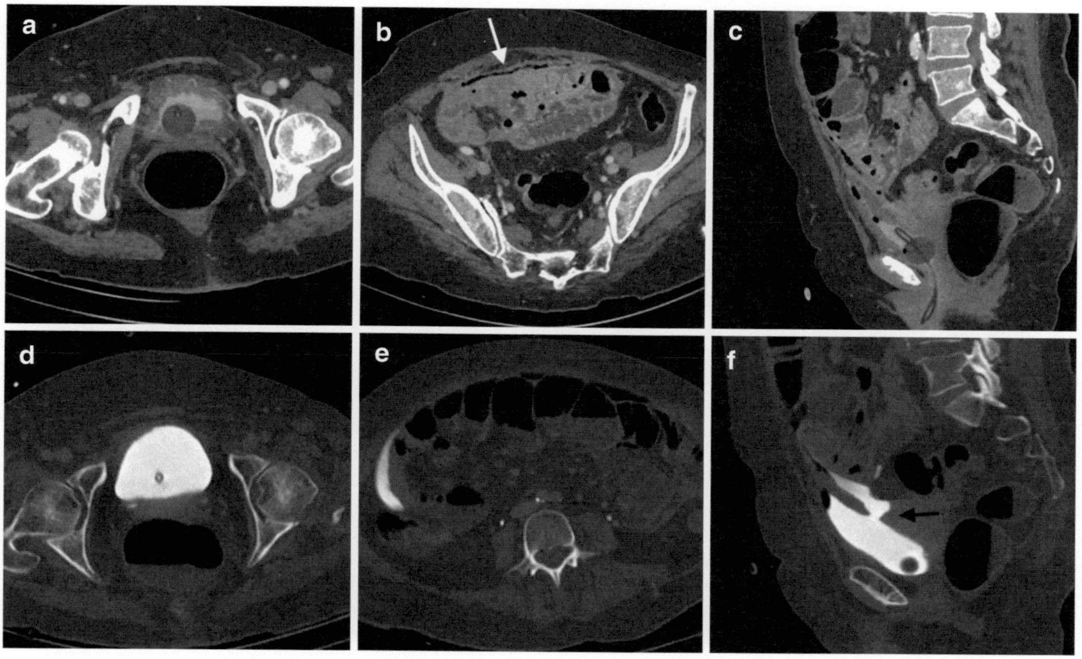

Fig. 26.7 A 58-year-old patient with neurogenic bladder. Contrast-enhanced CT evaluation shows a catheterized bladder (**a**), diffuse omental fat stranding with evidence of minimal pneumoperitoneum (white arrow) located in the submesocolic recesses (**b**, **c**). Contrast administration via the catheter (**d**) demonstrates peritoneal contrast extravasation (**e**) due to a bladder peritoneal lesion (**f**) (black arrow)

occasionally extends beyond the perivesical space to the thigh root, scrotum, and perineal region [24, 25]. Intraperitoneal and combined ruptures usually require surgical repair, while extraperitoneal perforations can be managed non-operatively by placing a Foley catheter [23].

References

1. Rishor-Olney CR, Hinson MR. Obstructive Uropathy. 2023 Jul 22. In: StatPearls [Internet]. Treasure Island (FL): StatPearls Publishing; 2024 Jan–. PMID: 32644347.
2. Yap E, Salifu M, Ahmad T, Sanusi A, Joseph A, Mallappallil M. Atypical causes of urinary tract obstruction. Case Rep Nephrol. 2019;2019:4903693.
3. Pérez-Aizpurua X, Cabello Benavente R, Bueno Serrano G, Alcázar Peral JM, Gómez-Jordana Mañas B, Tufet I, Jaumot J, Ruiz de Castroviejo Blanco J, Osorio Ospina F, Gonzalez-Enguita C. Obstructive uropathy: overview of the pathogenesis, etiology and management of a prevalent cause of acute kidney injury. World J Nephrol. 2024;13(2):93322. https://doi.org/10.5527/wjn.v13.i2.93322. PMID: 38983763; PMCID: PMC11229834
4. Mohebbi N. Wer bekommt Nierensteine? [Risk factors for urolithiasis]. Ther Umsch. 2021;78(5):223–7. German. https://doi.org/10.1024/0040-5930/a001264. PMID: 34032133.
5. Wagner CA. Etiopathogenic factors of urolithiasis. Arch Esp Urol. 2021;74(1):16–23. English, Spanish. PMID: 33459618.
6. Tamm E, Silverman P, Shuman W. Evaluation of the patient with Flank Pain and possible ureteral calculus. Radiology. 2003;228(2):319–29. https://doi.org/10.1148/radiol.2282011726.
7. Rucker CM, Menias CO, Bhalla S. Mimics of renal colic: alternative diagnoses at unenhanced helical CT. Radiographics. 2004;24(Suppl 1):S11–28; discussion S28–33. doi: https://doi.org/10.1148/rg.24si045505. PMID: 15486235.
8. Wang LJ, Ng CJ, Chen JC, Chiu TF, Wong YC. Diagnosis of acute flank pain caused by ureteral stones: value of combined direct and indirect signs on IVU and unenhanced helical CT. Eur Radiol. 2004;14(9):1634–40. https://doi.org/10.1007/s00330-004-2309-1. Epub 2004 Apr 2. PMID: 15060838.
9. Heneghan JP, McGuire KA, Leder RA, DeLong DM, Yoshizumi T, Nelson RC. Helical CT for nephrolithiasis and ureterolithiasis: comparison of conventional and reduced radiation-dose techniques. Radiology.

2003;229(2):575–80. https://doi.org/10.1148/radiol.2292021261. Epub 2003 Oct 2. PMID: 14526095.
10. Murray N, Darras KE, Walstra FE, Mohammed MF, McLaughlin PD, Nicolaou S. Dual-energy CT in evaluation of the acute abdomen. Radiographics. 2019;39(1):264–86. https://doi.org/10.1148/rg.2019180087. PMID: 30620698
11. Dhar M, Denstedt JD. Imaging in diagnosis, treatment, and follow-up of stone patients. Adv Chronic Kidney Dis. 2009;16(1):39–47. https://doi.org/10.1053/j.ackd.2008.10.005. PMID: 19095204
12. Craig WD, Wagner BJ, Travis MD. Pyelonephritis: radiologic-pathologic review. Radiographics. 2008;28(1):255–77; quiz 327–8. https://doi.org/10.1148/rg.281075171. PMID: 18203942
13. Goel RH, Unnikrishnan R, Remer EM. Acute urinary tract disorders. Radiol Clin North Am. 2015;53(6):1273–92. https://doi.org/10.1016/j.rcl.2015.06.011. Epub 2015 Aug 13. PMID: 26526438.
14. Majd M, Nussbaum Blask AR, Markle BM, et al. Acute pyelonephritis: comparison of diagnosis with 99mTc-DMSA, SPECT, spiral CT, MR imaging, and power Doppler US in an experimental pig model. Radiology. 2001;218(1):101–8.
15. Fukami H, Takeuchi Y, Kagaya S, Ojima Y, Saito A, Sato H, Matsuda K, Nagasawa T. Perirenal fat stranding is not a powerful diagnostic tool for acute pyelonephritis. Int J Gen Med. 2017;10:137–44. https://doi.org/10.2147/IJGM.S133685.
16. Kawashima A, Sandler C, Goldman S, Raval B, Fishman E. CT of renal inflammatory disease. Radiographics. 1997;17(4):851–66. https://doi.org/10.1148/radiographics.17.4.9225387.
17. Grayson DE, Abbott RM, Levy AD, Sherman PM. Emphysematous infections of the abdomen and pelvis: a pictorial review. Radiographics. 2002;22(3):543–61. https://doi.org/10.1148/radiographics.22.3.g02ma06543. PMID: 12006686.
18. Nepal P, Ojili V, Kaur N, Tirumani SH, Nagar A. Gas where it shouldn't be! imaging spectrum of emphysematous infections in the abdomen and pelvis. AJR Am J Roentgenol. 2021;216(3):812–23. https://doi.org/10.2214/AJR.20.23545. Epub 2021 Jan 13. PMID: 33439049.
19. Sharma R, Mitra SK, Choudhary A, Majee P. Emphysematous cystitis-gas in bladder: a rare urological emergency. BMJ Case Reports. 2015. https://doi.org/10.1136/bcr-2015-210836
20. Kawashima A, Sandler CM, Ernst RD, Tamm EP, Goldman SM, Fishman EK. CT evaluation of renovascular disease. Radiographics. 2000;20(5):1321–40. https://doi.org/10.1148/radiographics.20.5.g00se141321. PMID: 10992021.
21. Urban BA, Ratner LE, Fishman EK. Three-dimensional volume-rendered CT angiography of the renal arteries and veins: normal anatomy, variants, and clinical applications. Radiographics. 2001;21(2):373–86; questionnaire 549-55. https://doi.org/10.1148/radiographics.21.2.g01mr19373. PMID: 11259702
22. Mazhar HR, Aeddula NR. Renal Vein Thrombosis. 2023 Jun 12. In: StatPearls [Internet]. Treasure Island (FL): StatPearls Publishing; 2024 Jan–. PMID: 30725656.
23. Pan C, Nakrani S, Coneybeare D. Non-traumatic bladder rupture. Am J Emerg Med. 2023;63:179.e5–6. https://doi.org/10.1016/j.ajem.2022.09.043. Epub 2022 Sep 30. PMID: 36253214.
24. Gross JS, Rotenberg S, Horrow MM. Resident and fellow education feature bladder injury: types, mechanisms, and diagnostic imaging. RadioGraphics. 2014; https://doi.org/10.1148/rg.343140022.
25. Kivlin D, Ross C, Lester K, Metro M, Ginsberg P. A case series of spontaneous rupture of the urinary bladder. Curr Urol. 2015;8(1):53–6. https://doi.org/10.1159/000365690.

Part VII

The Extremities

Painful and Cold Limb

27

Francesco Verde, Monica Sicuranza,
Gaspare Oliva, Antonio Raucci, Marco Di Serafino,
and Gianluca Ponticiello

27.1 Introduction

A painful and cold limb represents a critical medical emergency that demands prompt diagnosis and intervention to prevent severe complications, including limb loss. This condition, also known as acute limb ischemia (ALI), is defined as the sudden loss or marked decrease in limb arterial perfusion causing a potential threat to limb viability. ALI is characterized by a symptom duration of fewer than two weeks, while chronic limb ischemia typically presents with symptoms lasting longer than two weeks [1]. Pathophysiology primarily relates to acute arterial ischemia, mainly due to an embolism or thrombosis obstruction associated with insufficient vascular collateralization. The lower limbs are more frequently involved, often caused by acute arterial thrombosis.

CT angiography provides detailed images of the arterial vascular extremities due to its widespread availability, rapid acquisition time, and high spatial resolution. This is particularly crucial in emergency settings where rapid diagnosis and initial management can significantly impact patient outcomes. The ability of CT angiography to generate isotropic datasets allows for advanced post-processing techniques, including multiplanar reformations (MPR), curved planar reformation (CPR), maximum intensity projection (MIP), and volume rendering (VR), which enhance the visualization of vascular anatomy and aid in accurate diagnosis and treatment planning of ALI providing accurate anatomic mapping disease and precise vascular lesion extension and severity.

This chapter aims to provide a diagnostic approach for assessing patients presenting with a painful and cold limb, focusing on the role of CT angiography in evaluating lower extremities arterial vascular emergencies. It covers relevant anatomy, clinical evaluation, and CT imaging protocol considerations, including technical pitfalls and insights into advancements. Additionally, it addresses the interpretation and reporting of CT angiography findings across various etiologies.

F. Verde (✉) · G. Oliva · A. Raucci · M. Di Serafino
G. Ponticiello
Department of General and Emergency Radiology, "Antonio Cardarelli" Hospital, Naples, Italy
e-mail: francesco.verde@aocardarelli.it; gaspare.oliva@aocardarelli.it; antonio.raucci@aocardarelli.it; marco.diserafino@aocardarelli.it; gianluca.ponticiello@aocardarelli.it

M. Sicuranza
Department of Cardiology, "San Giuliano" Hospital - Giugliano, Naples, Italy
e-mail: monica.sicuranza@aslnapoli2nord.it

L. Romano et al. (eds.), *CT of Non-Traumatic Body Emergencies*,
https://doi.org/10.1007/978-3-031-84849-0_27

27.2 Anatomy and Anatomical Variants

Recognition of the anatomical features and variants is crucial for accurate CT interpretation and effective planning of interventional procedures in patients presenting with painful and cold limbs [2].

The lower extremity vasculature can be categorized into "inflow" and "outflow" vessels. The inflow vasculature consists of the infrarenal abdominal aorta, common iliac arteries, and external iliac arteries. The outflow vasculature is further subdivided into two categories: runoff vessels, which provide inline flow to the foot, and musculoskeletal branches, which terminate in the structures of the limb. This distinction becomes particularly significant in cases of vascular occlusion. When runoff vessels are occluded, the musculoskeletal branches are the principal source of collateral blood supply.

The common femoral artery continues the external iliac artery and typically measures 6–9 mm in diameter. It extends from the inguinal ligament to the origins of the superficial femoral artery and profunda femoris artery, just distal to the inferior margin of the femoral head. A high bifurcation can occur in nearly 30% of individuals, where the artery divides while still anterior to the femoral head. This anatomical variation has significant implications for endovascular interventions, as an early division of the common femoral artery can complicate vascular access.

The profunda femoris artery gives rise to the medial femoral circumflex artery that supplies the femoral head and neck, the lateral circumflex artery that supplies the lateral portion of the thigh, and to the numerous perforating branches that contribute to the muscular supply in the medial and posterior thigh. These muscular branches anastomose with muscular branches of the superficial femoral and popliteal arteries. The origin and branching patterns of the profunda femoris artery can vary; the most common variants are independent origins of the medial or lateral circumflex femoral arteries from the common femoral artery.

The superficial femoral artery, typically 5–7 mm in diameter, is the continuation of the common femoral artery after the origin of the profunda femoris artery. It courses through the anterior thigh, transitioning into the popliteal artery as it passes through the adductor hiatus. The superficial femoral artery's numerous muscular branches play a crucial role as collateral pathways in cases of occlusive disease. A rare anatomical variant is the persistent sciatic artery (PSA), which occurs in approximately 0.025–0.04% of individuals. This embryonic vessel, a branch of the internal iliac artery, usually regresses as the external iliac artery takes over as the primary arterial supply to the lower limb. However, when it persists, the PSA can lead to complications such as occlusive disease or aneurysm formation due to its posterior course, which subjects it to repetitive trauma.

The popliteal artery, averaging 4–5 mm in diameter, descends along the posterior thigh and gives rise to genicular branches supplying the knee joint. At the lower border of the popliteus muscle, it bifurcates into the anterior tibial artery and the tibioperoneal trunk.

The anterior tibial artery runs anteriorly through the interosseous membrane between the tibia and fibula, proceeding down in the anterior fascial compartment of the calf to supply the anterior compartment of the leg by muscular branches. It continues below the ankle joint as the dorsalis pedis artery, providing the anterior circulation of the foot.

The tibioperoneal trunk is a short vessel of variable length, typically ranging from 2 to 3 cm, that extends some centimetres beyond the origin of the anterior tibial artery before dividing into the posterior tibial and peroneal arteries. The posterior tibial artery courses deep into the soleus muscle passes posterior and inferior to the medial malleolus and bifurcates into the medial and lateral plantar arteries. The peroneal artery descends posterior and medial to the fibula to terminate in the ankle, giving branches to supply the lateral and posterior surfaces of the calcaneus. Notably, the peroneal artery is usually spared in occlusive disease and serves as a crucial source of collateral supply due to its central

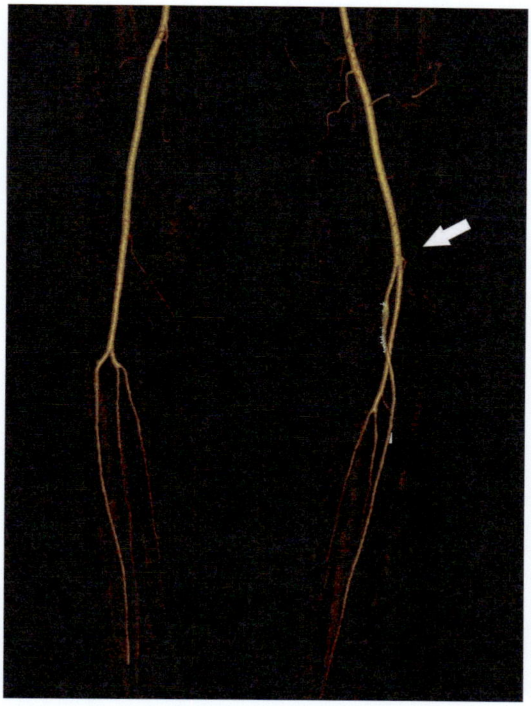

Fig. 27.1 Volume rendering of lower extremity arterial anatomy demonstrating a common anatomical variant. The left limb shows a high origin of the anterior tibial artery (white arrow), one of the most frequent variations in the branching pattern of the popliteal artery. Note the normal branching pattern in the right limb for comparison

location, where it can collateralize to both the distal anterior and posterior tibial arteries. Together, the branches from the posterior tibial and peroneal arteries constitute the posterior circulation of the foot.

Anatomical variations in the branching pattern of the popliteal artery are not uncommon, with CT angiography revealing such variations in approximately 10–11% of patients. The most frequently observed variations include a high origin of the anterior tibial artery (Fig. 27.1), a common origin of the anterior tibial and peroneal arteries, and a complete trifurcation of the popliteal artery without the presence of a tibioperoneal trunk. Additionally, hypoplastic or aplastic posterior tibial arteries are sometimes encountered. In cases where the anterior or posterior tibial artery is absent, the peroneal artery may extend its course to supply the foot, compensating for the missing vessel.

27.3 Etiology and Clinical Assessment of Acute Limb Ischemia

27.3.1 Etiology

ALI can be broadly categorized into two primary etiologies: thrombosis and embolism. Thrombosis is common in individuals with a significant underlying atherosclerotic disease, affecting native and reconstructed vessels such as bypass grafts and stents. Embolic events are frequently associated with atrial fibrillation or left ventricular mural thrombi following an acute myocardial infarction [3]. The most common and less frequent thrombotic and embolic causes of ALI are reported in Table 27.1.

27.3.2 Clinical Presentation

The clinical presentation of ALI varies significantly depending on several factors, including the location and duration of the arterial occlusion, the presence of collateral circulation, and the metabolic changes induced by tissue ischemia. Symptoms can manifest over a period of hours to days, ranging from new or worsening claudication to sudden paralysis of the affected limb. It is crucial to take a detailed patient history to determine if symptoms of chronic ischemia were present before the acute event to recognize two distinct presentations [4]:

- Acute exacerbation of chronic limb-threatening ischemia: in patients with known peripheral artery occlusive disease or prior revascularisation, symptoms may develop over hours to days. The sudden worsening of symptoms in a patient with a history of peripheral artery disease typically indicates arterial thrombosis. These patients typically present with a more gradual aggravation of symptoms because their pre-existing peripheral artery disease has allowed for the development of collateral circulation, which partially compensates for the occlusion [5].

Table 27.1 Etiology of acute limb ischaemia

Embolus	Thrombosis	Injury
Cardiac source Atrial fibrillation Myocardial infarction (with mural thrombus) Left ventricular aneurysm Valvular heart disease Prosthetic valves Endocarditis Cardiac tumor (atrial myxoma) Noncardiac source Aortic and peripheral arterial aneurysms Ulcerated atherosclerotic plaque with intraplaque hemorrhage Paradoxical (venous embolism in case of atrial or ventricular abnormal communication)	Thrombosis on atherosclerotic vessel disease atherosclerotic obstruction by-pass graft and stent occlusion aneurysm thrombosis Thrombosis on non-atheromatous pathological artery buerger disease vasculitis adventitial cystic disease post-actinic arteritis Thrombosis on healthy artery popliteal entrapment syndrome hyperviscosity systemic coagulation disorders drug-induced (heparin, chemotherapy) low cardiac output syndromes ischemic thrombophlebitis (phlegmasia cerulea dolens) Distal progression of aortic dissection	Iatrogenic Thromboembolism Closure devices Device embolization Traumatic

– Acute limb ischemia: in patients with otherwise normal vasculature, collateral vessels cannot be recruited quickly enough to bypass the occluded artery. Consequently, signs of acute ischemia develop rapidly. The sudden onset of ischemic symptoms in a previously asymptomatic patient is most consistent with an embolus, with patients often able to identify the exact time of symptom onset.

Differentiating between acute embolic and thrombotic occlusion can be challenging. Therefore, classifying the severity of arterial ischemia based on clinical presentation and physical examination is crucial for determining the urgency of intervention and predicting outcomes.

27.3.3 Severity Classification

A thorough examination of both lower extremities is necessary to detect signs of ischemia. The classic "six Ps"—pain, pallor, pulselessness, poikilothermia, paresthesia, and paralysis—are essential in the initial evaluation of the clinical severity of ischemia. A comprehensive vascular examination includes palpation of all pulses (femoral, popliteal, dorsalis pedis, and posterior tibial) and Doppler assessment of arterial and venous signals. The ankle-brachial index (ABI) should be obtained if Doppler signals are present, as an ABI of less than 0.7 is considered critical and predictive of poor outcomes [3].

The Society for Vascular Surgery/International Society for Cardiovascular Surgery (SVS/ISCVS) classification, also known as the Rutherford classification, is commonly used to stratify limb ischemia based on the presence and degree of sensorimotor deficits and Doppler findings (Table 27.2). This classification system guides clinicians in determining limb viability and appropriate management strategies, categorising limbs as viable, threatened, or irreversibly ischemic [1].

Table 27.2 Clinical categories of acute limb ischemia according to European Society for Vascular Surgery Classification

Category	Prognosis	Clinical findings	Doppler signals
I. Viable	Not immediately threatened	Sensory loss: none Muscle weakness: none	Arterial: audible Venous: audible
II. Threatened			
a. Marginally	Salvageable if promptly treated	Sensory loss: minimal (toes) or none Muscle weakness: none	Arterial: inaudible Venous: audible
b. Immediately	Salvageable with immediate revascularization	Sensory loss: more than toes, associated with rest pain Muscle weakness: mild, moderate	Arterial: inaudible Venous: audible
III. Irreversible	Major tissue loss or permanent nerve damage inevitable	Sensory loss: profound, anesthetic Muscle weakness: profound, paralysis (rigor)	Arterial: inaudible Venous: inaudible

27.4 CT Angiography Technique

27.4.1 Protocol Consideration

CTA protocol for acute limb ischemia typically involves a non-contrast baseline study followed by a biphasic contrast-enhanced examination. The contrast medium, ideally with a concentration of 400 mg/mL, is administered intravenously at a flow rate of 4–5 mL/sec, with a total volume of approximately 120 mL. This is followed by a saline flush (40 mL at 2 mL/s) to optimize bolus geometry. The arterial phase is initiated using the bolus tracking technique, while the portal venous phase is acquired with a 75-s delay. The venous phase allows for the evaluation of arterial segments that opacify late, potentially revealing occluded areas that might not have been well visualized earlier. Additionally, if necessary, an optional delayed phase can be acquired to assess venous return, which may be delayed or non-evaluable due to severe arterial stenosis or occlusions. By employing the multiphase technique approach, valuable information about the overall vascular status of the limb can be obtained, providing a complete understanding of vascular anatomy and pathology, even in complex cases of acute limb ischemia.

Extension of the study to include the entire aorta is certainly useful in cases of suspected embolic disease, but also in acute aortic occlusion, which can be caused by thrombosis of an atherosclerotic or aneurysmal aorta or by aortic dissection, most often as a result of compression of the true lumen..

Achieving high and homogeneous arterial enhancement is crucial in peripheral CTA to ensure synchronized image acquisition with optimal contrast timing, high resolution, and minimized radiation exposure. The primary goal in CTA image acquisition is to obtain clear and detailed images of the arterial tree, which requires precise timing of contrast injection and imaging [6].

Post-processing techniques are crucial in CTA interpretation, facilitating prompt reviewing of the peripheral vascular system [7]. Axial viewing serves as the basis for the vessel assessment, supplemented by reconstruction techniques (Fig. 27.2).

Volume Rendering (VR) and Maximum Intensity Projection (MIP): These techniques provide a rapid overview of the affected extremity and help localize significant vascular abnormalities that may require further localized analysis.

Multiplanar Reformations (MPR) and Curved Planar Reformations (CPR): These are well-suited for detailed evaluation of vascular segments, mainly when vessels take an oblique course through the axial plane or when areas of narrowing are eccentric. CPR is especially useful for evaluating longer segments of affected vessels. Both MPR and CPR techniques are invaluable in assessing calcified and non-calcified atherosclerotic plaque, mural wall thickening, native vessel stenosis, and stent patency.

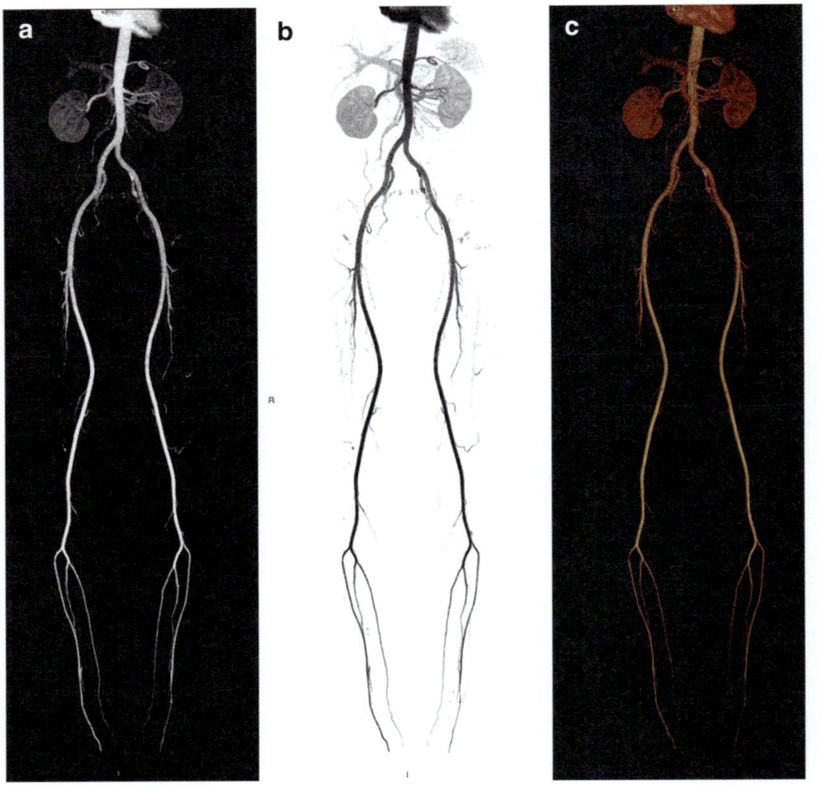

Fig. 27.2 Normal anatomy of the lower extremity arteries depicted using (**a**) coronal maximum intensity projection (MIP) with bone removal post-processing technique; (**b**) MIP inverted simulating angiographic view; (**c**) 3D-volume rendering algorithm

27.4.2 Pitfalls

CTA, in evaluating acute limb ischemia, is subject to several pitfalls that can affect the accuracy of the diagnosis and assessment. One of the primary challenges is the timing of the contrast bolus, which various factors can influence. If the scan is performed too early, a phenomenon known as 'outrunning the bolus' occurs, where the CT table moves faster than the contrast bolus (Fig. 27.3). This results in the distal arteries not being adequately opacified, leading to a gradual diminishment of arterial enhancement and eventual non-opacification. This issue is particularly pronounced in patients with poor cardiac output or low flow states, such as those with cardiomyopathy. Severe atherosclerotic disease can also significantly impact contrast flow. Additionally, aortic aneurysms can create turbulent blood flow, causing dilution of contrast media and delay in transit. In patients with peripheral arterial occlusive disease, arterial stenoses, occlusions, or aneurysms anywhere between the infrarenal abdominal aorta and the pedal arteries may substantially delay downstream vascular opacification. Conversely, if the scan is performed too late, venous contamination may occur, complicating the identification of arterial anatomy. Venous contamination can also be exacerbated by hyperemia of an extremity, often related to infection. These factors underscore the importance of considering multi-phase CT imaging protocol to capture early and delayed vascular opacification when necessary.

Dense vascular calcifications present another significant challenge. The "blooming" artefact, caused by calcifications or endovascular stents, can obscure the evaluation of the vessel lumen, leading to an overestimation of stenosis severity. This artefact is accentuated in settings with a narrow viewing window, where calcifications or stent struts appear overly bright and artificially larger, suggesting more severe steno-occlusive disease. To mitigate this, increasing the window

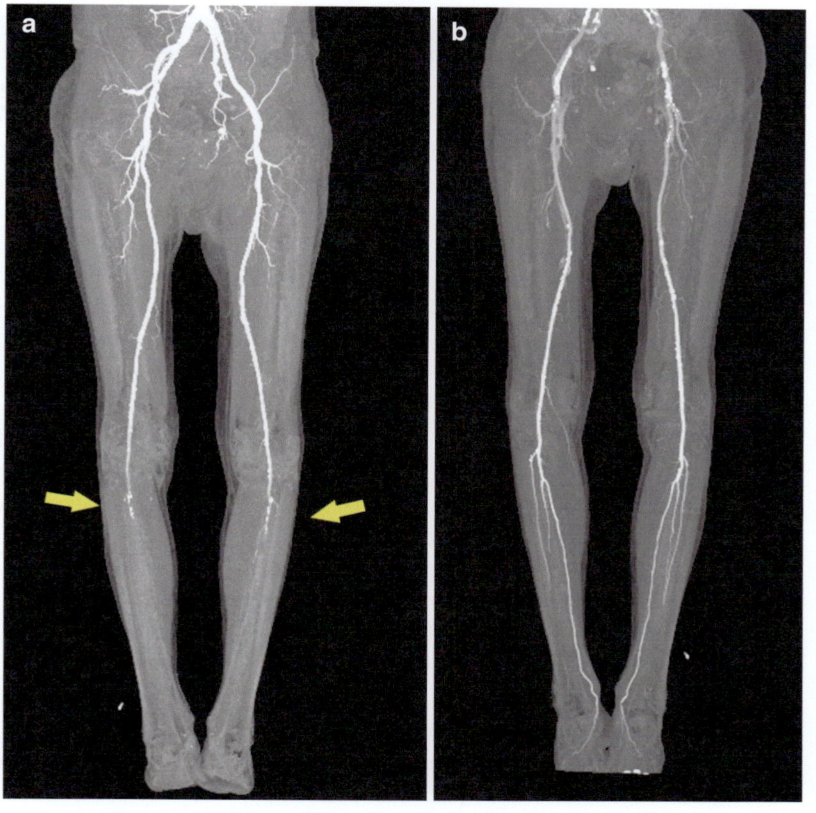

Fig. 27.3 Outrunning the contrast bolus in CT angiography of lower extremities. (**a**) Coronal MIP of arterial phase showing non-opacification of distal vessels (yellow arrows) due to scanning too fast relative to the contrast bolus in a patient with poor cardiac output. (**b**) Coronal MIP of venous phase demonstrating normal opacification of distal arterial vessels, confirming that the lack of enhancement in (**a**) was due to timing rather than occlusive disease

level and width can help diminish the brightness of calcifications and stents, allowing better visualization of the vessel lumen. Automated post-processing techniques can sometimes introduce artefacts and misrepresentations, particularly in the presence of calcifications and stents. Therefore, it is crucial to always review the source data, as 3D renderings can be misleading and may not accurately reflect the severity of the disease. Additionally, in patients with acute occlusions, vessels distal to the occlusion may fail to opacify, limiting the evaluation for potential distal revascularization targets. Repeating the scan acquisition through the non-opacified portion of the limb can sometimes overcome this limitation.

27.4.3 Advancement

Recent advancements in CT angiography have significantly enhanced diagnostic capabilities, particularly in complex cases where traditional techniques may fall short. Two notable innovations are the Dual-Energy CT (DECT) and dynamic computed tomography angiography (CTA) [8].

- DECT enhances the accuracy and speed of CTA analysis, particularly in the presence of significant vascular calcifications. By differentiating calcium and iodine-based on their attenuation differences at various kVp levels, DECT allows the automatic subtraction of mural calcifications and osseous structures from the images. This technique significantly improves image quality by reducing artefacts and providing better visualization of the vascular lumen.
- Time-resolved (dynamic) CTA of runoff vessels offers considerable improvements in diagnostic confidence and reduced venous contamination. However, these benefits come at the cost of increased radiation and contrast

doses. This advanced imaging method captures multiple phases of contrast passage through the vessels, allowing for a more detailed assessment of vascular anatomy and pathology, which is especially useful in evaluating complex cases where precise temporal resolution is crucial.

27.5 Emergent Peripheral Vascular Conditions: CT Findings and Interpretation

27.5.1 Arterial Embolism

Arterial embolism is a significant cause of acute limb ischemia, accounting for approximately 15% of cases. This condition typically results from cardiac dysrhythmias, with atrial fibrillation (AF) being the predominant etiology in about two-thirds of cases (Fig. 27.4), while ventricular thrombi account for another 20%. These emboli usually travel from the heart to the extremities, with lower extremities more frequently affected than upper extremities. Other potential sources include left ventricular dysfunction following myocardial infarction, prosthetic valve complications, and infected cardiac valves leading to septic emboli. Arterial-to-arterial embolization from aneurysms or atherosclerotic lesions contributes to about 20% of peripheral emboli (Fig. 27.5).

CT imaging plays a crucial role in diagnosing and characterizing arterial embolism [9]. Typical findings include:

- Abrupt focal occlusion: The hallmark of embolic disease is a sudden cutoff of contrast-enhanced blood flow, often visualized as a central arterial filling defect.
- Vessel expansion: The affected artery may appear slightly dilated proximal to the occlusion due to the impacted embolus.
- Predilection for bifurcations: Emboli tend to lodge at arterial bifurcations or areas of acute narrowing, such as atherosclerotic plaques. Common sites include the common femoral, common iliac, and popliteal artery bifurcations.
- Lack of collaterals: Unlike thrombotic occlusions, embolic events often occur in patients without pre-existing vascular disease, resulting in a paucity of collateral vessels.

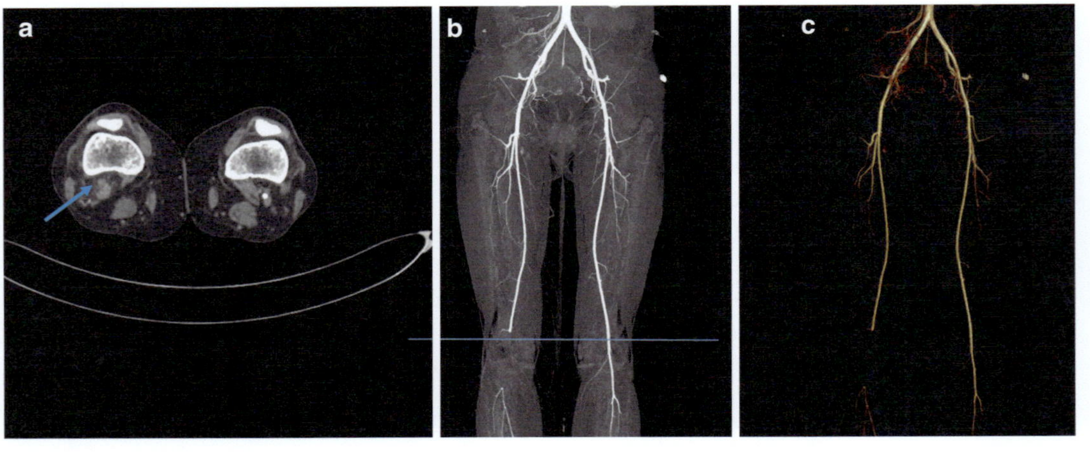

Fig. 27.4 54-year-old woman presenting with atrial fibrillation and right leg pain. (**a**) Axial Computed Tomography Angiography image showing an occlusive filling defect (arrow) in the suprageniculate segment of the right popliteal artery, extending for approximately 8 cm consistent with thromboembolism. (**b**) Coronal Maximum Intensity Projection (MIP) and (**c**) Volume Rendering (VR) images of the same finding. MIP allows for improved visualization of the extent of the occlusion and its relationship to adjacent vessels, while VR provides a three-dimensional representation that aids in understanding the overall vascular anatomy and the location of the occlusion in relation to key anatomical landmarks. These post-processing techniques complement the axial images, enhancing diagnostic confidence and facilitating treatment planning

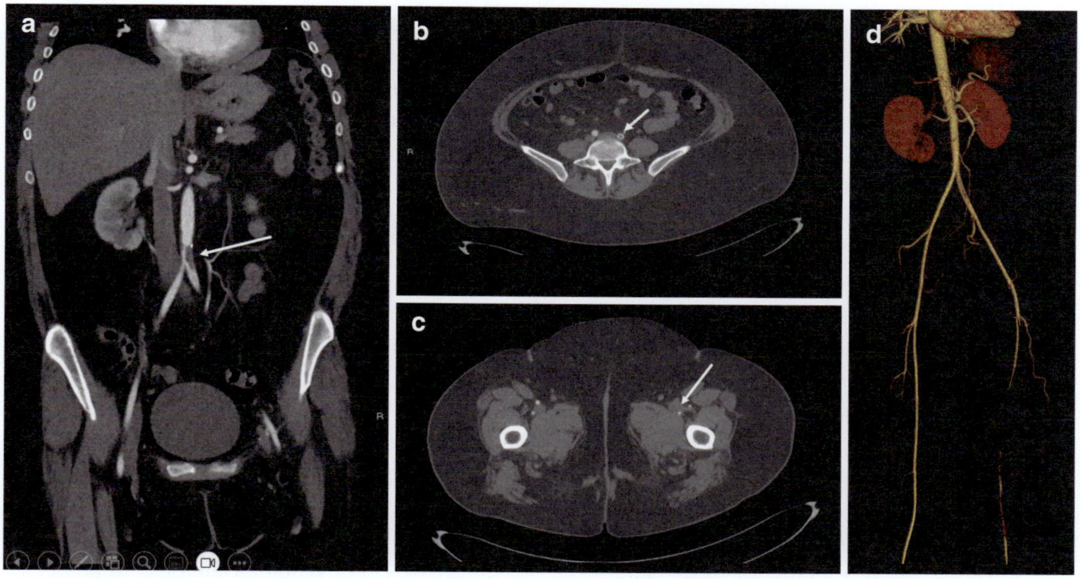

Fig. 27.5 CT angiography findings in a 53-year-old woman presenting with left leg pain. (**a**) Coronal image of the abdomen demonstrating an eccentric, non-occlusive filling defect in the distal infrarenal abdominal aorta (white arrow), representing mural thrombus. (**b**, **c**) Transaxial CT images revealing a subocclusive filling defect in the left common iliac artery (white arrow) and an occlusive defect in the left superficial femoral artery (white arrow), consistent with thromboembolism likely originating from the aortic mural thrombus. (**d**) 3D volume rendering providing a comprehensive overview of the vascular anatomy and embolic occlusions. This case illustrates the importance of evaluating the entire vascular tree in patients with acute limb ischemia, as proximal sources of embolism can lead to distal occlusions

- Multiple emboli: In some cases, multiple sites of embolic disease may be observed, potentially affecting other organs such as the kidneys, spleen, or bowel.

When reporting CTA findings of arterial embolism, it is essential to provide a comprehensive description that includes:

- Location: Specify the anatomical region (pelvis, thigh, knee, calf) and the exact arterial segment involved (above-knee and below-knee segments).
- Segmental reporting: Systematically describe the aorta, visceral arteries, and iliac arteries.
- Potential sources of embolism: Comment on possible embolic sources visible on the CT, such as cardiac chamber thrombi or aortic atherosclerotic plaques.

27.5.2 Arterial Thrombosis

Arterial thrombosis is the predominant cause of acute limb ischemia (ALI), accounting for approximately 85% of cases. This condition typically occurs in the setting of pre-existing vascular lesions, with thrombosis of bypass grafts now being the most frequent etiology. The clinical presentation of thrombosis on atherosclerotic stenosis, referred to as acute-on-chronic limb-threatening ischemia, may be less severe compared to embolic occlusions due to the presence of sufficient collateral circulation that has developed over time. Arterial thrombosis can manifest in three main scenarios:

- Thrombosis on Atherosclerotic Vessel Disease: This category encompasses the majority of acute limb ischemia cases.

Atherosclerotic obstruction is a common manifestation, where thrombosis typically occurs at sites of pre-existing atherosclerotic stenosis. In contemporary practice, bypass graft occlusion has emerged as the most frequent cause of acute limb ischemia, highlighting the importance of graft surveillance and management. Stent occlusion, characterized by thrombosis within previously placed arterial stents, represents another significant subset of cases. Lastly, popliteal aneurysm thrombosis, can lead to rapid onset of severe ischemia due to the sudden occlusion of a large-caliber vessel.

- Thrombosis on Non-atheromatous Pathological Artery: This can occur in patients with conditions such as Buerger disease, vasculitis, adventitial cystic disease, and post-actinic arteritis. The clinical presentation is similar to ALI occurring in patients with atherosclerotic plaques, as both involve chronic narrowing of the bloodstream.
- Thrombosis on Healthy Artery: A less frequent cause of ALI, this can be secondary to extrinsic compression (e.g., popliteal entrapment), hyperviscosity, systemic coagulation disorders, or drug-induced (e.g., estrogen-progestogen therapy, ergotism, drug addiction, chemotherapy). Heparin-induced thrombosis is another important cause in this category. Extreme low-flow states, such as in hypovolemic shock or cardiac failure, can also produce ALI, especially in patients with pre-existing peripheral arterial disease.

CTA plays a crucial role in the evaluation of patients presenting with deterioration of chronic limb-threatening ischemia due to thrombotic occlusion on atherosclerotic vessel disease [10].

In such emergent conditions, CTA can precisely delineate the extent and location of stenoses, often revealing the site of acute thrombosis superimposed on chronic atherosclerotic narrowing. It's important to distinguish between true luminal stenosis and simple reductions in vascular caliber when interpreting CTA images. Luminal stenosis is a pathological vessel lumen narrowing caused by atherosclerotic plaque, thrombus, or other vascular pathologies. This is characterized by irregular narrowing of the contrast-enhanced lumen, often associated with wall thickening, calcifications, or soft tissue components. In contrast, reductions in vascular caliber may be physiological or positional, such as vessel tapering at bifurcations or temporary narrowing due to external compression or vasospasm. True luminal stenosis is typically graded based on the percentage reduction of the vessel's normal lumen diameter: mild (1–49%), moderate (50–69%), severe (70–99%), and occlusion (100%).

For bypass graft occlusions, CTA not only identifies the thrombosed segment but also assesses the native vasculature and potential alternative conduits for revascularization (Fig. 27.6) [11]. When evaluating stent occlusions, CTA can demonstrate the extent of in-stent thrombosis and any associated complications such as stent fracture or migration (Fig. 27.7).

Given the critical role of CTA in diagnosing and managing arterial thrombosis, it is essential to recognize the hallmark imaging characteristics that aid in the accurate assessment of this condition. Key imaging findings include:

- Segmental non-opacification: The affected artery shows a lack of contrast enhancement, with an abrupt cutoff at the site of thrombosis.
- Associated atherosclerotic disease: Evidence of atherosclerotic disease is frequently observed in the peripheral vasculature, including calcified plaques and vessel wall irregularities.
- Collateral circulation: The presence of collateral vessels is a distinguishing feature of thrombotic occlusions, particularly in cases of acute-on-chronic limb-threatening ischemia.
- Graft or stent thrombosis: In cases involving bypass grafts or stents, the lumen fails to opacify after contrast administration, with variable reconstitution of flow distally depending on collateralization.

In the imaging assessment of chronic limb-threatening ischemia, CTA reports should include detailed information about the number and characteristics of stenotic or occlusive lesions, includ-

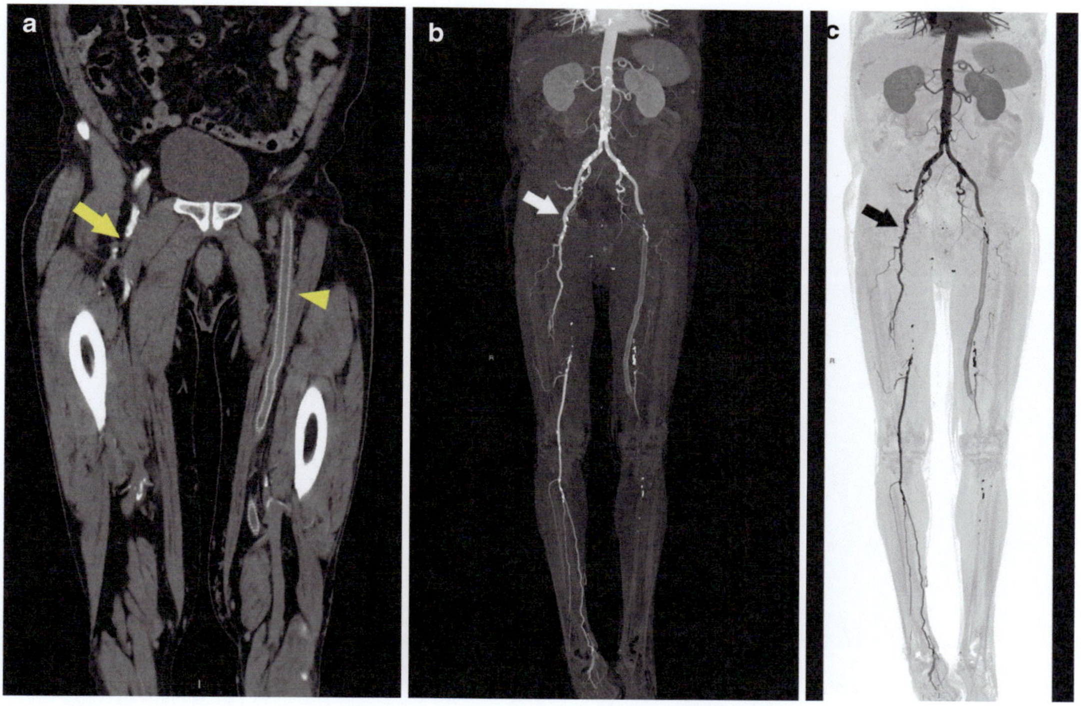

Fig. 27.6 67-year-old diabetic patient with advanced peripheral arterial disease presenting with left leg pain. (**a**) Coronal multiplanar reformation (MPR) CT image demonstrating thrombotic occlusion of the right superficial femoral artery (yellow arrow) and an occluded left femoropopliteal bypass graft (yellow arrow head). (**b**) Maximum Intensity Projection (MIP) and (**c**) inverted MIP reformations further delineate the occlusions and the extensive collateralization via branches of the right profunda femoris artery, revascularizing the popliteal artery (white arrow **b**, black arrow **c**). These post-processing techniques offer enhanced visualization of the vascular anatomy and pathology, aiding in the comprehensive evaluation of disease extent and collateral circulation, crucial for guiding management decisions in complex cases of acute-on-chronic limb ischemia

ing their length, diameter, and morphology, the degree of calcification, presence of non-calcified plaque, and status of inflow and outflow vessels. Additionally, CTA can reveal the extent of collateral circulation, which is well-developed in chronic atherosclerotic disease and can influence the severity of ischemia in acute thrombotic events [2].

The comprehensive assessment of the vascular lesions provided by CTA is crucial in guiding the selection of the most appropriate intervention strategy [12]. To standardize this decision-making process, two primary anatomic classification systems are used to stratify the severity of peripheral arterial disease and guide management decisions [5].

- Trans-Atlantic Inter-Society Consensus (TASC II) Classification: This system categorizes arterial lesions based on their anatomic distribution, number, and nature (stenosis or occlusion). TASC II primarily focuses on the aortoiliac and femoropopliteal segments, providing a widely used method to classify disease severity in these distributions [13]. However, it does not account for the extent of disease in more distal segments, particularly the tibial arteries.
- Global Limb Anatomic Staging System (GLASS): Proposed in the 2019 global vascular guidelines on chronic limb-threatening ischemia management, GLASS provides a more comprehensive anatomic scheme. It involves grading the level of disease in the femoropopliteal and infrapopliteal segments of the preferred target arterial path for revascularization.

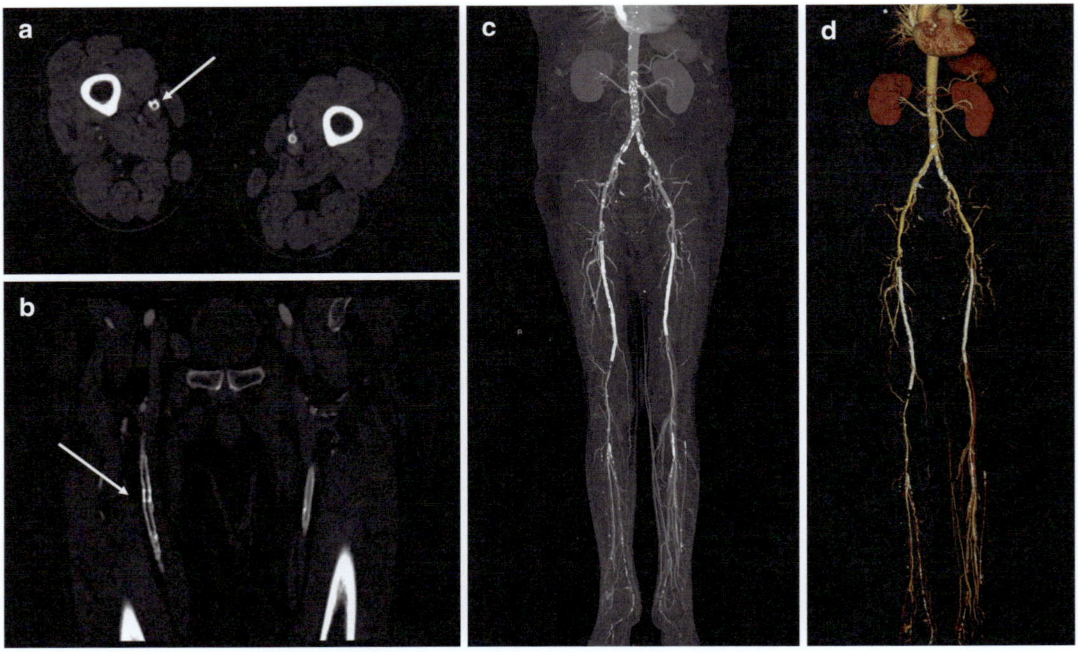

Fig. 27.7 CT angiography findings in a 71-year-old patient with chronic limb ischemia presenting with sudden right leg pain. (**a**) Axial and (**b**) coronal multiplanar reformation (MPR) CTA images demonstrating complete occlusion of the right superficial femoral artery from its origin, including thrombosis of a previously placed stent (white arrows). The right popliteal artery is reconstituted via collateral circulation from the profunda femoris artery . Note the patent left superficial femoral artery with a patent stent for comparison. (**c**) Maximum Intensity Projection (MIP) and (**d**) Volume Rendering (VR) images provide comprehensive visualization of the occlusions, collateral pathways, and overall vascular anatomy

27.5.3 Popliteal Artery Aneurysm

Popliteal artery aneurysms (Fig. 27.8) represent the most frequent peripheral arterial aneurysms and pose significant clinical concerns due to their potential complications such as distal embolization of mural thrombus and, less commonly, aneurysm rupture [14]. Defined as a focal dilatation of the artery greater than 50% of the normal adjacent vessel diameter (typically 0.7–1.1 cm), these aneurysms are predominantly degenerative in nature and often bilateral, occurring in 50–70% of cases. Their clinical significance stems from the high risk of acute limb ischemia (25%) due to thrombosis or distal embolization, with a small but noteworthy risk of rupture (3%).

The presence of a popliteal artery aneurysm should prompt consideration of concomitant aneurysms, particularly in the contralateral popliteal artery and the abdominal aorta, the latter being associated in up to 70% of cases. In younger patients, the finding of a peripheral artery aneurysm necessitates evaluation for connective tissue disorders such as Marfan, Ehlers-Danlos, and Loeys-Dietz syndromes.

CTA plays a pivotal role in the diagnosis, characterization, and treatment planning of popliteal artery aneurysms. Key imaging findings and reporting elements include:

- Dimensions: Accurate measurement in all three dimensions is crucial, with diameters exceeding 2 cm associated with an increased risk of thromboembolic events and typically indicating the need for intervention.
- Morphology: Description of the aneurysm shape (fusiform or saccular) and its relationship to arterial branches.

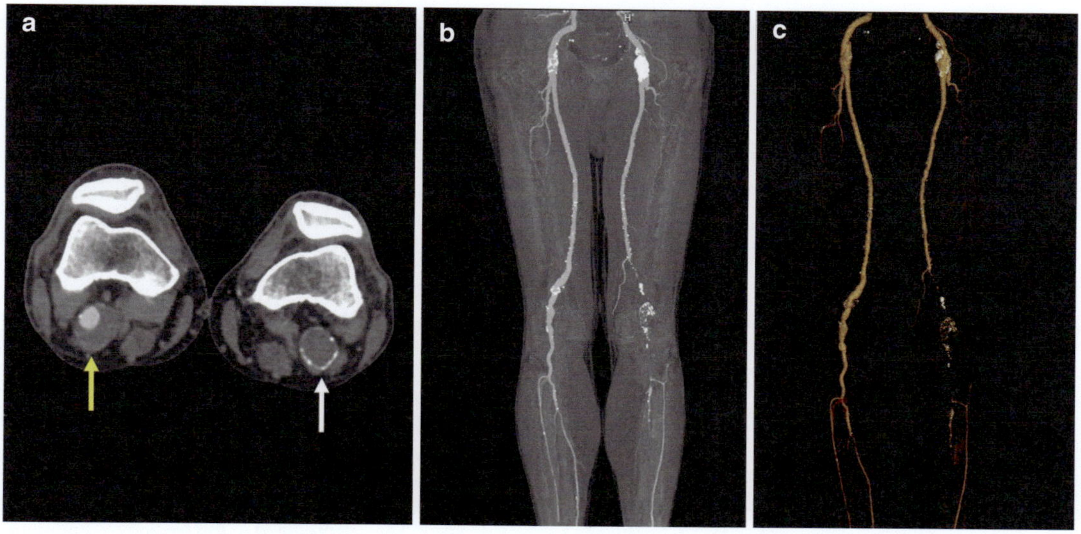

Fig. 27.8 CT angiography findings in a 77-year-old man presenting with a cold and painful left lower extremity (**a**) Axial CT image demonstrating occlusive thrombosis of a left popliteal artery aneurysm (white arrow) and a concomitant right popliteal artery aneurysm with mural thrombus (yellow arrow). (**b**) Maximum Intensity Projection (MIP) and (**c**) Volume-rendering images showing associated atherosclerotic calcification of both distal common femoral arteries with increased caliber, particularly on the left side. This case illustrates the importance of bilateral evaluation in popliteal artery aneurysms, as they are often bilateral. The combination of axial images and advanced post-processing techniques provides comprehensive visualization of aneurysmal disease, thrombosis, and associated atherosclerotic changes, crucial for accurate diagnosis and treatment planning in acute limb ischemia secondary to aneurysm complications

- Thrombus burden: Presence and extent of mural thrombus, which is associated with aneurysm growth and increased risk of complications.
- Inflow and outflow anatomy: Assessment of the entire length of the popliteal artery, including adequate segments of normal artery both proximal and distal to the aneurysm, is crucial for treatment planning, especially for endovascular approaches.
- Complications: Evidence of thrombosis, distal embolization (manifested as loss of tibial runoff), or rare cases of rupture.
- Associated findings: Status of the contralateral popliteal artery and the abdominal aorta, given the high incidence of bilateral and concurrent aneurysms.
- Surrounding structures: Evaluation of potential mass effect or compression on adjacent tissues.

27.6 Structured Reporting for Lower Extremity CT Angiography

By providing a detailed and structured report of these CT findings, radiologists can significantly contribute to the accurate diagnosis and appropriate management of acute limb ischemia, facilitating informed decision-making for potential endovascular or surgical interventions. A standardized reporting template for lower extremity CTA in the setting of acute limb ischemia should include the following elements:

A. Aorta and iliac arteries.
   - Presence of atherosclerotic disease, aneurysm, or dissection
   - Any significant stenosis or occlusion
B. Lower extremity arteries (report bilaterally and segmentally)

1. Above the knee (femoral and popliteal arteries)
2. Below the knee (tibial and peroneal arteries)

   For each segment, describe:

   Location of the lesion (pelvis, thigh, knee, calf)

   Type of lesion:

   - Stenosis (short <1 cm, long >1 cm, plaque morphology)
   - Chronic occlusion (atherosclerosis)
   - Acute occlusion (thromboembolic)

   Atherosclerotic plaque characteristics:

   - Length
   - Morphology (regular, irregular, ulcerated)
   - Composition (fibrolipidic, fibrocalcified, calcified)
   - Stenosis degree (mild 1–49%, moderate 50–69%, severe 70–99%, obstruction 100%)

   Presence and extent of collateral circulation

   For aneurysms: size, shape, presence of mural thrombus

   For bypass grafts: patency, thrombosis, stenosis, or occlusion

   For stents: in-stent thrombosis, stent migration, or fracture

C. Associated Findings

   Other relevant vascular or extra-vascular findings (lung, abdominal organs, bone and soft tissues)

References

1. Björck M, Earnshaw JJ, Acosta S, Bastos Gonçalves F, Cochennec F, Debus ES, et al. Editor's choice – European Society for Vascular Surgery (ESVS) 2020 clinical practice guidelines on the management of acute limb ischaemia. Eur J Vasc Endovasc Surg. 2020;59:173–218. https://doi.org/10.1016/j.ejvs.2019.09.006.
2. Keddie D, Abdulrehman Y, Shiau G. Reporting lower extremity CT angiography for treatment planning. Diagn Interv Imaging. 2022;103:387–93. https://doi.org/10.1016/j.diii.2022.06.010.
3. Santistevan JR. Acute limb ischemia: an emergency medicine approach. Emerg Med Clin North Am. 2017;35:889–909. https://doi.org/10.1016/J.EMC.2017.07.006.
4. Gornik HL, Aronow HD, Goodney PP, Arya S, Brewster LP, Byrd L, et al. 2024 ACC/AHA/AACVPR/APMA/ABC/SCAI/SVM/SVN/SVS/SIR/VESS guideline for the management of lower extremity peripheral artery disease. J Am Coll Cardiol. 2024;83:2497–604. https://doi.org/10.1016/j.jacc.2024.02.013.
5. Conte MS, Bradbury AW, Kolh P, White JV, Dick F, Fitridge R, et al. Global vascular guidelines on the management of chronic limb-threatening ischemia. J Vasc Surg. 2019;69:3S–125S.e40. https://doi.org/10.1016/J.JVS.2019.02.016.
6. Fleischmann D, Hallett RL, Rubin GD. CT angiography of peripheral arterial disease. J Vasc Interv Radiol. 2006;17:3–26. https://doi.org/10.1097/01.RVI.0000191361.02857.DE.
7. Cook TS. Computed tomography angiography of the lower extremities. Radiol Clin North Am. 2016;54:115–30. https://doi.org/10.1016/j.rcl.2015.08.001.
8. Rajiah P. Updates in vascular computed tomography. Radiol Clin North Am. 2020;58:671–91. https://doi.org/10.1016/J.RCL.2020.02.011.
9. Oweis Y, Viets Z, Shetty AS. Role of lower extremity run-off CT angiography in the evaluation of acute vascular disease. Abdom Radiol. 2017;42:1028–45. https://doi.org/10.1007/s00261-016-0907-4.
10. Met R, Bipat S, Legemate DA, Reekers JA, Koelemay MJW. Diagnostic performance of computed tomography angiography in peripheral arterial disease. JAMA. 2009;301:415. https://doi.org/10.1001/jama.301.4.415.
11. Willmann JK, Mayer D, Banyai M, Desbiolles LM, Verdun FR, Seifert B, et al. Evaluation of peripheral arterial bypass grafts with multi-detector row CT angiography: comparison with duplex US and digital subtraction angiography. Radiology. 2003;229:465–74. https://doi.org/10.1148/RADIOL.2292021123.
12. Itoga NK, Kim T, Sailer AM, Fleischmann D, Mell MW. Lower extremity computed tomography angiography can help predict technical success of endovascular revascularization in the superficial femoral and popliteal artery. J Vasc Surg. 2017;66:835–843.e1. https://doi.org/10.1016/J.JVS.2017.02.031.
13. Norgren L, Hiatt WR, Dormandy JA, Nehler MR, Harris KA, Fowkes FGR. Inter-society consensus for the management of peripheral arterial disease (TASC II). J Vasc Surg. 2007;45(Suppl S) https://doi.org/10.1016/J.JVS.2006.12.037.
14. Cellina M, Gibelli D, Martinenghi C, Oliva G, Floridi C. CT angiography of lower extremities from anatomy to traumatic and nontraumatic lesions: a pictorial review. Emerg Radiol. 2020;27:441–50. https://doi.org/10.1007/S10140-020-01770-9/METRICS.

Swollen Limb

28

Maria Laura Schillirò, Francesco Verde, Chiara D'Errico, Dario Grimaldi, Francesco Muto, and Gianluca Ponticiello

28.1 Introduction

In the emergency department, computed tomography (CT) represents a valuable diagnostic tool for evaluating patients with a swollen limb, offering detailed visualization of anatomical structures to aid in diagnosis and management. The clinical assessment in the emergency setting remains fundamental. CT imaging plays a crucial role when additional information is needed, due to its capability to provide detailed and accurate visualization of anatomical structures (bone, soft tissues, vessels) with high resolution. This property is essential in aiding diagnosis and management, particularly in cases of trauma, soft tissue injuries, infections/abscesses, thrombosis, neoplastic lesions, and vascular abnormalities. Moreover, contrast-enhanced CT enhances the visualization of vascular structures, facilitating the detection of vascular anomalies or occlusion, as well as in cases of trauma to identify any active bleeding. The swelling of the limbs represents a common clinical presentation and encompasses a wide range of possibilities in the realm of differential diagnosis. Swelling can be bilateral, (more often associated with systemic causes), or unilateral, (manifestation of multiple pathological situations that often require immediate evaluation). This chapter will focus on the application of computed tomography (CT) in evaluating patients with sudden limb swelling in emergency situations. Table 28.1 lists the main causes of bilateral and unilateral swelling.

Table 28.1 Main causes of bilateral and unilateral swelling

Bilateral swelling	Unilateral swelling
1. Lymphedema	1. Deep vein thrombosis (DVT)
2. Heart failure	2. Soft tissue injury
3. Nephrotic syndrome	3. Abscess
4. Hypothyroidism	4. Hematoma
5. Hepatic cirrhosis	5. Tumor

M. L. Schillirò (✉) · F. Verde · C. D'Errico
D. Grimaldi · F. Muto · G. Ponticiello
Department of General and Emergency Radiology, "Antonio Cardarelli" Hospital, Naples, Italy
e-mail: marialaura.schilliro@aocardarelli.it; francesco.verde@ao.cardarelli.it; Chiara.derrico@aocardarelli.it; Dario.grimaldi@aocardarelli.it; francesco.muto@aocardarelli.it; Gianluca.ponticiello@aocardarelli.it

L. Romano et al. (eds.), *CT of Non-Traumatic Body Emergencies*,
https://doi.org/10.1007/978-3-031-84849-0_28

28.2 Indications

Emergency CT is indicated for rapid and accurate evaluation of underlying causes. The main cause of limb swelling is represented by lymphedema; however, swelling can originate from various tissue components (fat, blood, muscle, collections). Essentially, the main causes in emergencies can be vascular, traumatic, inflammatory and infective, muscular, and articular, but this analysis also includes other less important causes such as Baker's cysts. In this chapter, we will examine the main causes of unilateral swelling, as they are more often of radiological interest and can be evaluated with imaging (Fig. 28.1).

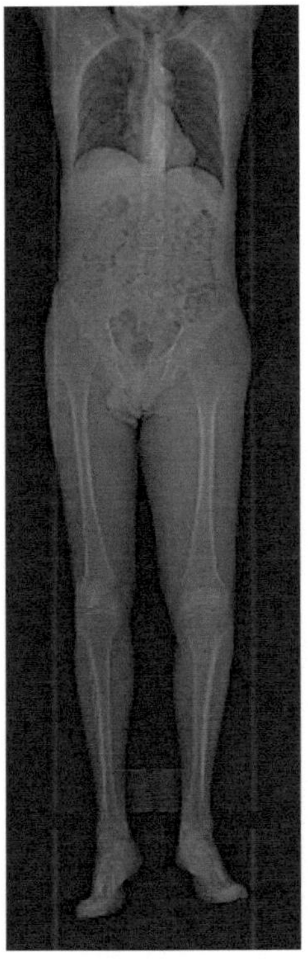

Fig. 28.1 Unilateral swelling of the left lower limb, clearly visible on the CT scanogram

28.3 Imaging Technique

CT must be performed rapidly and efficiently. The imaging technique should employ a specific protocol for limbs, with initial acquisitions without contrast medium, usually followed by intravenous injection of iodinated contrast medium. This allows for the evaluation of bone structures, soft tissues, vascular flow, identification of blood density material, and exclusion of any foreign bodies. Contrast medium is crucial for assessing vascular anomalies, active bleeding, opacification defects, and for characterizing tissue lesions. High-resolution scanning should be performed to acquire detailed images of anatomical structures. Maximum Intensity Projection (MIP) allows for better assessment of vascular structures, and with the aid of Multi-Planar Reconstruction (MPR) and Volume Rendering (VR) reconstructions, we are able to evaluate the image in three dimensions and provide exemplary and immediate images of the pathological nature.

28.4 Main Causes of Swollen Limb

28.4.1 Deep Vein Thrombosis

Deep vein thrombosis (DVT) is a common and serious medical condition characterized by the formation of blood clots within the deep veins of the body. This phenomenon occurs mainly in the lower limbs but can sometimes occur in the upper limbs as well. DVT primarily results from blood flow stagnation and shares common risk factors across upper and lower extremities, including trauma, cancer and its treatment, infections, previous clotting events, inherited disorders, hormone therapy, pregnancy, and varicose veins [1]. Upper extremity DVT has additional triggers like central venous catheters, pacemakers, and Paget-Schroetter syndrome [1]. Symptoms include unilateral limb pain, swelling, and redness, often accompanied by tenderness, warmth, and superficial vein dilation upon physical examination. Some patients may exhibit a positive Homan sign, experiencing pain during forceful dorsiflexion with the knee extended. It is important to note that DVT can occur without obvious symptoms and, if left untreated, can lead to pulmonary embolism in about 50–60% of cases, with consequent mortality of 25–30% [2]. Risk assessment for DVT is performed using the Wells score. Usually, ultrasound is the preferred diagnostic method for DVT, but CT plays a crucial role in cases with a high clinical suspicion or when ultrasound is not sufficiently accurate. CT is particularly useful for identifying DVT in the pelvis and inferior vena cava [3]. DVT most commonly occurs in the calf veins (peroneal veins and posterior tibial veins) and the gastrocnemius and soleus muscle vessels [4]. Upper extremity DVT refers to a thrombus occurring in veins such as the radial, ulnar, brachial, axillary, subclavian, internal jugular, and brachiocephalic veins. It is relatively rare, constituting less than 3% of all DVT cases. However, the incidence of pulmonary embolism (PE) associated with upper extremity DVT remains significant, at around 12% [1]. Clots are identified as filling defects or areas of non-opacification in the vein (Fig. 28.2). It is crucial to distinguish the location and extent of the clot, as infrapopliteal calf vein DVT often resolves spontaneously and rarely leads to pulmonary embolism. Conversely, DVT above the knee or proximally carries a higher risk of pulmonary embolism [5]. Contrast-enhanced CT (CE-CT) provides a comprehensive evaluation of the deep venous system, accurately detecting and characterizing clots (Fig. 28.3). In acute settings, CT can rapidly identify the presence and extent of thrombotic occlusions, facilitating prompt initiation of anticoagulant therapy. Additionally, CT can detect underlying conditions predisposing to DVT, such as venous compression or obstruction, congenital venous anomalies, or pelvic masses, which may require further management. CT pulmonary angiography (CTPA) is commonly performed to simultaneously evaluate both pulmonary arteries for emboli and lower extremity veins for DVT, providing a comprehensive assessment of venous thromboembolism.

28.4.2 Superficial Thrombophlebitis

Superficial thrombophlebitis, also known as superficial vein thrombosis (SVT), is characterized by the presence of a thrombus in the lumen of a superficial vein, accompanied by inflammation of adjacent tissues. Phlebitis, indicating vein inflammation, can occur even without a clot, often triggered by physical trauma or IV insertions. Predominantly seen in women and increasing with age in both genders [6], SVT is often associated with varicose veins, present in up to 62% of cases [7]. Other predisposing factors include prolonged immobilization, trauma, obesity, hypercoagulable states, and hormonal therapy [7]. SVT manifests as thrombosis and inflammation, commonly affecting the great saphenous vein (60–80% of cases), followed by the small saphenous vein and upper extremity veins [8]. Thrombosis arises from vein inflammation, external trauma, direct endothelial damage, and primary hematologic changes. Asymptomatic

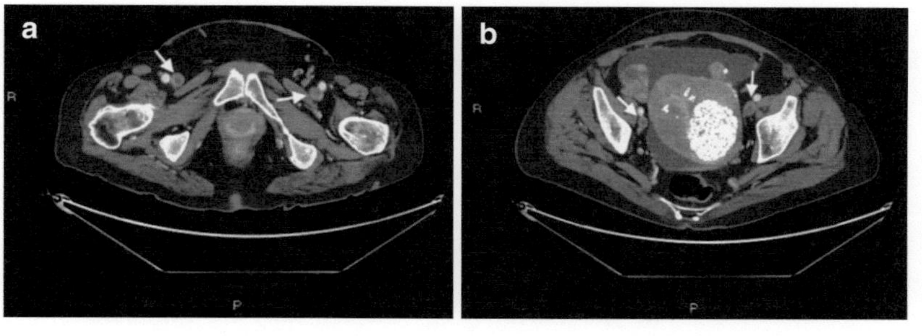

Fig. 28.2 In the CT image, a defect in opacification is observed in both common femoral veins (arrows, **a**) and external iliac veins (arrows, **b**). This opacification defect indicates the presence of a blood clot within the blood vessels and is therefore indicative of extensive bilateral deep vein thrombosis

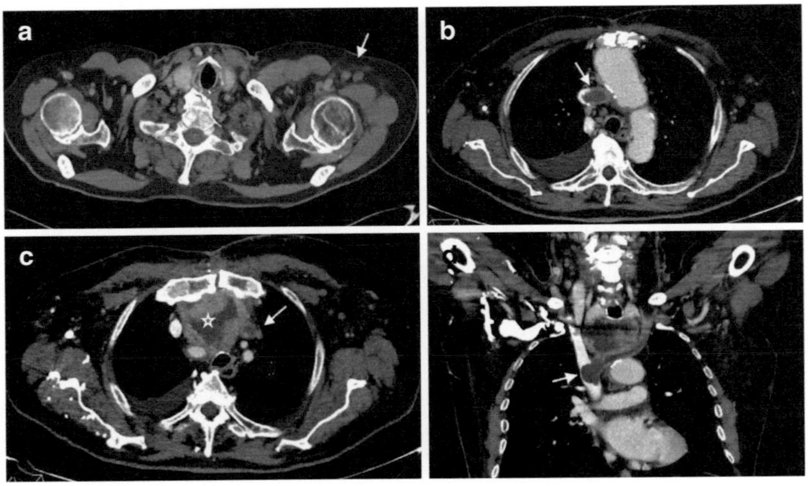

Fig. 28.3 The patient presented to the emergency room with upper limb edema (arrow, **a**), which was the primary reason leading to medical attention. Image **b** reveals an opacification defect at the junction of the superior vena cava and the brachiocephalic trunks (arrow, **b**), indicating venous obstruction. The thrombus originates from an anaplastic thyroid carcinoma (star, **c**) infiltrating the left brachiocephalic trunk, resulting in extensive neoplastic thrombosis (arrows, **c**, **d**) extending through the venous system, with significant impact on blood flow and lymphatic drainage in the region

pulmonary embolism can be observed in up to one-third of patients with SVT [8]. In cases where ultrasound is inconclusive or unavailable, CT may offer valuable information, especially if there's concern for extension into deeper veins or concurrent DVT. CE-CT can outline the extent and involvement of superficial veins and identify associated complications like abscess formation or septic thrombophlebitis.

28.4.3 Venous Thoracic Outlet Syndrome

Venous thoracic outlet syndrome (TOS) is a condition where blood flow through the veins in the thoracic outlet, the space from the cervical spine and the superior border of the mediastinum to the lateral border of the pectoralis minor muscle, is restricted. This can lead to symptoms such as swelling, pain, and discoloration of the arm, as well as potential complications like spontaneous axillosubclavian thrombosis (effort thrombosis or Paget-Schroetter syndrome), while some exhibit symptoms of intermittent venous compression without thrombosis, known as McCleery syndrome [9].

Venous TOS often results from anterior costoclavicular shears mechanism, narrowing the space due to muscular hypertrophy. This raises vein damage potential, leading to wall thickening, fibrosis, and thrombosis. Patients typically present with rapid onset of discoloration, swelling, and pain, with collateral vessel engorgement [10]. Symptoms often follow vigorous upper extremity use, occasionally preceded by herald events, and pulmonary emboli may occur in 10% of cases [11]. CT can be valuable in diagnosing venous TOS by visualizing the anatomy of the thoracic outlet and identifying any compression or obstruction of the veins. Imaging findings of TOS include bone and soft-tissue abnormalities, axillosubclavian vein thrombosis, enlarged collateral veins, fixed axillosubclavian vein stenosis at the site of dynamic narrowing, and axillosubclavian vein narrowing with arm abduction [10].

CE-CT may be particularly useful in highlighting areas of vascular compression or abnormalities, aiding in treatment planning. To avoid streak artifacts caused by dense contrast material, it is important to place the intravenous catheter on the unaffected side, preserving vasculature visibility.

28.4.4 Acute Arterial Ischemia

In cases of acute arterial ischemia, CT can help differentiate between embolic and thrombotic occlusions, assess collateral circulation, and identify any associated vascular pathology such as aneurysms or arterial dissections. Additionally, CT can detect signs of tissue ischemia, such as muscle necrosis or edema, which may impact clinical management decisions. For further insights, please refer to the dedicated chapter.

28.4.5 Joint Effusion or Hemarthrosis

CT permits to swiftly evaluate joint effusion or hemarthrosis, particularly when there's a pressing need to assess traumatic injuries or suspected intra-articular bleeding. Hemarthrosis, stemming from trauma, bleeding disorders, or other medical conditions, can prompt the use of CT to visualize fluid accumulation within joint spaces. This not only helps gauge the extent of bleeding but also aids in ruling out associated injuries, thereby informing emergent management decisions. CE-CT further enhances its utility by pinpointing active bleeding or vascular injuries contributing to hemarthrosis, thus facilitating the localization of the bleeding source and guiding decisions on urgent interventions like angiography or surgical exploration.

28.4.6 Hematoma

CT plays a crucial role in the evaluation of patients presenting with a swollen limb and suspected hematoma, particularly in cases of trauma or acute bleeding. CT can accurately localize and quantify the extent of hematoma formation within the affected limb, providing valuable information for treatment planning and guiding immediate interventions. On CT, hematomas typically appear as well-defined areas of increased attenuation compared to surrounding tissues. Acute hematomas typically appear hyperdense on CT scans due to the presence of fresh blood. Over time, as the hematoma undergoes changes such as clot retraction and breakdown of red blood cells, it may become less dense and eventually appear isodense or hypodense compared to surrounding tissues. CE-CT can further enhance the detection of active bleeding sources contributing to hematoma formation, facilitating prompt identification of vascular injuries that may require urgent intervention (Fig. 28.4). In cases of trauma, CT can assess for associated injuries such as fractures or vascular damage that may be contributing to the hematoma. Additionally, CT can help differentiate between various types of hematomas, such as subcutaneous, intramuscular, or intra-articular hematomas, based on their characteristic imaging features. A significant concern is that hematomas may obscure the presence of an underlying hemorrhagic tumor [12]. CT is particularly valuable in emergency settings where rapid assessment and decision-making are critical and permits to promptly identify and prioritize patients at higher risk of complications from hematoma, such as those with ongoing bleeding or potential neurovascular compromise.

28.4.7 Compartment Syndrome

Compartment syndrome is a serious condition characterized by increased pressure within a muscle compartment, leading to insufficient blood supply to the muscles and nerves. It can result from trauma, burns, overuse, extravasation of contrast agents, surgery, and other causes. Acute compartment syndrome frequently accompanies fractures, especially those of the tibia, and soft tissue injuries. Chronic compartment syndrome typically arises from exertional factors like exercise or overuse or causes such as mass lesions, anomalous muscles, or infections [13]. If left untreated, compartment syndrome can lead to critical dysfunction, muscle necrosis, permanent damage, or even limb amputation. The compartment most prone to acute compartment syndrome

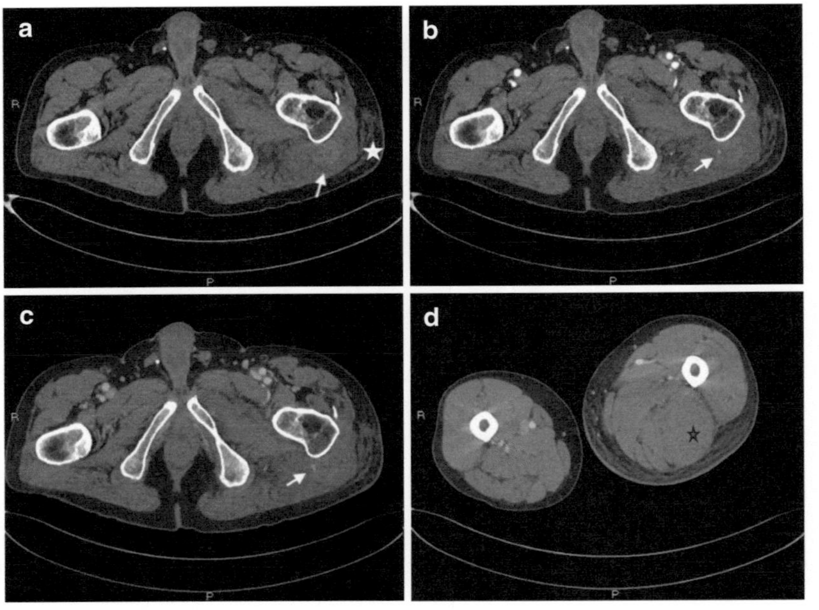

Fig. 28.4 Swollen and infiltrated appearance of the subcutaneous fat (star, **a**) with evidence of a spontaneously hyperdense muscular hematoma at baseline (arrow, **a**). Active arterial phase bleeding (arrow, **b**) is observed in the region of the lesser trochanter, more prominently visible in the venous phase (arrow, **c**). Non-bleeding muscular hematoma is also present in the posterior region of the left thigh (blue star, **d**)

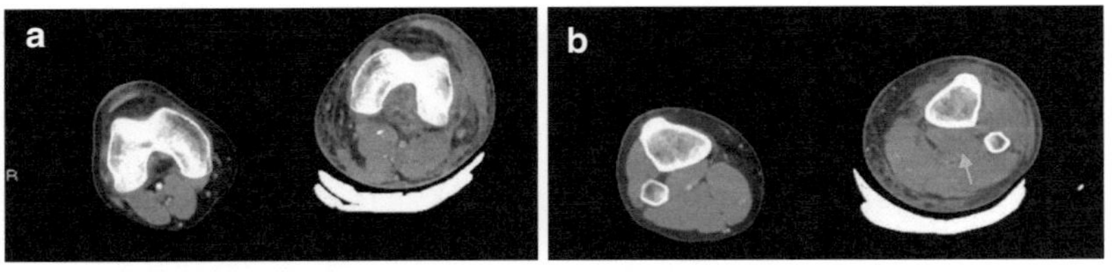

Fig. 28.5 The posterior compartment of the left lower leg appears markedly swollen due to blood infiltration (**a**), with no opacification of the distal popliteal artery (yellow arrow, **b**). The right popliteal artery is normally opacified

is the lower leg below the knee, followed by the forearm, thigh, and upper arm [14]. CT can help in visualizing muscle swelling, fluid accumulation, and changes in muscle density indicative of edema or hemorrhage. CT scans, particularly when enhanced with contrast, can show decreased muscle perfusion, which may indicate compromised blood flow due to increased compartmental pressure (Fig. 28.5).

28.4.8 Arthritis

One potential reason for limb swelling is arthritis, which can manifest as an inflammatory joint condition. Involvement of a single joint may suggest infectious arthritis, while multiple joint involvement often prompts a rheumatologic evaluation. While CT isn't typically the initial diagnostic choice, it can provide valuable insights into bone erosions, joint effusions, soft tissue involvement, and the presence of lesions or foreign bodies within the joint, potentially triggering arthritis. CE-CT is particularly beneficial for assessing infectious or inflammatory arthritis, allowing detection of synovial enhancement, joint space widening, and inflammation of surrounding soft tissues, potentially indicating inflammation or abscess in adjacent areas.

28.4.9 Soft Tissue Infections

In assessing a swollen limb with suspected soft tissue infection, it is crucial to first understand the underlying process and its severity to promptly administer the best-targeted treatment. This ranges mainly from simple cellulitis to abscess formation and, in severe rare cases, necrotizing fasciitis. Distinguishing between a localized accumulation of pus (abscess) and widespread skin infection (cellulitis) is crucial, as the former requires incision and drainage, while the latter is managed with antibiotics alone [15]. Chao et al. classified the spectrum of infection, ranging from cellulitis to abscess formation, into four categories: (1) subcutaneous thickening without pus accumulation, (2) disruption of subcutaneous tissues without pus accumulation, (3) disruption of subcutaneous tissues with pus accumulation, and (4) abscess formation [16].

CT is not typically the primary modality for diagnosing cellulitis, as clinical assessment, physical examination, and ultrasound often suffice for diagnosis. However, in certain cases of diagnostic uncertainty or suspicion of complicating factors, CT may be utilized to provide additional information. CT imaging can be valuable in cases where cellulitis is severe, extensive, or complicated by factors such as abscess formation, necrotizing fasciitis, or deep tissue involvement. CT shows skin thickening, underlying fat stranding or subcutaneous edema, and thickening of underlying fascia [17]. It can accurately delineate the extent of soft tissue inflammation, identify areas of abscess formation, and assess for deeper tissue involvement or spread of infection beyond the subcutaneous layers. Enhancement of the septations and an asymmetric distribution distinguish it from bland edema, which can occur with cardiac or renal failure. If present, an abscess appears as a ring-enhancing fluid collection [18]. CE-CT may be particularly useful in identifying areas of vascular compromise or thrombosis, which can occur in severe cases of cellulitis.

Soft tissue abscesses are typically encased by a peripheral membrane and can occur in various body regions within the soft tissues. These abscesses encompass subcutaneous, intramuscular, and intermuscular types, which may develop within the fascial planes. CT is particularly valuable in cases where there is suspicion of deep-seated or extensive abscess formation, as it can accurately delineate the size, location, and extent of the abscess. Contrast-enhanced CT is often used to enhance visualization of the abscess cavity and surrounding tissues, aiding in the differentiation of necrotic tissue from viable tissue and helping identify potential complications such as adjacent vascular involvement or abscess extension into neighboring compartments. The surrounding tissues may also exhibit edema, cellulitis, and mild enhancement [18]. Prompt identification and drainage of abscesses are essential to prevent complications such as sepsis, tissue necrosis, or systemic spread of infection. CT-guided percutaneous drainage may be performed under image guidance to drain the abscess, providing rapid symptomatic relief and facilitating resolution of the infection safely and effectively. Additionally, CT can help identify underlying causes or predisposing factors for abscess formation, such as traumatic injuries, foreign bodies, or underlying medical conditions, preventing recurrence of abscesses in the future.

Necrotizing fasciitis (NF) is a rare potentially life-threatening soft tissue infection characterized by rapid tissue destruction. Clinical presentations vary widely, but patients often exhibit signs and symptoms resembling cellulitis [18]. As the disease progresses, the skin becomes discolored, and bullae (often hemorrhagic) form and slough off as gangrene advances. These changes are accompanied by signs of systemic infection, which can escalate to shock with hypotension and multiorgan failure [19]. CT can accurately delineate the affected soft tissue planes, increased density and stranding in subcutaneous fat, tissue edema or inflammation extending beyond the initially affected area, thickening and enhancement of the fascial plain, fluid collection, muscle thickening and enhancement, aid in the differentiation of necrotic tissue from viable tissue, and detect gas within the soft tissues (crepitus), which are characteristic findings of NF (Fig. 28.6). Although CE- CT is recommended, it may not be feasible in cases of acute renal failure [18]. For suspected NF, prompt surgery is crucial. CT assists surgical planning by detailing tissue involvement and guiding debridement or fasciotomy.

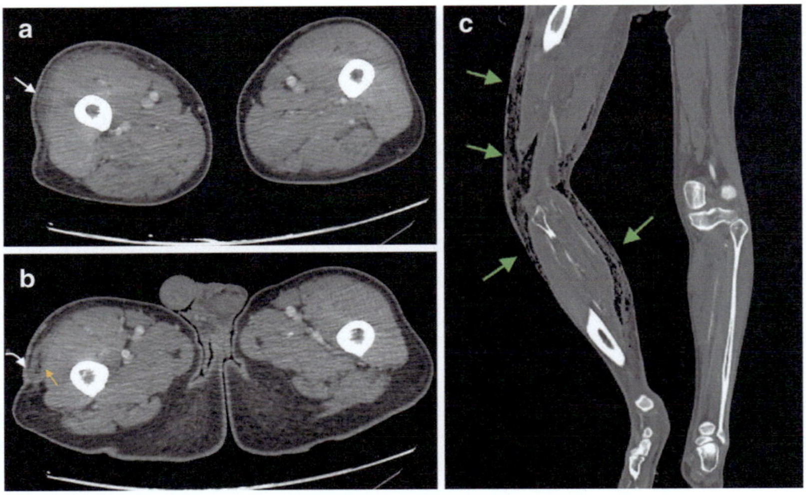

Fig. 28.6 On the right, there is a subcutaneous fluid collection (straight arrow, **a**) on the anterolateral aspect of the thigh (**a**) extending to the middle third of the leg with air bubbles in the proximal part (yellow arrow, **b**), where a cutaneous fistula (curved array, **b**) appears to be present (**b**). After three weeks (**c**), the collection has significantly increased, involving the entire lower limb with a notable increase in the air component (green arrows, **c**). It extends into the subcutaneous soft tissues, nearly circumferentially in the distal third of the thigh and along the leg

28.4.10 Osteomyelitis

Osteomyelitis is a severe infection of the bone that is often associated with soft tissue involvement and complications such as abscess formation and then it should be considered in case of swollen limb. CT plays a crucial role in accurately delineating affected bone structures, identifying areas of cortical erosion/destruction, sequestra, involucre, and intraosseous gases, periosteal reaction, increased density of fatty marrow, and blurring of fat planes [20]. CE-CT further enhances visualization of the infected bone and surrounding soft tissues, aiding in the differentiation between infected and non-infected tissues. It also helps identify areas of reduced vascularity that suggest ischemic necrosis. Some limitations of CT include its inability to reliably detect marrow edema, meaning that a normal CT scan cannot rule out early osteomyelitis, and image degradation due to streak artifacts when metallic implants are present [21].

28.4.11 Muscle Injury

Currently, ultrasonography and magnetic resonance imaging (MRI) are the most commonly used modalities for assessing muscular injuries [22]. Nevertheless, CT can accurately delineate the extent and severity of muscle injury, including the location and size of the tear, as well as any associated soft tissue damage or hematoma formation. Additionally, CT can assess for potential complications such as muscle herniation, avulsion fractures, or abscessual complications (Fig. 28.7). CE-CT may be particularly useful in cases where there is concern for vascular injury or significant hemorrhage associated with the muscle tear.

28.4.12 Rhabdomyolysis

Rhabdomyolysis, characterized by the breakdown of skeletal muscle tissue and release of muscle cell contents into the bloodstream [23],

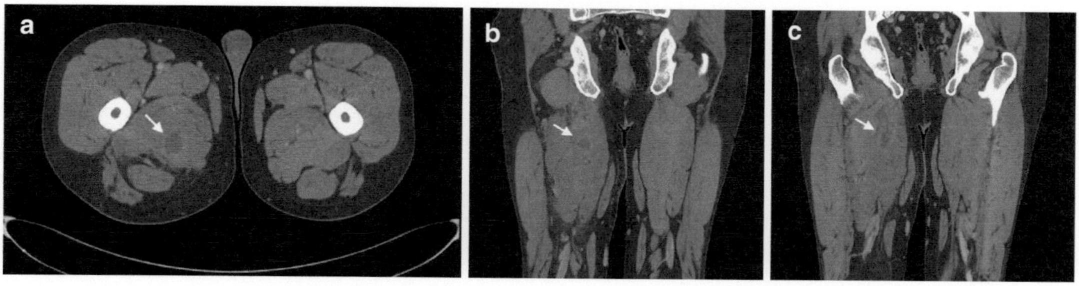

Fig. 28.7 In the proximal third of the posterior aspect of the right thigh, within the muscles of the adductor compartment, particularly in the belly of the semimembranosus muscle, multiple fluid-filled and particulate collections (arrows, **a**, **b**, **c**) with thick, hyperemic margins and a multiloculated appearance are observed, indicating abscess formation from a previous muscle injury

typically relies on clinical findings and laboratory tests for diagnosis. However, CT imaging can be instrumental in assessing complications or underlying causes of muscle injury. It can identify signs of muscle injury and assess complications such as compartment syndrome or soft tissue necrosis, which may occur in severe cases of rhabdomyolysis. Furthermore, CT can evaluate associated injuries, such as fractures or vascular damage, which may contribute to muscle ischemia or exacerbate tissue damage. CE-CT is particularly beneficial in cases with suspected underlying causes of rhabdomyolysis, such as trauma, vascular occlusion, or compartment syndrome. CT angiography can detect vascular abnormalities or thrombosis that contribute to muscle ischemia, while CE-CT of the abdomen and pelvis can identify signs of visceral injury or underlying conditions predisposing to rhabdomyolysis.

28.4.13 Baker's Cyst

One cause of a swollen limb can be the presence of a Baker's cyst. While ultrasound is generally used for diagnosis, CT becomes valuable when the presentation is atypical or complications such as DVT are suspected [24]. CT imaging provides a detailed anatomical assessment of the knee joint and surrounding structures, enabling accurate detection and characterization of Baker's cysts. CT can visualize the cystic lesion, its size, location, and any associated intra-articular pathology such as meniscal tears or osteoarthritis. Additionally, CT can identify complications such as cyst rupture, which may lead to synovial fluid leaking into the surrounding soft tissues or calf muscles. CE-CT is particularly useful when concomitant DVT or other vascular pathologies are suspected to be contributing to lower limb swelling. CT venography can evaluate the deep venous system for thrombus formation and assess compression or displacement of vascular structures caused by the Baker's cyst.

28.5 Conclusion

Although the clinical approach remains crucial, CT imaging of swollen limbs in emergency situations is a fundamental diagnostic tool for a rapid and accurate assessment of the underlying causes, which can be numerous. A timely and precise diagnosis is essential to initiate appropriate treatment and reduce the risk of serious complications. Correct interpretation of CT images requires an in-depth understanding of normal anatomy and the various pathologies that can affect the limbs. The ability of CT to visualize bones, soft tissues, and blood vessels with high resolution is critical across a wide spectrum of conditions, from traumatic injuries to vascular and infectious pathologies (Table 28.2). The use of contrast media further enhances the visualization of blood vessels, facilitating the detection of

Table 28.2 Main causes, signs and symptoms, and CT findings of unilateral swelling

Main causes of swollen limb	Main signs and symptoms	Main CT findings
Deep vein thrombosis	Swelling, tenderness, or sudden and persistent pain in a limb—Feeling of warmth, redness, or changes in skin temperature.	Clots identified as filling defects or areas of non-opacification in the vein
Superficial thromboflebitis	Swelling, redness, tenderness, and pain along the course of a superficial vein—May have a hard lump or palpable cord under the skin.	Signs of local inflammation in the superficial vein—Dilation of the involved vein
Venous Thoracic Outlet Syndrome	Pain and swelling in the arm, shoulder, or chest—Upper limb paresthesia—Presence of visible edema and venous distension	Venous stenosis and dilatation of thoracic veins
Hematoma	Swelling, pain, tenderness, and bruising in the affected area	Collection of blood—Possible displacement or compression of surrounding tissues—Evaluate for active bleeding
Infections	Swelling, redness, pain, and warmth in the affected area—Fever—Pus discharge.	Signs of local infection on CT (e.g., inflamed tissue, pus collections) Possible signs of bone or muscle involvement
Necrotizing fascitiis	Intense pain in the affected area—Swelling, redness, and warmth—Fever and general malaise	Signs of inflammation and necrosis of soft tissues—Increased tissue density and signs of gas

anomalies and active bleeding. CT remains indispensable in guiding treatment decisions and surgical interventions. With its capacity to delineate tissue involvement, identify complications, and aid in surgical planning, CT contributes significantly to improving patient outcomes by facilitating timely and appropriate management strategies. Therefore, integrating CT into the diagnostic algorithm for swollen limb presentations enhances the efficiency and effectiveness of emergency care, ultimately benefiting patient care and prognosis.

References

1. Karande GY, Hedgire SS, Sanchez Y, Baliyan V, Mishra V, Ganguli S, Prabhakar AM. Advanced imaging in acute and chronic deep vein thrombosis. Cardiovasc Diagn Ther. 2016;6:493–507. https://doi.org/10.21037/cdt.2016.12.06.
2. Hamper UM, DeJong MR, Scoutt LM. Ultrasound evaluation of the lower extremity veins. Radiol Clin North Am. 2007;45:525.
3. Ravenel JG, Ackerman SJ. Sonography in ICU Patients. 2005:457–62.
4. Sapp B, Craddock G, Sapp J. Patterns and distribution of deep vein thrombus in the lower extremity. J Vasc Ultrasound. 2015;39:71–7. https://doi.org/10.1177/154431671503900201.
5. Hanley M, Steigner ML, Ahmed O, Azene EM, Bennett SJ, Chandra A, Desjardins B, Gage KL, Ginsburg M, Mauro DM, et al. ACR appropriateness criteria® suspected lower extremity deep vein thrombosis. J Am Coll Radiol. 2018;15:S413–7. https://doi.org/10.1016/j.jacr.2018.09.028.
6. Marchiori A, Mosena L, Prandoni P. Superficial vein thrombosis: risk factors, diagnosis, and treatment. Semin Thromb Hemost. 2006;32:737–43. https://doi.org/10.1055/s-2006-951459.
7. Meissner MH, Wakefield TW, Ascher E, Caprini JA, Comerota AJ, Eklof B, Gillespie DL, Greenfield LJ, He AR, Henke PK, et al. Acute venous disease: venous thrombosis and venous trauma. J Vasc Surg. 2007;46 Suppl S:25S–53S. https://doi.org/10.1016/j.jvs.2007.08.037.
8. Litzendorf ME, Satiani B, Litzendorf M. Vascular health and risk management dovepress superficial venous thrombosis: disease progression and evolving treatment approaches. Vasc Health Risk Manag. 2011:7–569.
9. Tubbs RS, Shoja MM. Embryology of the thoracic outlet; 2021; ISBN 9783030550738.
10. Raptis CA, Sridhar S, Thompson RW, Fowler KJ, Bhalla S. Imaging of the patient with thoracic outlet syndrome. Radiographics. 2016;36:984–1000. https://doi.org/10.1148/rg.2016150221.
11. Thompson JF, Winterborn RJ, Bays S, White H, Kinsella DC, Watkinson AF. Venous thoracic outlet compression and the Paget-Schroetter syndrome: a review and recommendations for management. Cardiovasc Intervent Radiol. 2011;34:903–10. https://doi.org/10.1007/s00270-011-0148-4.

12. Bhangle DS, Sun K, Wu JS. Imaging features of soft tissue tumor mimickers: a pictorial essay. Indian J Radiol Imaging. 2022;32:381–94. https://doi.org/10.1055/s-0042-1756556.
13. Fraipont MJ, Adamson GJ. Chronic exertional compartment syndrome. J Am Acad Orthop Surg. 2003;11:268–76. https://doi.org/10.5435/00124635-200307000-00006.
14. Cone J, Inaba K. Lower extremity compartment syndrome. Trauma Surg Acute Care Open. 2017;2:1–6. https://doi.org/10.1136/tsaco-2017-000094.
15. Gaspari R, Dayno M, Briones J, Blehar D. Comparison of computerized tomography and ultrasound for diagnosing soft tissue abscesses. Crit Ultrasound J. 2012;4:1–7. https://doi.org/10.1186/2036-7902-4-5.
16. Chao HC, Lin SJ, Huang YC, Lin TY. Sonographic evaluation of cellulitis in children. J Ultrasound Med Off J Am Inst Ultrasound Med. 2000;19:743–9. https://doi.org/10.7863/jum.2000.19.11.743.
17. Chang C-D, Wu JS. Imaging of musculoskeletal soft tissue infection. Semin Roentgenol. 2017;52:55–62. https://doi.org/10.1053/j.ro.2016.10.001.
18. Spinnato P, Patel DB, Di Carlo M, Bartoloni A, Cevolani L, Matcuk GR, Crombé A. Imaging of musculoskeletal soft-tissue infections in clinical practice: a comprehensive updated review. Microorganisms. 2022;10 https://doi.org/10.3390/microorganisms10122329.
19. Stevens DL, Bryant AE. Necrotizing soft-tissue infections. N Engl J Med. 2017;377:2253–65. https://doi.org/10.1056/NEJMra1600673.
20. Pineda C, Espinosa R, Pena A. Radiographic imaging in osteomyelitis: the role of plain radiography, computed tomography, ultrasonography, magnetic resonance imaging, and scintigraphy. Semin Plast Surg. 2009;23:80–9. https://doi.org/10.1055/s-0029-1214160.
21. Lee YJ, Sadigh S, Mankad K, Kapse N, Rajeswaran G. The imaging of osteomyelitis. Quant Imaging Med Surg. 2016;6:184–98. https://doi.org/10.21037/qims.2016.04.01.
22. Guermazi A, Roemer FW, Robinson P, Tol JL, Regatte RR, Crema MD. Imaging of muscle injuries in sports medicine: sports imaging series. Radiology. 2017;282:646–63. https://doi.org/10.1148/radiol.2017160267.
23. Kodadek L, Carmichael SP, Seshadri A, Pathak A, Hoth J, Appelbaum R, Michetti CP, Gonzalez RP. Rhabdomyolysis: an American Association for the Surgery of Trauma Critical Care Committee Clinical Consensus Document. Trauma Surg Acute Care Open. 2022;7:1–7. https://doi.org/10.1136/tsaco-2021-000836.
24. Arumilli BRB, Babu VL, Paul AS. Painful swollen leg – think beyond deep vein thrombosis or Baker's cyst. World J Surg Oncol. 2008;6:1–5. https://doi.org/10.1186/1477-7819-6-6.

Sepsis

29

Roberto Ronza, Camilla Russo, Francesco Verde,
Maria Laura Schillirò, Francesco Muto,
and Marco Di Serafino

29.1 Introduction

Sepsis is a critical condition triggered by an excessive immune response to infections, which can lead to organ dysfunction, death, or persistent disabilities. It can be caused by various infections, including bacterial, fungal, and viral, as well as injuries [1]. Sepsis impacts individuals of all ages, with the highest rates observed in the very young (neonates and children) and the elderly [1]. Globally, sepsis affects around 50 million people each year, leading to 11 million deaths, and leaves more than half of the survivors with lasting physical or mental health issues [1].

Septic shock is identified as a specific category within sepsis, characterized by severe circulatory, cellular, and metabolic abnormalities. It is linked to a significantly increased mortality rate of approximately 40%, in contrast to the 10% mortality rate associated with sepsis [2]. According to the revised Septic 2016 criteria, also known as Sepsis-3, patients with septic shock are identified by the simultaneous presence of sepsis symptoms and continuous hypotension necessitating vasopressors to sustain a mean arterial pressure of 65 mmHg or more. Additionally, this condition is characterized by serum lactate levels, exceeding 2 mmol/L (18 mg/dL), despite sufficient fluid resuscitation [3–6]. Prompt diagnosis and early treatment are crucial in managing its high mortality risk. Given its high mortality rate, swiftly recognizing and managing sepsis is essential for improving patient outcomes, akin to the urgency in handling cases like polytrauma or heart attacks. Timely treatment of septic shock involves quick detection, administering appropriate antibiotics, supporting hemodynamics, and pinpointing and addressing the infection's source [7, 8]. Diagnostic imaging, especially total-body computed tomography (CT), plays a key role here due to its accuracy in detecting sepsis and examining multiple body parts simultaneously, providing comprehensive images for diagnosis [9].

The aim of this chapter is to examine septic shock from a diagnostic imaging standpoint, focusing on characteristics beyond its root causes. It underscores the utility of CT scans in detecting a range of septic shock-associated indicators collectively referred to as CT hypoperfusion complex. These findings, frequently observed in trauma-induced hypovolemic shock, can also be helpful in identifying septic shock. Timely iden-

R. Ronza (✉) · F. Verde · M. L. Schillirò
F. Muto · M. Di Serafino
Department of General and Emergency Radiology, "Antonio Cardarelli" Hospital, Naples, Italy
e-mail: roberto.ronza@aocardarelli.it; francesco.verde@aocardarelli.it; marialaura.schilliro@aocardarelli.it; francesco.muto@aocardarelli.it; marco.diserafino@aocardarelli.it

C. Russo
Neuroradiology Unit, Department of Pediatric Neurosciences, Santobono-Pausilipon Children's Hospital, Naples, Italy

L. Romano et al. (eds.), *CT of Non-Traumatic Body Emergencies*,
https://doi.org/10.1007/978-3-031-84849-0_29

tification, diagnosis, and treatment of septic shock carry significant implications for both prognosis and therapy [9].

29.2 Etiopathogenesis and Pathophysiology

The occurrence of septic shock is linked to a wide range of infection pathologies affecting various parts of the body. Gram-negative bacilli (such as *Escherichia coli*, *Klebsiella pneumoniae*, *Enterobacter* spp., *Acinetobacter baumannii*, and *Pseudomonas aeruginosa*) and nosocomial gram-positive cocci (including Staphylococcus aureus and coagulase-negative Staphylococcus) are the most common culprits [9–11]. Septic shock is often observed in immunocompromised individuals and those with chronic debilitating illnesses. Infections caused by antimicrobial-resistant bacteria like methicillin-resistant Staphylococcus aureus and vancomycin-resistant Enterococci are prevalent in septic patients with nosocomial infections. Uncommon pathogens like invasive candidiasis may need consideration, especially in neutropenic patients [9–11]. Common infection sites encompass the lungs (pneumonia, empyema, and lung abscess), urinary tract (obstructive urosepsis), biliary tract (cholangitis), gallbladder (acute cholecystitis), gastrointestinal tract (acute appendicitis and colic abscesses), skin/soft tissue, intravascular catheters, central nervous system, and endocardium. In specific situations, subtle signs like septic thrombosis of vascular access, mycotic aneurysms, abscess formations, and Fournier's gangrene may also be present [5–10].

The pathogenesis of septic shock is intricate, involving complex interactions between the inflammatory process and coagulation. The initial phase is characterized by transient arterial and arteriolar dilation, reduced peripheral arterial resistance, and an increase in cardiac output, termed "hot shock" or "high-range shock." Subsequently, cardiac output decreases, blood pressure drops (with or without increased peripheral resistance), and typical shock symptoms emerge, leading to decreased perfusion. This sequence of events can result in organ dysfunction, disseminated intravascular coagulation (DIC), and ultimately, death [3, 9, 11, 12].

29.3 Signs and Symptoms

Sepsis presents with a wide range of signs and symptoms, and clinical diagnosis often precedes culture results [13]. Typical sepsis indicators include high fever (>38 °C), chills, profuse sweating, rapid heart rate, increased respiratory rate, reduced urine output, confusion, edema, and overall malaise, in addition to infection-related symptoms. Headaches, rashes, bruising, or bleeding may also occur [3–6]. If left untreated, septic shock can progress to refractory hypotension, characterized by paradoxically warm skin, reduced urine production, lactic acidosis, altered consciousness, and signs of organ dysfunction associated with the underlying septic process. It's important to note that sepsis can manifest with subtle symptoms that may mimic other conditions like delirium, heart failure, and pulmonary embolism [3–6].

29.4 Clinical Diagnosis and Therapy Strategy

The clinical diagnosis of septic shock involves assessing various parameters like blood pressure, heart rate, O_2 levels, blood tests, and monitoring potential infection sites. Sepsis is suspected in patients with an infection showing systemic inflammation or organ dysfunction [3–6]. Currently, there is no definitive diagnostic test for identifying septic shock. However, the quick Sequential Organ Failure Assessment (qSOFA) score has emerged as a new tool for the early identification of patients with potential infections who are not in critical care settings but are at risk of extended intensive care unit stays or mortality [3, 14]. The qSOFA score is determined by the presence of at least two out of three criteria: a respiratory rate of 22 breaths per minute or more, a systolic blood pressure of 100 mmHg or less, and altered mental status [3–14]. This assessment, which does not rely on lab tests, allows for straightforward and repeated evaluations [3–14].

Sepsis leads to vasodilation, capillary leakage, and a decrease in the effective volume of circulating blood, which diminishes venous return. This results in compromised blood flow to tissues and organ malfunction. While specific signs and symptoms of organ dysfunction might be observed, organ under-perfusion or shock could occur without clear knowledge of the underlying cause [13]. The primary objectives in treating sepsis and septic shock are to replenish intravascular volume, enhance the supply of oxygen to tissues, and reverse organ damage. Although administering fluids can notably boost cardiac output, treatment should be tailored to the individual needs of each patient, considering their fluid requirements and pre-existing health conditions [3, 15]. It is crucial to start diagnosing promptly to pinpoint the source of infection, focusing simultaneously on stabilizing hemodynamics and essential bodily functions. Early detection and quick treatment of the infection source are critical to effectively manage septic patients [3, 15].

29.5 Diagnostic Imaging

The significance of imaging in determining the source of infection in sepsis and septic shock is widely acknowledged. There's an array of imaging options, with the choice dependent on the patient's overall condition and specific symptoms. CT scans are particularly noted for their effectiveness in quickly providing detailed views of various body areas, aiding in pinpointing the source of septic shock. The procedure for CT involves specific techniques and technologies to enhance image quality while minimizing radiation exposure. In emergency scenarios, the recommended procedure for a CT multiphasic protocol involves an initial pre-contrast scan of the abdomen and pelvis, followed by dynamic imaging of the chest, abdomen, and pelvis during the arterial and portal venous phases, without using oral contrast agents. Administering intravenous contrast medium with high iodine concentrations (370–400 mg I/mL) in volumes ranging from 80 to 130 mL, based on the patient's weight, is recommended. This should be injected at a rate of 3.5–4 mL/s using an 18-gauge needle into the antecubital vein. Following this, a 40 mL saline bolus should be administered at the same injection rate [9]. It is advised to acquire the abdomen and pelvis scans during the arterial phase with bolus tracking mode and scans of the chest, abdomen, and pelvis during the portal venous phase. An additional scan of the abdomen and pelvis may be performed 3–5 min later to investigate various shock causes such as urinary sepsis [9]. In patients with a confused or altered mental state, an initial non-contrast head CT should be conducted to rule out any intracranial bleeding. After the full-body scan, a subsequent head CT in the late phase is advisable to investigate the presence of any intracranial abscesses or tumors [9, 16, 17]. For adequate analysis and post-processing, with maximum intensity projection (MIP) and multiplanar reconstruction (MPR), an effective slice thickness of 2.5 mm, with reconstruction at 0.625 mm, is advisable [9, 16]. Institutions are encouraged to periodically evaluate the quality of their images, reassess their protocols concerning radiation dose, and explore opportunities to minimize the use of contrast media [16].

29.6 CT Hypoperfusion Complex

Beyond identifying the root cause of a septic condition, CT is crucial for the early detection of signs related to shock, known as the CT hypoperfusion complex. This complex, which can enhance patient prognosis and treatment plans, is often linked to low blood pressure. It's important to note that such signs are not exclusive to sepsis and may appear in various other medical scenarios, including trauma-related shock, cardiac arrest, and diabetic emergencies [18–21]. The CT hypoperfusion complex is significant for both prognosis and treatment in septic shock and needs to be quickly identified [9]. While the causes of hypotensive and septic shock differ, the CT signs for both conditions are similar [9].

Table 29.1 Summary of the most common vascular, visceral, and parenchymal signs of septic shock that can be documented on CT examination

CT hypoperfusion complex			
Type	Sign	Definition	Incidence (if severe hypoperfusion)
Vascular features	Flattening of the inferior vena cava	IVC fattening with anterior-posterior diameter <9 mm in three consecutive segments, 20 mm above and below the renal veins, at the level of the perihepatic portion	77–100%
	The halo sign	Presence of low-density fluid <20HU surrounding the IVC	77%
	Small calibre aorta	Small-calibre abdominal aorta with anterior–posterior diameter <13 mm detected 20 mm above and below renal arteries	20–48%
Visceral features	Shock bowel	Small bowel fluid-filled dilated loops with thickened walls (>3 mm) due to oedema of the submucosa and increased mucosal enhancement	40–70%
	Mucosal enhancement of the gallbladder	Mucosal enhancement, without thickened gallbladder walls	33.3%
Parenchymal features	Peripancreatic oedema and abnormal pancreatic enhancement (shock pancreas)	Abnormal post-contrast attenuation (20HU greater than liver and spleen), often associated with peripancreatic low density fluid (<20HU)	44%
	Splenic hypoperfusion	Extremely decreased enhancement in contrast early CT phase	11–29.6%
	Abnormal liver enhancement	Reduced hepatic enhancement (25HU lower than the spleen)	4–11.1%
	Abnormal renal enhancement	Increased and prolonged parenchymal enhancement	55%
	Abnormal adrenal hyperenhancement (adrenal stress)	Bilateral hyperenhancement of the adrenal gland	> 60%
	Abnormal thyroid enhancement (shock thyroid)	Heterogeneous contrast hyperenhancement, like a multinodular gland, with the presence of low-density fluid surrounding the thyroid (5–10 HU)	Not detected
Other features	Ascites	Fluid collects in peritoneal spaces	Not detected

These signs, previously documented in the case of trauma-related shock, fall into categories like vascular, visceral, and parenchymal changes (Table 29.1) [9, 18–21]. These signs encompass a variety of changes, such as reduced visceral contrast, enhanced mucosal layers and expansion of the small intestine, wall thickening, and fluid accumulation in the small intestine, along with the halo effect and the flattering of the inferior vena cava (IVC). They also include a narrowed aorta, swelling around the pancreas, and other less consistent changes in the organ and tissue structure, including fluid accumulation in the abdominal cavity [9]. These signs are often reversible in the early stages and identifying two or more of these changes is critical for diagnosing the CT hypoperfusion complex [9, 16–21].

CT hypoperfusion complex *vascular signs* include flattering of the IVC, the IVC halo sign, and small caliber aorta.

29.7 Flattening of the IVC

IVC flattening is characterized by a decrease in its anterior-posterior measurement to less than 9 mm across three sequential segments—20 mm above and below the renal veins and at the seg-

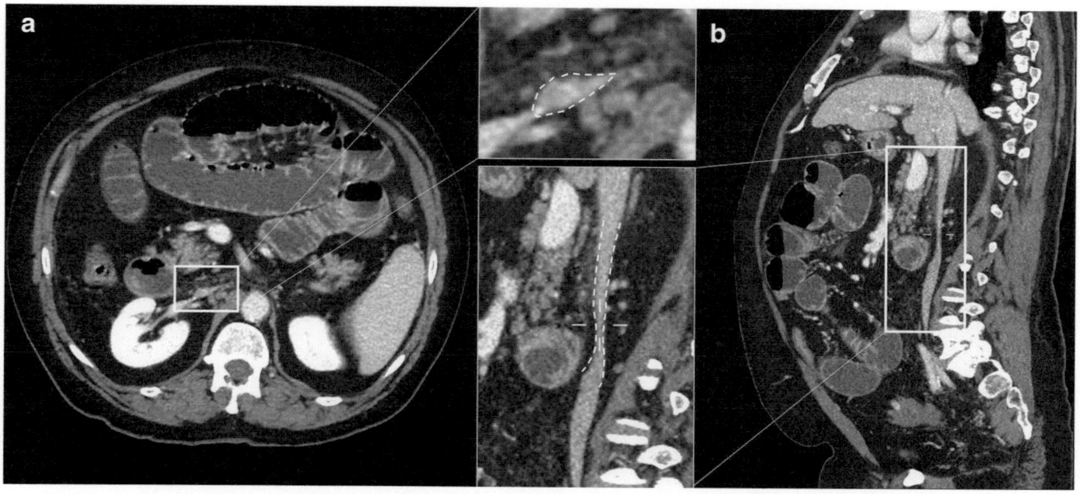

Fig. 29.1 Multiphasic CT examination of venous phase showing collapsed inferior vena cava (details, dashed lines) on axial (**a**) and sagittal (**b**) reconstructions, in a patient with hemodynamically unstable large bowel obstruction causing hypovolemia and shock

ment of perihepatic portion (Fig. 29.1) [9]. This decrease is indicative of a diminished circulating blood volume, suggesting a decrease in venous return, which can occur in patients with systemic low blood pressure and may go undetected due to large-volume fluid resuscitation. Furthermore, changes in intra-abdominal pressure and the respiratory cycle may influence the diameter of the IVC. Moreover, a ratio of 2.5 or more between the transverse and anteroposterior dimensions at the suprarenal IVC level may suggest flattening. The flatness index or IVC diameter ratio is determined by dividing the maximum transverse diameter by the anteroposterior diameter of the IVC [16]. The specificity and sensitivity of IVC flattening in detecting hypo-perfusion shock in spontaneously breathing patients are 90% and 84%, respectively [9, 16]. The IVC diameter ratio, as measured by CT scans, is found in predicting in-hospital mortality among patients with septic shock, where a ratio of 1.3 cm or greater offers 75% sensitivity and 42% specificity [9, 16]. Additionally, this measurement is valuable for estimating the required volume of blood transfusions and evaluating the volume status [9, 16].

29.8 The Halo Sign

A low-density fluid surrounding the IVC, also called halo sign, measuring less than 20 Hounsfield Units (HU) (Fig. 29.2), is detectable in about 80% of patients experiencing severe low blood pressure [9]. This halo indicates the accumulation of extracellular fluid and may be a consequence of increased vascular permeability associated with the systemic inflammatory response syndrome [18]. The halo is most commonly seen at intra- and retro-hepatic IVC. However, the presence of the IVC halo is not exclusive to hypoperfusion shock resulting from sepsis; it can also be present in other conditions like liver cirrhosis, cardiac congestion, hepatitis, or other diseases that obstruct lymphatic drainage at the porta hepatis [9, 16, 18].

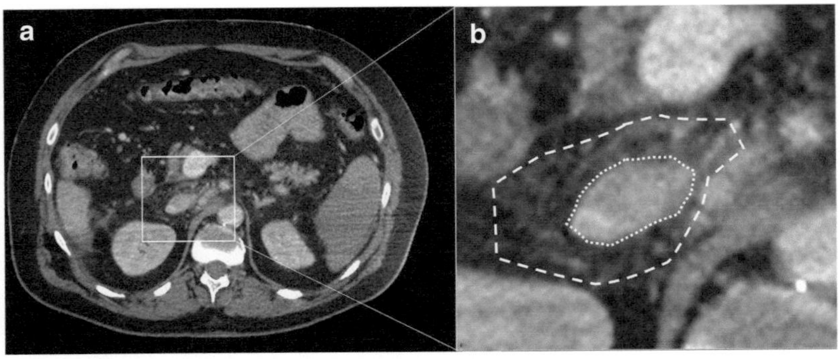

Fig. 29.2 «Halo sign», or rather a low-density fluid (<20HU) surrounding a partly flattened inferior vena cava, as a sign of shock complex in a patient with complicated diverticulitis (**a**); detail (**b**) showing inferior vena cava (white dotted) surrounded by fluid halo (white dashed line)

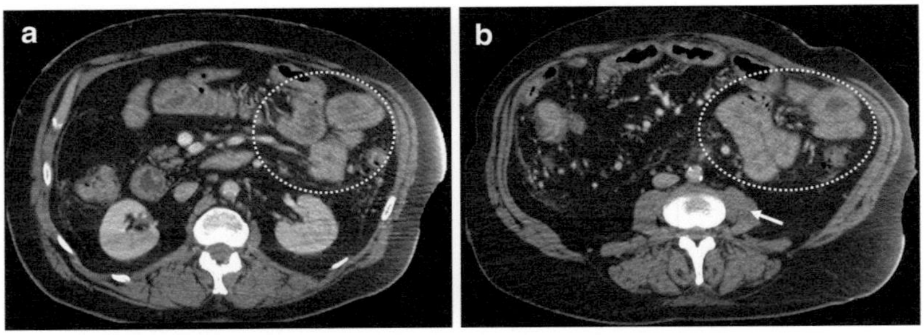

Fig. 29.3 Multiphasic CT examination of venous phase showing shock bowel (**a**–**b**), with fluid-filled partly dilated intestinal loops, thickened walls due to mucosal-submucosal edema (dotted lines) and mucosal enhancement compared to psoas muscle (white arrow)

29.9 Small-Caliber Aorta

An abdominal aorta of small diameter is characterized by an antero-posterior measurement of less than 13 mm, observed 20 mm above and below the renal arteries [9]. This feature is found in around 30% of patients with systemic low blood pressure and is not unique to hypoperfusion shock resulting from sepsis, since it can also be seen in individuals without any medical conditions. The reduced diameter of the aorta is typically linked to vasoconstriction triggered by the adrenergic system as a response to shock [9, 18–22].

CT hypoperfusion complex *visceral signs* consist of decreased blood flow to the bowels, also known as shock bowel, and increased contrast visibility of the gallbladder lining.

29.10 Bowel Hypoperfusion (Shock Bowel)

Common CT findings indicative of shock bowel are loops of bowel filled with fluid and dilated, with wall thickening greater than 3 mm due to submucosal edema and pronounced mucosal enhancement in comparison to the psoas muscle (Fig. 29.3) [9]. These alterations in the small intestine are typically the most prominent signs of shock on a CT scan [9]. The small intestine is usually extensively affected in cases of hypotensive shock, while the colon is less frequently involved [18–21]. Shock bowel occurs as a result of systemic low blood pressure leading to sympathetic nervous system activation, which in turn causes splanchnic blood vessel constriction and diminished blood flow to the intestines. This leads to a lack of oxygen in the tissues, increased permeability, and consequent mucosal hyperenhancement and edematous thickening of the intestinal wall and submucosa [9]. Fluid reabsorption is compromised, causing the bowel loops to become distended. Recognizing shock bowel is critical to differentiate it from other conditions like intestinal ischemia due to a vascular blockage, which presents with different CT features [9, 18]. The most difficult differential diagnosis is widespread bowel ischemia resulting from a vascular blockage, which may also manifest as bowel wall thickening and dilation of the lumen. However, unlike shock bowel, ischemia caused by arterial blockage does not involve mucosal hyperenhancement or wall congestion [18]. Mesenteric venous occlusion might display similar CT findings, along with a filling defect in the superior mesenteric vein or its branches, mesenteric congestion, and surrounding fat stranding. CT signs linked with hypotensive complex can be crucial in identifying systemic low blood pressure, aiding in the differential diagnosis. The mortality rate for shock bowel can reach up to 70% [9, 18–21, 23–26].

29.11 Mucosal Enhancement of the Gallbladder

Enhanced visibility of the gallbladder mucosa, without accompanying wall thickening, may be seen in cases of hypotensive shock complex, although this sign is not highly specific (Fig. 29.4).

CT hypoperfusion complex *parenchymal signs* include abnormal pancreatic enhancement, associated with peripancreatic fluid, the hypoperfusion of the spleen and liver, and the abnormal perfusion of the adrenal glands, kidneys, and thyroid.

29.12 Peripancreatic Edema and Abnormal Pancreatic Enhancement (Shock Pancreas)

The "shock pancreas" manifests through an unusual increase in post-contrast density, showing values 20 HU higher than those of the liver and spleen, and accompanied by low-density peripancreatic fluid (less than 20 HU) (Fig. 29.5). This condition often occurs alongside mesenteric and other retroperitoneal fluid accumulations, with a prevalence of up to 44% [9, 18–22, 27, 28]. Such changes may stem from cytokine release triggered by the systemic inflammatory response syndrome and pancreatic ischemia. This leads to heightened capillary leakage and a reduction in intravascular oncotic pressure. Although this indicator may also be observed in cases of pancreatitis, its presence is a notable sign in the assessment of shock-induced organ effects [9, 18–22, 27, 28].

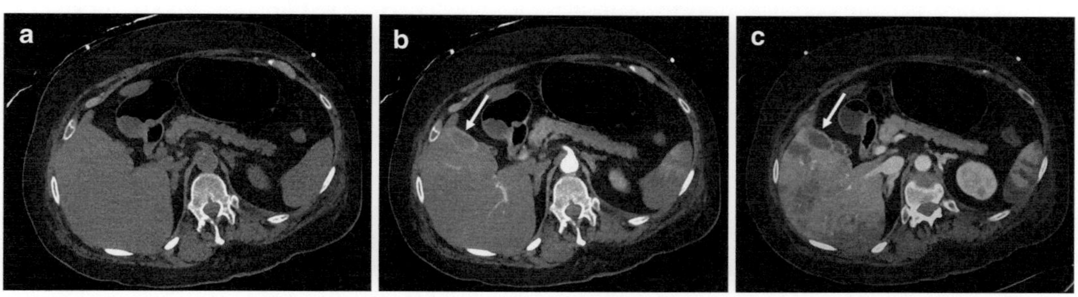

Fig. 29.4 Multiphasic CT examination with non-contrast (**a**), arterial (**b**), and venous (**c**) phases showing mucosal enhancement of the gallbladder (white arrows) in a patient with septic shock due to endocarditis; inhomogeneous enhancement of liver and spleen parenchyma can also be observed

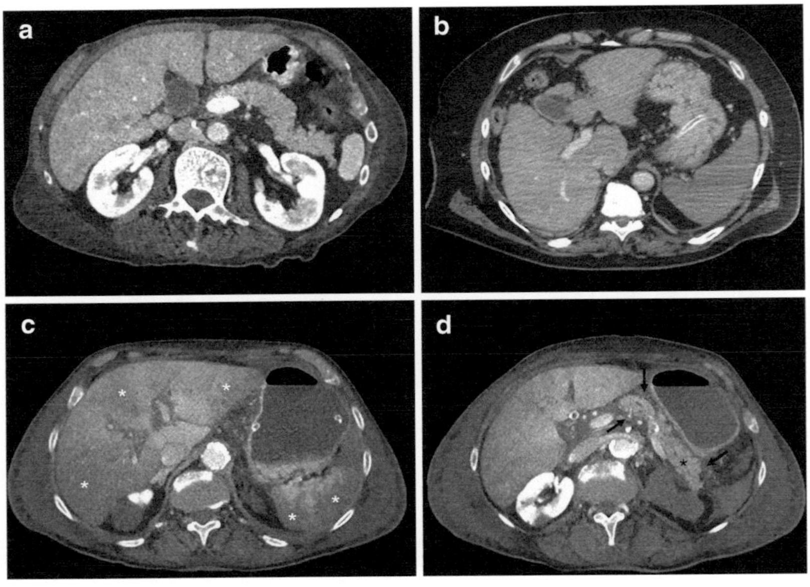

Fig. 29.5 Multiphasic CT examination of venous phase in a case of liver (**a**) and splenic (**b**) hypoperfusion in two different patients diagnosed with septic shock due to complicated pneumonia. Companion case showing liver and splenic hypoperfusion (**c**, white asterisks) associated with milder pancreatic hypoperfusion (**d**, black asterisk) and peripancreatic edema (black arrows), in a patient undergone nephrectomy and right hemicolectomy due to double primary malignancies; surgery was complicated by a leak at the point of anastomosis

29.13 Splenic Hypoperfusion

The spleen is one of the abdominal organs most susceptible to hypotensive shock, frequently exhibiting significantly reduced contrast enhancement in early-phase CT scans [9]. The diminished enhancement and decrease in splenic size are indicative of severe blood flow reduction (Fig. 29.5). The extent of this reduced enhancement is considered to correlate directly with the level of shock-induced hypoperfusion, particularly because the splenic artery lacks autoregulatory capabilities. The latter may result in reduced blood flow to the spleen and reduced enhancement, generally exhibiting a contrast of at least 20 HU lower than that of the liver [16] As such, splenic hypoperfusion is viewed as a valuable indicator for predicting adverse outcomes in patients experiencing systemic low blood pressure [9, 18–22, 26].

29.14 Liver Hypoperfusion

During hypotensive shock complex, liver contrast enhancement is often uneven. A notable decrease in liver enhancement, showing 25 HU less than the spleen, is believed to be a key indicator of edema (Fig. 29.5) [9, 18]. This phenomenon of delayed and uneven enhancement of the liver, due to its dual blood supply, is a well-acknowledged indicator of shock linked to increased sympathetic activity [16]. The increased permeability of parenchymal capillaries can lead to contrast pooling in the dependent right liver parenchyma, giving it a gravitationally dense appearance. Additionally, a demarcation line might be observed between the enhancing dependent parenchyma and the non-enhancing non-dependent parenchyma corresponding to the height of the feeding vein [16]. This specific CT finding is less frequently observed compared to other abnormalities in solid organ tissues. However, caution is advised as misinterpretations may arise in individuals with widespread liver conditions, including fatty liver disease or congestive hepatic venous stasis [9, 18–22].

29.15 Abnormal Renal Enhancement

Abnormal kidney perfusion often results in heightened and extended enhancement of the parenchyma also called "white kidney." A decrease in systolic blood pressure leads to significant constriction of the efferent arterioles of the glomeruli, enhancing glomerular filtration. This reaction causes stagnation of contrast media within the renal parenchyma, manifesting as an extended period of heightened cortical enhancement in the kidneys (Fig. 29.6) [9, 16, 18–22, 26]. The degree of renal enhancement is influenced by various factors, such as cardiac output and the timing of the scan in relation to when the contrast agent is administered, making it a non-specific sign [9, 16]. Nonetheless, the extent of kidney enhancement can differ based on the level of systemic low blood pressure. In certain instances, instead of an increased enhancement, a reduction in the enhancement of the renal medulla may be noted during the venous phase. This is likely due to hindered movement of the contrast medium from the renal cortex to the medulla, a consequence of acute renal tubular dysfunction, and is often associated with a negative prognosis [9, 16, 21].

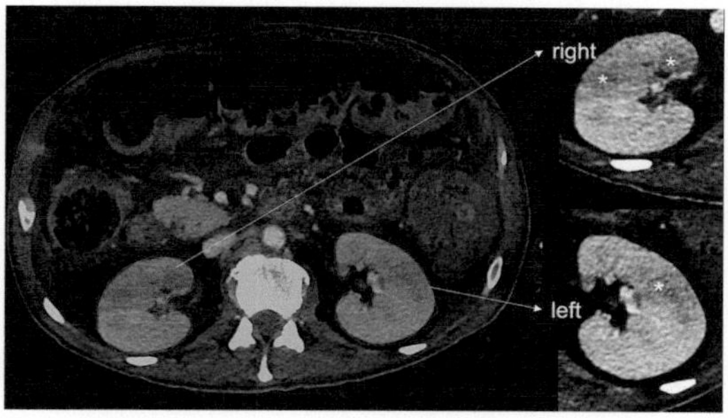

Fig. 29.6 Multiphasic CT examination of venous phase in a case of bilateral abnormal patchy renal enhancement (white asterisks, details) in a patient with septic shock

29.16 Abnormal Adrenal Enhancement (the Adrenal Stress)

Enhanced bilateral adrenal gland visibility is more frequently observed in children than in adults and may occur alongside acute adrenal bleeding, which typically impacts the right gland on one side. This condition is characterized by uniform enlargement of the gland and diffusion of fat surrounding it. Such phenomenon can also be seen in adults, stemming from the redirection of blood flow to the adrenal glands in hypotensive states [9, 18–21, 28–30]. During the arterial phase, the central part of the adrenal gland exhibits less pronounced enhancement compared to its outer region, the so-called "hollow adrenal gland sign", or it might display a patchy pattern due to uneven enhancement of the central area (Fig. 29.7) [30]. By the venous phase, however, the enhancement of the entire adrenal gland becomes uniform [30]. This phenomenon is likely linked to specific pathophysiological alterations occurring during septic shock. Research has pointed out dysfunctions in the hypothalamic-pituitary-adrenal axis, heightened resistance to glucocorticoids, and damage to the adrenal glands caused by inflammatory mediators in the context of septic shock. These factors can lead to a state of overcompensation, ischemia, swelling, and even microhemorrhages and necrosis within the adrenal glands that underscores the critical function of the adrenal glands in the body's sympathetic response to hypotensive shock indicating a negative outcome [9, 16, 18–21, 28–30].

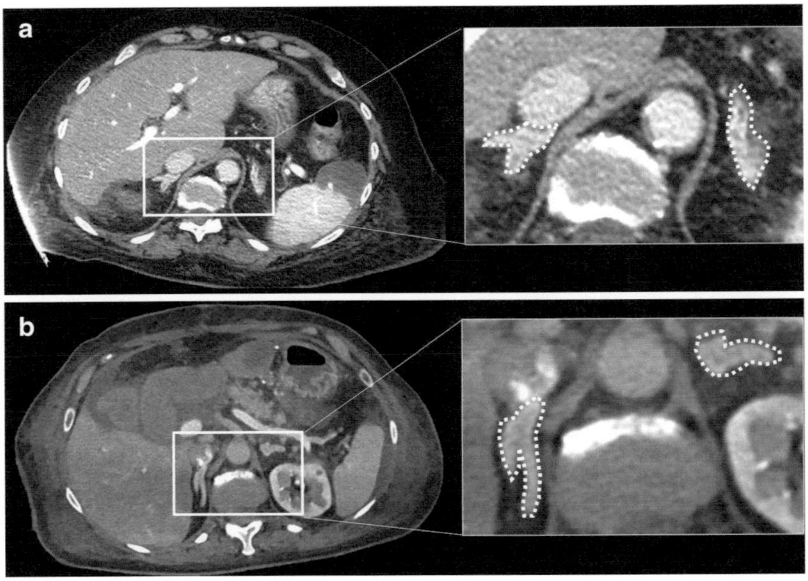

Fig. 29.7 Two companion cases of abnormal adrenal enhancement in a patient with nephritis (**a**) and in a patient with post-operative sepsis (**b**); in detail, bilateral adrenal enhancement (dotted lines)

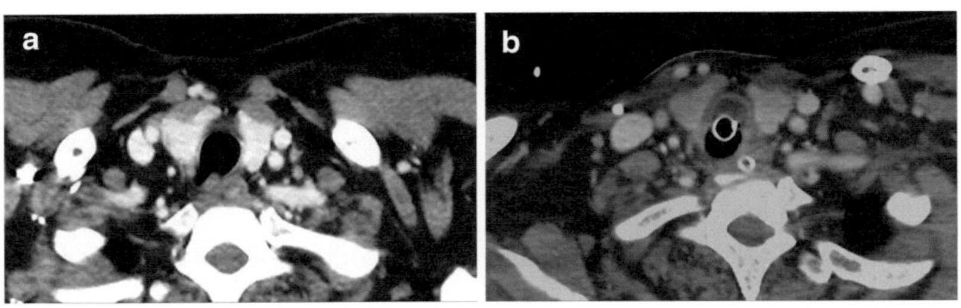

Fig. 29.8 Multiphasic CT examination of venous phase in the same patient with pelvic collections due to complicated sigmoid diverticulitis at diagnosis (**a**) and 2 days later (**b**), showing progressive inhomogeneous thyroid enhancement due to septic shock

29.17 Abnormal Thyroid Enhancement (Shock Thyroid)

Shock thyroid, also known as "transient thyroid," is characterized by swelling of the thyroid gland and the surrounding tissues. It presents as a uniform area of fluid accumulation around the thyroid, displaying a density measure of −5 to 10 HU, accompanied by irregular enhancement patterns within the thyroid gland itself (Fig. 29.8) [9, 16]. This condition, known as thyroid shock, is a less common observation linked with hypotensive shock complex and occurs without any direct or indirect damage to the thyroid itself. The suggested underlying process involves the highly vascular thyroid gland undergoing hypoperfusion, potentially leading to cellular swelling or necrosis, along with the leakage of fluid from within cells [9, 16, 18–22, 31, 32]. Alternative theories suggest that the accumulation of fluid administered during resuscitation in the third space and a significant reaction of the thyroid, which leads to temporary thyrotoxicosis and gland enlargement, are to preserve cardiac output. These changes in the gland can be reversed if hypovolemia and hypotension are effectively treated [9, 16, 18–22, 31, 32].

29.18 Ascites

Ascites is associated with multiorgan dysfunction and is considered a general indicator, not specific to any single condition [9, 16, 33].

29.19 Conclusion

Previous research has primarily focused on the CT hypoperfusion complex in the context of trauma-induced hypotensive shock, with only a limited number of studies examining its relationship with prognosis. Identifying findings from CT hypoperfusion complex offers crucial biomarkers and indicators of prognosis, allowing for efficient risk categorization and enhanced patient outcomes in cases of shock [9, 16]. It has been indicated that signs such as IVC flattening, shock bowel, decreased renal enhancement, and splenic hypoperfusion are key indicators of the hypoperfusion complex, often associated with a negative prognosis in cases of trauma-related hypovolemic shock [18–21, 26]. In the case of septic shock, however, only adrenal hyperenhancement has been linked to a poor outcome [30]. Despite these mixed findings, recognizing these signs can lead to the exploration of new methods for early diagnosis and treatment of septic shock in emergency situations [9]. Therefore, beyond using CT to identify the cause of sepsis, healthcare providers should also be skilled in detecting various CT signs indicative of hypotension. From this perspective, CT imaging emerges as a valuable diagnostic tool for the comprehensive, quick, and thorough evaluation of septic shock suspected clinically, potentially enhancing patient outcomes.

References

1. Giamarellos-Bourboulis EJ, the European Sepsis Alliance (ESA), Zinkernagel AS, et al. Sepsis, a call for inclusion in the work plan of the European Center for Disease Prevention and Control. Intensive Care Med. 2023;49:1138–42. https://doi.org/10.1007/s00134-023-07127-3.
2. Font MD, Thyagarajan B, Khanna AK. Sepsis and septic shock – basics of diagnosis, pathophysiology and clinical decision making. Med Clin North Am. 2020;104(4):573–85. https://doi.org/10.1016/j.mcna.2020.02.011. Epub 2020 May 12
3. Singer M, Deutschman CS, Seymour CW, et al. The third international consensus definitions for sepsis and septic shock (Sepsis-3). JAMA. 2016;315(8):801–10. https://doi.org/10.1001/jama.2016.0287.
4. Dellinger RP, Levy MM, Rhodes A, et al. Surviving sepsis campaign: international guidelines for management of severe sepsis and septic shock 2012. Intensive Care Med. 2013;39(2):165–228. https://doi.org/10.1007/s00134-012-2769-8.
5. Levy MM, Fink MP, Marshall JC, et al. SCCM/ESICM/ACCP/ATS/SIS international sepsis definition conference. Intensive Care Med. 2001;29(4):530–8. https://doi.org/10.1007/s00134-003-1662-x.
6. Shankar-Hari M, Phillips GS, Levy ML, et al. Developing a new definition and assessing new clinical criteria for septic shock: for the third international consensus definitions for sepsis and septic shock (Sepsis-3) (2016).
7. Levy MM, Evans LE, Rhodes A. The surviving sepsis campaign bundle: 2018 update. Intensive Care Med. 2018;44(6):925–8. https://doi.org/10.1007/s00134-018-5085-0.
8. Dugar S, Choudhary C, Duggal A. Sepsis and septic shock: guideline-based management. Clevel Clin J Med. 2020;87(1):53–64. https://doi.org/10.3949/ccjm.87a.18143.
9. Di Serafino M, Viscardi D, Iacobellis F, Giugliano L, Barbuto L, Oliva G, Ronza R, Borzelli A, Raucci A, Pezzullo F, De Cristofaro MG, Romano L. Computed tomography imaging of septic shock. Beyond the cause: the "CT hypoperfusion complex". A pictorial essay. Insights Imaging. 2021;12(1):70. https://doi.org/10.1186/s13244-021-01006-5. PMID: 34089401; PMCID: PMC8178660
10. Vendemiato AV, von Nowakonski A, Marson FA, Levy CE. Microbiological characteristics of sepsis in a university hospital. BMC Infect Dis. 2015;14(15):58. https://doi.org/10.1186/s12879-015-0798-y.
11. Angus DC, van der Poll T. Severe sepsis and septic shock. N Engl J Med. 2013;369(9):840–51. https://doi.org/10.1056/NEJMra1208623.
12. Gruartmoner G, Mesquida J, Ince C. Microcirculatory monitoring in septic patients: where do we stand? Med Intensiva. 2017;41(1):44–52. https://doi.org/10.1016/j.medin.2016.11.011.
13. Gauer RL. Early recognition and management of sepsis in adults: the first six hours. Am Fam Physician. 2013;88(1):44–53.
14. Rhee C, Zhang Z, Kadri SS, et al. CDC prevention epicenters program. Sepsis surveillance using adult sepsis events simplified eSOFA criteria versus sepsis-3 sequential organ failure assessment criteria. Crit Care Med. 2019;47(3):307–14. https://doi.org/10.1097/CCM.0000000000003521.

15. Thompson K, Venkatesh B, Finfer S. Sepsis and septic shock: current approaches to management. Intern Med J. 2019;49(2):160–70. https://doi.org/10.1111/imj.14199.
16. Valente T, Bocchini G, Massimo C, Rea G, Lieto R, Guarino S, Muto E, Abu-Omar A, Scaglione M, Sica G. Multidetector CT imaging biomarkers as predictors of prognosis in shock: updates and future directions. Diagnostics (Basel). 2023;13(13):2304. https://doi.org/10.3390/diagnostics13132304. PMID: 37443697; PMCID: PMC10341185.
17. Pescatori LC, Brambati M, Messina C, Mauri G, Di Leo G, et al. Clinical impact of computed tomography in the emergency department in non-traumatic chest and abdominal conditions. Emerg Radiol. 2018;25(4):393–8. https://doi.org/10.1007/s10140-018-1592-0.
18. Tarrant AM, Ryan MF, Hamilton PA, Benjaminov O. A pictorial review of hypovolaemic shock in adults. Br J Radiol. 2008;81(963):252–7. https://doi.org/10.1259/bjr/40962054.
19. Ames JT, Federle MP. CT hypotension complex (shock bowel) is not always due to traumatic hypovolemic shock. AJR Am J Roentgenol. 2009;192(5):W230–5. https://doi.org/10.2214/AJR.08.1474.
20. Higashi H, Kanki A, Watanabe S, et al. Traumatic hypovolemic shock revisited: the spectrum of contrast-enhanced abdominal computed tomography findings and clinical implications for its management. Jpn J Radiol. 2014;32:579–84. https://doi.org/10.1007/s11604-014-0354-5.
21. Wang J, Liang T, Louis L, Nicolaou S, McLaughlin PD. Hypovolemic shock complex in the trauma setting: a pictorial review. Can Assoc Radiol J. 2013;64(2):156–63. https://doi.org/10.1016/j.carj.2013.03.002.
22. Shin MS, Berland LL, Ho KJ. Small aorta: CT detection and clinical significance. J Comput Assist Tomogr. 1990;14(1):102–3.
23. Hara H, Babyn PS, Bourgeois D. Significance of bowel wall enhancement on CT following blunt abdominal trauma in childhood. J Comput Assist Tomogr. 1992;16(1):94–8. https://doi.org/10.1097/00004728-199201000-00017.
24. Macari M, Balthazar EJ. CT of bowel wall thickening: significance and pitfalls of interpretation. AJR Am J Roentgenol. 2001;176(5):1105–16. https://doi.org/10.2214/ajr.176.5.1761105.
25. Sugi MD, Menias CO, Lubner MG, et al. CT findings of acute smallbowel entities. Radiographics. 2018;38(5):1352–69. https://doi.org/10.1148/rg.2018170148.
26. Kanki A, Ito K, Tamada T, et al. Dynamic contrast-enhanced CT of the abdomen to predict clinical prognosis in patients with hypovolemic shock. AJR Am J Roentgenol. 2011;197(6):W980–4. https://doi.org/10.2214/AJR.10.5736.
27. Ryan MF, Hamilton PA, Sarrazin J, et al. The halo sign and peripancreatic fluid: useful CT signs of hypovolaemic shock complex in adults. Clin Radiol. 2005;60(5):599–607. https://doi.org/10.1016/j.crad.2004.02.012.
28. Venkatanarasimha N, Roobottom C. Intense adrenal enhancement: a feature of hypoperfusion complex. AJR Am J Roentgenol. 2010;195(1):W82. https://doi.org/10.2214/AJR.09.3829.
29. Di Serafino M, Severino R, Coppola V, Gioioso M, et al. Nontraumatic adrenal hemorrhage: the adrenal stress. Radiol Case Rep. 2017;12(3):483–7. https://doi.org/10.1016/j.radcr.2017.03.020.
30. Peng Y, Xie Q, Wang H, et al. The hollow adrenal gland sign: a newly described enhancing pattern of the adrenal gland on dualphase contrast-enhanced CT for predicting the prognosis of patients with septic shock. Eur Radiol. 2019;29:5378–85. https://doi.org/10.1007/s00330-019-06172-1.
31. Han DH, Ha EJ, Sun JS, Jung SL. Remarkable CT features of shock thyroid in traumatic and non-traumatic patients. Emerg Radiol. 2017;24(3):319–24. https://doi.org/10.1007/s10140-016-1475-1.
32. Brochert A, Rafoth JB. Shock thyroid: a new manifestation of the hypovolemic shock complex in trauma patients. J Comput Assist Tomogr. 2006;30(2):310–2. https://doi.org/10.1097/00004728-200603000-00028.
33. Rossaint J, Zarbock A. Pathogenesis of multiple organ failure in sepsis. Crit Rev Immunol. 2015;35(4):277–91. https://doi.org/10.1615/critrevimmunol.2015015461.

30 Emergencies in Pregnancy

Luigia Romano, Tiziana Capussela, Sonia Fulciniti, Francesco Muto, and Silvana Nicotra

30.1 Introduction

Knowledge of the dose of exposure to ionizing radiation on the fetus, determined by Computed Tomography (CT), in the different gestational stages, facilitates the most appropriate choices for diagnostic imaging of pregnant patients, with acute non-obstetric and non-traumatic clinical conditions, such as respiratory distress from pulmonary embolism and abdominal pain. Imaging modalities that do not use ionizing radiation (Ultrasound and Magnetic Resonance) are preferred. However, Ultrasound (US) has limitations such as dependence on the operator, the restricted field of vision, and the presence of viscera overlying the pregnant uterus.

In 30% of pregnant patients with abdominal pain, in which US was substantially negative, subsequent imaging produced significant positive results, which required urgent surgery in 64% of cases [1]. There is no doubt that CT is the most conclusive method of emergency diagnostic imaging, with an undeniable advantage due to the short examination time associated with a high informative value. Therefore, if it is necessary to resort to CT, the principle of using the lowest and reasonably obtainable dose must be followed, after having analyzed the risk compared to the patient's benefit. According to the latest American College of Obstetricians and Gynecologists (ACOG) guidelines, the use of CT in pregnancy should not be denied whenever its use is deemed to be of high benefit to the patient, despite the potential risks of ionizing radiation and contrast medium (CM) on the fetus [2].

L. Romano (✉) · T. Capussela · S. Fulciniti
F. Muto · S. Nicotra
Department of General and Emergency Radiology, "Antonio Cardarelli" Hospital, Naples, Italy
e-mail: tiziana.capussela@aocardarelli.it; sonia.fulciniti@aocardarelli.it

30.2 Assessment of the Risk of Exposure of the Fetus to Ionizing Radiation

The CT examination of a pregnant patient is a source of concern for both the patient and the Radiologist due to the potential risk of adverse effects on the fetus due to exposure to ionizing radiation. However, if the CT examination is necessary and is performed with modern and adequate equipment, with careful technique, then the potential benefit for the health of the mother and fetus will be greater than the exposure risk [3].

As demonstrated by studies conducted on animals and by the observation of human exposures at high doses, the potential effects of radiation on the fetus include prenatal death, congenital malformations, growth retardation, reduced intelligence quotient (IQ), and an increase in childhood cancers. The severity and the effect on the tissues

L. Romano et al. (eds.), *CT of Non-Traumatic Body Emergencies*,
https://doi.org/10.1007/978-3-031-84849-0_30

Table 30.1 Summary of suspected in utero-induced deterministic radiation effects [4, 5]

Menstrual or Gestational age	Conception age	<50 mGy (<5 rad)	50–100 mGy (5–10 rad)	>100 mGy (>10 rad)
0–2 weeks (0–14 days)	Prior to conception	None	None	None
3rd and 4th weeks (15–28 days)	1st–2nd weeks (1–14 days)	None	Probably none	Possible spontaneous abortion.
5th–10th weeks (29–70 days)	3rd–8th weeks (15–56 days)	None	Potential effects are scientifically uncertain and probably too subtle to be clinically detectable.	Possible malformations increasing in likelihood as dose increases
11th–17th weeks (71–119 days)	9th–15th weeks (57–105 days)	None	Potential effects are scientifically uncertain and probably too subtle to be clinically detectable.	Risk of diminished IQ or of mental retardation, increasing in frequency and severity with increasing dose
18th–27th weeks (120–189 days)	16th–25th weeks (106–175 days)	None	None	IQ deficits not detectable at diagnostic doses

of the fetus depend on the stage of gestation in which the exposure occurs and on the radiation dose (Table 30.1) [4, 5]. The International Scientific Societies (International Commission on Radiation Protection [5], American College of Radiology [6], American College of Obstetricians and Gynecologists [7]) consider the risk of spontaneous abortion and serious malformations in fetuses exposed to a lower radiation dose, to be negligible or just above 50 mGy [8, 9].

During the first two weeks of gestation, the greatest risk is pregnancy loss; the "all or nothing" phenomenon is assumed to occur and could potentially result in miscarriage or an unharmed embryo. During the 3rd to 8th weeks, which correspond to the period of organogenesis, the fetus is most vulnerable to congenital malformations, while from the 9th to 15th weeks, the fetus has the highest risk of mental retardation. For most of these deterministic effects, a threshold dose of 100 mGy is observed. Stochastic effects, however, do not have a threshold, and data on risk are controversial [10]. Assuming the threshold-free linear model of radiation risk, as recommended in various reports [10, 11], the incidence of radiation-induced childhood cancer is generally low: an absorbed fetal dose of 20 mGy corresponds to a cancer risk of 1/125, in addition to the natural background.

The European Directive 2013/59/Euratom [12] adopted by the European Union (EU) Member States, indicates specific provisions for the radiation protection of women of childbearing age, including:

- find out whether the patient subjected to medical exposure is pregnant, unless this cannot be excluded for obvious reasons, or is not relevant for the radiological examination;
- pay particular attention to the justification of the examination, in particular in urgent clinical conditions and to the optimization of the exposure dose of both the mother and the unborn child;
- evaluate the dose that will be administered to the unborn child following the diagnostic process which exposes the fetus to doses potentially higher than 1 mSv;
- inform the pregnant woman about the potential risks and benefits of any medical procedure involving radiation exposure, in order to make informed decisions regarding her care.

Not all radiological tests exceed the threshold of 100 mGy and not all tests are greater than 1 mSv, in which case an estimate of the fetal dose by the Medical Physicist is not necessary.

CT exams must be classified according to whether the fetus is positioned inside or outside the scan volume. When the study volume includes the fetus, the radiation dose depends on the thickness of the patient, the depth of the conceptus with respect to the skin surface, and the CT technique adopted. If the CT scan does not directly irradiate the fetus, the fetal dose is mainly due to dispersion within the mother's body volume. In this case, the use of lead shields has been shown to potentially increase internal leakage. Therefore, the use of protective shields for the pelvis is not recommended [13]. In general, reducing the length of the study volume is the most effective means of reducing the doses absorbed by the fetus [14].

Chest CT showed a significantly low fetal absorbed dose, typically ranging from 0.01 mGy to 0.15 mGy. As the threshold of 1 mSv is not exceeded, formal dose estimates are not necessary. The most significant fetal exposure occurs during abdominal and pelvic CT [15]. The average fetal dose for single-phase abdomino-pelvic CT is approximately 20 mGy and is rarely greater than 50 mGy, unless multiple phases are used. Therefore, optimization of patient dose is essential to obtain diagnostically acceptable image quality at the lowest possible radiation dose and a preliminary formal estimate of the dose by the medical physicist is necessary. For the process of optimizing the exposure dose [16] it is advisable to define a "dose team" composed of the Radiologist, the Medical Physicist, and the Radiology Technician who, by analytically evaluating the examination protocol, ensures the best benefit/risk ratio for the patient and the fetus [17].

Estimated radiation exposure is low for CT when the fetus is outside the study volume. Therefore, chest CT is considered a low-dose examination provided that the fetus is excluded from the primary beam. It is necessary to reduce the exposure dose as much as possible for performing abdominal and pelvic CT, reducing the milliampere-second value, applying modulation along the axis, and increasing the pitch.

The exposure algorithm is based on the following principles:

1. if an imaging study is necessary to evaluate a pregnant patient, it is best to use a modality that does not use ionizing radiation (US or MRI);
2. if it is necessary to use CT, the radiation dose to the fetus must be kept as low as possible;
3. all CT protocols, even for emergency exams, aimed at pregnant patients, must be preliminarily evaluated by Radiologists and Medical Physicists to estimate the dose to the fetus. The protocols will be based on experience gained and literature reviews;
4. both the scanning parameters and the acquisition technique must be optimized to obtain a significant reduction in the fetal dose, without sacrificing the quality of the diagnostic image;
5. automatic dose control software must be used that limits exposure to a preset noise level, or uses iterative reconstruction techniques that improve image quality and reduce the radiation dose compared to filtered back projection techniques;
6. it is necessary to reduce the number of images and the CT acquisition phases of the abdomen/pelvis scan, limiting the study volume as much as possible;
7. each pregnant patient to be examined must be evaluated individually. The dose absorbed by the conceptus (embryo or fetus) and not by the mother must always be considered and this will be expressed in gray (Gy) or milligray (mGy). Dose limits will be given in Sv. In most medical applications using X-rays, the numerical value of the absorbed dose in Gy is essentially the same as the numerical value of the equivalent dose in Sv.

The International Commission on Radiological Protection (ICRP) [5] states: "fetal doses less than 100 mGy should not be considered a reason for terminating the pregnancy. At fetal doses above this level, decisions should be made based on individual circumstances" [18].

30.3 Use of Contrast Medium (CM)

The American College of Radiology (ACR) recommends not to deprive the use of iodinated cm in pregnant or potentially pregnant patients, when it is considered necessary for diagnostic purposes

[19, 20] as there are no data that suggest potential harm to the fetus.

In 2016, the American College of Obstetricians and Gynecologists (ACOG) published guidelines on diagnostic imaging during pregnancy and breastfeeding. The use of iodized cm is recommended only if necessary to obtain diagnostic information that will positively influence the mother's care. Its use entails a low risk of adverse effects and anaphylactic reactions, the incidence of which is the same for all individuals [21]. The CM crosses the placenta by diffusion and, after entering the fetal bloodstream, is excreted through urine into the amniotic fluid and subsequently ingested by the fetus [22]. Animal studies have not reported teratogenic or mutagenic effects resulting from the use of iodinated CM during pregnancy. There is no evidence that CM is teratogenic in humans [23]. The use of non-ionic CM in pregnant women does not affect neonatal thyroid-stimulating hormone (TSH), probably because the overall amount of excess iodide in the fetal circulation is minimal and short-lived [24]. Atwell et al. [25] 2007 evaluated the thyroid function of the newborn after exposure to CM during gestation and, based on TSH measurements, found no negative effects. The volume of CM should be kept as limited as possible [26]. Although screening for hypothyroidism is standard practice for all newborns, it is recommended to carry it out during the first week of life for newborns exposed to CM during gestation [26]. Plasma volume increases with pregnancy. Cardiac output increases by up to 50% due to increased stroke rate and volume [27]. These physiological changes begin to occur already in the first trimester and increase in the last trimester and determine a dilution of the CM with a reduction in enhancement. To compensate for the increase in cardiac output it is necessary to increase the flow rate of the cm to 3–4 ml/s and choose a high concentration product. To minimize the amount of cm injected, the injection time will need to be adapted to the duration of the scan. Given the hyperdynamic state of pregnant patients, a short delay of 4–5 s after reaching the trigger level is appropriate [27]. Reducing the voltage from 140 kVp to 100 kVp increases the average enhancement of the aorta by 40% and increases the enhancement of the small arteries even more [28].

30.4 Venous Thromboembolism and Pulmonary Thromboembolism

According to data from the World Health Organization, venous thromboembolism (VTE) is responsible for 3% of all maternal deaths worldwide. A recent analysis of maternal mortality in the United States showed that VTE between 2003 and 2011 caused 15% of all deaths during pregnancy [29]. Pregnant patients have an incidence of venous thromboembolism approximately five times higher than non-pregnant patients [30].

The increased incidence of thrombosis derives from hyperestrogenemia, hypercoagulability due to an increase in coagulation factors, and the compressive effects of the uterus on the inferior vena cava, which cause a reduction in venous return [31].

Unlike VTE in the general population which mostly affects the lower limbs, VTE in pregnant women most frequently begins in the pelvis. Risk factors unrelated to pregnancy include age over 35, obesity, varicose veins, sickle cell anemia, and heart disease. Those associated with antepartum VTE include immobility, assisted reproductive techniques, smoking, and antepartum hemorrhage [32].

Pulmonary embolism (PE) is associated with high pregnancy mortality (up to 15%); unjustified treatment with anticoagulants causes maternal and fetal morbidity [33], with teratogenic effects. Therefore, it is crucial to confidently diagnose or exclude PE in pregnant patients. Unfortunately, the clinical symptoms and signs are not specific and D-dimer values cannot be used for screening, due to the physiological progressive increase during pregnancy [34]. CT pulmonary angiography (CTA) is the most accurate method for the diagnosis of PE [35] and has the advantage of not directly exposing the fetus to the radiation beam. It has high sensitivity (81–91%) and specificity

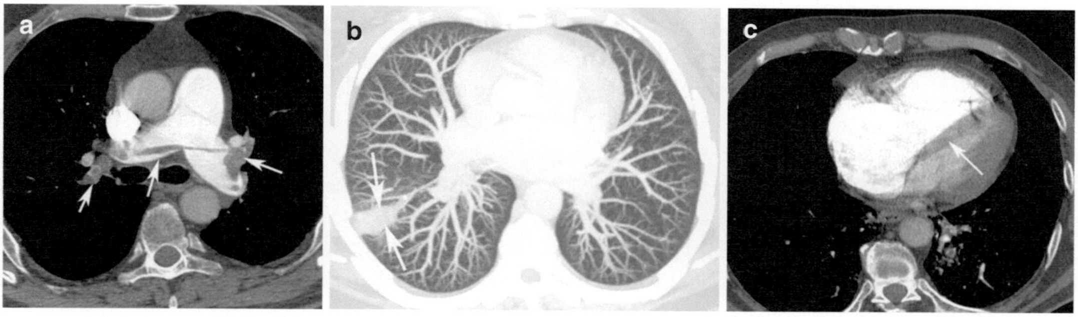

Fig. 30.1 Pulmonary thromboembolism in a pregnant patient at the 20th week. (**a**) the axial ACT scan at the pulmonary hilar level, documents a linear and incomplete opacification defect in the pulmonary arterial lumen and complete opacification defects of the lumen of its main arterial branches (arrows). (**b**) the window for the lung parenchyma, documents the presence of an infarct area with triangular morphology (arrows) affecting the apical segment of the right lower lung lobe. (**c**) the axial ACT scan at the cardiac level, documents a volumetric increase in the right cardiac chambers with dislocation of the interventricular septum to the left (arrow) resulting in overload of the right heart

(93–97%) for the detection of emboli in the main, lobar, segmental, and subsegmental pulmonary arteries, which present as opacification defects of the CM-enhanced arterial lumen, eventually associated with pulmonary infarct (Fig. 30.1). Furthermore, using a low kVp protocol [36], the radiation dose can be further reduced and the vascular contrast increased.

30.5 Acute Abdominal Pain

The diagnosis of the causes of abdominal pain in pregnant women is particularly complex, due to the difficulty of the clinical examination in the presence of the pregnant uterus and misleading symptoms usually present, such as nausea, vomiting, and non-specific leukocytosis [37]. However, diagnosis and timely treatment are crucial for the well-being of the mother and fetus. US and MRI are the basic imaging investigations in pregnancy, due to the absence of exposure to ionizing radiation. US can clarify the cause of the pain particularly if it is due to an obstetric or gynecological condition. The US evaluation of the digestive system, pancreas, urinary excretory tracts, and mesenteric vascular system, is severely limited due to the patient's body habitus, reduced visual field, and the presence of overlying visceral structures [38]. MRI is often used when US is inconclusive. Gadolinium-based CM is classified as a category C drug by the Food and Drug Administration (FDA) and should be administered only if the benefit justifies the potential risk to the fetus [39].

Unfortunately, access to MRI can be limited by the unavailability of the equipment and the frequent intolerance of the pregnant patient towards this type of investigation, burdened by long execution times and discomfort. Therefore, CT may be justified in pregnancy, in selected cases, when the study is in the best interest of the mother's health and the patient is informed of the minimal risks to the fetus. However, it is the investigation of choice when there is a particularly compromised clinical situation and a very rapid diagnosis is necessary [40].

30.6 Non-obstetric Clinical Conditions Causing Acute Abdomen in Pregnancy

Acute abdomen affects 1 in 500–635 pregnancies [41].

Various clinical conditions may be responsible such as gastrointestinal, urinary, hepatic, and gynecological pathologies. The pregnant uterus causes compression and displacement of the surrounding viscera and, consequently, there is often a delay in the clinical diagnosis of acute abdominal pathologies due to their atypical localization and the often delayed peritoneal signs.

30.6.1 Acute Appendicitis

Acute appendicitis affects 1 in 1500 pregnancies and is the most common cause of acute abdomen [42] with a higher rate of viscera perforation in pregnant women compared to the general population (43% vs 4–19%). It occurs more frequently in the second trimester of gestation and causes premature birth. Since the site of the appendix migrates some centimeters upwards, in the third trimester of gestation the pain can be localized to the upper right abdominal quadrant [43]. Since there is no direct contact between the area of periappendiceal inflammation and the parietal peritoneum, there is less pain during clinical compression. The pregnant uterus may also prevent contact between the omentum and the inflamed appendix, which facilitates the spread of sepsis, with quick development of diffuse peritonitis [44]. The frequent delay in diagnosis is due to the anomalous position of the appendix, the lack of typical painful characteristics, the presence of pregnancy nausea/vomiting, and non-specific leukocytosis which makes laboratory values unreliable.

Non-perforated appendicitis results in fetal mortality of 3–5%, with little effect on maternal mortality. On the contrary, in perforated appendicitis, the percentage of fetal death is between 20% and 25% [45]. These data highlight the need for early and accurate diagnosis and timely surgical intervention. In suspected diagnostic cases, if US is not exhaustive, MRI cannot be performed, CT of the abdomen and pelvis with intravenous CM should be used. A retrospective study including 78 pregnant women suffering from abdominal pain reported a sensitivity of 92%, a specificity of 99%, and a negative predictive value of 99% of CT for the diagnosis of appendicitis [34].

CT signs of non-perforated appendicitis are: appendix diameter greater than 6 mm.; wall thickness greater than 2 mm with marked CM enhancement and inflammatory edema of the adjacent adipose tissue. The presence of a phlegmon or an abscess collection, that may contain a calcified appendicolith, are signs of perforation (Fig. 30.2) [46].

30.6.2 Bowel Obstruction

Intestinal obstruction (BO) in pregnancy is uncommon (1 in 2500 to 1 in 3500 pregnancies) and is usually due to small intestinal adhesions (60–70%), less commonly to volvulus (25%) [47]. It occurs more frequently in the third trimester, probably due to the mechanical effects of the pregnant uterus on the intestine. The maternal mortality rate can reach 6% and the fetal mortality rate can exceed 25% [48]. The dilation of the intestine upstream of the obstruction increases

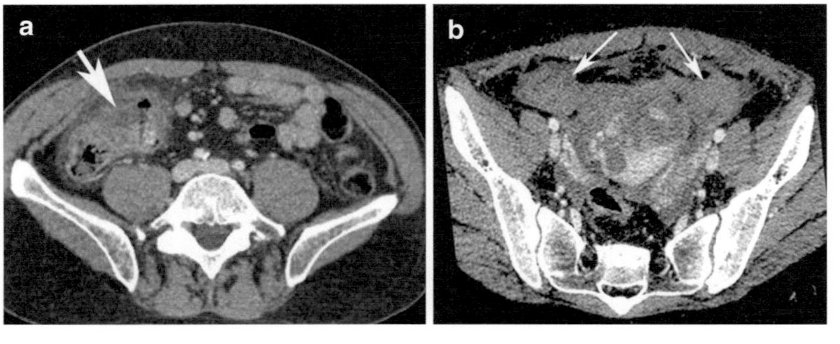

Fig. 30.2 Acute perforated appendicitis in a pregnant patient in the 14th week. (**a**) post-CM axial CT scan documents a phlegmon in the right iliac fossa (arrow) with relief of an appendicolith in the context. (**b**) Axial pelvic CT scan documents the presence of free fluid in the lower peritoneal recesses (arrows)

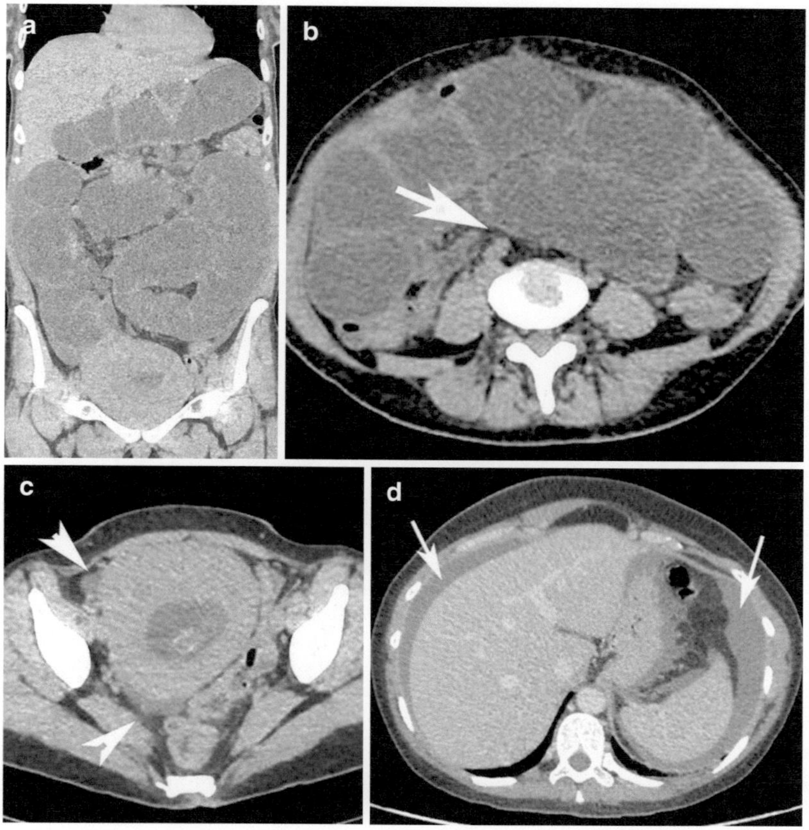

Fig. 30.3 Intestinal obstruction due to "adhesive bridle" in a pregnant patient at the 10th week. (**a**) the coronal reconstruction of the abdominal CT exam without CM documents a marked fluid overdistention of the lumen of the small bowel loops, with smoothing of the mucous folds. (**b**) axial CT scan without CM documents the collapse of the lumen of an ileal loop in the center of the abdomen at the site of the obstruction (arrow). The downstream ileal loop is collapsed. (**c**) Axial CT scan without CM at the pelvic level, highlights the presence of a free fluid layer in the lower peritoneal recesses (arrowheads). (**d**) axial CT scan without CM at the subdiaphragmatic level highlights the presence of free fluid in the supramesocolic peritoneal recesses (arrows)

wall tension, causes edema of the loop wall, decreases mucosal perfusion, causes bacterial proliferation with further development of intraluminal gas, and reduces tensile strength with the risk of perforation. The perforation usually occurs in correspondence with an intestinal segment that is particularly dilated and/or particularly compromised by ischemia. There is a transudative loss of fluid from the intestinal lumen which spreads into the mesentery and peritoneal cavity [49].

CT plays a fundamental role in the diagnosis of BO and in the detection of signs of occlusion, ischemia, and perforation. It has a sensitivity of 94%, a specificity of 96%, and an accuracy of 95% in detecting BO and its complications [50].

CT findings suggestive of SO include: loops proximal to the site of occlusion dilated and overdistended by fluid and gas; collapsed, gas-free distal bowel loops, with an abrupt transition point between these two segments (Fig. 30.3).

CT usually fails to identify intestinal adhesions, but their presence is suspected by an abrupt transition from dilated to collapsed intestinal loops, without a detectable cause at the point of passage (Fig. 30.4). The accuracy in identifying the location of the transition point on CT varies from 63% to 93% [51]. Air bubbles distributed

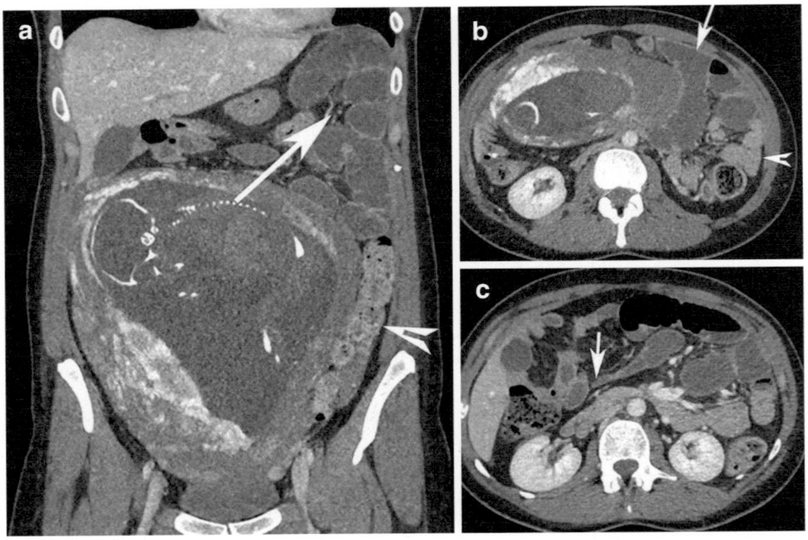

Fig. 30.4 Intestinal obstruction due to "adhesive bridle" in a pregnant patient at the 36th week. (**a**) the coronal reconstruction of the abdominal CT exam with CM documents a fluid overdistention of the lumen of the loops of the small intestine located in the left quadrants (arrow) from the pregnant uterus. The colon is collapsed (arrowhead). (**b**) the abdominal axial CT scan documents that in the left quadrants, there are loops of the small intestine overdistended by fluid (arrow) and others collapsed (arrowhead). (**c**) the central-abdominal axial CT scan highlights the transition point (arrow) at the site of the mechanical occlusion of the ileum

between the folds of the mesentery, possibly mixed with fluid effusion, or in the peritoneal recesses, indicate intestinal perforation.

In the case of BO due to volvulus, both the mesenteric vessels and the affected intestinal loops are twisted. The intestinal loops at the fulcrum of rotation show a narrowing of the lumen with a "beak" appearance. The "whirl" sign occurs when the intestinal loops, and their meso, afferent, and efferent mesenterial vessels rotate around a fixed point of obstruction. The efferent mesenterial venous vessels are typically congested and the mesenteric fat thickened [52]. Fluid effusion accumulates in the mesenteric folds due to transudation of fluid through the serosa due to obstruction of mesenteric venous outflow.

During pregnancy, a dilation of the right colon can occur, which predisposes patients to cecal volvulus [35]. In half of patients with cecal volvulus, the cecum twists in the axial plane, rotating along its long axis, appearing in the right lower quadrant.

The other half of patients present with a "loop" type cecal volvulus, with the cecum twisting and inverting, resulting in the apex of cecal torsion in the left upper quadrant. The terminal ileum usually entwines with the cecum. Identification of the gas-displaced and distended appendix confirms the diagnosis.

30.6.3 Urolithiasis

During pregnancy, ureteral dilatation on a compressive basis is associated with a decrease in peristalsis due to the relaxing effects of the smooth muscles of the ureters, caused by progesterone, with an increase in the risk of stone formation and the development of pyelonephritis [53].

Urolithiasis is the most common abdominal pain condition of non-obstetric origin, with an incidence ranging from 1 in 200, to 1 in 1500 [54].

The pain usually occurs after the second trimester of gestation, when the ureteral dilation is more marked. Diagnosis of obstructive uropathy is difficult during pregnancy, as differentiation between symptomatic urolithiasis and painful hydronephrosis is often difficult. Differential diagnoses include appendicitis, diverticulitis, and placental abruption. If misdiagnosed or late, it can be complicated by pyelonephritis, preterm labor, fetal death, hypertension, and gestational diabetes [55]. US is the first diagnostic test for suspected urolithiasis in pregnancy but has a sensitivity of only 34% [56]. Renal and urinary tract US findings may be nonspecific and may not be able to distinguish between ureteral obstruction secondary to stones and physiologic hydronephrosis. False positives are therefore frequent due to the dilation of the collecting system that occurs physiologically during pregnancy. MRI is also useful for highlighting complications, such as pyelonephritis.

In unresolved cases, CT remains a very reliable method for highlighting stones obstructing the urinary tract in pregnant women. Low-dose CT has a sensitivity of 95% and a specificity of 98% for the detection of urinary tract stones and related complications [57].

30.6.4 Liver Pathologies

A rare liver disease of pregnancy that can present with acute abdominal pain is Haemolysis, Elevated Liver Enzymes, and Low Platelet count (HELLP) syndrome [58]. The incidence is 0.2–0.6% of all pregnancies and 10–20% of pregnancies complicated by preeclampsia [59].

It usually develops in the third trimester or immediately after birth and is associated with maternal complications (placental abruption, disseminated intravascular coagulation, hematoma and spontaneous rupture of the liver, acute renal failure) and neonatal complications (prematurity and low birth weight). It is a serious and rare variant of preeclampsia, manifesting itself after the 20th week of gestation with high blood pressure, proteinuria, or with organ dysfunction in the absence of proteinuria. It manifests as hemolysis, elevated liver enzyme levels, and low platelet counts. Clinically, the patient complains of intense pain in the right upper abdominal quadrant radiating to the shoulder, hepatomegaly, nausea, vomiting, jaundice, and confusion.

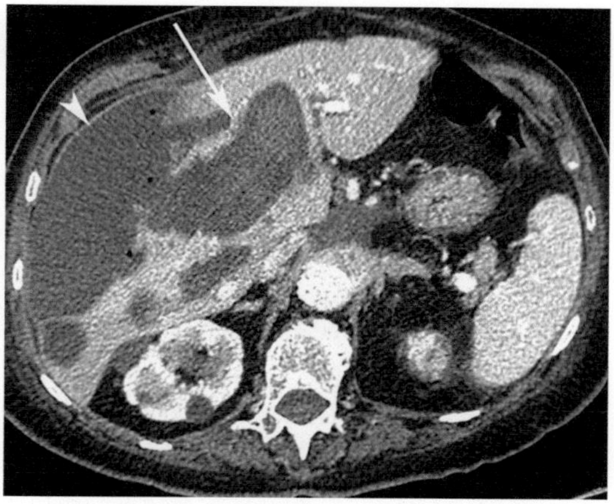

Fig. 30.5 HELLP syndrome in full-term pregnant women. At the end of the pregnancy, the patient develops HELLP syndrome for which birth is induced by cesarean section. CT with CM performed immediately after delivery documents a centroparenchymal hematoma of the liver (arrow) communicating with a large subcapsular hematoma (arrowhead)

Although the etiopathogenesis remains unclear, histopathological findings of the liver highlight intravascular fibrin deposits with hepatic sinusoidal obstruction, intrahepatic vascular congestion, and increased intrahepatic pressure with consequent diffuse hepatocyte necrosis, intraparenchymal and subcapsular hemorrhage (Fig. 30.5) and eventual rupture of the liver capsule with hemoperitoneum [60].

30.6.5 Uterine Rupture

The clinical presentation of uterine rupture is dominated by abdominal pain associated with hypotension, due to large peritoneal and intrauterine blood losses [61]. It indicates complete separation of the uterine layers with rupture of the membranes and intramniotic contents.

It most commonly originates from a spontaneous rupture of a cesarean or a myomectomy scar (Fig. 30.6) or is caused by trauma to an intact uterus. It can occur preferentially in the third trimester of pregnancy or during labor and can cause severe uterine and peritoneal bleeding, fetal distress, and expulsion of the placenta and/or fetus into the abdominal cavity [62].

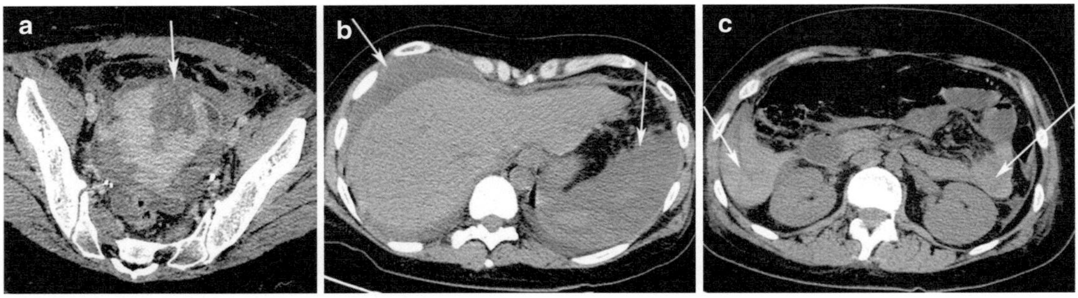

Fig. 30.6 Rupture of the uterus in correspondence with the cesarean section scar, in a pregnant woman at the 12th week. (**a**) axial CT scan with CM shows a large hypodense breach of the myometrium (arrow) of the anterior wall of the uterus. The embryo is aborted. (**b**) baseline axial CT scan documents a fair amount of hemoperitoneum in the subphrenic spaces (arrows). (**c**) central-abdominal basal CT axial scan highlights the blood overdistention of the parieto-colic spaces (arrows)

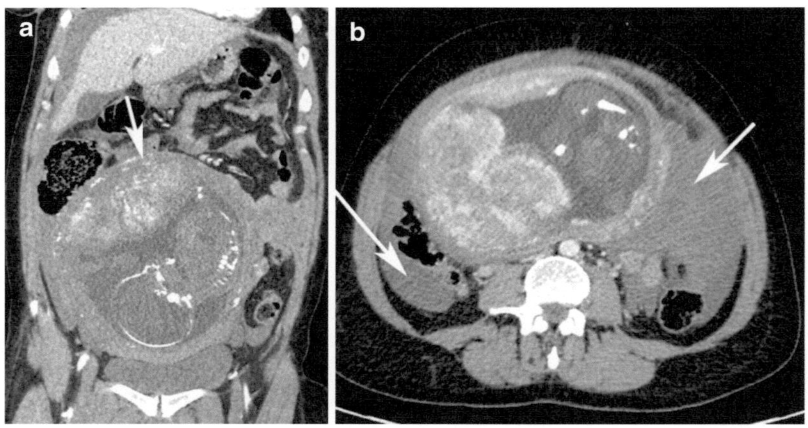

Fig. 30.7 Rupture of the uterus in a pregnant woman at the 27th week. (**a**) coronal reconstruction of the abdominal CT with CM demonstrating an interruption of the myometrium at the level of the uterine fundus (arrow). (**b**) Abdominal axial CT scan documents abundant hemoperitoneum (arrows)

Uterine dehiscence instead indicates the separation of the myometrium with preservation of the internal fetal membranes and the peritoneal serosa that lines the uterus; occurs due to a functional weakening of the myometrium [63]. It is generally asymptomatic and rarely causes potentially lethal complications [64].

The incidence of uterine rupture reported for a scarless uterus is 5 per 10,000 patients, while it is 20–80/10,000 patients in the presence of a scar.

The site of the uterine rupture appears on CT as a hypodense post-contrast enhancement defect, sometimes with air bubbles in the context, with complete interruption of myometrial continuity, with collections of blood in its context and hemoperitoneum (Fig. 30.7).

Risk factors contributing to uterine rupture during labor, include advanced gestational age, multiparity, and inadequate cervical preparation [65].

References

1. Lazarus E, Mayo-Smith WW, Mainiero MB, et al. CT in the evaluation of nontraumatic abdominal pain in pregnant women. Radiology. 2007;244(3):784–90. https://doi.org/10.1148/radiol.2443061634.
2. Jain C. ACOG committee opinion no. 723: guidelines for diagnostic imaging during pregnancy and lactation. Obstet Gynecol. 2019;133:186. https://doi.org/10.1097/AOG.0000000000003049.
3. Mainprize JG, Yaffe MJ, Chawla T, et al. Effects of ionizing radiation exposure during pregnancy. Abdom

Radiol. 2023;48:1564–78. https://doi.org/10.1007/s00261-023-03861-w.
4. ICRP. Biological effects after prenatal irradiation (embryo and fetus). ICRP Publication 90. Ann ICRP. 2003;33(1–2)
5. ICRP. Pregnancy and medical radiation. ICRP Publication 84. Ann. ICRP (2000), 30.
6. Council, N. R. Health risks from exposure to low levels of ionizing radiation: BEIR VII phase 2. Retrieved from https://www.nap.edu/catalog/11340/health-risks-from-exposure-to-low-levels-of-ionizing-radiation.
7. ACOG Committee Opinion n.299. Guidelines for Diagnostic Imaging During Pregnancy. Obstet Gynecol. 2004;104(3):647. https://doi.org/10.1097/00006250-200409000-00053.
8. ACR–SPR practice parameter for imaging pregnant or potentially pregnant patients with ionizing-radiation-resolution 31 Revised 2023. Retrieved from https://www.acr.org/media/acr/files/practice-parameters/pregnant-pts.pdf.
9. Wiles R, Hankinson B, Benbow E, et al. Making decisions about radiological imaging in pregnancy. BMJ. 2022;377:e070486. https://doi.org/10.1136/bmj-2022-070486.
10. National Council on Radiation Protection and Measurements. Statement No. 13: NCRP Recommendations for Ending Routine Gonadal Shielding During Abdominal and Pelvic Radiography. Retrieved from https://ncrponline.org/wp-content/themes/ncrp/PDFs/Statement13.pdf.
11. United Nations Scientific Committee on the Effects of Atomic Radiation (UNSCEAR). Report to general assembly volume II: scientific annex B: effects of radiation exposure of children. New York: United Nations; 2013.
12. Council Directive 2013/59/EURATOM of 5 December 2013. Official Journal of the European Union, L 013, 17 January 2014.
13. Ye Z, Qi M, Zhao Y, et al. Estimation of fetal and pediatric doses from chest CT examinations using virtual dose software. Radiat Prot Dosim. 2023;199(1):52–60. https://doi.org/10.1093/rpd/ncac225.
14. Begano D, Soderberg M, Boleiko A. To use or not use patient shielding on pregnant woman undergoing CT pulmonary angiography: a phantom study. Radiat Prot Dosim. 2020;189(4):458–65. https://doi.org/10.1093/rpd/ncaa059.
15. Lazarus E, Debenedectis C, North D, et al. Utilization of imaging in pregnant patients: 10-year review of 5270 examinations in 3285 patients 1997–2006. Radiology. 2009;251(2):517–24. https://doi.org/10.1148/radiol.2512080736.
16. Tsapaki V. Radiation dose optimization in diagnostic and interventional radiology: current issues and future perspectives. Phys Med. 2020;79:16–21. https://doi.org/10.1016/j.ejmp.2020.09.015.
17. Ratnapalan S, Bona N, Chandra K, et al. Physicians' perceptions of teratogenic risk associated with radiography and CT during early pregnancy. AJR. 2004;182:1107–9. https://doi.org/10.2214/ajr.182.5.1821107.
18. Flanagan E, Bell S. Abdominal imaging in pregnancy (maternal and foetal risks). Best Pract Res Clin Gastroenterol. 2020;44–45:101664. https://doi.org/10.1016/j.bpg.2019.101664.
19. American College of Radiology. Manual on contrast media version 10.2. Reston: American College of Radiology; 2016. p. 55–103.
20. Wang CL, Asch D, Cavallo J, et al. Statement from the ACR Committee on drugs and contrast media on the intravenous iodinated contrast media shortage. J Am Coll Radiol. 2022;19:834–5. https://doi.org/10.1016/j.jacr.2022.05.006.
21. American College of Obstetricians and Gynecologists' Committee on Obstetric Practice. Committee Opinion No. 656: guidelines for diagnostic imaging during pregnancy and lactation. Obstet Gynecol. 2016;127(2):e75–80. https://doi.org/10.1097/AOG.0000000000001316.
22. Morrison JC, Boyd M, Friedman BI, et al. The effects of renografin-60 on the fetal thyroid. Obstet Gynecol. 1073;42(1):99–103. Retrieved from http://www.ncbi.nlm.nih.gov/pubmed/4720211.
23. Calado AM, Dos Anjos PM. An overview of teratology. Methods Mol Biol. 2018;1797:3–32. https://doi.org/10.1007/978-1-4939-7883-0_1.
24. Kochi MH, Kaloudis EV, Ahmed W, et al. Effect of in utero exposure of iodinated intravenous contrast on neonatal thyroid function. J Comput Assist Tomogr. 2012;36(2):165–9. https://doi.org/10.1097/RCT.0b013e31824cc048.
25. Atwell TD, Lteif AN, Brown DL, et al. Neonatal thyroid function after administration of IV iodinated contrast agent to 21 pregnant patients. Am J Roentgenol. 2008;191(1):268–71. https://doi.org/10.2214/AJR.07.3336.
26. Webb JAW, Thomsen HS, Morcos SK. Members of contrast media safety Committee of European Society of Urogenital Radiology (ESUR). The use of iodinated and gadolinium contrast media during pregnancy and lactation. Eur Radiol. 2005;15:1234–40. https://doi.org/10.1007/s00330-004-2583-y.
27. Mabie WC, Disessa TG, Crocker LG, et al. A longitudinal study of cardiac output in normal human pregnancy. Am J Obstet Gynecol. 1994;170:849–56. https://doi.org/10.1016/s0002-9378(94)70297-7.
28. Schueller-Weidekamm C, Schaefer-Prokop C, Weber M. CT angiography of pulmonary arteries to detect pulmonary embolism: improvement of vascular enhancement with low kilovoltage settings. Radiology. 2006;241:899–907. https://doi.org/10.1148/radiol.2413040128.
29. Kuriya A, Piedimonte S, Spence AR, et al. Incidence and causes of maternal mortality in the USA. J Obstet Gynaecol Res. 2016;42:661–8. https://doi.org/10.1111/jog.12954.

30. Winer-Muram HT, Boone JM, Brown, et al. Pulmonary embolism in pregnant patients: fetal radiation dose with helical CT. Radiology. 2002;224:487–92. https://doi.org/10.1148/radiol.2242011581.
31. Brenner B. Haemostatic changes in pregnancy. Thromb Res. 2004;114:409–14. https://doi.org/10.1016/j.thromres.2004.08.004.
32. Bates SM, Middeldorp S, Rodger M, et al. Guidance for the treatment and prevention of obstetric-associated venous thromboembolism. J Thromb Thrombolysis. 2016;41:92–128. https://doi.org/10.1007/s11239-015-1309-0.
33. Nijkeuter M, Ginsberg JS, Huisman MV. Diagnosis of deep vein thrombosis and pulmonary embolism in pregnancy: a systematic review. J Thromb Haemost. 2006;4:496–500. https://doi.org/10.1111/j.1538-7836.2005.01779.x.
34. van Mens TE, Scheres LJ, de Jong PG, et al. Imaging for the exclusion of pulmonary embolism in pregnancy. Cochrane Database Syst Rev. 2017;1:CD011053. https://doi.org/10.1002/14651858.CD011053.pub2.
35. Tromeur C, van der Pol LM, Le Roux PY, et al. Computed tomography pulmonary angiography versus ventilation-perfusion lung scanning for diagnosing pulmonary embolism during pregnancy: a systematic review and meta-analysis. Haematologica. 2019;104:176–88. https://doi.org/10.3324/haematol.2018.196121.
36. Litmanovich D, Boiselle PM, Bankier AA. Dose reduction in cardiothoracic CT: review of currently available methods. Radiographics. 2009;29:981–93. https://doi.org/10.1148/rg.346140084.
37. Taylor A. The pediatric dosage handbook. 3rd ed. American Pharmaceutical Association; 1996.
38. Greene MF. Teratogenicity of recently introduced medications in human pregnancy. Obstet Gynecol. 2003;102(2):409–10. https://doi.org/10.1016/s0029-7844(02)02122-1.
39. Ufuk F, Kaia F, Sagtas E, et al. Non thrombotic pulmonary embolism in Emergency CT. Emerg Radiol. 2020;27(3):343–50. https://doi.org/10.1007/s10140-020-01755-8.
40. Kirsch J, Wu CC, Bolen MA, Henry TS, Rajiah PS, Brown RKJ, Galizia MS, Lee E, Rajesh F, Raptis CA, Rybicki FJ, Sams CM, Verde F, Villines TC, Wolf SJ, Yu J, Donnelly EF, Abbara S. ACR appropriateness criteria® pulmonary embolism in pregnancy. J Am Coll Radiol. 2018;15:S258–67.
41. The National Institute for Health and Care Excellence. Venous thromboembolic diseases: diagnosis, management and thrombophilia testing. NICE clinical guidelines, No. 144. (2012). Retrieved from https://www.ncbi.nlm.nih.gov/books/NBK385316/.
42. Makowska A, Treumann T, Venturini S. Pulmonary embolism in pregnancy: a review for clinical Practioners. J Clin Med. 2024;13(10):2863. https://doi.org/10.3390/jcm13102863.
43. Righini M, Robert-Ebadi H, Elias A, et al. Diagnosis of pulmonary embolism during pregnancy: a multicenter prospective management outcome study. Ann Intern Med. 2018;169:766–73. https://doi.org/10.7326/M18-1670.
44. Hendriks BM, Schnerr RS, Milanese G, et al. Computed tomography pulmonary angiography during pregnancy: radiation dose of commonly used protocols and the effect of scan length optimization. Korean J Radiol. 2019;20(2):313–22. https://doi.org/10.3448/kji.2017.0779.
45. McLean D, Delfino O, Moorin R. Estimation of maternal and foetal risk of radiation-induced cancer from a survey of computed tomography pulmonary angiography and ventilation/perfusion lung scanning for diagnosing pulmonary embolism during pregnancy. J Med Imaging Radiat Oncol. 2024;68(4):385–92. https://doi.org/10.1111/1754-9485.13661.
46. Bourjeily G, Levinson A. Pulmonary disease and critical illness in pregnancy. Semin Respir Crit Care Med. 2017;38(2):121–2. https://doi.org/10.1055/s-0037-1602168.
47. Al-Rammah TY, Alohaly A, Albatsh K. Reducing computed tomography radiation dose in diagnosing pulmonary embolism. Pak J Med Sci. 2016;32(6):1444–8. https://doi.org/10.12669/pjms.326.11347.
48. Royal College of Obstetricians and Gynaecologists (RCOG). Guidelines for the diagnosis and management of pulmonary embolism in pregnancy. (2015). Retrieved from https://www.rcog.org.uk/globalassets/documents/guidelines/gtg-37b.pdf.
49. The European Society of Cardiology. Guidelines on the diagnosis and management of acute pulmonary embolism. Eur Heart J. 2014;35:3033–69. https://doi.org/10.1093/eurheartj/ehu283.
50. Mazze RI, Kallen B. Reproductive outcome after anesthesia and operation during pregnancy: a registry study of 5405 cases. Am J Obstet Gynecol. 2001;161(5):1178–85. https://doi.org/10.1016/0002-9378(89)90659-5.
51. Goodacre S, Hunt BJ, Nelson-Piercy C. Diagnosis of suspected pulmonary embolism in pregnancy. N Engl J Med. 2019;380(25):e49. https://doi.org/10.1056/NEJMc1905283.
52. Dado CD, Levison AT, Bourjieily G. Pregnancy and pulmonary embolism. Clin Chest Med. 2018;39(3):525–37. https://doi.org/10.1016/j.ccm.2018.04.007.
53. Ridge CA, McDermott S, Freyne BJ, et al. Pulmonary embolism in pregnancy: comparison of pulmonary CT angiography and lung scintigraphy.AJR. Am J Roentgenol. 2009;193(5):1223–7. https://doi.org/10.2214/AJR.09.2360.
54. Scarsbrook AF, Gleeson FV. Investigating suspected pulmonary embolism in pregnancy. BMJ. 2007;24; 334(7590):418–9. https://doi.org/10.1136/bmj.39071.617257.80.
55. Simcox L, Ormesher L, Tower C, et al. Pulmonary thrombo-embolism in pregnancy: diagnosis and management. Breathe (Sheff). 2015;11(4):282–9. https://doi.org/10.1183/20734735.008815.

56. International Commission on Radiological Protection. ICRP Publication 103. The 2007 Recommendations of the International Commission on Radiological Protection (2007). Ann ICRP.
57. Rivera-Lebron B, Mc DM, Ahrar K, et al. Diagnosis, treatment and follow up of acute pulmonary embolism: consensus practice from the PERT consortium. Clin Appl Thromb Hemost. 2019;25 https://doi.org/10.1177/1076029619853037.
58. The Royal College of Radiologists. Guidance on imaging for suspected pulmonary embolism in pregnancy. (2015). Retrieved from https://www.rcr.ac.uk/publication/guidance-imaging-suspected-pulmonary-embolism-pregnancy.
59. Bourjieily G, Paidas M, Khali H, et al. Pulmonary embolism in pregnancy. Lancet. 2010;6;375(9713):500–12. https://doi.org/10.1016/S0140-6736(09)60996-X.
60. Lowe S. Diagnostic imaging in pregnancy: making informed decisions. Obstet Med. 2019;12(3):116–22. https://doi.org/10.1177/1753495X19838658.
61. Albakri AA, Alzahrani MM, Alghamdi S. Medical imaging in pregnancy: safety, appropriate utilization, and alternative modalities for imaging pregnant patients. Cureus. 2024;16(2):e54346. https://doi.org/10.7759/cureus.54346.
62. Loren AW, Mangu PB, Beck LN, et al. Fertility preservation for patients with cancer: American Society of Clinical Oncology clinical practice guideline update. J Clin Oncol. 2013;1;31(19):2500–10. https://doi.org/10.1200/JCO.2013.49.2678.
63. Applegate KE, Findlay U, Fraser L, et al. Radiation exposures in pregnancy, health effects and risks to the embryo/foetus information to inform the medical management of the pregnant patient. J Radiol Prot. 2021:41 S522. https://doi.org/10.1088/1361-6498/ac1c95.
64. Public Health England. Ionising Radiation (Medical Exposure) Regulations 2017. (2017). Retrieved from https://assets.publishing.service.gov.uk/government/uploads/system/uploads/attachment_data/file/682480/Ionising_Radiation_Medical_Exposure_Regulations_2017.pdf.
65. Al-Zirqi I, Stray-Pedersen B, Forsén L, et al. Uterine rupture: trends over 40 years. BJOG Int J Obstet Gynaecol. 2015;123:780–7. https://doi.org/10.1111/1471-0528.13394.

31 Tips and Tricks for Reading CT Body Emergency Examinations

Francesca Iacobellis, Gianluca Ponticiello, Costanza Camillo, Martina Caruso, Amelia Sparano, and Luigia Romano

31.1 Introduction

Computed tomography (CT) has revolutionized the field of diagnostic imaging, especially in emergency settings where timely and accurate diagnosis is crucial. CT body emergency examinations play a pivotal role in assessing various non-traumatic emergencies ranging from the more common acute abdominal pain, to systemic critical conditions, to particular conditions, as emergencies in pregnancy. This chapter aims to provide radiologists with practical tips and tricks for interpreting CT scans effectively and efficiently in emergency settings.

31.2 CT Machine and Protocol Familiarity

Understanding the diagnostic advantages of a *wide CT protocol* used for emergency body imaging, as suggested in the dedicated chapter, is important, as well as the knowledge of the available CT scanners and their different potentialities, technical parameters, post-processing software (including computed-aided diagnosis (CAD) and artificial intelligence (AI) software), contrast agent typology and injection parameters, CT phases to acquire and images reconstruction modalities. This aids in optimizing imaging protocol and obtaining good-quality CT images that helps in identifying key structures and abnormalities quickly. Furthermore, this familiarity helps in adapting and extending the protocol in specific circumstances, such as in case of suspicion of late bleeding, or in case of suspicion of pathologies of the urinary system (Figs. 31.1 and 31.2).

F. Iacobellis (✉) · G. Ponticiello · C. Camillo
M. Caruso · A. Sparano · L. Romano
Department of General and Emergency Radiology, "Antonio Cardarelli" Hospital, Naples, Italy
e-mail: Francesca.iacobellis@aocardarelli.it; Gianluca.ponticiello@aocardarelli.it; Costanza.camillo@aocardarelli.it; martina.caruso@aocardarelli.it; amelia.sparano@aocardarelli.it; luigia.romano1@gmail.com

L. Romano et al. (eds.), *CT of Non-Traumatic Body Emergencies*,
https://doi.org/10.1007/978-3-031-84849-0_31

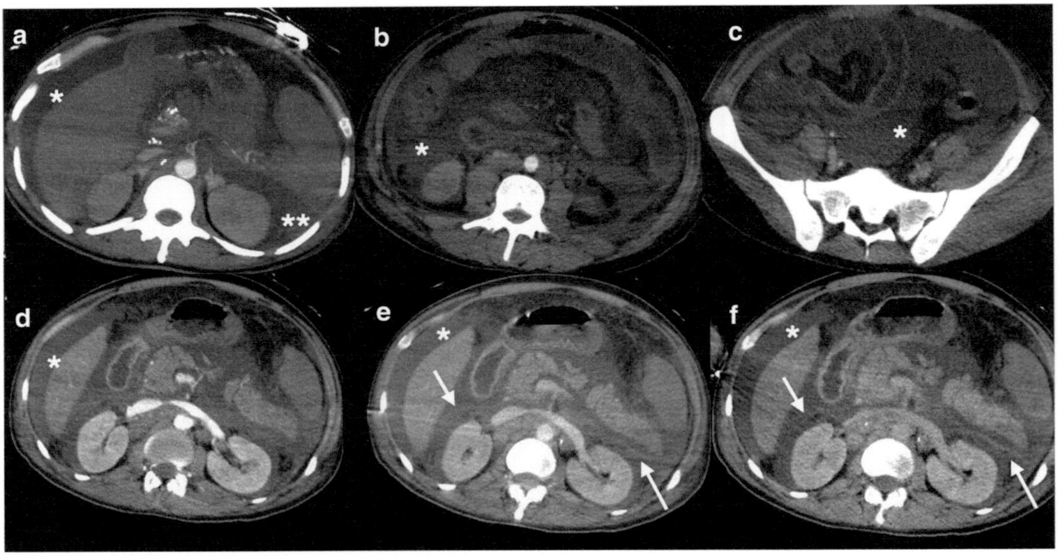

Fig. 31.1 Shock in a young patient with hematological malignancy. The previous CT examination, carried out 5 days earlier, did not detect fluid in the peritoneal cavity. At the current examination (**a-c** arterial phase, **d** portal phase, **e** late phase, **f** ultra-late phase acquired 10 minutes after the administration of the intravenous contrast medium, axial planes) the presence of hemoperitoneum (*) and a retroperitoneal fluid layer (**) is detected, the density of which is difficult to assess due to the presence of artifacts. Organ lesions cannot be defined (the spleen shows inhomogeneous enhancement due to the state of shock). It was necessary to acquire a late (**e**) and ultra-late phase (**f**) in view of hypotension and the paucity of the splanchnic vascular representation, to search for sources of bleeding visible in the late and ultra-late phase along the anterior pararenal bands (**e**, **f,** arrows) in the presence of disseminated intravascular coagulation (DIC)

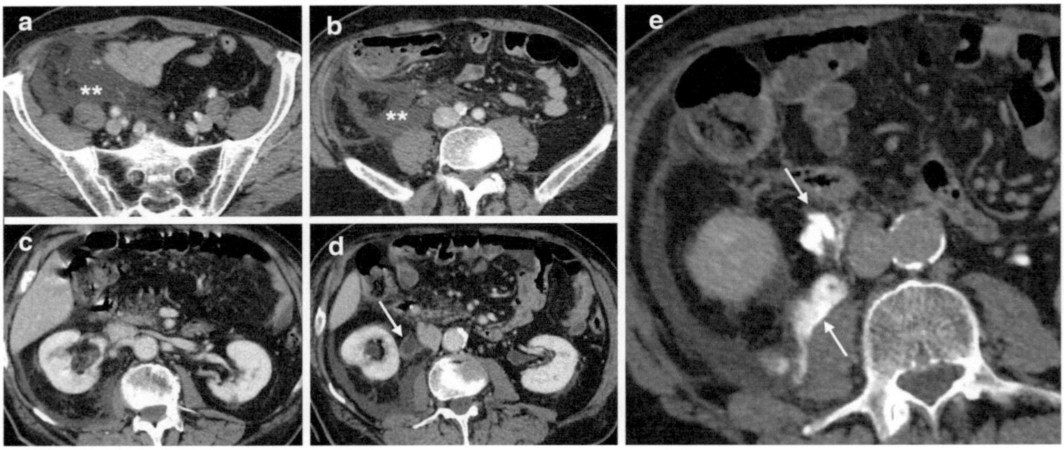

Fig. 31.2 Patient with persistent right flank pain after operative cystoscopy (**a–d** venous phase, **e** late phase, axial planes). There is a right retroperitoneal fluid collection (**a**, **b** **) and a dilation of the right ureter (**d**, arrow). Due to the patient's clinical history, it is appropriate to complete the examination with a late excretory phase (**e**) demonstrating a urinary leak from the proximal ureter (**e**, arrows) probably related to the high intraluminal pressure during cystoscopy

31.3 Contrast Enhancement

Pay close attention to areas with contrast enhancement, as it highlights vascular structures, perfusion abnormalities, and enhances lesion detection. In this sense, the knowledge of the different contrast agent properties [1] and the use of dual-energy technology [2, 3] may offer further help to increase the conspicuity of enhancing findings, particularly in critically ill patients, in which venous access and contrast injection flow may be suboptimal (Fig. 31.3). In this sense, new perspectives are opening up with photon counting technology and will need to be carefully evaluated in the future [4, 5].

31.4 Windowing and Reconstruction

Always look to the unenhanced scans searching for spontaneous hyperdensities. Optimize window settings to appreciate different tissue densities on the pre and post-contrast acquisitions. Adjust window width and level to enhance contrast resolution for specific conditions, e.g., use the lung window to look for free abdominal air (Fig. 31.4), and adapt the window to look for endoluminal vascular abnormalities (Fig. 31.5). Use multiplanar reconstruction (MPR) to visualize anatomical structures or devices from various perspectives

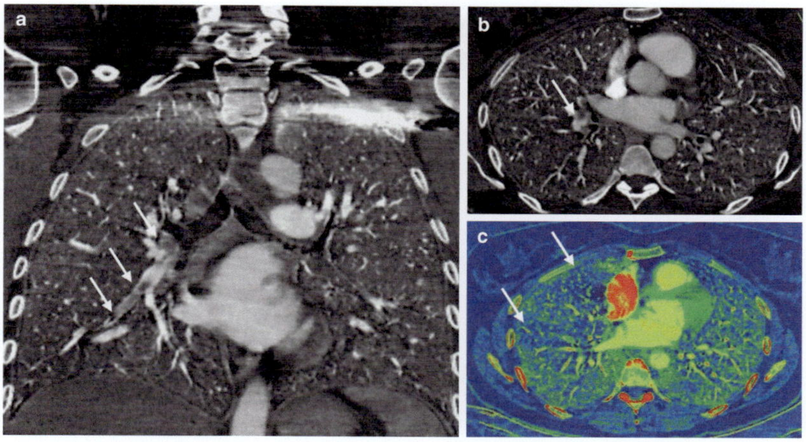

Fig. 31.3 Elderly patient with pulmonary embolism. Dual-energy CT acquisition helps in detecting the thrombotic defects in the lumen of the right pulmonary arteries (**a**,**b** arrows) despite using a low intravenous contrast injection flow rate (2 ml/sec). Color-coded iodine perfusion maps further assist in identifying areas of hypoperfused lung parenchyma (**c**, arrows) depicted in blu in comparison with green areas of the normal perfused lung

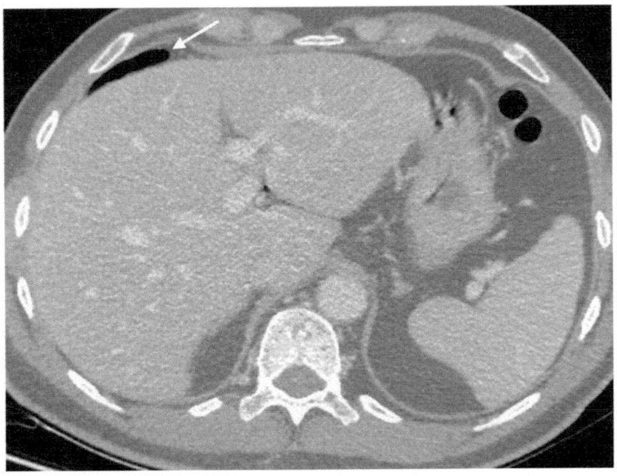

Fig. 31.4 Patient with acute abdomen. Evaluating the abdomen with lung window helps in detecting intraperitoneal free air (arrow)

(Fig. 31.6), to properly define organ origin and margins of any lesion, as well as to adequately study intestinal loops and vascular structures. Indeed, MPR can elucidate subtle abnormalities, improve lesion characterization, and facilitate accurate measurements. Incorporate axial, sagittal, and coronal views into your analysis for comprehensive assessment. Maximum Intensity Projection (MIP) may also be useful, particularly in the evaluation of lung nodules and vascular structures; Minimum Intensity Projection (MinIP) helps in the evaluation of low-density structures as bronchus, biliary tree, and similar. Volume rendering (VR) reconstruction provides three-dimensional (3D) visualization of anatomical structures and

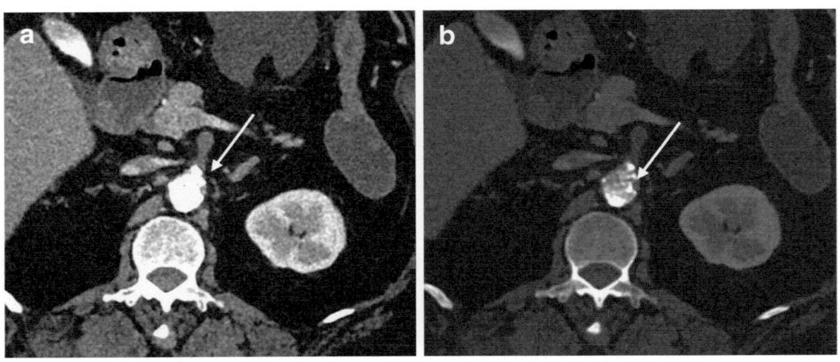

Fig. 31.5 Patient with acute abdomen. Manually changing the window level and width from standard abdominal value (**a**) to **b,** helps in distinguishing between endoluminal hyperdensity due to calcified plaque to those due to luminal opacification from intravenous contrast agent

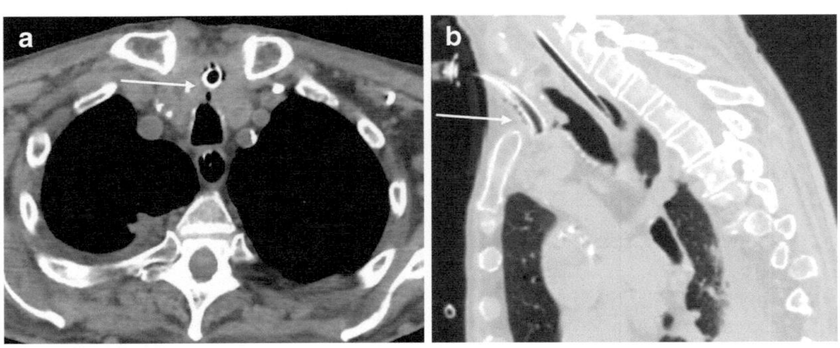

Fig. 31.6 Patient staying in intensive care unit with respiratory impairment (**a**, axial plane, soft tissue, **b**, sagittal plane, lung window). Multiplanar Reconstructions (MPR) help in evaluating the position of the endotracheal tube, displaced outside the tracheal lumen (**a**, **b** arrows)

pathological findings from computed tomography (CT) imaging data. This may help in providing a comprehensive understanding of complex spatial relationships and in communicating imaging findings to referring clinicians, surgeons, and other healthcare providers as VR is visually striking and easily interpretable, making them valuable tools.

31.5 Systematic Approach

Developing a systematic approach helps avoid oversight and ensures a comprehensive evaluation of the entire scan. In this sense, the adoption of a structured report helps to be complete and exhaustive in the reporting. Structured reporting provides a standardized framework for documenting imaging findings, ensuring consistency, clarity, and completeness in radiological reports. In the fast-paced environment of the emergency department, structured reports facilitate rapid interpretation, streamline communication between radiologists and referring clinicians, and expedite patient management decisions. Additionally, structured reporting enhances report comprehensibility for non-radiology healthcare providers, thereby improving interdisciplinary collaboration and patient care coordination. By incorporating structured templates tailored to emergency radiology scenarios, institutions can enhance efficiency, accuracy, and quality in the interpretation and communication of imaging findings, ultimately leading to improved patient outcomes [6, 7].

However, even with the help of a structured report, it's crucial to grasp the clinical context, set up and follow diagnostic reasoning, starting from the clinical question, patient's history, presenting symptoms, and any relevant laboratory findings, when available, attempting to correlate the identified findings with each other, while considering the possibility of collateral findings or of coexistent pathological conditions in the same patient. This is supported by several studies demonstrating that appropriate clinical informations improve the reports of diagnostic examinations, indeed, having access to clinical informations improve the accuracy of reading CT scans, possibly because radiologists either consciously or unconsciously make diagnostic prediction of diseases [8, 9].

31.6 Recognize Critical Findings

Identify critical and unexpected findings promptly to facilitate timely intervention [10] (Figs. 31.7 and 31.8) . These may include:

- *Massive pneumotorax or massive pleural effusion*: these conditions impair respiration and cardiovascular function.
- *Aortic type A dissection or aneurism rupture*: these conditions cause ischemia or bleeding and needs to be promptly treated.
- *Active bleeding*: look for spontaneous hyperdensity areas in the unenhanced scan and contrast medium extravasation in the following acquisitions. The bleeding site, the etiology and the entity orient the following management.
- *Acute vascular occlusion*: look for signs of arterial or venous occlusion, such as vessel cutoff or absence of contrast flow. Vascular occlusion impairs organ perfusion.

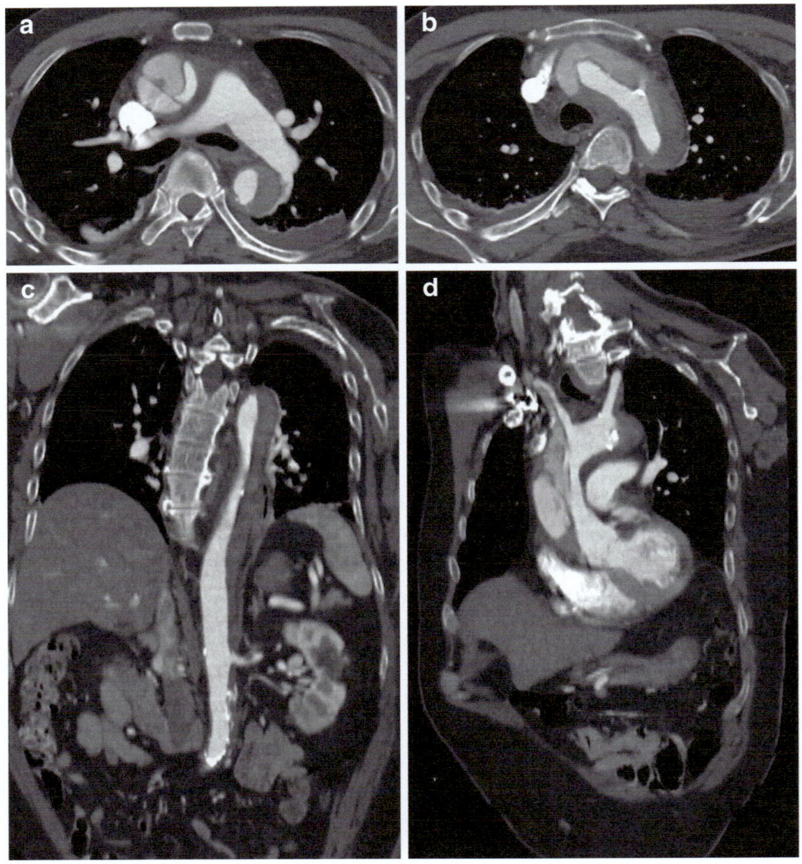

Fig. 31.7 Sixty-four-year-old male patient with acute abdominal pain (**a**,**b** arterial phase, axial planes, c,d, arterial phase, coronal plane). Note the type A aortic dissection starting from the aortic valve plane, involving the brachiocephalic artery and extending caudally to the abdominal aorta

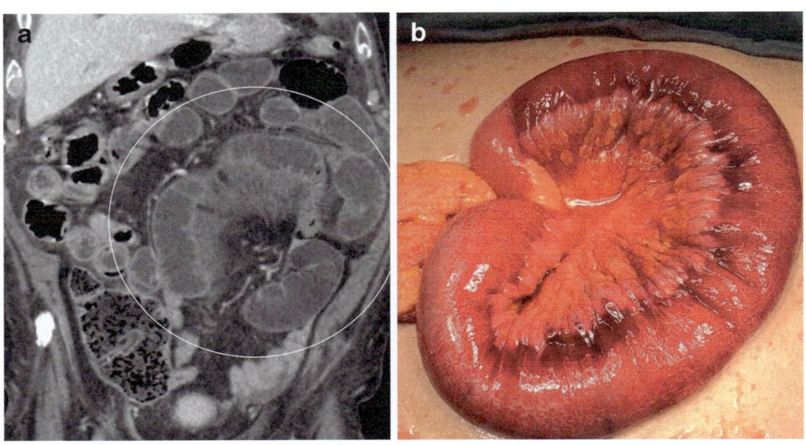

Fig. 31.8 Sixty-year-old female patient with acute abdominal pain. Note the closed loop bowel obstruction (**a**, circle) causing mixed vascular impairment that needs to be promptly surgically treated (**b**, intraoperative finding of the involved ischemic bowel). The authors would like to thank Colleagues of the Department of Emergency Surgery, "A. Cardarelli" Hospital, Naples, Italy, directed by Dr. Maurizio Castriconi, for figure **b**

- *Bowel perforation*: signs of organ perforation, such as free intraperitoneal or retroperitoneal air or fluid, indicate urgent surgical management.
- *Ischemic bowel*: look for alterations in bowel wall enhancement.

31.7 Recognize Normal Variants

Familiarize yourself with common anatomical variants to avoid misinterpretation. Distinguish between normal variants and pathological findings to prevent misdiagnosis. Regular exposure to different cases improves your ability to differentiate between variants and abnormalities.

31.8 Utilize Comparative Analysis

Comparative analysis with prior imaging studies can elucidate interval changes and disease progression. Evaluate current findings in conjunction with prior examinations to identify new or evolving abnormalities, assess treatment response, and guide clinical management effectively.

31.9 Communication and Collaboration

Effective communication with referring clinicians is vital for accurate diagnosis and patient management [11]. Be cooperative with referring clinicians and provide clear and concise reports highlighting critical findings and, when indicated, recommendations for further instrumental evaluation.

31.10 Know the Possibilities of Error

Especially in an emergency setting, there are many triggering factors, such as carrying out multiple simultaneous activities (following multiple patients and related imaging examinations at the same time), the need to make decisions quickly on patients with an incomplete medical history often with multiple pathologies and in compromised conditions, as well as the emotional pressure caused by all of this [12–17]. In Table 31.1 several causes of errors are listed, with possible solutions.

Table 31.1 Causes of errors and possible solutions

Causes of errors in emergency CT	Possible solution
Pre-procedural error:	
Incomplete or inconsistent clinical question in the examination request that limits the understanding of the clinical context	Don't underestimate the importance of medical history and to discuss it with the referring physician
Request for examination	
Patient identification, especially in unconscious or uncooperative patients	Check that strict procedures are followed in your workflow
Failure to inform the patient (acquisition of informed consent, when possible)	When possible, speak with the patient
Error in execution:	
Patient positioning	Pay attention to the imaging protocol as reported in the paragraph 1.
Technical parameters	
Patient movement	
Examination protocol	
Intra-procedural error:	
Perception error	Stay focused on the patients conditions, limit distractions, help yourself with the available software (image reconstructions, computer-aided diagnosis (CAD) systems, artificial intelligence (AI) systems) and with structured report
Interpretation error	Study and stay updated
Transcription error	Limit distractions
Post-procedural error:	
Delay in diagnosis due to untimely delivery of the report	Ensure that the referring physician receives the report and, if possible, agrees on the use of a pre-report highlighting the key findings
Failure of the clinician to understand the report	Use clear and concise language throughout the report, and include a detailed diagnostic conclusion at the end to support optimal patient management

31.11 Continuous Learning

Radiology is an evolving field with constant advancements and new discoveries. Stay updated with the latest advancements in CT imaging and emergency radiology through continuous learning and participation in relevant educational activities, conferences, and case discussions in national and international emergency radiology scientific societies such as the Italian Society of Medical and Interventional Radiology (https://sirm.org), European Society of Emergency Radiology (https://www.eser-society.org), American Society of Emergency Radiology (https://aser.org/), and similar organizations. Embrace new technologies and techniques to stay updated about the latest developments and refine your diagnostic skills.

31.12 Conclusion

Interpreting CT body emergency examinations requires a systematic approach, protocol familiarity, and attention to detail. By employing the tips and tricks outlined in this chapter, radiologists can optimize their diagnostic accuracy and contribute to improving patient outcomes in emergency settings.

References

1. Bae KT. Intravenous contrast medium administration and scan timing at CT: considerations and approaches. Radiology. 2010;256(1):32–61. https://doi.org/10.1148/radiol.10090908. PMID: 20574084.
2. Machida H, Tanaka I, Fukui R, Shen Y, Ishikawa T, Tate E, Ueno E. Dual-energy spectral CT: vari-

ous clinical vascular applications. Radiographics. 2016;36(4):1215–32. https://doi.org/10.1148/rg.2016150185. PMID: 27399244.
3. Abu-Omar A, Murray N, Ali IT, Khosa F, Barrett S, Sheikh A, Nicolaou S, Tamburrini S, Iacobellis F, Sica G, Granata V, Saba L, Masala S, Scaglione M. Utility of dual-energy computed tomography in clinical Conundra. Diagnostics (Basel). 2024;14(7):775. https://doi.org/10.3390/diagnostics14070775. PMID: 38611688; PMCID: PMC11012177.
4. Onishi H, Tsuboyama T, Nakamoto A, Ota T, Fukui H, Tatsumi M, Honda T, Kiso K, Matsumoto S, Kaketaka K, Enchi Y, Kawabata S, Nakasone S, Tomiyama N. Photon-counting CT: technical features and clinical impact on abdominal imaging. Abdom Radiol (NY). 2024;49:4383. https://doi.org/10.1007/s00261-024-04414-5
5. Toia GV, Mileto A, Borhani AA, Chen GH, Ren L, Uyeda JW, Marin D. Approaches, advantages, and challenges to photon counting detector and multi-energy CT. Abdom Radiol (NY). 2024. https://doi.org/10.1007/s00261-024-04357-x. Epub ahead of print. PMID: 38744702.
6. Ganeshan D, Duong PAT, Probyn L, et al. Structured reporting in radiology. Acad Radiol. 2018;25(1):66–73. https://doi.org/10.1016/j.acra.2017.08.005.
7. Granata V, Fusco R, Cozzi D, Danti G, Faggioni L, Buccicardi D, Prost R, Ferrari R, Trinci M, Galluzzo M, Iacobellis F, Scaglione M, Tonerini M, Coppola F, Bortolotto C, Caruso D, Ciaghi E, Gabelloni M, Rengo M, Giacobbe G, Grassi F, Romano L, Pinto A, Caranci F, Bertelli E, D'Andrea P, Neri E, Giovagnoni A, Grassi R, Miele V. Structured reporting of computed tomography in the polytrauma patient assessment: a Delphi consensus proposal. Radiol Med. 2023;128(2):222–33. https://doi.org/10.1007/s11547-023-01596-8. Epub 2023 Jan 19. PMID: 36658367; PMCID: PMC9938818.
8. Shikino K, Ikusaka M, Ohira Y, Miyahara M, Suzuki S, Hirukawa M, Noda K, Tsukamoto T, Uehara T. Influence of predicting the diagnosis from history on the accuracy of physical examination. Adv Med Educ Pract. 2015;6:143–8. https://doi.org/10.2147/AMEP.S77315. PMID: 25759604; PMCID: PMC4345897.
9. Suzuki S, Ikusaka M, Ohira Y, Miyahara M, Noda K, Kajiwara H, Shikino K, Kondo T. Effect of diagnostic predictions combined with clinical information on avoiding perceptual errors of computed tomography. Jpn J Radiol. 2013;31(11):731–6. https://doi.org/10.1007/s11604-013-0244-2. Epub 2013 Sep 14. PMID: 24037534.
10. European Society of Radiology (ESR). ESR guidelines for the communication of urgent and unexpected findings. Insights Imaging. 2012;3(1):1–3. https://doi.org/10.1007/s13244-011-0135-y. Epub 2011 Nov 22. PMID: 22695992; PMCID: PMC3292650.
11. Moore CL, Baskin A, Chang AM, Cheung D, Davis MA, Fertel BS, Hans K, Kang SK, Larson DM, Lee RK, McCabe-Kline KB, Mills AM, Nicola GN, Nicola LP. White paper: best practices in the communication and management of actionable incidental findings in emergency department imaging. J Am Coll Radiol. 2023;20(4):422–30. https://doi.org/10.1016/j.jacr.2023.01.001. Epub 2023 Mar 13. PMID: 36922265.
12. Scaglione M, Iaselli F, Sica G, Feragalli B, Nicola R. Errors in imaging of traumatic injuries. Abdom Imaging. 2015;40(7):2091–8. https://doi.org/10.1007/s00261-015-0494-9. PMID: 26099475.
13. Sica G, Guida F, Bocchini G, Codella U, Mainenti PP, Tanga M, Scaglione M. Errors in imaging assessment of polytrauma patients. Semin Ultrasound CT MR. 2012;33(4):337–46. https://doi.org/10.1053/j.sult.2012.01.012. PMID: 22824123
14. Mandato Y, Reginelli A, Galasso R, Iacobellis F, Berritto D, Cappabianca S. Errors in the radiological evaluation of the alimentary tract: part I. Semin Ultrasound CT MR. 2012;33(4):300–7. https://doi.org/10.1053/j.sult.2012.01.011. PMID: 22824120.
15. Reginelli A, Mandato Y, Solazzo A, Berritto D, Iacobellis F, Grassi R. Errors in the radiological evaluation of the alimentary tract: part II. Semin Ultrasound CT MR. 2012;33(4):308–17. https://doi.org/10.1053/j.sult.2012.01.016. PMID: 2282412.
16. Pinto A, Lanzetta MM, Addeo G, Bonini MC, Grazzini G, Miele V. Errors in MDCT diagnosis of acute mesenteric ischemia. Abdom Radiol (NY). 2022;47(5):1699–1713. https://doi.org/10.1007/s00261-020-02732-y. Epub 2020 Sep 11. PMID: 32918107.
17. Pinto A, Caranci F, Romano L, Carrafiello G, Fonio P, Brunese L. Learning from errors in radiology: a comprehensive review. Semin Ultrasound CT MR. 2012;33(4):379–82. https://doi.org/10.1053/j.sult.2012.01.015. PMID: 22824127.

Correction to: Urologic Emergencies

Dario Grimaldi, Pierantonio Grimaldi,
Chiara Rinaldo, Giuliana Giacobbe,
Vittorio Sabatino, and Marco Di Serafino

Correction to:
Chapter 26 in: L. Romano et al. (eds.), *CT of Non-Traumatic Body Emergencies*,
https://doi.org/10.1007/978-3-031-84849-0_26

In Chapter 26, the author name Pierantonio Grimaldi was incorrectly spelled as "Pietrantonio Grimaldi." This has now been updated—from "Pietrantonio Grimaldi" to "Pierantonio Grimaldi."

The updated version of this chapter can be found at
https://doi.org/10.1007/978-3-031-84849-0_26

L. Romano et al. (eds.), *CT of Non-Traumatic Body Emergencies*,
https://doi.org/10.1007/978-3-031-84849-0_32

MIX
Papier aus verantwortungsvollen Quellen
Paper from responsible sources
FSC® C105338

If you have any concerns about our products,
you can contact us on
ProductSafety@springernature.com

In case Publisher is established outside the EU,
the EU authorized representative is:
Springer Nature Customer Service Center GmbH
Europaplatz 3, 69115 Heidelberg, Germany

Printed by Libri Plureos GmbH
in Hamburg, Germany